Concepts in Immunology and Immunotherapeutics

Fourth Edition

BLAINE T. SMITH, R.Ph., Ph.D.

WHITTIER LONG TERM
REHABILITATION CENTER

Westborough, Massachusetts

American Society of Health-System Pharmacists®

Bethesda, Maryland

Any correspondence regarding this publication should be sent to the publisher, American Society of Health-System Pharmacists, 7272 Wisconsin Avenue, Bethesda, MD 20814, attention: Special Publishing.

The information presented herein reflects the opinions of the contributors and advisors. It should not be interpreted as an official policy of ASHP or as an endorsement of any product.

Because of ongoing research and improvements in technology, the information and its applications contained in this text are constantly evolving and are subject to the professional judgment and interpretation of the practitioner due to the uniqueness of a clinical situation. The editors, contributors, and ASHP have made reasonable efforts to ensure the accuracy and appropriateness of the information presented in this document. However, any user of this information is advised that the editors, contributors, advisors, and ASHP are not responsible for the continued currency of the information, for any errors or omissions, and/or for any consequences arising from the use of the information in the document in any and all practice settings. Any reader of this document is cautioned that ASHP makes no representation, guarantee, or warranty, express or implied, as to the accuracy and appropriateness of the information contained in this document and specifically disclaims any liability to any party for the accuracy and/or completeness of the material or for any damages arising out of the use or non-use of any of the information contained in this document.

Director, Special Publishing: Jack Bruggeman
Senior Editorial Project Manager: Dana Battaglia
Production Editor: Johnna Hershey
Page Design: Carol Barrer

Library of Congress Cataloging-in-Publication Data

Concepts in immunology and immunotherapeutics/ [edited by] Blaine T. Smith.—4th ed.
    p. ;cm.
  Includes bibliographical references and index.
  ISBN: 978-1-58528-127-5
  1. Immunotherapy. 2. Immunology. I. Smith, Blaine T. II. American
Society of Health-System Pharmacists.
[DNLM: 1. Immune System—Programmed Instruction.
2. Immunity—Programmed Instruction. 3. Immunotherapy—Programmed Instruction.
QW 518.2 C744 2008]

RM275.C66 2008
616.0'9—dc22

                                                                 2007045458

ISBN: 978-1-58528-127-5

To Jim Krieger, a skilled pharmacist and teacher . . .

His vision helped to make this edition possible.

Acknowledgments

It is a wonder in itself how a book can be created when contributors, staff, and publishers are in disparate physical locations, most having never met face-to-face. Yet it came to pass through the tireless efforts of many people.

I would like to thank the writers of each chapter. All of you assumed your role like true professionals. Thank you all for putting up with my cajoling and badgering—your product is superb. We finished what we started, and can be proud of it.

And to Jack Bruggeman, Dana Battaglia, and all the staff at ASHP: I thank you for having confidence in me when you did not even know me. Thank you for letting me step in, and showing me how things work when making this thing called a "book"! My part in it was to be the captain of a ship that ran itself.

Blaine Smith

Preface

Concepts in Immunology and Immunotherapeutics, fourth edition, is not simply a textbook—nor just a reference—but both. The book is designed for students new to the field of immunology and serves as a reference for those already in practice. Therefore, the text begins with basic concepts in immunology and then covers current clinical applications in the field of pharmacy.

This book is divided into two parts: overview of the immune system and clinical applications of immunology. Chapters 1–3 in Part I provide foundational knowledge on the complex topics of basic immunology. Part II opens with Chapter 4, which discusses mechanisms of hypersensitivity and drug allergy, and begins the transition from basic immunology to applied immunology. Chapter 5 discusses inflammatory diseases and autoimmunity. Chapters 6–11 discuss topics in clinical practice, where the application of immunodiagnosis and immunotherapy is becoming more of an everyday experience for pharmacists, even those who do not consider themselves to be in a "clinical" setting. These chapters include the immunological background and current treatment practices for infectious diseases. Two chapters cover HIV/AIDs from two perspectives: immunology and treatment. Other chapters cover transplantation and cancer therapies. The information should be of interest to all health care professionals, especially those whose practice settings include patients in these categories.

The authors of these chapters are experts in their respective fields. Thousands of hours of experience enrich their writing. For instructors, learning objectives and self-assessment questions are included to enhance the learning experience of their students.

If you are a student, welcome to the intriguing field(s) of immunology and immunotherapeutics. You may ask, as many of my students ask, "How are immunology and immunotherapeutics related to the current practice of pharmacy?" The answer is that every day it is becoming more and more commonplace to see these drugs and treatments in practice.

If you are already in practice, you surely noticed the introduction of biotechnological drugs into your setting. Many of these are immunologically based. This trend will accelerate in the near future, since many immunomodulators and immunotherapeutic drugs are seeking FDA approval.

This project was begun and inspired by Jim Kreiger, whose outgoing personality and friendly enthusiasm were contagious. It is his memory that drove this book to completion.

We, the authors, and I, as editor, hope you gain enrichment from this text that will help you in your professional endeavors.

Blaine T. Smith
July 8, 2007

Contributors

Arezoo Campbell, Ph.D.
Assistant Professor, Pharmaceutical Sciences
Western University of Health Sciences
Pomona, California

Lindsay Corporon, Pharm.D., BCOP
Clinical Oncology Pharmacist
Magee Women's Hospital
Assistant Professor
Department of Pharmacy and Therapeutics
University of Pittsburgh School of Pharmacy
Pittsburgh, Pennsylvania

Karen M. Fancher, Pharm.D., BCOP
Clinical Pharmacist, Blood and Marrow
    Transplantation
H. Lee Moffitt Cancer Center & Research Institute
Tampa, Florida

Andrea K. Hubbard, Ph.D.
Associate Professor, School of Pharmacy
University of Connecticut
Storrs, Connecticut

Christopher W. James, Pharm.D.
Clinical Pharmacy Specialist, HIV Community
    Program
Christiana Care Health Services
Wilmington, Delaware

Stephen O'Barr, Ph.D.
Associate Professor of Pharmaceutical Sciences,
    Immunology
College of Pharmacy
Western University of Health Sciences
Pomona, California

Gina Peacock, Ph.D.
Associate Professor, Biopharmaceutical Sciences
Shenandoah University
Winchester, Virginia

Beulah Perdue Sabundayo, Pharm.D., M.P.H.
Research Associate
Johns Hopkins University School of Medicine
Baltimore, Maryland

Rowena Schwartz, Pharm.D., BCOP
Director of Oncology Pharmacy
The Johns Hopkins Hospital
Baltimore, Maryland

Debra Tucker Sierka, Pharm D.
Transplant Consultant
Norristown, Pennsylvania

Nicole Sifontis, Pharm.D., BCPS
Clinical Associate Professor
Specialist, Organ Transplantation
Temple University School of Pharmacy
Philadelphia, Pennsylvania

Blaine T. Smith, R.Ph., Ph.D.
Whittier Long Term Rehabilitation Center
Westborough, Massachusetts

Douglas Smith, Pharm.D., BCNSP, BCOP
Associate Professor, Department of Pharmacy
    Practice
Bernard J. Dunn School of Pharmacy
Shenandoah University
Winchester, Virginia

Gail Goodman Snitkoff, Ph.D.
Associate Professor, Department
    of Pharmaceutical Sciences
Albany College of Pharmacy
Albany, New York

Brad L. Stanford, Pharm.D, BCOP
Assistant Professor of Pharmacy Practice—
    Oncology
Texas Tech University Health Sciences Center
School of Pharmacy
Lubbock, Texas

Marc G. Sturgill, Pharm.D.
Associate Professor, Ernest Mario School of
    Pharmacy
Rutgers, The State University of New Jersey
Adjunct Associate Professor and Assistant
    Director
Pediatric Clinical Research Center
Department of Pediatrics
UMDNJ—Robert Wood Johnson Medical School
New Brunswick, New Jersey

Contents

Part I—Basic Immunology

Overview of the Immune System

Marc G. Sturgill

INTRODUCTION

The human immune system is a highly efficient and complicated network of antigen-specific and antigen-nonspecific tissue barriers, cellular components, and soluble factors that can recognize and eliminate a vast array of microbial pathogens. Initial exposure to a pathogen triggers a rapid antigen-nonspecific inflammatory response that isolates the invader and activates the antigen-specific arm of the immune system. Antigen-specific immune cells then remove the pathogen and generate memory cells that respond faster and more effectively to repeated exposure.

Not all immune responses are beneficial to the host. Inflammatory responses identical to those that destroy foreign pathogens also cause transplant rejection. Many autoimmune diseases, such as rheumatoid arthritis and type 1 diabetes mellitus, result from a loss of normal immune system tolerance of host tissues. Dysregulation of normal inflammatory responses is also associated with allergic rhinitis and other hypersensitivity disorders. Finally, several types of human cancer are associated with suppressed normal immune surveillance functions.

This chapter gives the pharmacist a brief introduction to the cells and tissues that make up the human immune system, the mechanisms responsible for normal immune responses, and the potential consequences of immune dysfunction. The reader will be referred to review articles or book chapters for a more thorough discussion of each topic.

After completing this introductory chapter, the reader should be able to:

1. Describe the general organization and function of the immune system.
2. Understand the coordinated role of innate and adaptive immune responses in host defense.
3. Describe the cells and soluble mediators responsible for innate and adaptive immune responses.
4. Understand the process of antigen recognition and how the immune system differentiates "self" from "nonself."
5. Describe the four basic types of hypersensitivity.
6. Describe the potential consequences of immune dysfunction or suppression.

INNATE AND ADAPTIVE IMMUNE RECOGNITION

Discrimination between "self" and "nonself" is a central characteristic of the immune system. It permits efficient removal of invading pathogens without excessive damage to surrounding normal tissue and prevents autoimmune reactions. An *immunogen* is any substance that can provoke immune system recognition and response.[1] The molecular sequence of an immunogen that is actually recognized and bound by immune receptors is called an *antigen*. Most antigens are microbial cell surface proteins not expressed by normal host cells, although some lipids and polysaccharides with large molecular weights can also be antigenic. *Lymphocytes* are responsible for adaptive immune responses; B lymphocytes and T lymphocytes express antigen-specific receptors.[2] A unique characteristic of adaptive immune responses is the clonal expansion of an antigen-specific lymphocyte that greatly increases the number of antigen-specific lymphocytes and the efficiency of antigen removal. These cells both destroy the pathogen directly and orchestrate the overall response by recruiting and activating antigen-nonspecific (innate) immune cells. Adaptive responses also produce immunologic memory. On repeated exposure to the same pathogen, memory lymphocytes orchestrate an even faster and more efficient response.

In contrast, innate immune responses cannot adapt to invading pathogens[2] and are identical upon repeated exposure. Innate immunity includes physical barriers to invasion; soluble inflammatory mediators, such as complement;

antigen-nonspecific cellular responses mediated by a third type of lymphocyte called a natural killer (NK) cell; and a number of myeloid cells including monocytes, dendritic cells, and granulocytes. These cells all express pattern recognition receptors (PRRs) that bind to microbial cells' unique molecular sequences, or pathogen-associated molecular patterns (PAMPs).[3] PAMPs are not considered true antigens because they are neither specific to a particular microbial species nor recognized by a specific immune cell. For example, the lipid A side chain of lipopolysaccharide (LPS) is relatively conserved among all species of gram-negative bacteria. This motif is recognized by special types of PRRs called *toll-like receptors* (TLR2 and TLR4), expressed by neutrophils, macrophages, dendritic cells, and mast cells.[3] Viral infections are often associated with infected host cell production of viral peptides, many of which are ultimately expressed on the surface of the infected cell. The presence of double-stranded viral RNA (dsRNA) activates TLR3, expressed by macrophages, certain dendritic cells, and surface epithelial cells.[3] PRR recognition and signaling can activate the innate immune cell, initiating an inflammatory response and resulting in an antigen-specific response by lymphocytes. Innate immunity is responsible for the initial activation of the adaptive immune response through a process called *antigen presentation*.[2]

INNATE IMMUNITY

Physical Barriers

Physical barriers such as skin and mucous membranes serve as the innate immune system's first line of defense.[4] Most microorganisms cannot penetrate intact skin because of the relative impermeability of the outer keratin-rich epidermal layer and the low pH generated by lactic acid and unsaturated fatty acids in the underlying dermis. Inner epithelial surfaces such as the nasopharynx, lungs, and gut are protected by a layer of mucous that can trap microorganisms until they are removed by ciliary movement, coughing, or peristalsis. These surfaces are also exposed to a variety of bactericidal chemicals, such as gastric acid in the stomach. Few microorganisms are able to survive both the acidic pH of the stomach and the alkaline pH of the small intestine. The normal commensal bacterial flora of the intestine compete with pathogenic microorganisms for essential nutrients and produce bactericidal metabolic by-products such as lactic acid. The bactericidal enzyme lysozyme, which cleaves microbial cell wall peptidoglycan, is present in saliva and tears as well as nasal and most other body secretions.

Complement

Once physical barriers have been breached, a number of circulating mediators rapidly bind to the invading microbial cells. Although direct cellular destruction can follow, most of these mediators enhance antigen-nonspecific cell activity by serving as potent homing signals (chemotaxis) or by binding to the surface of invading cells to facilitate phagocytic destruction by macrophages and neutrophils (opsonization). The *complement cascade* is a network of more than 35 circulating and cell surface proteins that play each of these vital roles in maintaining host defense during the early stages of microbial invasion.[5]

Activation of the complement cascade. Complement can be activated by the classical pathway, the lectin pathway, or the alternative pathway, all resulting in the formation of the C3 convertase enzyme complex (**Figure 1.1**).[4,5] Complement protein C1 circulates as a complex of six C1q, two C1r, and two C1s molecules. The classical pathway is initiated when a C1q molecule

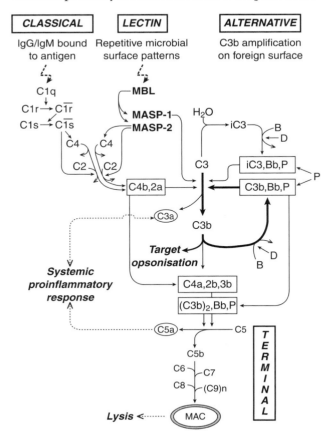

Figure 1.1. The classical, mannan-binding lectin, and alternate pathways of complement activation. (Adapted from Paul WE, ed. *Fundamental Immunology.* 5th ed. Philadelphia, PA: Lippincott Williams & Wilkins; 2003:1079.)

binds to at least two adjacent Fc (constant region) antibody fragments on an immune complex (a single immunoglobulin M [IgM] or two IgG antibodies bound to an antigen). C1q activation cleaves and activates C1r, which in turn cleaves and activates C1s. Activated C1s then sequentially cleaves complement proteins C4 (into C4a and C4b fragments) and C2 (into C2a and C2b fragments). The C4b and C2b fragments then bind to form the classical C3 convertase (C4b,2b). C4b,2b cleaves C3 into the C3a and C3b fragments. Some of the C3b fragments bind to C4b,2b to form the C5 convertase enzyme, but most randomly deposit on, and bind to, nearby cell surfaces, including both normal host cells and invading pathogens. Host cells are called inactivator surfaces because C3b is rapidly bound and inactivated by factor H. C3b acts as a powerful opsonin and plays a prominent role in the alternative complement pathway once it binds to an activator surface (bacterial, fungal, or viral cell surface). The classical pathway can be activated only if the host has been previously exposed to the pathogen and has already generated antigen-specific memory B lymphocytes.

The lectin and alternative pathways play critical roles in innate host defense because activation is not dependent on pre-formed IgM or IgG antibodies.[5] Human plasma contains a mannose-binding lectin (MBL) that circulates complexed to MBL-associated serine protease enzymes (MASP-1, MASP-2, and MASP-3). MBL binds to the mannose or N-acetylglucosamine carbohydrate motifs expressed on the cell surface of most bacteria, fungi, parasites, and viruses. In contrast, MBL does not bind to the sialic acid or galactose molecules expressed on human cells. Binding activates MASP, which directly cleaves C4 and C2 in the absence of activated C1, again forming C4b,2b and producing the C3b fragments described earlier.

Alternative complement pathway activation is based on the continual spontaneous hydrolysis of serum C3 into C3(H_2O).[5] In the presence of magnesium, C3(H_2O) can bind to factor B, subsequently activating factor D, which in turn cleaves factor B to form the alternative pathway C3 convertase C3(H_2O)Bb(Mg). C3(H_2O)Bb(Mg) binds to membrane-bound C3b in the presence of properdin (P) to form the C5 convertase enzyme. However, C3(H2O)Bb(Mg) can also cleave several molecules of circulating C3 to generate additional C3b fragments and serve as a positive feedback loop.

Cellular lysis. The classical, lectin, or alternative pathway C5 convertase enzymes all cleave complement protein C5, releasing the C5b fragment, which rapidly interacts and binds to

C6, C7, and C8 to form a strongly hydrophobic complex. This complex inserts itself into the lipid bilayer of the target cell membrane, then binds to multiple molecules of C9 to form an osmotically active pore through the cell membrane called the membrane attack complex (MAC). Cell death ensues secondary to osmotic lysis.[5]

Opsonization and chemotaxis. Several complement fragments have biological activity. Membrane-bound C3b is an important opsonin for antigen-nonspecific phagocytic cells expressing the appropriate complement receptors (CR1 through CR4).[5] CR1, CR3, and CR4 are expressed by macrophages, neutrophils, and certain dendritic cells, while CR1 and CR2 are expressed by B lymphocytes. The C5a complement fragment is a potent chemotactic signal for monocytes and granulocytes.

Generation of inflammatory mediators. Complement fragments C3a, C4a, and C5a are referred to as anaphylatoxins because they are potent inducers of histamine release by mast cells and basophils.[5,6] They also have direct inflammatory effects including smooth muscle contraction, increased vascular permeability, and expression of vascular adhesion molecules. The anaphylatoxins also induce expression of adhesion molecules on circulating monocytes and neutrophils, facilitating the migration of these cells out of the bloodstream, through the endothelial wall, and toward the infected tissue.

Cellular Components of Innate Immunity

Cells with a prominent role in innate immunity include granulocytes, monocytes, dendritic cells, and NK cells.[3] Three primary results of this antigen-nonspecific cellular response are phagocytosis, direct target cell cytotoxicity (cell death), and antigen presentation to T lymphocytes.

Phagocytosis. *Phagocytosis* is the process by which a target cell is engulfed and enzymatically destroyed.[7] Neutrophils, macrophages, and dendritic cells are the major phagocytic cells. Target-cell PAMPs can be recognized directly by TLRs, although phagocytosis generally is enhanced by opsonization, such as CR1 recognition of membrane-bound C3b. Phagocytic cells also express Fc receptors for the constant region of IgG and IgA antibody molecules, which (also) serve as potent opsonins. Receptor ligand-binding initiates sequential membrane fusion events allowing the membrane of the phagocyte to enclose the target (**Figure 1.2**).[7] Eventually the target cell is

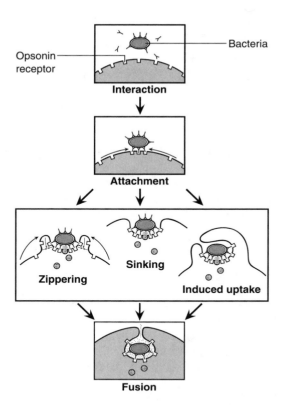

Figure 1.2. Phagocytosis begins with interaction and attachment of the target cell, mediated by phagocytic receptors (Fc receptor binding to opsonizing antibody molecules is shown). The phagocyte then engulfs the target cell by one of three mechanisms to form a cytoplasmic phagosome. Fc receptor-mediated phagocytosis (left) exhibits a "zipper-like" pattern, in which the phagocytic membrane actively extends around the target cell. In contrast, during complement receptor-mediated phagocytosis, the target cell "sinks" into the phagocytic cell in the absence of membrane extensions (center). Phagocytosis can also take place by macropinocytosis (right), a process similar to zippering in which signals generated by the target cell induce phagocytic membrane fusion events and target cell uptake. Enzymatic destruction of the microbial target cell follows once the phagosome fuses with cytoplasmic endosomes and lysosomes. (Adapted from Paul WE, ed. *Fundamental Immunology*. 5th ed. Philadelphia, PA: Lippincott Williams & Wilkins; 2003:1108.)

surrounded and internalized to form an intracellular vacuole, or phagosome. Cytoplasmic storage granules called lysosomes fuse with the phagosome and release degradative lysosomal enzymes. Phagocytic cells possess different types of hydrolytic enzymes, but enzymes such as neutrophil myeloperoxidase can convert molecular oxygen into bactericidal reactive oxygen intermediates. Lysosomal degranulation is often referred to as the "respiratory burst" because oxidative enzyme activity causes a temporary increase in oxygen consumption by the phagocyte.

Phagocytic enzymes can also damage normal tissue, because some degraded cellular debris and enzymes are released extracellularly following phagocytosis.[7] In some cases the phagocyte is too small to totally engulf the target, leading to the secretion of lysosomal enzymes onto the surface of the target cell and into the surrounding microenvironment. Also, some phagocytes die during a prolonged or highly intense inflammatory response. Ensuing lysis of these cells exposes surrounding tissues to the effects of lysosomal enzymes. Pus formation during infection with pyogenic bacteria is the result of these processes. It is composed of cellular debris generated by liquefaction of surrounding tissue.

Phagocytic granulocytes. Granulocytes get their name from the morphologic appearance of the cell cytoplasm, which contains numerous lysosomal storage granules.[3] Both neutrophils and eosinophils are capable of phagocytosis. Eosinophils, however, are ineffective phagocytes that secrete their lysosomal enzymes into the extracellular microenvironment. On the contrary, neutrophils are highly efficient phagocytes that play the primary role in early innate immune responses.[3,7] Also called polymorphonuclear leukocytes (PMNs) because of their unique multilobed nucleus, neutrophils normally account for approximately 60% of all circulating white blood cells and 95% of all granulocytes. Neutrophils mature fully in the bone marrow over a period of 6 days and enter the circulation as terminally differentiated quiescent cells with a lifespan of only 1–2 days. During this brief time, they continually circuit the bloodstream until the appropriate chemotactic signal is received. Because all neutrophils respond to the same limited set of chemotaxins, they are the most rapidly mobilized cells after acute tissue injury. Important chemotaxins for neutrophils include complement fragment C5a, CXCL8 (secreted at the site of tissue injury by endothelial and epithelial cells as well as by activated macrophages), and tumor necrosis factor-alpha (TNF-α), which is secreted primarily by activated macrophages.[8] CXCL8, also called interleukin-8 (IL-8), is a chemokine, a secreted chemical that induces leukocyte chemotaxis. TNF-α is a cytokine, a secreted chemical that induces growth, differentiation, and biologic activity in target leukocytes. Each of these signals causes neutrophil activation, inducing the expression of vascular adhesion molecules called selections and integrins, chemotaxis, and the subsequent release of lysosomal enzymes once phagocytosis has occurred.[3,7] TNF-α also induces the expression of intercellular cell adhesion molecules (ICAMs) on the surface of endothelial cells close to the injured tissue. Activated neutrophils migrate toward the source of the chemotactic signals, adhere to local blood vessel walls, and migrate between endothelial cells into the outlying injured tissue.

Neutrophils are highly efficient phagocytes well adapted to destroy target cells enzymatically.[7] Once they arrive at the inflammatory site, phagocytosis follows. Primary storage granules contain a number of enzymes including lysozyme, nicotinamide adenine dinucleotide phosphate (NADPH) oxidase, and myeloperoxidase. NADPH oxidase and myeloperoxidase are responsible for the respiratory burst. NADPH oxidase catalyzes the conversion of molecular oxygen to the reactive oxygen intermediate superoxide anion, which in turn is converted to hypochlorous acid by myeloperoxidase. Among the enzymes secreted by secondary granules is lactoferrin, which is microbicidal via iron sequestration.

Mononuclear phagocytes. Monocytes develop in the bone marrow but enter the circulation as immature cells capable of further differentiation.[3,7] They remain in the circulation for less than a day, then enter tissues and differentiate into tissue-resident cells called macrophages and immature dendritic cells (DCs).[9] Macrophages are located strategically in tissues particularly vulnerable to antigen exposure,[2,3] such as Kuppfer cells in the sinusoids of the liver, alveolar macrophages in the lung, and microglial cells in the brain. Collectively, tissue-resident macrophages form the mononuclear phagocytic or reticuloendothelial system. Immature DCs, including the Langerhans cells of the skin, are primarily responsible for antigen processing and presentation to T lymphocytes, which will be discussed below.[9]

Macrophages are more effective phagocytes than neutrophils.[7] They are larger cells that can ingest larger particles, express a wider variety of PRRs, and contain sufficient intracellular organelles to manufacture and replenish spent lysosomal enzymes. Also, activated macrophages secrete a wider array of lysosomal enzymes and other products, including inflammatory cytokines such as TNF-α, IL-1, IL-6, IL-8 (CXCL8), and IL-12.[7,8] Macrophages therefore can initiate other components of the inflammatory response, such as neutrophil recruitment and activation (TNF-α and IL-8). IL-1 and IL-6 also play a crucial role in early host protection by inducing fever (many bacteria are temperature-labile) and initiating the hepatic acute phase response.[8] Acute phase proteins synthesized by the liver include C-reactive protein (CRP), which effectively opsonizes microbial cells and initiates the classical complement cascade. IL-1 and IL-6 also exert important effects on the bone marrow, stimulating the production of additional neutrophils. IL-12 plays a central role in T lymphocyte differentiation, discussed more fully under Adaptive Immunity.

NK cells. NK cells represent a third lineage of lymphocytes that differ from T lymphocytes and B lymphocytes by the absence of normal cell surface markers of lymphocyte lineage and differentiation called cluster of differentiation (CD) molecules.[10,11] NK cells also lack an antigen-specific receptor and are therefore classified as part of the innate immune system. These cells develop in the bone marrow and enter the circulation as activated cells. NK cells play the predominant role in immune surveillance, the continual scanning of host tissues for infected or malignant cells.

NK cells respond to many of the same chemotactic signals that recruit neutrophils.[10,11] Opsonization by C3b or IgG antibodies enhance target cell contact. *Antibody-dependent cell-mediated cytotoxicity* (ADCC) is used to describe NK cell destruction of antibody-coated target cells. Once contact is made with a target cell, a number of stimulatory and inhibitory receptors scan the cell surface to determine its "nonself" and "missing self" characteristics. Normal host cells express the appropriate complement of class I major histocompatibility complex (MHC) molecules, discussed more fully under Adaptive Immunity.[12] Class I MHC expression is often down-regulated by viral infection or malignant transformation.[10,11] Inhibitory receptors such as the killer cell immunoglobulin-like receptor (KIR) prevent target cell lysis if class I MHC expression is normal. At the same time, stimulatory receptors on the NK cell, such as NKG2D, search for molecules unique to malignant or infected cells.

The overall mix of inhibitory and stimulatory signals determines the ultimate response to the target cell.[10,11] NK cells are not phagocytic; target-cell destruction is mediated by direct and indirect mechanisms. NK cells secrete interferon-gamma (IFN-γ) and TNF-α, activating local tissue macrophages. NK cells exert direct cytotoxic effects by secreting an enzyme called perforin onto the target cell, which induces lysis by forming osmotic pores in the cell membrane. NK cells also induce the target cell to undergo apoptosis (programmed cell death), in which activation of cellular caspase enzymes leads to the systematic destruction of DNA. NK cells induce apoptosis by secreting enzymes called granzymes into the target cell and by binding Fas molecules on the NK cell surface to Fas ligand (FasL) on the target cell.

Nonphagocytic granulocytes. Eosinophils are produced in the bone marrow and, after entering the circulation, rapidly distribute into peripheral tissues, particularly in the respiratory, intestinal, and genitourinary tracts.[6] Eosinophils play a prominent pro-inflammatory role during allergic reactions, and also respond to helminthic parasitic infections. The inflammatory effects of eosinophils result from the degranulation of lysosomal storage granules, and the secretion of cytokines, major basic protein, eosinophil-derived neurotoxic protein, and other inflammatory mediators. Initial eosinophil activation is largely mediated by activated macrophages, which secrete macrophage inflammatory protein (MIP-1α). Activated T lymphocytes can also activate eosinophils via secretion of cytokines such as IL-5.[2]

Mast cells and basophils are unique among the cells of the immune system because of their expression of high-affinity IgE receptors (FcεRI) and their capacity for degranulation and release of histamine and other inflammatory mediators.[2] Members of the granulocyte lineage produced in the bone marrow will be discussed under Acute Allergic Inflammation.

ADAPTIVE IMMUNITY

The antigen-nonspecific inflammatory response plays a vital role in host protection, but it has some important disadvantages.[3,4] Antigen destruction tends to occur only after tissue damage has already taken place, because chemotaxins are generated by the same processes that produce potent inflammatory mediators. The response to an antigen does not change with repeated exposure because monocytes and granulocytes cannot adapt. And through mutation, many microorganisms are able to devise strategies that can render a rigid defense system ineffective. These shortcomings are addressed by the antigen-specific immune response, mediated by T and B lymphocytes.[10] The two primary advantages of this response are clonal expansion of antigen-specific cells and the development of immunologic memory.

Antigen Presentation to T Lymphocytes

T lymphocytes recognize an antigen through membrane-bound T cell receptors (TCRs).[10,13] A mature T cell expresses thousands of TCRs, each identical in specificity for the same antigen. TCRs are constructed in a random process of gene splicing and combinatorial uniting of variable (V), diversity (D), and joining (J) segments, each existing in multiple allelic forms.[13] Gene rearrangement is catalyzed by enzymes encoded by recombination activation genes (RAG-1 and RAG-2). It is estimated that more than 10^7 unique TCR antigen-binding sites can be constructed. Because each mature T lymphocyte (or its clone of progeny cells) expresses a unique TCR repertoire, the host can recognize a vast array of different antigens. Most T lymphocytes express TCRs composed of an α subunit and a β subunit (α/β TCRs), with about 10% of T cells expressing γ/δ TCRs.[10] TCRs are not capable of cytoplasmic signal transduction, which is carried out by an associated transmembrane CD3 molecule.

TCRs cannot bind to whole or "unprocessed" antigens.[10,13] α/β TCRs recognize linear fragments of the original protein antigen that are 10–12 amino acids long. Similarly, γ/δ TCRs recognize fragments of lipid antigens. Furthermore, the antigenic fragment can only be recognized if presented to the TCR while bound to a surface MHC molecule, also called human leukocyte antigen (HLA). The human MHC is located on the short arm of chromosome six and is divided into three gene classes, each containing multiple loci in a wide variety of allelic forms.[12] Class I genes are comprised of the HLA-A, HLA-B, and HLA-C loci, while class II genes contain the HLA-DP, HLA-DQ, and HLA-DR loci. We each inherit one MHC haplotype (one allele from each of the six gene loci) from each parent, and the two haplotypes are codominant. Depending on the cell type, up to 12 genes can be expressed. The wide variety of alleles at each gene locus makes it highly unlikely that any two individuals, except monozygotic twins, would share identical sets of HLA antigens. In a given individual, the particular constellation of class I and/or class II HLA antigens is identical on the surface of all body cells, allowing T lymphocytes to discriminate between "self" and "nonself." HLA recognition by T lymphocytes is pivotal to transplant rejection and graft-versus-host disease.

Class II HLA antigens are normally expressed only by professional antigen-presenting cells (APCs), which include macrophages, DCs, and B lymphocytes.[10] These cells are specialized to process and present antigens derived from exogenous proteins, such as microbial antigens generated by phagocytosis. The class II HLA antigen processing pathway is depicted in **Figure 1.3**.[14] Helper T lymphocytes express CD4 molecules, which bind to class II HLA antigens and stabilize the simultaneous binding of the TCR to the microbial antigen.[10] Because CD4 molecules cannot bind to class I HLA molecules, helper T lymphocytes are class II HLA-restricted. In contrast, cytotoxic T lymphocytes express CD8 molecules, which can only bind to class I HLA antigens. Class I HLA antigens are normally expressed by all somatic host cells, including APCs. APCs therefore express class I and class II HLA molecules.[10] The class I HLA antigen-processing pathway is specialized to process and present antigenic peptides derived from internally synthesized endogenous proteins such as unique viral peptides or tumor-associated antigens (see Figure 1.3).[14]

APCs are therefore keenly adapted to activate helper T lymphocytes, which in turn activate and regulate all other components of the adaptive immune response.[10] Class I HLA antigens allow potential targets of cytotoxic T lymphocytes to display the cell surface markers that stimulate cytotoxic attack and destruction. This process, *cell-mediated immunity*, is particularly crucial for effective host responses to intracellular infections such as viruses and to newly transformed tumor cells.

Cell-Mediated Immunity

Cell-mediated immune responses are regulated by helper T lymphocytes, with effector functions (destruction of target cells) provided by cytotoxic T lymphocytes and antigen-nonspecific macrophages, NK cells, and granulocytes.[10] Individuals with selective deficiencies of T lymphocyte–mediated immune responses are prone to severe infections with viruses, mycobacteria, or other intracellular organisms.

Helper T lymphocytes. Cell-mediated immunity is initiated and orchestrated by cytokines secreted by antigen-activated CD4+ helper T lymphocytes.[10] As mentioned previously, helper T cells can only be activated by APCs expressing the antigen bound to a class II HLA molecule. Mature lymphocytes are concentrated in secondary lymphoid organs, whereas microbial invasion generally takes place in peripheral tissues. DCs are ideal APCs that can effectively link the secondary lymphoid organs to the periphery because they migrate and mature.[9,10] Immature DCs, which are highly active and efficient phagocytes, reside primarily in the periphery. Activation secondary to PRR recognition and phagocytosis transforms DCs into migratory cells that can move toward draining lymph nodes (where helper T lymphocytes are located). During their journey, DCs mature, losing their phagocytic characteristics but gaining expression of class II HLA molecules and costimulatory molecules, and beginning to secrete IL-12.

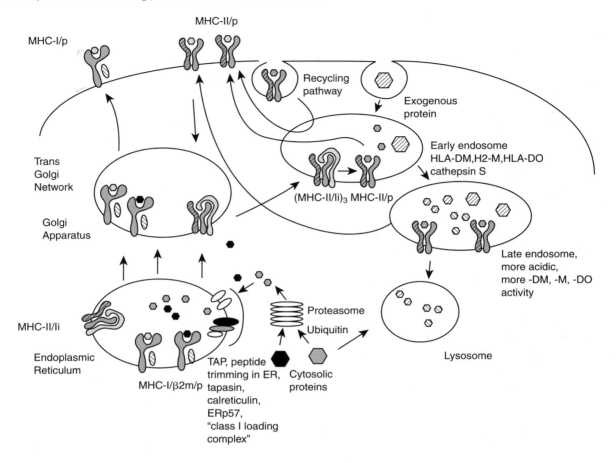

Figure 1.3. The HLA (or MHC) antigen-processing pathways. Endogenous (cytosolic) antigenic peptides (shaded hexagon) are transported to the cell surface and displayed by class I HLA molecules, with subsequent recognition by a complementary cytotoxic T lymphocyte triggering cell death. Examples include viral peptides (virally infected cells) and tumor-associated antigens. In contrast, exogenous proteins (barred hexagon) are taken up by professional antigen-presenting cells and processed by the class II HLA antigen processing pathway. The resulting cell surface antigen/class II HLA complex can activate a complementary helper T lymphocyte. (Adapted from Paul WE, ed. *Fundamental Immunology*. 5th ed. Philadelphia, PA: Lippincott Williams & Wilkins; 2003:578.)

Helper T-cell activation requires two signals (**Figure 1.4**).[14,15] The first is provided when the TCR binds to the microbial antigen/class II HLA complex on the APC surface. The second or costimulatory signal is provided by the binding of CD28 (T lymphocyte) to B7 (APC). If the costimulatory signal is not received, the helper T cell becomes anergic (unable to activate and proliferate). T-cell anergy is a pivotal part of peripheral immune tolerance, discussed under Autoimmunity.[16] Once both signals are received, the helper T cell becomes activated and begins to secrete IL-2, leading to clonal expansion of antigen-specific CD4+ T lymphocytes, all expressing identical TCRs and all able to recognize the same specific antigen that activated the parent cell. Clonal expansion temporarily increases the percentage of antigen-specific T lymphocytes in the total T cell pool from about 0.001% to more than 30%.[10]

Two subclasses of activated CD4+ T lymphocytes have been described, based on the profile of cytokines these cells secrete after activation.[10] The Th2 phenotype may represent the default pathway for activated CD4+ T lymphocyte differentiation. Th2 cells primarily secrete IL-3, IL-4, and IL-5, which promote activation of antigen-specific B lymphocytes. Th2 cells also secrete IL-10, which suppresses cell-mediated immunity. The presence of IL-12 (secreted by activated DCs) promotes the differentiation of activated CD4+ lymphocytes into Th1 cells, which secrete IL-2, IFN-γ, and TNF-β. These cytokines promote cell-mediated immunity by activating macrophages and antigen-specific CD8+ cytotoxic T lymphocytes.

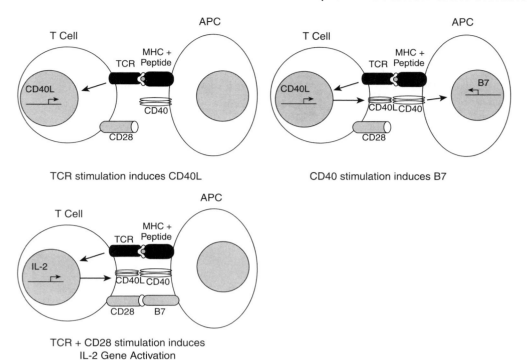

Figure 1.4. Helper T-cell activating signals. The first signal is delivered once the T cell receptor (TCR) binds to the antigen/class II HLA (or MHC) complex on the antigen-presenting cell (APC) surface. This binding induces the expression of CD40L on the T-cell surface, which binds to CD40 on the APC. CD40/CD40L binding then induces the expression of B7 (or CD80/86) on the APC membrane, which binds to CD28 on the T cell, delivering the second or costimulatory signal needed for helper T cell activation. (Adapted from Paul WE, ed. *Fundamental Immunology*. 5th ed. Philadelphia, PA: Lippincott Williams & Wilkins; 2003:330.)

Cytotoxic T lymphocytes. CD8⁺ T lympho-cytes are class I HLA-restricted; like naive helper T cells, they require two signals for activation.[10] The first signal is provided by the binding of the TCR to an antigen/class I HLA complex. The second is provided by the costimulating B7, whose source is somewhat controversial.[17] As mentioned earlier, B7 is normally expressed only by profes-sional APCs, which express both class I and class II HLA molecules. Although all somatic cells can process and present endogenous antigens via the class I HLA pathway, only professional APCs can provide the costimulatory signal that prevents inappropriate T-cell activation in peripheral tis-sues. However, exogenous antigens normally enter the class II HLA pathway and are not available for CD8⁺ T-lymphocyte recognition. Current evidence suggests that certain populations of DCs can pro-cess and present exogenous antigens through the class I HLA pathway, a mechanism called *cross-presentation*.[17] Cross-presentation is enhanced by antigen-activated CD4⁺ T lymphocytes, implying that mature DCs complete the process of antigen-specific helper and cytotoxic T-cell activation simultaneously. Clonal expansion secondary to

IL-2 release results in a clone of antigen-specific cytotoxic T cells.

Similar to helper T cells, cytotoxic T cells also differentiate into at least two subpopulations.[10] Tc1 cells secrete IFN-γ, with effects similar to those described earlier. Tc2 cells secrete IL-4 and IL-5, and are thought to help stimulate B lymphocyte function. Tc1 and Tc2 cells are equally effective at destroying target cells bearing the corresponding antigen/class I HLA complex. Because Tc1 and Tc2 cells are effector cells already in an activated state, a costimulatory signal is no longer needed. Once the TCR binds to an antigen/class I HLA complex on an infected or malignant target cell, a cytotoxic response follows. The cytotoxic mechanisms are very similar to those described earlier for NK cells, including perforin and granzyme secretion and Fas/FasL binding.[18] Each cytotoxic T cell can kill multiple target cells.

Memory T lymphocytes. About 95% of the helper and cytotoxic T-cell clones produced during a primary adaptive immune response die within a few days of antigen removal. The surviving 5% differentiate into memory T cells and can survive for long periods, in some cases for the life of the host.[19] Reexposure to the same antigen results in a faster activation of cell-mediated immunity than initial exposure. Distinct subpopulations of CD8[+] and CD4[+] memory T cells called central and effector memory cells have been identified.

Central CD4[+] memory T cells do not exhibit effector activity.[19] Additionally, these cells express the same homing receptors (CD62L and CCR7) that are expressed by naive CD4[+] T cells. As a result, these cells continually migrate through secondary lymphoid organs and the bloodstream but cannot enter peripheral tissues. Effector CD4[+] memory T cells no longer express these homing receptors and tend to migrate into peripheral tissues such as the skin, lungs, and gastrointestinal tract. These cells have effector capability (cytokine secretion), strongly express the Th1 or Th2 phenotype, and are considered more differentiated than central memory cells. CD8[+] memory T cells exist in similar central and effector subpopulations.

The mechanism of memory T-cell differentiation is poorly understood. One hypothesis relates to the limited capacity for normal T-cell replication.[19] Naive T cells appear to live for about 6 months after they exit the thymus. These cells proliferate rapidly after antigen activation, followed inevitably by apoptosis once a threshold number of cell divisions occurs. Accordingly, memory T cells may represent a subpopulation of cells that were stimulated less intensely or perhaps in a unique manner during the initial primary response. Central memory cells are more primitive than effector memory cells because of fewer replications. It is known that CD62L and CCR7 expression is down-regulated as replication continues. Finally, IL-15 (secreted by mononuclear phagocytes) promotes the differentiation of CD8[+] T cells into central memory cells, a sharp contrast to the proliferative effects of IL-2.[19] CD8[+] memory cell formation may also depend on the microenvironment in which naive cytotoxic T-cell activation occurs, and therefore whether these cells are predominantly exposed to IL-2 or IL-15.

Suppressor T lymphocytes. T lymphocytes with immune suppressive activity are critical to maintaining peripheral tolerance and preventing excessive normal tissue damage during adaptive immune responses.[10,20] Both naturally occurring and induced populations have been identified. CD4[+]/CD25[+] suppressor T cells (Tregs) develop in the thymus as a distinct third T-lymphocyte lineage.[20,21] Tregs appear to enter the circulation in a perpetually activated state, because they express a number of surface markers normally expressed by other T cells only after antigen activation. These surface molecules include CD25 (the alpha chain

of the IL-2 receptor) and cytotoxic T-lymphocyte–associated antigen (CTLA-4). Tregs inhibit IL-2 secretion and clonal expansion of helper T cells. The precise mechanism is still unknown, but initial suppression appears to require direct cell contact and TCR recognition. Following activation, small numbers of Tregs can suppress up to 90% of total T-lymphocyte proliferation, illustrating the importance of immunosuppressive cytokines secreted by Tregs such as IL-10 and transforming growth factor-beta (TGF-β). Because Tregs constitutively express the IL-2 receptor, they are also hypothesized to competitively inhibit helper T-cell proliferation by acting as IL-2 "traps." Tregs may also exert indirect inhibitory effects on helper T cells by binding to DCs via CTLA-4, which binds to B7 costimulatory molecules and down-regulates their expression.

Suppressor T cells can also be induced from normal helper and cytotoxic T-cell populations.[20] T-regulatory 1 (Tr1) cells (also called CD4[+]/CD25− Tregs) are generated in vitro from antigen-activated helper T cells cultured with IL-10 and IFN-α. They inhibit helper T cells by secreting large amounts of IL-10 and variable amounts of TGF-β. Tr1 cells also induce apoptosis of mature DCs. Cytotoxic T cells can also acquire suppressor activity.[22] Normal murine helper T-cell activation leads to brief expression of an HLA variant called Qa-1, which binds to a variety of self-peptides. Cytotoxic T cells expressing TCRs specific for these Qa-1/self-peptide complexes bind, and are transformed into Qa-1 CD8[+] Tregs. The precise mechanism of suppression is not known, but Qa-1 CD8[+] Tregs only inhibit helper T cells expressing the complementary Qa-1/self-peptide complexes.

Antigen Recognition by B Lymphocytes

B cells recognize whole (unprocessed) antigen by membrane-bound IgM and IgD immunoglobulin (antibody) molecules, which effectively serve as B-cell receptors.[10,23] Antigens do not require prior processing to be recognized by antibodies. In fact, alteration of the native tertiary or quarternary structure of an antigen (denaturation of a protein antigen, for example) generally renders the molecule nonantigenic.[1] The antigen-binding site of an antibody molecule (paratope) actually binds to a 6–8 amino acid or oligosaccharide sequence called the epitope.[24] The shape of the epitope (determined by the overall structure of the antigen) determines the required shape of the corresponding paratope.[1] The epitope is not always a sequential sequence, but instead may be composed of individual sequences from varying parts of the antigen brought together by the folding of the protein chain. Each antigen molecule can express a number of unique epitopes, each recognized by a different antibody molecule.

Each individual antibody molecule (monomer) is made up of two identical heavy chains and two identical light chains, held together by interchain disulfide bonds (**Figure 1.5**).[24,25] Five classes of heavy chains (α, δ, ε, γ, and μ) and one type of light chain (either κ or λ) can be constructed by each developing B cell or its clone of progeny cells. Each chain is made up of folded regions (domains). Light chains contain one variable region (V_L) and one constant region (C_L), while heavy chains contain one variable (V_H) and three or four constant regions (C_H1-C_H4). Variable regions are so named because the amino acid sequence is highly variable among antibodies from different B cell lineages. Constant regions are relatively conserved within a given antibody subclass (IgA, IgD, IgE, IgG, or IgM) among different B cell lineages. Paired V_L and V_H regions form the antigen-binding site, so each antibody monomer carries two identical antigen-binding sites. With the exception of IgE, antibodies are hinged between the C_H1 and C_H2 regions. The paired regions above the hinge are referred to as the antigen-binding fragment (Fab). Each antibody monomer has two identical Fab fragments. The paired constant regions below the hinge form a single constant fragment (Fc).

The V_L and V_H regions are constructed in a random gene-splicing and combinatorial-joining process analogous to that used to construct TCRs.[26] V_L regions consist of a variable (V) and a joining (J) segment; V_H regions consist of V, J, and diversity (D) segments. As with the diversity of TCR antigen-binding sites, more than 10^7 V_L or V_H regions can be constructed. B lymphocytes develop in the bone marrow, with each cell programmed to produce antibody monomers (regardless of class) of only one antigen specificity (idiotype).[24,25] Should this cell subsequently be activated by its complementary antigen and cloned, all of its progeny would share the identical idiotype.

Humoral Immunity

Humoral immunity is conferred by soluble antibody molecules, and can be transferred from one individual to another through serum transfusion. B lymphocytes synthesize and display antibodies on their cell surface, but large quantities of soluble antibody can only be secreted by a specialized type of B lymphocyte called the plasma cell.[2]

B lymphocytes complete several maturation steps in the bone marrow.[27] Pro-B cells express RAG-1 and RAG-2 genes and begin synthesizing the μ V_H chain. Early pre-B cells then synthesize a temporary (surrogate) light chain, assemble surrogate IgM monomers, and transport them to the cell surface. Pre-B cells then replace the surrogate light chains with true λ or κ light chains, completing the surface expression of true IgM monomers. Once surface IgM is expressed, the cells enter the bloodstream as immature B cells and migrate to secondary lymphoid organs where they begin to synthesize δ heavy chains. Mature B cells express IgM and IgD monomers on their surface, all of identical idiotype. These quiescent cells are referred to as naive B cells prior to antigen encounter. They continually migrate through the bloodstream and secondary lymphoid organs, where they die after about 6 months unless activated by their complementary antigen.

B-cell activation. Naive B lymphocytes can become activated two ways: direct activation and cognate activation.[10,23] Antigens that express multiple copies of the same epitope can activate B cells directly by cross-linking surface IgM monomers. Examples include bacterial capsular polysaccharides and envelope proteins expressed by a variety of circulating viruses. Direct activation is enhanced by prior opsonization with C3b, which binds to complement receptor CR2 on the B-cell surface. Most commonly, B-cell activation needs help from antigen-activated helper T lymphocytes, a process called *cognate activation*.[23] Three critical events follow B-cell activation: antibody class switch

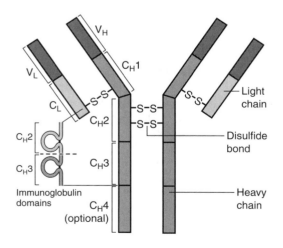

Figure 1.5. Basic structure of an antibody monomer. An antibody monomer contains two identical light and heavy chains, each made up of variable (dark gray) and constant (light gray) regions. (Adapted from Doan T, Melvold R, Waltenbaugh C, eds. *Concise Medical Immunology*. Philadelphia, PA: Lippincott Williams & Wilkins; 2005:48.)

recombination (CSR), variable chain somatic hypermutation (SHM), and development of B-cell memory. These generally occur only when B-cell activation involves cognate T-cell help.

B lymphocytes are concentrated in primary B-cell follicles found in secondary lymphoid organs such as the spleen or lymph nodes.[23] T cells are concentrated in adjacent T-cell zones such as the paracortex of lymph nodes. Primary B-cell follicles consist of naive B cells clustered around follicular DCs (FDCs). Thought to be derived from stromal cells, FDCs differ from the migratory DCs that present antigen to helper T cells. FDCs are specialized to activate B cells, because they express CD40L and can secrete IL-2. B cells likely first encounter antigen as it is carried through the lymphoid tissue by blood or lymph. The antigen is bound by surface antibody, internalized, and processed; and the antigenic peptide is subsequently displayed on the B-cell surface complexed to a class II HLA molecule. Putative B cell activation or "priming" is completed by the binding of CD40 (B cell) and CD40L (FDC) and the secretion of IL-2.[23] These antigen-primed B cells then migrate to the border separating the B-cell and T-cell regions, where they receive cognate signals. Cognate signaling can only occur between B cells and helper T cells that have already been activated by the same antigen. Migratory DCs from the periphery carry the antigenic peptide to the T-cell zones of draining lymph nodes and activate antigen-specific helper T cells, as previously described. In response to homing signals secreted by antigen-primed B cells, some members of the resulting activated helper T-cell clone migrate to the B-cell/T-cell border.[23]

Primed B-cell/activated T-cell contact is initially mediated through binding the TCR and complementary antigen/class II HLA complex, but costimulatory signals appear to be crucial for subsequent CSR, SHM, and memory B-cell development.[23] CD40-CD40L signaling seems necessary for all three processes. CSR is also thought to be induced through binding OX-40 (activated helper T cell) to OX-40L (primed B cell). Finally, the activated helper T cell secretes a variety of cytokines (IL-2, IL-4, IL-5, IL-6, and IFN-γ) that also contribute to B-cell proliferation and CSR.

Once the primed B cell is fully activated and cloned, two subpopulations emerge.[23] One population stays in the T-cell zone and undergoes terminal differentiation (including CSR) to form plasma cells, large cells incapable of further mitosis. These cells secrete large quantities of soluble antibodies but no longer express typical B-cell markers, such as surface antibody monomers or class II HLA molecules. As a result of CSR, these cells secrete a variety of antibody classes, including IgM and IgG. Since SHM has not taken place, however, the affinity of these antibodies (the degree to which the antibody is attracted to its complementary antigen) is highly variable. T-cell zone plasma cells typically live no longer than 2 or 3 days, but the antibodies produced mediate the early phase of a primary humoral immune response.

Germinal center reaction. The other subpopulation of antigen-activated B cells migrates back to primary B-cell follicles and proliferates rapidly.[23] The intense proliferation crowds naive B cells to the periphery, forming a germinal center. The germinal center polarizes into a dark zone and light zone, with the dark zone adjacent to the B-cell/T-cell border. The dark zone is packed with rapidly proliferating centroblasts—activated B cells that have undergone differentiation and lost surface expression of IgM and IgD. Both CSR and SHM take place in these cells.[28] During SHM, variable chain gene segments (particularly the V segments that form the antigen-binding sites) are randomly rearranged.[23] SHM leads to *affinity maturation*, the production of antibody monomers with higher antigen affinity. Continued CSR favors a switch to IgG antibody production. After these processes, nonproliferating centroblasts express the new antibody, migrate to the light zone, and become centrocytes.[23] Light zones, rich in FDCs that express high-affinity IgG receptors (FcγR) and complement receptor CR-1, are adapted to present antigen to light zone centrocytes. Centrocytes are selected for survival based on antigen-binding affinity, with cells expressing surface antibody of lower affinity removed by apoptosis. Affinity maturation develops as successive cycles of centroblast proliferation, SHM, and selection take place. Most of these cells differentiate into larger plasma cells.

Antigen destruction by soluble antibodies. High-affinity B cells that survive germinal center selection exist in two subpopulations.[23] One population differentiates into long-lived plasma cells that secrete high-affinity IgG monomers. These plasma cells migrate to the bone marrow, where they are thought to survive for as long as a year after the primary humoral response has ended. Circulating antibodies are the primary effectors of humoral immunity, binding to antigen and forming immune complexes.[25] Antibody binding alone can inactivate some infectious processes, such as the effects of released bacterial toxins or the binding of certain viruses to host cells. But in most cases, immune complexes initiate destruction by antigen-nonspecific mechanisms discussed earlier, such as the classical complement cascade, opsonization, or ADCC.

B-cell memory. The other post–germinal center B cells become long-lived memory cells.[19,23] Memory B cells and plasma cells appear to have distinct differentiation pathways. Whereas plasma cells are large cells and lack surface antibody or class II HLA expression, memory B cells are small and express both surface markers. Memory B cells have successfully completed CSR, SHM, and selection, and express high-affinity IgG, IgA, or IgE antibodies. On subsequent exposure to the same antigen, a faster and more effective secondary humoral response will follow.

TISSUES OF THE IMMUNE SYSTEM

The immune system is organized into primary lymphoid organs (bone marrow and thymus), where new immune cells grow and mature, and secondary lymphoid organs, where antigen-specific immune responses are generated.[29] A network of blood vessels and lymphatic channels connects these organs to each other and to the peripheral tissues, where microbial invasion typically begins.

Primary Lymphoid Organs

Bone marrow. The bone marrow is the site of *hematopoiesis*, the process by which all lymphoid and myeloid blood cells develop from common, self-renewing progenitors called pluripotent stem cells (**Figure 1.6**).[29] The bone marrow microenvironment contains a network of stromal cells, connective tissue, adipocytes, and macrophages that form a mesh for physical support and supply stem cells and developing hematopoietic precursors with essential nutrients. Stromal cells also secrete

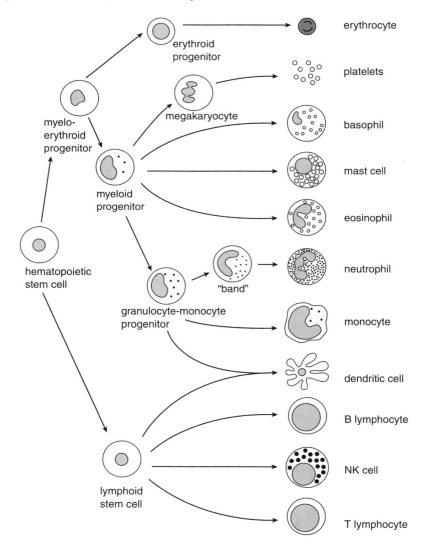

Figure 1.6. Hematopoiesis. (Adapted from Parslow TG, Stites DP, Imboden JB, eds. *Medical Immunology*. 10th ed. New York, NY: McGraw-Hill Companies; 2001:3.)

a variety of cytokines (IL-3, IL-7, IL-11) and growth factors such as granulocyte-macrophage colony-stimulating factor (CSF), granulocyte-CSF, and stem cell growth factor (c-kit). It is hypothesized that different microenvironments exist in the bone marrow. Each is adapted to support the development of a particular hematopoietic lineage, based in part on the relative availability and mixture of these highly pleiotropic growth factors.

Many hematopoietic cells live only for days. To maintain homeostasis, the bone marrow produces billions of new cells daily, of which about 60% are neutrophils.[29] Activated helper T cells and macrophages can (also) secrete hematopoietic growth factors, and during infection can stimulate a rapid expansion of hematopoietic activity.

Thymus. The thymus is a bilobed organ located above the heart that serves as the site of T-lymphocyte differentiation and lineage commitment.[29,30] Immature T-cell precursors migrate from the bone marrow to the outer subcapsular zone of the thymus.[30] These cells do not express TCRs and are referred to as double-negative (DN) thymocytes because they also do not express CD4 or CD8 molecules. At this point they begin to proliferate and initiate TCR rearrangement, synthesizing TCRβ, TCRδ, and TCRγ chains. Thymocytes that successfully synthesize functional γ/δ TCRs appear to undergo no subsequent selection steps, and typically mature without expressing CD4 or CD8 molecules. In contrast, DN thymocytes that successfully synthesize a TCRβ chain begin a process of positive and negative selection prior to maturation.

Once the TCRβ chain is formed, it is complexed to a surrogate TCRα chain and CD3 molecule, then transported to the cell surface to begin β selection.[30] Further TCRβ rearrangement stops, TCRα rearrangement begins, and both CD4 and CD8 are expressed, transforming the cell into a double-positive (DP) thymocyte. Independent of ligand binding, the putative TCR attempts to signal the nucleus. If the TCR is not functional, the cell undergoes apoptosis. If signaling succeeds, the cell completes β selection and migrates beneath the subcapsular zone into the thymic cortex. In the cortex, the DP thymocyte must now produce a viable TCRα chain, replace the surrogate chain to produce a true α/β TCR, and complete the process of positive selection.[30] Not only must the TCR be capable of successful nuclear signaling, it must also recognize and bind to self-HLA molecules with a minimum threshold affinity. Surviving cells commit to the CD4 or CD8 lineage based on the affinity of their α/β TCRs for class I or class II HLA molecules. Single-

positive (CD4+ or CD8+) thymocytes then migrate into the inner medulla of the thymus, where they must survive negative selection.[30] Medullary DCs present a variety of self-antigens bound to class I and class II HLA molecules. If the affinity of TCR binding exceeds a maximum threshold, the cell dies. Fewer than 5% of the T-cell precursors that enter the thymus survive positive and negative selection. Mature CD4+ or CD8+ T cells then enter the circulation and migrate to secondary lymphoid organs.

Secondary Lymphoid Organs

Secondary lymphoid organs include lymph nodes, the spleen, and mucosal-associated lymphoid tissue (MALT)—clusters of lymphoid tissue that drain mucosal surfaces.[29] These tissues are strategically located to trap antigens entering the body through the blood or other tissues. Secondary lymphoid organs are home to most of the body's lymphocytes, and are therefore the sites in which adaptive immune responses develop.

Lymph nodes. Lymph nodes are small, round, encapsulated organs situated at the major junctions of lymphatic vessels.[29] Lymphatic vessels drain interstitial fluid from the tissues, ultimately returning it to the bloodstream at the thoracic duct after having circulated it through secondary lymphoid organs. Lymph nodes are therefore especially suited to trapping antigens that invade peripheral tissues. Prominent collections of lymph nodes include the cervical, axillary, intercostal, mesenteric, and inguinal nodes.

Lymph nodes are fed by afferent lymphatic vessels and drained on the opposite side by an efferent lymphatic channel. Efferent lymphatics merge to form the thoracic duct.[29] The afferent lymphatics enter the node and empty into the subcapsular sinus, which overlies the cortex. Soluble antigen and migratory DCs carrying antigen enter draining lymph nodes through the afferent lymphatic vessels. The inner cortex contains primary B-cell follicles, secondary B-cell follicles (with active germinal centers), and the T-cell zone (paracortex). Immediately adjacent to the efferent lymphatic vessel is the medulla, which consists of medullary cords and medullary sinuses. The medullary sinuses merge to form the efferent lymphatic channel. The medullary cords contain activated B cells, activated T cells, and plasma cells in the process of exiting the lymph node.

Naive lymphocytes enter lymph nodes from the bloodstream.[29] Nodal arteries empty into the paracortex by way of high endothelial venules. These specialized postcapillary endothelial cells express cell adhesion molecules that effectively promote the transmigration of naive T cells and B cells from blood to paracortex.

Spleen. While lymph nodes are efficient filters of antigens that enter the body in peripheral tissues, they can trap blood-borne antigens only if they extravasate into outlying tissues. This potential void in the host defense system is corrected by the spleen, which is adapted to filter and trap blood-borne antigens.[29]

This encapsulated organ, located in the left abdominal cavity, is fed by the splenic artery and is divided into compartments designated as red pulp and white pulp.[29] Red pulp contains aged red blood cells (RBCs), stromal cells, macrophages, NK cells, and plasma cells; it serves as the primary site of RBC degradation and removal. Antigen processing takes place in the lymphocyte-rich white pulp, made up of B-cell follicles and T-cell zones analogous to those found in lymph nodes.

Both blood-borne antigens and naive lymphocytes enter the spleen through the splenic artery.[29] Arterial branches feed each white pulp nodule, connecting by way of central arterioles surrounded by a T-lymphocyte– and DC-rich periarticular lymphoid sheath (PALS). The PALS is surrounded by the marginal zone, containing macrophages and a collection of naive, activated, and memory B cells. As with lymph nodes, these B cells are arranged in primary and secondary follicles. Blood initially enters the marginal sinus, then travels into the T-cell zones of the PALS. Blood exits the spleen through the venous sinusoids of the red pulp.

MALT. These nonencapsulated lymphoid tissues include organized networks of primary lymphoid follicles and other immunocompetent cells (the tonsils, adenoids, appendix, and Peyer's patches of the intestine) and loosely organized collections of lymphoid cells that populate the intestinal villi.[29] These tissues adjoin mucosal surfaces, such as the gastrointestinal and respiratory tracts, and are specially adapted to filter and trap antigens that invade these surfaces. MALT immune responses generate plasma cells that primarily secrete IgA antibody.

THE IMMUNE SYSTEM IN HUMAN DISEASE

The same innate and adaptive immune responses that protect the host from infection can cause significant tissue injury if normal regulatory mechanisms are lost. Hypersensitivity reactions result from abnormal or dysregulated extensions of the acute inflammatory response.

Inflammation

The typical result of an innate immune response is inflammation at the site of tissue injury or infection.[31] Acute inflammation is characterized clinically by swelling, pain, warmth, and erythema. Symptoms can develop quite rapidly following changes in local vascular endothelial cells and the recruitment and activation of innate immune cells, particularly neutrophils and eosinophils. Local vasodilation increases blood flow to the area, causing warmth and redness. Endothelial cells also contract (increased vascular permeability), allowing an exudate of fluid and plasma proteins to accumulate and contribute to local pain and swelling. A number of rapidly liberated inflammatory mediators direct this process.

The lectin and alternative complement cascades discussed earlier play a major role in neutrophil activation and chemotaxis.[5] Tissue damage initiates the kinin cascade.[31] Bradykinin contributes to local vascular changes including increased permeability. Bradykinin and complement fragment C3a also induce the release of prostaglandins (PGs) such as PGD2 from local tissue macrophages, endothelial cells, and platelets. PGs contribute to pain, fever, and increased vascular permeability. Neutrophils and eosinophils arriving at the inflammatory site also contribute to inflammation by releasing leukotrienes such as LTA4, LTB4, and LTC4. Leukotrienes promote a further increase in vascular permeability, and accelerate neutrophil recruitment by inducing the expression of endothelial adhesion molecules and acting as potent chemotaxins. Tissue damage can also trigger the degranulation of local tissue mast cells, which liberates histamine, one of the most potent inducers of local vasodilation and increased vascular permeability.

Acute inflammation is vital to host defense since it helps limit the spread of bacteria, cellular debris, or toxic by-products of phagocytosis and mast cell degranulation. On initial exposure to an antigen, the innate immune response is the only defense until adaptive immunity develops. Disordered regulation of normal inflammatory mechanisms in genetically prone individuals can lead to hypersensitivity reactions or certain types of autoimmune disorders.

Hypersensitivity

Hypersensitivity is an uncontrolled inflammatory response leading to significant or even fatal local or systemic organ damage.[32] Four distinct patterns of hypersensitivity are recognized, based on the type of immune cells that mediate the response. The underlying mechanisms of B-cell and/or T-cell activation are identical to those previously described. All four types of hypersensitivity require an initial asymptomatic sensitization exposure to an antigen; clinical symptoms appear on subsequent exposure.

Acute allergic inflammation (Type I hypersensitivity). Allergic inflammation is often called immediate hypersensitivity or anaphylaxis because clinical symptoms can appear within seconds to minutes of allergen exposure.[32] Allergens are typically ubiquitous proteins (ragweed pollen, for example) that elicit an immune response in only a small percentage of the population. *Atopy* describes individuals genetically prone to immediate hypersensitivity reactions. The cause of these reactions is poorly understood, but seems to involve dysregulation of normal cell-mediated immune responses, leading to excessive Th2 development and subsequent production of circulating IgE antibodies.

Type I hypersensitivity is mediated by the degranulation of circulating basophils and tissue mast cells bearing allergen-specific IgE antibodies.[6,32] Mast cells and basophils both develop in the bone marrow as members of the granulocyte lineage; they are unique among all hematopoietic cells because of their expression of high-affinity IgE receptors (FcεRI). Basophils enter the circulation as mature cells, normally about 1% of circulating white blood cells. Mast cells leave the bone marrow as immature cells, circulating briefly before entering tissues and differentiating into mature, tissue-resident cells. Tissue mast cells are concentrated in connective and mucosal tissues adjacent to blood and lymphatic channels. Initial allergen exposure is asymptomatic, but the host is sensitized by production of allergen-specific IgE antibodies that rapidly bind to basophils and mast cells.

On subsequent exposure, the allergen rapidly binds to IgE and cross-links FcεRI receptors causing mast cell and basophil degranulation and histamine release.[6,32] Histamine rapidly causes local smooth muscle contraction, increased vascular permeability, and mucus secretion. Neutrophils and eosinophils are activated and recruited, further amplifying the inflammatory response. Examples of Type I hypersensitivity include allergic rhinitis and allergic asthma.

Acute immunoglobulin-mediated inflammation (Type II hypersensitivity). As discussed earlier, both IgM and IgG immune complexes can "fix" complement (initiate the classical complement cascade). Target cell destruction can follow directly (MAC formation), or can occur secondary to opsonization and chemotaxis of phagocytes.

Type II hypersensitivity reactions are most commonly associated with transfusion reactions, as antibodies form immune complexes with foreign antigens on the surface of mismatched red blood cells or platelets.[32] A number of autoimmune disorders are mediated by Type II hypersensitivity, including Goodpasture's syndrome, myasthenia gravis, autoimmune hemolytic anemia, and idiopathic thrombocytopenic purpura.

Acute immune complex–mediated inflammation (Type III hypersensitivity). IgM and IgG immune complexes are formed during all normal humoral immune responses, and are efficiently removed by tissue-resident macrophages. Excess immune complexes can form during certain chronic or repeated infections, preventing efficient removal by phagocytosis.[32] These complexes can become deposited in small blood vessels or well-perfused organs; this can lead to acute inflammatory reactions within hours. As with Type II hypersensitivity reactions, immune complexes fix complement and recruit activated phagocytic neutrophils. However, Type III hypersensitivity reactions take place on tissue surfaces. Neutrophils are unable to phagocytose the target, resulting in extracellular release of lysosomal enzymes and extensive tissue damage.

Type III hypersensitivity can be localized (arthus reactions in the skin secondary to an insect bite) or systemic (serum sickness).[32] Autoimmune diseases mediated by Type III hypersensitivity include systemic lupus erythematosus and rheumatoid arthritis.

Chronic inflammation (Type IV hypersensitivity). Chronic inflammation (delayed-type hypersensitivity) is an example of cell-mediated immunity.[32] Th1 effector cells called T_{DTH} cells (delayed-type hypersensitivity helper T cells) mediate Type IV hypersensitivity by activating and recruiting macrophages and cytotoxic T cells. Large numbers of activated macrophages and cytotoxic T cells accumulate at the inflammatory site within 48–72 hours, classically producing induration or swelling.

A positive tuberculin skin test and contact dermatitis are examples of Type IV hypersensitivity.[32] Type IV hypersensitivity is also responsible for acute allograft rejection, discussed below.

Autoimmunity

Because the antigen-binding regions of TCRs and antibody variable chains are synthesized in random chromosomal rearrangement, self-reactive lymphocytes inevitably are produced. Autoimmune disorders result from poorly understood disruptions in normal immune tolerance. Immune tolerance consists of central tolerance, peripheral tolerance, and suppressor T-cell activity.[16]

Central tolerance. T cells must survive positive and negative selection in the thymus prior to full maturation.[30] The negative selection of DP thymocytes is an example of central tolerance. Developing B cells are also subject to negative selection before they leave the bone marrow.[16] Once pre–B cells express surface IgM monomers, the cells are exposed to a variety of self-antigens. If the antigens are bound with excess affinity, the cell undergoes reversible maturational arrest. Through receptor editing, the pre–B cell rearranges the VDJ segments of the variable chain to produce a new antigen-binding site, which is retested. Self-reactive cells eventually undergo apoptosis if receptor editing fails.

Peripheral tolerance. Only a small fraction of developing lymphocytes fully mature and enter the circulation. Even so, central tolerance is not foolproof. Peripheral tolerance addresses this problem by rendering autoreactive B cells and T cells anergic, or functionally inert.[16] Anergic lymphocytes are unable to activate even if they encounter their true complementary foreign antigen.

Peripheral tolerance is driven by lymphocytes' need to receive the appropriate costimulatory signals during activation.[16] For example, helper T cells can only be activated by professional APCs via expression of class II HLA and costimulatory B7 molecules. Anergy results from TCR binding in the absence of B7-CD28 signaling. Cytotoxic T cells are thought to require the same signals as those provided by APCs via cross presentation. Naive self-reactive CD8[+] T cells that bind to self-antigen/class I HLA complexes on host cells (non-APCs) are rendered anergic since B7-CD28 signaling does not occur. Anergy is also induced in self-reactive B cells that bind to antigen in the absence of cognate helper T-cell CD40-CD40L signaling.

Loss of tolerance. A number of autoimmune disorders appear to be associated with infection.[33] Through *molecular mimicry*, antigenic microbial peptides closely resemble peptides displayed by normal host cells. The adaptive immune response to infection sets in motion an autoimmune response to the affected host tissues. Rheumatic fever is thought to be an example of molecular mimicry. Group A, β-hemolytic *Streptococcus pyogenes* produces an antigen called M protein, which closely mimics the peptide sequence of sarcolemmal molecules on normal heart valves.

Autoimmunity clearly has a genetic link that is not fully understood. The expression of certain HLA molecules seems to predispose individuals to particular autoimmune disorders.[34] For example, the class I HLA molecule B27 greatly increases the risk of ankylosing spondylitis. Other HLA molecules associated with autoimmunity include HLA-DR2 (Goodpasture's syndrome) and HLA-DR3 (systemic lupus erythematosus).

Congenital Immunodeficiency Disorders

Acquired immunodeficiency is well documented as a result of myelosuppressive or immunosuppressive drug therapy or infections caused by agents such as the human immunodeficiency virus (HIV-1). Equally profound immune suppression can also result from a variety of autosomal recessive or X chromosome-linked, inherited disorders.[35,36] Autosomal recessive disorders are expressed only if the mutated gene is inherited from both parents; they tend to affect both genders equally. X-linked disorders affect males more commonly, since only a single X chromosome is inherited from the mother. These disorders can selectively affect the development and function of a single component of the immune system or many coordinated pathways. Such disorders not only predispose affected individuals to a variety of infections, but may also increase the risk of certain types of malignancies caused by a failure of normal immune surveillance. Much of the knowledge concerning the role of B cells, T cells, and other immune system components in host protection has been gained through studying individuals with hereditary immunodeficiency disorders.

Severe combined immune deficiency (SCID). SCID can be X-linked or autosomal recessive, the latter due to a mutation in chromosome 11 that prevents the normal development of RAG-1 and RAG-2 enzymes.[35,36] The inability to construct viable antigen-binding sites results in a severe deficiency of T cells, B cells, and immunoglobulin. Individuals suffer severe early morbidity because of repeated infections by extracellular and intracellular organisms. X-linked SCID results from a mutation on the X chromosome that prevents synthesis of the common cytokine receptor γ chain, preventing IL-2, IL-4, IL-7, IL-9, and IL-15 signaling. Although B cells develop normally, T-cell development is severely inhibited, preventing normal B-cell activation and immunoglobulin secretion.

Isolated T-cell deficiencies. As mentioned, these disorders not only affect T-cell development or function but also B-cell activation and immunoglobulin production. Bare lymphocyte syndrome is an autosomal recessive disorder with a mutation on chromosome 1 that inhibits class II HLA expression by APCs. Because helper T cells cannot be properly activated, it affects the activation of B cells and cytotoxic T cells.[35,36] In DiGeorge syndrome, the thymus gland fails to develop fully, preventing the maturation of all T-cell lineages. This syndrome is thought to involve deletions on chromosome 22.

Isolated B-cell deficiencies. These disorders tend to selectively affect B-cell function and immunoglobulin production, while T-cell–mediated immune responses remain normal.[35,36] Those affected are highly susceptible to infection with encapsulated bacteria, since polysaccharide capsules, in the absence of opsonization, effectively prevent phagocytosis. Bruton's agammaglobulinemia is an X-linked disorder with a mutation on the Bruton tyrosine kinase gene that prevents proper B cell development. Individuals display severe deficiencies of B cells and all classes of immunoglobulin. Hyper-IgM syndrome, also X-linked, results from the inability of B cells to express CD40L. Lack of CD40-CD40L signaling during cognate helper T-cell activation prevents immunoglobulin class switch reactions.

Complement deficiencies. Inherited deficiencies of complement proteins are generally autosomal recessive disorders.[35,36] Selective deficiencies of virtually all complement proteins have been identified, as have deficiencies of complement receptors and regulatory proteins. Deficiencies of key regulatory proteins can permit inappropriate activation of the complement cascade on host cells, leading to disorders such as paroxysmal nocturnal hemoglobinuria. Because the lectin and alternative complement pathways are critical to innate immune responses, deficiencies can also predispose the host to a variety of infections.

Deficiencies of phagocytic effector cells. These disorders can be X-linked or autosomal recessive, typically affecting the synthesis or secretion of lysosomal enzymes.[35,36] X-linked chronic granulomatous disease prevents macrophages and neutrophils from producing superoxide metabolites. Individuals with the autosomal recessive disorder Chediak-Higashi disease inherit a mutation on chromosome 1 that prevents neutrophil lysosomes from fusing to phagosomes and releasing lysosomal enzymes.

Allograft Transplant Rejection

The rejection of transplanted allogeneic grafts—transplants between individuals who are not monozygotic twins—is a natural extension of the T-cell–mediated response to invasion by nonself antigens.[37] Rejection is initiated by recognition of foreign HLA molecules on the transplanted tissue. Donor and recipient matching at class I and class II HLA alleles is vital, but non-HLA or minor antigens also are likely to be involved in initiating rejection. Other factors that may lead to transplant rejection include the normal expression of class II HLA molecules on the grafted tissue, the degree to which the tissue is perfused (corneal transplants are protected from invasion by blood-borne T cells), and the competence of the recipient's immune system (post-transplant therapeutic immunosuppression is vital to preventing rejection).

Hyperacute rejection. Hyperacute rejection, occurring within minutes of transplantation, is characterized by vascular thrombosis and destruction in the transplanted tissue.[37] It occurs when preformed antibodies in the recipient target HLA molecules on donor endothelial cells. Antibodies bind rapidly to the vascular endothelium, activating the complement and coagulation cascades. Hyperacute rejection is prevented by testing for the presence of antibodies prior to transplantation and avoiding ABO blood group mismatches.

Acute rejection. Acute rejection, generally evident within 10 days of transplantation, is T-cell–mediated, with helper T cells directing the response and cytotoxic T cells providing the effector functions.[37] Recipient T-cell activation is thought to occur in three ways (**Figure 1.7**). Immediately after transplantation, donor DCs expressing foreign class I and class II HLA molecules begin to migrate out of the graft and into draining lymph nodes, while recipient DCs migrate into the graft. Recipient helper T cells in the draining lymph nodes can be directly activated by recognition of foreign class II HLA on donor DCs. Activated T cells then complete the activation of recipient cytotoxic T cells, which have recognized foreign class I HLA molecules on the donor DCs. Activated cytotoxic T cells then migrate into the graft and begin tissue destruction. Indirect activation of helper T cells also occurs, by which recipient DCs migrate into the graft, process foreign antigens, then migrate back to lymph nodes for helper T-cell presentation and activation. Finally, some cytotoxic T cells are thought to be capable of direct activation by foreign class I HLA-bearing donor DCs in the absence of helper T-cell signaling.

Chronic rejection. Chronic rejection, occurring months or years after transplantation, is responsible for the continual risk of graft loss over time (a rate of 3% to 5% per year). This occurs

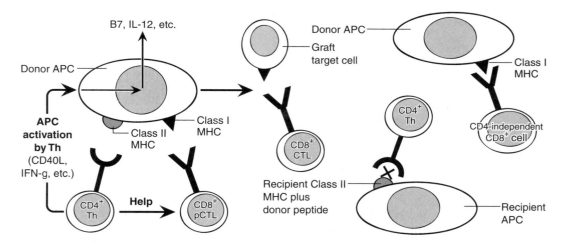

Figure 1.7. T-cell–mediated acute allograft rejection. (Adapted from Paul WE, ed. *Fundamental Immunology*. 5th ed. Philadelphia, PA: Lippincott Williams & Wilkins; 2003:1504.)

despite immunosuppressive drug therapy that effectively prevents acute rejection.[37] The cause of chronic rejection is still debated, with both T-cell–mediated and humoral (antibody) responses being suspected. Chronic rejection primarily leads to vascular fibrotic changes in the allograft. For example, accelerated atherosclerosis of coronary arteries can occur after cardiac transplantation, and renal arteries can undergo fibrosis after kidney transplantation.

Graft-versus-host disease. Acute graft versus host disease results from recognition of recipient class II HLA antigens by donor helper T cells.[37] These reactions are generally seen in a severely immunocompromised host, and are most commonly associated with allogeneic bone marrow transplantation. Reactions most commonly involve the skin, intestine, and liver (tissues having especially prominent expression of class II HLA antigens).

Malignancy

A number of human cancers, such as squamous cell carcinoma of the skin, cervical carcinoma, Kaposi's sarcoma, and non-Hodgkin's lymphoma, occur more commonly in patients with congenital or acquired immunodeficiency. Insights into the role of normal immune surveillance and adaptive immune responses to tumor cells help explain this phenomenon.[38]

The immune response to tumor cells is largely a T-cell–mediated response.[38] Since cancer begins with the malignant transformation of a single host cell, a tumor cell can theoretically be likened to a virally infected cell bearing unique surface

antigens complexed to class I HLA molecules. Researchers studying immune surveillance theorize that tumor-associated antigens (TAAs) should provoke a vigorous innate and adaptive immune response, and much evidence supports this theory. Clearly, however, immune surveillance often fails.

The vast majority of TAAs are self-antigens that may be overexpressed by the tumor but can also be expressed by normal cells.[38] As a result, most human tumor cells are only weakly immunogenic. It is increasingly apparent that tumor cells are not passive targets. They are genetically unstable. As the tumor grows, repeated mutations result in many different clones, some of which adapt to evade normal immune responses. Tumors are typically infiltrated with a mixture of CD4+ and CD8+ T cells, referred to as tumor-infiltrating lymphocytes (TILs).[38] Rather than indicating a vigorous cell-mediated immune response, most of these T cells have been rendered nonfunctional through apparent tumor-induced defects in TCR signaling pathways. Many tumor cells appear immune to the cytotoxic effects of NK cells, known to play a pivotal role in the elimination of newly transformed cells. NK cells need IL-2, normally provided by helper T cells, for activation and maintenance. The inactivation of TILs may also render NK cells ineffective in the tumor microenvironment. Macrophages also frequently infiltrate tumors and apparently acquire unique immunosuppressive properties. Tumor-associated macrophages (TAMs) may contribute to TIL inhibition by secreting reactive oxygen intermediates such as superoxide anion.[38]

SUMMARY

The coordinated actions of the innate and adaptive immune systems efficiently detect and destroy an enormous variety of environmental pathogens. The adaptive immune response is also responsible for immunologic memory, permitting an even faster and more effective response upon subsequent exposure. Inherited or acquired deficiencies in one or more components of the immune system increase the risk of infection and may also predispose the host to certain malignancies.

Immune responses can also result in significant tissue injury if normal control mechanisms are lost. Loss of central or peripheral tolerance leads to a variety of autoimmune disorders. Atopic individuals are prone to intense inflammatory responses or allergic reactions to common environmental antigens. Rejection of transplanted allografts is mediated by immune mechanisms identical to those operating in a normal response to infection.

REFERENCES

1. Berzofsky JA, Berkower IJ. Immunogenicity and antigen structure. In: Paul WE, ed. *Fundamental Immunology*. 5th ed. Philadelphia, PA: Lippincott Williams & Wilkins; 2003:631–683.
2. Chaplin DD. Overview of the immune response. *J Allergy Clin Immunol*. 2003; 111:S442–459.
3. Medzhitov R. The innate immune system. In: Paul WE, ed. *Fundamental Immunology*. 5th ed. Philadelphia, PA: Lippincott Williams & Wilkins; 2003:497–517.
4. The innate immune response. In: Doan T, Melvold R, Waltenbaugh C, eds. *Concise Medical Immunology*. Philadelphia, PA: Lippincott Williams & Wilkins; 2005:28–45.
5. Prodinger WM, Wurzner R, Stoiber H, et al. Complement. In: Paul WE, ed. *Fundamental Immunology*. 5th ed. Philadelphia, PA: Lippincott Williams & Wilkins; 2003:1077–1103.
6. Prussin C. IgE, mast cells, basophils, and eosinophils. *J Allergy Clin Immunol*. 2003; 111:S486–494.
7. Brown EJ, Gresham HD. Phagocytosis. In: Paul WE, ed. *Fundamental Immunology*. 5th ed. Philadelphia, PA: Lippincott Williams & Wilkins; 2003:1105–1126.
8. Borish LC, Steinke JW. Cytokines and chemokines. *J Allergy Clin Immunol*. 2003; 111:S460–475.
9. Moser M. Dendritic cells. In: Paul WE, ed. *Fundamental Immunology*. 5th ed. Philadelphia, PA: Lippincott Williams & Wilkins; 2003:455–480.
10. Alam R, Gorska M. Lymphocytes. *J Allergy Clin Immunol*. 2003; 111:S476–485.
11. Raulet DH. Natural killer cells. In: Paul WE, ed. *Fundamental Immunology*. 5th ed. Philadelphia, PA: Lippincott Williams & Wilkins; 2003:365–391.
12. Margulies DH, McCluskey J. The major histocompatibility complex and its encoded proteins. In: Paul WE, ed. *Fundamental Immunology*. 5th ed. Philadelphia, PA: Lippincott Williams & Wilkins; 2003:571–612.
13. Davis MM, Chien YH. T-cell antigen receptors. In: Paul WE, ed. *Fundamental Immunology*. 5th ed. Philadelphia, PA: Lippincott Williams & Wilkins; 2003:227–258.
14. The adaptive immune response. In: Doan T, Melvold R, Waltenbaugh C, eds. *Concise Medical Immunology*. Philadelphia, PA: Lippincott Williams & Wilkins; 2005:67–97.
15. Weiss A, Samelson LE. T-lymphocyte activation. In: Paul WE, ed. *Fundamental Immunology*. 5th ed. Philadelphia, PA: Lippincott Williams & Wilkins; 2003:321–363.
16. Schwartz RH, Mueller DL. Immunological tolerance. In: Paul WE, ed. *Fundamental Immunology*. 5th ed. Philadelphia, PA: Lippincott Williams & Wilkins; 2003:901–934.
17. Jenkins MK. Peripheral T-lymphocyte responses and function. In: Paul WE, ed. *Fundamental Immunology*. 5th ed. Philadelphia, PA: Lippincott Williams & Wilkins; 2003:303–319.
18. Henkart PA, Sitkovsky MV. Cytotoxic T lymphocytes. In: Paul WE, ed. *Fundamental Immunology*. 5th ed. Philadelphia, PA: Lippincott Williams & Wilkins; 2003:1127–1150.
19. Tough DF, Sprent J. Immunological memory. In: Paul WE, ed. *Fundamental Immunology*. 5th ed. Philadelphia, PA: Lippincott Williams & Wilkins; 2003:865–899.
20. Shevach EM. Regulatory/suppressor T cells. In: Paul WE, ed. *Fundamental Immunology*. 5th ed. Philadelphia, PA: Lippincott Williams & Wilkins; 2003:935–963.
21. Fehervari Z, Sakaguchi S. CD4+ Tregs and immune control. *J Clin Invest*. 2004; 114:1209–1217.
22. Jiang H, Chess L. An integrated view of suppressor T cell subsets in immunoregulation. *J Clin Invest*. 2004; 114:1198–1208.
23. McHeyzer-Williams M. B-cell signaling mechanisms and activation. In: Paul WE, ed. *Fundamental Immunology*. 5th ed. Philadelphia, PA: Lippincott Williams & Wilkins; 2003:195–225.
24. Kolar GR, Capra JD. Immunoglobulins: structure and function. In: Paul WE, ed. *Fundamental Immunology*. 5th ed. Philadelphia, PA: Lippincott Williams & Wilkins; 2003:47–68.
25. Molecules of the adaptive immune system. In: Doan T, Melvold R, Waltenbaugh C, eds. *Concise Medical Immunology*. Philadelphia, PA: Lippincott Williams & Wilkins; 2005:46–66.
26. Gellert M. V(D)J recombination: RAG proteins, repair factors, and regulation. *Annu Rev Biochem*. 2002; 71:101–132.
27. Hardy RR. B-lymphocyte development and biology. In: Paul WE, ed. *Fundamental Immunology*. 5th ed. Philadelphia, PA: Lippincott Williams & Wilkins; 2003:159–194.

28. Li Z, Woo CJ, Iglesias-Ussel MD, et al. The generation of antibody diversity through somatic hypermutation and class switch recombination. *Genes Dev.* 2004; 18:1–11.
29. Chaplin DD. Lymphoid tissues and organs. In: Paul WE, ed. *Fundamental Immunology.* 5th ed. Philadelphia, PA: Lippincott Williams & Wilkins; 2003:419–453.
30. Rothenberg EV, Yui MA, Telfer JC. T-cell developmental biology. In: Paul WE, ed. *Fundamental Immunology.* 5th ed. Philadelphia, PA: Lippincott Williams & Wilkins; 2003:259–301.
31. Rosenberg HF, Gallin JI. Inflammation. In: Paul WE, ed. *Fundamental Immunology.* 5th ed. Philadelphia, PA: Lippincott Williams & Wilkins; 2003:1151–1169.
32. Wills-Karp M, Khurana Hershey GK. Immunological mechanisms of allergic disorders. In: Paul WE, ed. *Fundamental Immunology.* 5th ed. Philadelphia, PA: Lippincott Williams & Wilkins; 2003:1439–1479.
33. Cohen PL. Systemic autoimmunity. In: Paul WE, ed. *Fundamental Immunology.* 5th ed. Philadelphia, PA: Lippincott Williams & Wilkins; 2003:1371–1399.
34. Autoimmunity and tolerance. In: Doan T, Melvold R, Waltenbaugh C, eds. *Concise Medical Immunology.* Philadelphia, PA: Lippincott Williams & Wilkins; 2005:153–166.
35. Buckley RH. Primary immunodeficiency diseases. In: Paul WE, ed. *Fundamental Immunology.* 5th ed. Philadelphia, PA: Lippincott Williams & Wilkins; 2003:1593–1620.
36. Immune deficiency. In: Doan T, Melvold R, Waltenbaugh C, eds. *Concise Medical Immunology.* Philadelphia, PA: Lippincott Williams & Wilkins; 2005:119–136.
37. Sykes M, Auchincloss H, Sachs DH. Transplantation immunology. In: Paul WE, ed. *Fundamental Immunology.* 5th ed. Philadelphia, PA: Lippincott Williams & Wilkins; 2003:1481–1555.
38. Schreiber H. Tumor immunology. In: Paul WE, ed. *Fundamental Immunology.* 5th ed. Philadelphia, PA: Lippincott Williams & Wilkins; 2003:1557–1592.

SELF-ASSESSMENT QUESTIONS

1. Antigen-specific receptors are expressed by which of the following cell types?
   A. Macrophages
   B. Neutrophils
   C. Cytotoxic T lymphocytes
   D. A and C

2. Double-stranded viral RNA activates a pattern recognition receptor expressed by macrophages, certain dendritic cells, and surface epithelial cells called:
   A. TLR3
   B. TLR4
   C. CD3
   D. CD7

3. The classical complement pathway can be initiated by all of the following except:
   A. Binding of C1q to at least two adjacent Fc antibody fragments on an immune complex
   B. Binding of C1q to an immune complex containing a single IgM pentamer
   C. Binding of C1q to an immune complex containing a single IgG monomer
   D. Binding of C1q to an immune complex containing two IgG antibodies

4. Which of the following is a characteristic of the innate immune system?
   A. Immunologic memory
   B. Adaptation
   C. Formation of an immune complex
   D. Recognition of gram-negative bacterial lipopolysaccharide by TLR2

5. Antigen presentation to helper T lymphocytes can be carried out by all of the following cell types except:
   A. B cells
   B. T cells
   C. Dendritic cells
   D. Liver Kuppfer cells

6. Clonal expansion is a characteristic of:
   A. Innate immunity
   B. Adaptive immunity
   C. Acute solid organ transplant rejection
   D. B and C

7. Signals required for helper T lymphocyte activation include all of the following except:
   A. Binding of the T-cell receptor to the microbial antigen/class II HLA complex
   B. Binding of CD28 to B7
   C. Binding of interleukin 2 to the IL-2 receptor
   D. A and B

8. All of the following statements are true regarding suppressor T lymphocytes except:

A. Tregs require the same two activation signals as do helper T lymphocytes.
B. Tregs inhibit the clonal expansion of activated helper T lymphocytes.
C. Tregs enter the circulation in a perpetually activated state.
D. Tregs constitutively express IL-2 receptors.

9. All of the following statements are true regarding B lymphocyte activation except:

A. Cognate activation requires the assistance of antigen-activated helper T lymphocytes.
B. B cells can be directly activated by antigens that express multiple copies of the same epitope.
C. Cognate activation can also be completed by follicular dendritic cells, without the assistance of antigen-activated helper T lymphocytes.
D. Fully activated B cells can undergo terminal differentiation to form antibody-secreting plasma cells.

10. Which of the following is an example of acute immune complex-mediated or Type III hypersensitivity?

A. Allergic rhinitis
B. Rheumatoid arthritis
C. Immune thrombocytopenic purpura
D. Contact dermatitis

Monoclonal Antibodies and Antibody Fragments

Blaine T. Smith

CHAPTER OUTLINE

LEARNING OBJECTIVES

After completing this chapter, the reader should be able to:

1. Differentiate the meanings of "antibody"; "monoclonal antibody"; "antibody fragments"; "bispecific antibodies"; and "chimeric," "humanized," and "human" antibodies.
2. Outline the basic methods of preparation for each of the above.
3. Discuss the advantages and disadvantages of each of the above, when applied to diagnostic and therapeutic uses in humans.
4. Identify antibody products by their nomenclature.

MONOCLONAL ANTIBODIES

The body secretes antibodies in response to foreign (nonself) stimuli. This occurs through the B-cell lineage, with direct interaction from T cells, stromal cells, dendritic cells, other environmental cells, and cytokines. The resulting antibody-secreting cell is a plasma cell, geared for prolific production of a single-epitope-specific antibody. Plasma cells normally secrete antibodies for several days before undergoing apoptosis and elimination. Researchers interested in harnessing a single-specificity antibody for clinical application initially faced two basic problems: (1) the brief time that the single-specificity antibody was produced and (2) that only polyclonal antibodies could be obtained from a culture of stimulated B-cells.

Antibodies themselves offer possibilities afforded by proteins having specific targets with which they can combine (complex). Possibilities include in vitro diagnostics (used as indicators) and in vivo diagnostic and therapeutic agents. With in vivo exposure, the normal response to a particular immunogen is polyclonal, meaning—the antibodies appearing in the immunized individual's serum have different binding conformations and affinities for the same immunogen. For the body's defense, this overlap in reactivity is quite effective and reassuring. But for the more exacting diagnostic and therapeutic investigation, where superior accuracy and reproducibility are important, only one of the many potential antibody products is desired.

Typically, an immunogen selects multiple B-cell lineages with varying combining specificities through a process called *clonal selection*. Multiple clonal lineages of B cells are simultaneously stimulated to differentiate into plasma cells (or into memory cells) over 4–5 days for a combined polyclonal antibody response. For study and use, though, only one clonal lineage (or a very few) is desired. It is maintained and expanded, so that only one antibody type, with one combining characteristic, is secreted. This monoclonal antibody—derived from a single clonal lineage, and identical to any other antibody from the same lineage—acts predictably in vitro and in vivo.

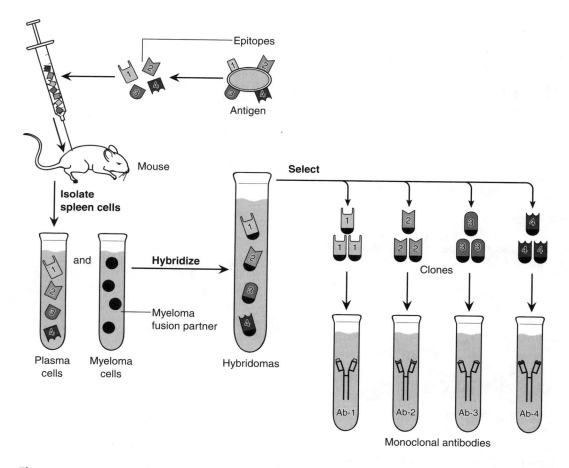

Figure 2.1. The method of producing murine antibodies by fusing immunized mouse splenocytes with mouse myeloma cells, then separating the cultures that secrete monoclonal antibodies.

The original problem was how to keep a plasma cell secreting the desired antibody alive past its natural time of demise—at most a few generations. In 1975, Köhler and Milstein[1] successfully fused a cancerous (immortal) mouse B-cell myeloma with a mouse plasma cell from an immunized mouse spleen. The resulting hybrid's immortality was provided by the myeloma cell and the specific, monoclonal antibody secretion from the selected plasma cell. These hybrid cells could be maintained indefinitely in culture, establishing a method of obtaining a potentially unlimited supply of a desired (monoclonal) antibody—always with exactly the same isotype and combining region—for study and use. These cell lines are called *hybridomas*.

General Procedures for Producing Monoclonal Antibodies

Originally, murine (mouse) hybridomas were the only way to procure monoclonal antibodies. Generally they were, and are still, made as shown in **Figure 2.1.** Myeloma cells are immortalized B lymphocytes able to secrete homogeneous, single-specificity antibodies. Myeloma fusion partners are unable to synthesize the enzyme hypoxanthine guanine-phosphoribosyl transferase (HGPRT), a salvage pathway for nucleotide synthesis. As a result, myeloma cells are sensitive to HAT medium, made up of hypoxanthine, thymidine (a pyrimidine), and aminopterin. Aminopterin blocks the main biosynthetic pathway for nucleic acids. Normal cells can continue to grow in the presence of aminopterin, if they are also given hypoxanthine and thymidine. HGPRT enables (normal) cells to synthesize purines using the extracellular source of hypoxanthine as a precursor. Normally, absence of HGPRT is not a problem for the cells because they have an alternate pathway they can use to synthesize purines, but when cells are exposed to aminopterin (a folic acid analog), they are unable to use this other (salvage) pathway and are fully dependent on HGPRT for survival.

Generation and Selection of Hybrid Cells (Hybridomas)

For murine hybridomas, the mouse is immunized and usually boosted with the immunogen. Sometimes adjuvants are used to increase the mouse's inflammatory response, improving immunogen exposure to the mouse immune system. Antibody titers can be monitored to be sure the mouse is producing the desired antibodies. A few days after a final boost, plasma cells in the spleen can be caught at the optimum rate of stimulation and division. The spleen is removed, and its cells are separated gently by passing the spleen through a sieve or by some other method. The spleen cells are mixed with an appropriate myeloma cell line and fusion-enhancing agent such as polyethylene glycol. After allowing time for the cells to fuse, they are dispersed into tissue culture plates and left to grow in HAT medium. Unfused myeloma cells cannot grow; they lack HGPRT, and are killed by the aminopterin. Unfused spleen cells have a limited natural lifespan and will not grow past a few days. Only the hybridized cells can grow. The spleen cell partner supplies the HGPRT gene and the myeloma partner supplies immortality (**Figure 2.2**).

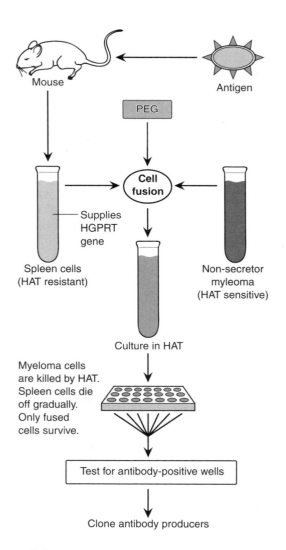

Figure 2.2. Murine hybridomas are produced by allowing HGPRT genes to be supplied by the murine spleen cells.

After the fused cells have grown 1–2 weeks, the supernatant is screened for the desired antibody. (This includes screening against immunogen or hapten.) Testing, normally by ELISA (enzyme-linked immunosorbent assay), identifies antibodies binding to the desired epitope or antigen. Positive culture wells are diluted to one cell per well and placed in new plates, so that new colonies will be expanded single-lineage colonies. Each colony is again screened for antigen reactivity, and positive colonies—now secreting monoclonal antibodies—are expanded further for use. Some of the colonies are stored. Growth is scaled up to yield enough antibodies for scientific or commercial use. Antibodies can be frozen, as can aliquots from actively growing hybridoma cultures, so culture and product can be revived at any time.

A predictable problem with murine antibodies for in vivo use is the human against mouse antibody (HAMA), an undesirable human immune response to the unique epitopes on the mouse antibody. Though repertoires of mammals for combining sites are enormous, some immunogens simply do not stimulate the same immune response in one mammal that they do in another. These immunological "holes" present the potential inability to create an antibody useful to humans. Further, once introduced into humans, antibodies of foreign origin do not always follow the same pharmacokinetics (distribution, elimination) as their human counterparts. These obstacles inevitably led to research in making antibodies more human, and more human-like in regard to all the concerns discussed. The steps in creating a more human-like antibody include creation of chimeric antibodies, humanized antibodies, antibodies prepared through bacteriophage display, and using transgenic animals to produce essentially human antibodies. These newer monoclonal antibodies use recombinant DNA methods to achieve a product not available naturally.

Production of Monoclonal Antibodies by Recombinant DNA (rDNA) Methods

Recombinant DNA methods incorporate human and, to varying degrees, animal immunoglobulin DNA into a gene employed in a transfection system, from which the desired protein can be derived. Other approaches to deriving more human-like monoclonal antibodies include (1) the use of transgenic mice, which, upon immunization, produce human antibodies, and (2) the creation of heterohybridomas (fusions of murine and human

cells). Chimeric and humanized technologies also make extensive use of this technology (see below).

From a therapeutic standpoint, the more human an antibody, the less likely it will present problems such as HAMA. Murine monoclonal antibodies are a reproducible and relatively simple and reliable method of producing antibodies for a desired epitope. But the human body normally detects murine monoclonal antibodies as nonself, with two direct effects. First, adverse hypersensitivity reactions in the patient may occur as a HAMA reaction evolves; the risk increases with each exposure of the patient to the antibody. Second, dangers to the patient aside, the HAMA response tends to capture the murine monoclonal antibodies introduced into the patient, and either decrease or inhibit their access to the target, leading to decreased efficacy upon repeated use.

With the HAMA response in mind, investigators turned to methods to make antibodies appear more "human" to the immune system of the patient and still be reactive toward the desired epitopes. Investigators hoped this would circumvent the HAMA response, its dangers to the patient, and diagnostic and therapeutic failures due to rapid clearance.

For both chimeric and humanized antibodies, a new gene is expressed in cells grown in tissue culture. But because *Escherichia coli* and other bacteria normally cannot glycosylate the antibodies properly, their Fc-related actions in vivo are adversely affected.

Chimeric Antibodies

The first revolution beyond murine monoclonal antibodies was the creation of chimeric antibodies. Whereas murine antibodies are obviously 100% murine protein, chimeric antibodies are typically only about 33% murine protein, with the remainder human.[2] Chimeric antibodies are made by fusing murine variable region genes with human constant region genes, resulting in the chimeric antibody. Chimeric antibodies are produced by isolating the variable region genes from a hybridoma secreting an antibody of interest, followed by use of polymerase chain reaction (PCR) to amplify the genes, and providing a copy DNA (cDNA) product, which may be ligated into a plasmid. cDNA for human heavy chain constant regions is amplified and ligated into a separate plasmid. Alternatively, the murine variable region cDNA can be ligated into immunoglobulin expression vectors, so that only one transfection into a host cell line is needed. If the cDNAs are kept separate, they are cotransfected into a host cell line containing a suitable vector (such as COS, a plasmid commonly used for transfections and grown for expression). In either case, the intact chimeric antibody is normally expressed in inclusion bodies in the host cell line, from which it is extracted and purified. Even with this rather radical modification, there often can still be a human response—human against chimeric antibody (HACA)—to the murine portion of the antibody.

Humanized Antibodies

To attempt to further decrease immunogenicity, humanized monoclonal antibodies were created. Humanized monoclonal antibodies typically retain only the hypervariable regions (complementarity-determining regions [CDRs]) of a murine antibody, while the remainder of the antibody is human. Thus, humanized antibodies typically contain only 5% to 10% murine composition. Humanized antibodies are prepared in much the same way as chimerics, and have shown little or no adverse human immunological response.

A typical "humanization" grafts mouse CDRs to a human antibody.[3] Human immunoglobulin G (IgG) light and heavy chains can be amplified by PCR, and a human lymphoid or genomic cDNA library can be created and used as a template. Occasionally, one or a few amino acids are altered in an effort to maintain, or improve upon, the original murine affinity. These are *framework residues*. Likewise, the CDRs are cloned and grown. These genes are spliced into vectors and incorporated into bacteria for growth. Multiple vectors can be incorporated into the same cell, as a cotransfection, and an intact monoclonal antibody can be secreted.

One problem with chimeric and humanized monoclonal antibodies is that sometimes a remote framework amino acid has a large bearing on whether the antibody retains combining region conformation integrity. A consequence can be lower binding efficiency than the native murine antibody. Minor alterations are sometimes made in the DNA of human framework residues to optimize antibody-epitope binding. Further slight modifications must be made in the amino acid sequence of the monoclonal antibody, so that it retains the desired affinity and avidity. Also, the artificial means of expressing antibodies often leads to improper or nonexistent glycosylation.

One final step currently being investigated is the creation of fully human monoclonal antibodies. Approaches include using Epstein-Barr virus to immortalize lymphocytes, and using transgenic animals and plants; new methods are constantly being attempted. Human monoclonal antibodies are fully human, generated from transgenic mice such as the XenoMouse (Abgenix, Inc.), Trans-Chromo mouse (Kirin Brewing Company, Japan), or the HumAb-Mouse (Medarex, Inc.).[4–7] XenoMouse's antibody-producing genes have been replaced by about 90% of the human genes for immunoglobulin IgG_1, IgG_2, or IgG_4 isotypes, and the human κ light chain. The XenoMouse is immunized with a human or nonhuman antigen, and the monoclonal antibodies produced are fully human and have high-affinity binding. Kirin Brewing Company has created Trans-Chromo mouse, a transgenic mouse that can produce human subtypes IgG_1, IgG_2, IgG_3, IgG_4, IgA, and IgM.[7] Mice and humans often have antibody glycosylation differences, a concern for in vivo applications with these engineered human monoclonal antibodies.[8] The role played by glycosylation of antibodies has not been completely explained; the absence or incorrectness of glycosylation alters the solubility and serum clearance of antibodies, and the efficient interaction between antibodies and Fc receptors.[9] Correct or nearly correct glycosylation of the Fc portion of the antibody is very important if the antibody action depends on complement activation or antibody-dependent cell-mediated cytotoxicity (ADCC). Human monoclonal antibodies engineered from transgenic mice strains have been reported to (1) have affinity values rivaling those of human antibodies against human antigens, (2) exhibit kinetics comparable to human immunoglobulin, and (3) have a nearly nonexistent hypersensitivity response compared to murine, chimeric and humanized monoclonal antibodies.[4–6,8,10]

Intact monoclonal antibody fragments have also been expressed in plant cells, perhaps soon to be followed by secretion of whole antibodies.[11] Humanized antibodies show much less propensity to induce an immune response. This reduced response normally is seen as acceptable, although the drive toward purely human monoclonal antibodies goes on. Much work is being done in the synthesis of the component pieces of monoclonal antibodies: antibody fragments.

ANTIBODY FRAGMENTS

For some applications, only certain portions of an intact monoclonal antibody are needed. In therapeutic applications, the smaller fragments penetrate tissue better and faster, clear the general circulation faster, and are eliminated more completely, with less hepatic binding. Depending on the proposed use, fragments are either made from intact antibodies or synthesized through genetic engineering using recombinant DNA technology.[12] Through genetic engineering we are able to create antibody fragments that combine the targeting regions of monoclonal antibodies into small functional proteins. The smallest antibody fragments are the minimal recognition units derived from the peptide sequence of the single CDR. These can be acquired from small segments of DNA cloned into plasmids or bacteriophage, producing single-chain variable section fragment (Fv) (scFV) units, up to larger DNA, cloned into yeast and bacteria in attempts to artificially complete entire antibody molecules (chimeric and humanized antibodies). Antibody genes from one animal are amplified by PCR and expressed in various formats, such as Fab (antigen-binding portion fraction), Fv (scFv), and the variable fragment (V_{HH}) of single-domain heavy chain antibodies (HCAb) from camelids. These small fragments are easier to manipulate genetically and express in bacterial systems. They can also be displayed on bacteriophage surfaces, allowing affinity selection of the fragments (and their coding sequences) from a diverse library of displayed antibodies.[12] Fragments are often useful when specific tissue penetration and rapid clearance are needed, as in tumor imaging.[13] Antibody fragments can also effectively treat specific diseases, like rheumatoid arthritis.[14]

Antibody fragments generally include the Fab, F(ab')$_2$ (divalent antigen-binding fragment), Fc (crystalizable fragment), and scFv. These smaller molecules tend to have better penetration into solid tumors than whole antibodies. The pharmacokinetics, in general, favor faster clearance than that of monoclonal antibodies—a desirable feature for fragments used as antitoxins. And fragments are easier to produce through genetic engineering and molecular biology, circumventing hybridoma technicalities. Because these fragments normally are composed entirely of human peptide sequences, immune responses are negligible. Fragments without an Fc portion obviate interactions with Fc receptors, which may be a desired characteristic.[15] The fragment portions used are not normally glycosylated proteins, so they can be expressed in bacteria. Glycosylation for fragments is not as much a consideration as it is for whole antibodies, and the Fc portion is the major area of glycosylation. High yields of fragments can be obtained using bacteria, which is a scientific and economic advantage.

Production is based more on a genetic engineering approach, rather than the molecular biology approach used with chimeric and humanized antibodies. Fragments often are made using PCR, plasmid inserts, and bacteriophage ("phage") display, followed by phage or plasmid expression of the fragment for harvesting and use. Production also is much faster, sometimes allowing designed fragments to be produced in a few days, not the weeks or months needed for hybridoma techniques. The particle produced can be used as is, or molecules can be attached for use as in vitro or in vivo diagnostic products, or even in vivo therapeutic agents.

Preparation

Originally, Fab, F(ab')$_2$, and Fc fragments of antibodies were derived by enzymatic cleavage of existing whole antibodies (**Figure 2.3**). Pepsin cleaves the antibody on the carboxy-terminal side of the antibody disulfide bonds, providing one F(ab')$_2$ and many small parts of the Fc fragment. Papain cleaves the antibody on the amino-terminal side of the disulfide bonds, providing two identical Fab fragments and an Fc fragment. These enzymatic digests were useful for existing antibodies, but not for antibodies needing custom design, so scientists developed methods to produce fragments without first producing the whole antibody.

Synthetic Fragments

The Fab is about 50 kDa in size, and can be derived enzymatically from existing antibodies or genetically engineered.[7,16] A cell type or tissue is isolated from an area of plentiful antibody-producing cells (plasma cells) or B cells, then actively stimulated by an antigen. The RNA is extracted from these cells, and is reverse-transcribed to create cDNA. The cDNA in turn is subjected to and amplified by PCR. Primers for the PCR are chosen to amplify only the V_H and V_L regions of the cDNA, and these reactions are run separately. Sometimes the entire κ or λ chain is amplified. After amplification, this V_H and V_L DNA is inserted (ligated) into a plasmid or phage (**Figure 2.4**), and the plasmid or phage is inserted into a host bacteria (usually *E. coli*) and grown. A phage and helper phage can later be added, if the fragments are to be displayed on the phage. Helper phage superinfection allows for packaging of single-stranded phagemid and leads to expression of two forms of cpIII, a bacteriophage coat gene. Normal phage morphogenesis is altered by competition between the Fab-cpIII fusion, which codes for the Fab protein for display, and the native cpIII, needed for infection.[17] The N-terminal part of cpIII normally binds F' pili, allowing infection of *E. coli*. The C-terminal part caps the

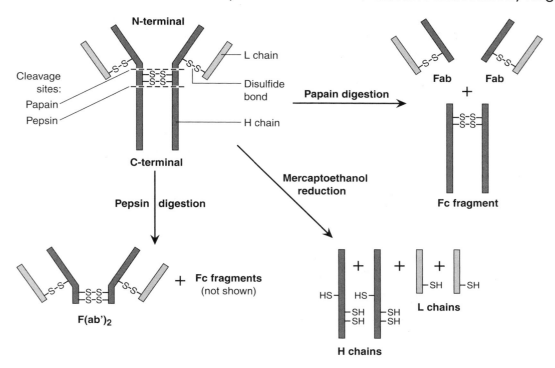

Figure 2.3. Results of cleavage of antibodies with different enzymes. Note the different fragments produced.

trailing end of the filament. After the phage has been assembled, it is extruded from the host. The phage has the gene of interest ligated into gene III (gIII) or gene VIII (gVIII), which normally code for phage coat proteins (cpIII and cpVIII).

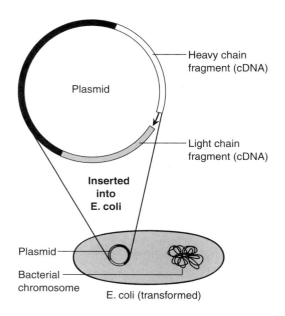

Figure 2.4. Propagation of cDNA of variable and light-chain fragments and plasmids.

The Fab fragments are displayed on the outside of the phage, which can be selected by reactivity with the original antigen. This selection process is called panning, and often uses ELISA methods to detect positive- and negative-presenting phage. Panning can enrich the percentage of positive-reacting phage by repeating the procedure several times. All the possible combining conformations for a human can be recreated and displayed by phage, then screened for reactivity against the antigen (**Figure 2.5**).

Even though cDNA from activated cells has been described for this procedure, Fab fragments that can bind a desired antigen/epitope can be made this way without ever immunizing any animal or hybridizing any cells. When a colony with a reactive phage/Fab is found, it can be expanded, and the bacteria induced to secrete the Fab for harvest and purification (**Figure 2.6**).

Fab products include those designed against digoxin, digitoxin, other related cardiotoxins, *Nerium* and *Thevetia* (oleander), *Bufo* (toads), crotalid snake venoms, paraquat, and phencyclidine. Some have been developed, though not marketed, including those against colchicine and tricyclic antidepressants.

The F(ab')$_2$, about 100 kDa, can also be derived enzymatically or through genetic engineering. Its

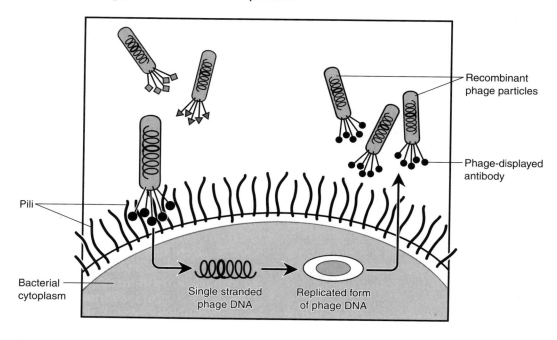

Figure 2.5. Bacteriophage normally infect specific bacterial cells, replicate, and continue infecting bacterial cells. This process can be harnessed to use the phage to also propagate antibody fragments from cDNA pieces inserted into the phage DNA.

main advantage is its bivalency, for better binding and a higher probability of binding the target.

scFV are engineered and consist of the V_H and V_L connected by a flexible peptide linker. They are

about 25 kDa, or roughly half the size of Fab fragments. Phage display library techniques are also used in scFV synthesis, but making only a single chain, rather than a double (or more) chain as needed for Fab and whole antibody production (**Figure 2.7**). Stability can be an issue for scFV, so insertion of a disulfide bridge between the V_H and V_L regions helps stabilize the chain. The steps for

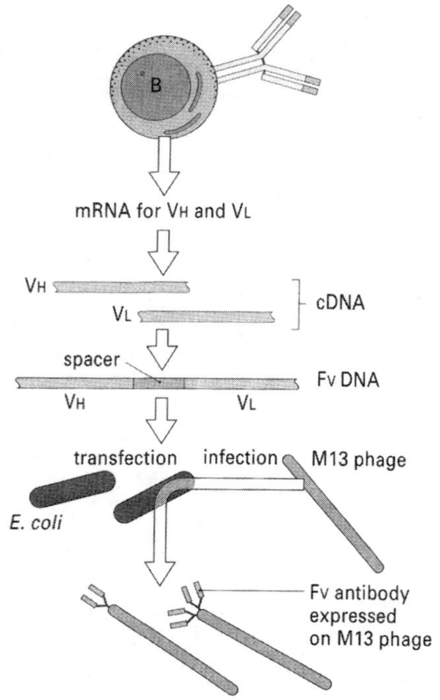

Figure 2.6. Production of F_v antibody fragments. (Reprinted, with permission, from Roitt I, Brostoff JH, Male D. *Immunology,* 5th ed. Oxford, England: Blackwell Publishing; 1998.)

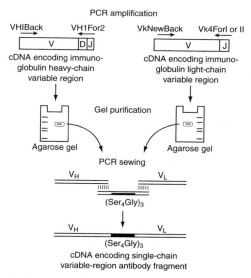

Figure 2.7. Method of producing single-chain variable fragments of antibodies using linker segments. (Reprinted, with permission, from Cyr JL, Hudspeth AJ. A library of bacteriophage-displayed antibody fragments directed against proteins of the inner ear. *PNAS.* 2000; 97(5): 2276–2281.)

display are similar to those for Fab. A linker segment (such as $(Gly_4Ser)_3$, $(Ser_4Gly)_3$, or $(Gly_4Ser)_4$) is added between the V_H and V_L regions—"PCR sewing"—so a single-chain peptide results. Again, the cDNA is inserted into phage, although for scFv there is only one DNA insert: the V_H and V_L with the linker. Positive phages are then used to infect *E. coli*, the phagemid DNA is isolated, and the genes of interest amplified from the positive phage DNA and cloned into a vector for expression (**Figure 2.8**).

Similar to scFv, there are diabodies (noncovalent dimers of scFv), minibodies (scFv-C_H3 dimers), and other combinations, as the creativity of biochemists and immunologists expands (**Figure 2.9**).

The Fc fragment has been used as Fc linked to drugs, such as erythropoietin, for delivery to the lungs. In this specialized case, a unique type of Fc receptor (FcRn, in the lung) is available. The drug is linked to an Fc on either end, and, through the FcRn in the lung, delivered by an active carrier mechanism. These were grown in Chinese hamster ovary (CHO) cells transfected with plasmids containing the Fc DNA. The Fc fragment also has been used to produce unique molecules vaguely falling into the category of antibodies. These molecules use the Fc portion of the antibody for its ability to bind to effector cells, for its recruitment of complement, and for its effects on circulating half-life, normally prolonging it. Smaller fragments without the Fc do not have long circulating half-lives.

CONJUGATED ANTIBODIES
Immunotoxins

Immunotoxins are chimeric, or hybrid, molecules—a fusion of a toxin (or portion of a toxin) with an antibody (or antibody fragment). If a fragment is used, typically it is the Fv portion. The antibody or fragment portion serves for targeting the overall conjugate. By design, antibody-based immunotoxins have a specific mechanism that allows them to use the antibody or antibody fragment specificity and deliver some sort of toxin to the desired site. This lowers exposure of healthy, nontarget tissues to the toxin. The objective is to target the toxin to a novel, or nearly novel, epitope on a tumor cell: a differentiation marker, overexpressed receptor, or altered receptor. Internalization of the toxin leads to cell death.

If the Fv portion is used instead of the parent whole antibody, its smaller size may give it superior tumor penetration. The heavy and light chains of a recombinant fragment may be linked chemically after they are expressed, and the linker chain composition may be varied to optimize the Fv binding properties.

Examples of toxins that have been used for targeting cancer and other diseases include diphtheria toxin, *Pseudomonas* exotoxin, the α-chain of ricin, saporin, and pokeweed antiviral protein. The most commonly used are diphtheria toxin and *Pseudomonas* exotoxin. Once successfully delivered to the target cell, these toxins are internalized, where they ADP-ribosylate elongation factor two, inhibit protein synthesis, and cause target cell death.[18] Since the toxin is targeted using an antibody or fragment, the natural toxin-binding domain is removed and replaced with the antibody or fragment.

Originally, toxins were chemically attached to the targeting fragment. More recently genetic engineering techniques allow fragments and toxins to be created in one process, normally in *E. coli*, by inserting a gene that codes for the toxins' domains into an expression plasmid.[18] Recombinant immunotoxins are often produced in *E. coli* for two reasons. Newer methods use recombinant technology to coexpress both portions

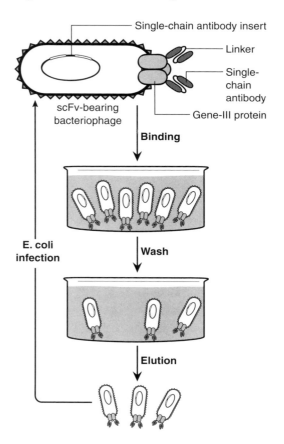

Figure 2.8. Use of bacteriophage to express the single-chain antibody variable regions.

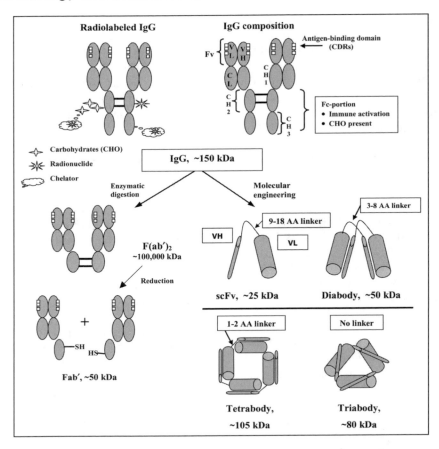

Figure 2.9. Many unique molecules that retain immunologic activity can be created using phage technology. (Reprinted, with permission, from Sharkey RM, Goldenberg DM. Perspectives on cancer therapy with radiolabeled monoclonal antibodies. *J. Nucl. Med.* 2005; 46 (Suppl 1): 1155–1275.)

of the conjugate, and expression of the toxin in eukaryotic cells often kills the expressing cell, just as it would the human cell. One or two plasmids are used to express a finished construct or one whose two components are later easily combined.

So far there are two main problems with immunotoxin therapy using monoclonal antibodies, bispecific antibodies, or other variations. The first problem is the tendency for at least the conjugated portion to induce an immune response against the agent. Another is vascular leak syndrome (VLS), often a dose-limiting toxicity. VLS, which includes hypoalbuminemia, hypotension, and edema, has been observed in almost all clinical trials. Studies are being performed with anti-inflammatory agents to see if they can prevent immunotoxin-induced VLS by inhibiting immunotoxin binding to endothelial cells. The mechanisms responsible for VLS are not well understood so it is difficult to develop methods to prevent it.[19]

Targets for antibody-based immunotoxins have thus far included such epitopes as CD22, expressed on the surface of B-cell malignancies, and the interleukin (IL)-2 receptor (IL-2R, Tac, p55, CD25)

which is expressed on activated T cells, such as those associated with adult T-cell leukemia. Fv and scFv fragments have also been used, though these are often murine in origin.

Bispecific Monoclonal Antibodies

Bispecific monoclonal antibodies (bsmAbs) are directed toward two different targets. They have a unique two-arm structure, with each variable region of the antibody being distinct, making them attractive for therapeutic targeting. Because this does not occur in nature, these antibodies must be synthesized with two different variable regions as part of the same intact antibody. Each arm is designed through chemical reactions, hybridization, or genetic engineering to have a different antigen affinity.

There are three general methods for producing bsmAbs. The first bsmAb was made about 40 years ago, before the advent of hybridoma and genetic engineering technologies. At that time chemical methods were used, and only polyclonal antibodies were available. Polyclonal antibodies were chemically dissociated then linked together, producing bispecific polyclonal antibodies. The chemical cross-linking of the different antibodies is a quick and relatively simple way to produce high-yield bsmAbs. Because of the randomness of the process, though, each batch of product varies greatly. Another drawback to the chemical production of bsmAbs is the potential for protein denaturation, resulting in an unusable antibody product. Fab and/or $F(ab')_2$ fragments can also be cross-linked chemically to make unique immunologically based molecules.[20] Production of bsmAbs was improved by using disparate hybridoma antibodies for dissociation and relinkage as bifunctional reagents.

Hybridoma technology led to a departure from chemical linkage and resulted in purer and more predictable products. Biological manufacture of bsmAbs today uses somatic hybridization to produce either quadromas (hybrid hybridomas) or triomas (lymphoma cells fused to a hybridoma). Quadromas are created by fusing two known hybridomas, and triomas are made by fusing one known hybridoma with mouse lymphocytes.[21]

After fusion, vectors with selectable features can be added, but—as with traditional hybridomas—these hybrid hybridomas undergo selection pressure resulting in cell lines that secrete a potential variety of combinations of heavy and light chains. Because they are derived from separate hybridomas, each variable region can bind its own epitope, distinct from each other (with the proper chain and specificity arrangement).

A more precise method of producing bsmAbs uses fluorescein cell labeling and fluorescence-activated cell sorter selection to accurately match hybridomas based on the two antibody reactivities. This results in fewer hybrids with undesirable chain combinations. It is difficult to isolate correct hybrids secreting the desired chain configuration using the biological method. All biologically produced bsmAbs are synthesized and secreted the same as hybridoma antibodies; therefore, only a fraction of the fusions secrete the desired bsmAbs.

Genetic engineering is the most advanced way to produce bispecific monoclonal antibodies. It is less expensive and easier to fine-tune than the chemical or biological methods. This method uses recombinant DNA technology to produce recombinant bsmAbs appropriate for a variety of clinical applications. Yet even the advanced genetic engineering technique still has imperfections. Because the engineered proteins contain foreign peptides, the human body may produce an immune response against the antibodies.[21]

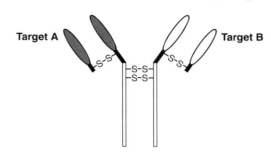

Figure 2.10. Schematic of bispecific antibody. The arm on the right is specific for one target (Target B), while the arm on the left is specific for a different target (Target A).

Even tetravalent antibodies have been created using molecular engineering techniques similar to those used for chimeric and humanized monoclonal antibodies. The molecular engineering approach will likely become the most predictable and dependable method for making bsmAbs (**Figure 2.10**).

The introduction of bifunctional/bispecific (bsmAb) antibodies is an exciting innovation in immunology. The bsmAb can bring two targets into close proximity or stimulate two receptors simultaneously; or one arm can be directed toward a target epitope, while the other is specific for a toxin, enzyme, or linker molecule. These toxins, enzymes, and linkers can be added to the antibody before or after introduction into the body. They are powerful tools with many uses including targeted delivery of drugs, toxins, cytokines, and enzymes. They can also activate the humoral and cellular immune branches, causing them to act against tumors and other target cells. Bispecific antibodies will be used more widely as new technologies are developed for their production.[21]

bsmAbs can react with the T-cell receptor (TCR)/CD3 complex to initiate cytotoxicity, bypassing the TCR complex requirement for stimulation. The second signal needed for T-cell activation—normally provided by the interaction of the TCR/CD3 complex with major histocompatibility complex (MHC)-peptide—instead is provided by the bsmAb.[22] Bispecific monoclonal antibody therapy with cytotoxic T lymphocytes (CTLs) is somewhat difficult because it does not provide enough of the many costimulatory signals needed to fully activate effector T cells. Because of these complications, other immune effector cells, specifically natural killer (NK) cells, may be better choices in bsmAb immunotherapy.

bsmAbs can be used for immunoassays, immunohistochemistry, and immunotherapy. bsmAbs excel at directing cytotoxic agents to specific sites of action. Monoclonal antibodies, which are chemically conjugated to the cytotoxic agent, generate complex aggregates, which results in batch-to-batch variation. bsmAbs can have intrinsic binding sites to any two antigens, eliminating the need for chemical conjugation to the cytotoxic agent and reliably improving the compound purity. A specific example is Mylotarg, a humanized bsmAb approved by the Food and Drug Administration (FDA) for treatment of acute myeloid leukemia (AML). One arm of this antibody binds to the CD33 antigen, which is expressed on myeloid leukemia cells. The other arm is linked to calicheamicin, a potent antibiotic with an antitumor effect on cells. bsmAbs have also been designed and constructed to deliver drugs such as doxorubicin, epirubicin, methotrexate, and alkaloids, successfully treating a variety of cancers and lymphomas.[21]

bsmAbs offer an alternative to conventional radioimmunotherapy, in which monoclonal antibodies linked to radionuclides deliver a toxin to a tumor site. Radiolabeled monoclonal antibody use can lead to damage of critical organs through exposure to high radiation levels and the nonspecific accumulation of the toxin in nontargeted organs. By using bsmAbs, the isotope can be delivered quickly to the site of action with minimal nontarget radiation exposure. This is done by designing a bsmAb with one affinity for the tumor antigen and another affinity for a small, rapidly excreted radionuclide. After the antibody has targeted the tumor, a clearing agent can be given to clear the excess antibody.

bsmAbs can also target and activate the cellular immune system, often leading to the destruction of tumor cells and viruses. These antibodies can induce effector mechanisms, including cell-mediated cytotoxicity, by targeting CTLs, NK cells, and neutrophils, while also targeting an infected cell or tumor.

Monoclonal Antibody Imaging and Radioimmunotherapy

Monoclonal antibodies and fragments offer unique targeting specificity not only for delivery of toxins but also for carrying radioisotopes to specific sites. Depending on the isotope used, the antibody or fragment can be used for imaging or for therapy. Ideal imaging isotopes emit gamma photons at energies detectable by a scintillation camera. The gamma-emitting isotopes considered potentially useful in imaging include ^{67}Ga, ^{111}In, ^{123}I, ^{131}I, ^{99m}Tc, ^{201}Tl, ^{133}Xe, and ^{11}C. Alternatively, positron-emitting isotopes annihilate upon contact with an electron and emit two 511 KeV gamma photons at a 180-degree angle. They are therefore valued for positron emission tomography (PET). PET radionuclides include ^{62}Cu, ^{18}F, ^{68}Ga, ^{13}N, ^{15}O, ^{38}K, and ^{82}Rb. Gamma photon emission is not very useful for therapeutic purposes; isotopes that release alpha and beta particles upon decay are preferred. Particles are much more damaging to cells, especially the DNA of cells, than gamma photons. The isotopes with therapeutic potential include ^{211}At, ^{212}Bi, ^{213}Bi, ^{131}I, ^{90}Y, ^{111}In, ^{186}Re, ^{188}Re, ^{67}Cu, and ^{177}Lu.

Not only the radionuclide or toxin affixed to the antibody is responsible for the target cell death; the Fc portion of the whole antibody also plays an important role. The Fc is responsible for the induction of ADCC and complement-mediated target cell death. So there is good reason for using whole antibodies as well as fragments and smaller constructs. Fragments and constructs tend to have better solid tumor penetration and clear the general circulation faster than whole antibodies, which is beneficial when carrying a diagnostic or therapeutic payload. Using fragments tends to promote more rapid elimination of unbound material, which may be desirable. Even so, whole antibodies will remain important in radioimmunodetection and radioimmunotherapy, especially as we move toward totally human antibodies.

Originally, whole radiolabeled murine monoclonal antibodies were used for imaging and radioimmunotherapy. In addition to causing HAMA responses, whole antibodies did not penetrate solid tumors as well as antibody fragments nor did they clear the circulation as quickly to limit exposure to normal tissues. Thus, not only has there been a move toward chimeric and humanized/human antibodies but also toward antibody fragments.

Radiolabels are attached by different means. Many isotopes are metals that must be chelated and attached to the proteinaceous antibody. Choice of isotope also depends on whether a diagnostic (photon) or therapeutic (particulate, α or β) emission is desired. Therapeutic antibodies are not always radiolabeled, but they sometimes initiate the complement cascade or ADCC to induce target cell death.

MONOCLONAL ANTIBODY NOMENCLATURE

Because of the growing importance of monoclonal antibodies in the medical fields, the United States Adopted Name (USAN) Council has provided guidelines for their nomenclature. All monoclonal antibody generic names end with the suffix *mab*. Preceding this suffix is a one- or two-letter identifier of the animal source of the product, and preceding the animal source is the general disease or target identifier, usually three letters. To simplify pronunciation, the last consonant of the disease- or target-identifier syllable is often removed. If the antibody is radiolabeled or has a toxin affixed, a separate word is used to identify this portion. For toxins, *tox* is included in the name. Finally, a unique prefix is used to identify the product.[23] To summarize and illustrate, the name will be composed as a unique prefix-target-source-suffix (**Table 2.1**).

For example, the product rituximab (Rituxan) was the first monoclonal antibody approved in the United States for treatment of malignancy. The name can be deciphered as follows: ri = unique prefix, tu = tumor, xi = chimeric, mab = monoclonal antibody. This is a chimeric (human/ mouse) monoclonal antibody that targets CD20 on B cells. It is used to treat non-Hodgkin's lymphomas

Table 2.1. Nomenclature for Antibodies and Antibody Fragments

Sources (thus far) are:	
Human	u
Mouse	o
Rat	a
Humanized	zu
Hamster	e
Primate	I
Chimera	xi
Diseases or targets (thus far) are:	
Viral	vir
Bacterial	bac
Immune	lim
Infectious lesions	les
Cardiovascular	cir
Colon tumors	col
Melanoma	mel
Mammary tumors	mar
Testicular tumors	got
Ovarian tumors	gov
Prostate tumors	pr(o)
Miscellaneous tumors	tum

Table adapted from reference 22.

and pre-B-cell acute lymphoblastic leukemias. Another example is ^{90}Y-ibritumomab tiuxetan. Ibri = unique prefix, tum = tumor, o = murine, mab = monoclonal antibody, tiuxetan = the conjugate (the chelator site for ^{90}Y, and also ^{111}In).

DIAGNOSTIC AND THERAPEUTIC MONOCLONAL ANTIBODIES

The rapid introduction of in vivo diagnostic and therapeutic antibodies renders any discussion of current or prospective products out of date, even at the time of publication, because many products move through Phase I, II, and III trials rather quickly. Others are withdrawn at various stages. Any products described that are in the testing phases may, in fact, be either fully approved products by the time this book is published, or may have been withdrawn. Even after initial approval, many products are assessed for uses not originally approved by the FDA, due to common target epitopes found in other diseases. Some of the antibodies, bivalent antibodies, and fragments will be discussed below, many in disparate proximity of approval. The general order is from murine monoclonal antibodies to chimerics; humanized, human, and bispecific antibodies; then immunotoxins and fragments. The bispecific antibodies and immunotoxins have had the least development of all the categories, so fewer are on the market. Several of the products and possible future products are shown in **Table 2.2**.

^{90}Y-Ibritumomab Tiuxetan (Zevalin) and ^{131}I-Tositumomab (Bexxar)

Ibritumomab tiuxetan was the first radioimmunoconjugate approved as an anticancer agent. It is a murine monoclonal antibody attached to the linker tiuxatan, which provides a chelator site for the beta-emitter ^{90}Y. Like rituximab, ibritumomab binds to CD20 surface antigens on B-cell precursors and mature B cells. The beta particle emission induces cellular damage in both target cells and surrounding cells. Because it is a murine monoclonal antibody, ibritumomab allows for more efficient clearing of the radioactivity, which, in this situation, is a desirable characteristic.[24] In treating relapsed or refractory, low-grade, or follicular B-cell non-Hodgkin's lymphoma (NHL), ibritumomab tiuxetan is administered in two separate doses and in conjunction with rituximab. In the first dose, preadministration of rituximab saturates nonmalignant B cells, so ^{111}In radiolabeled ibritumomab

Table 2.2. Current and Possible Future Monoclonal Antibody Products

Trade Name	Generic Name	Application	Origin	Specifics
OKT3	Muromonab	Acute organ rejection	Murine IgG2a	Anti-CD-3 Orthoclone/ Johnson & Johnson
Remicade	Infliximab	Anti-inflammatory rheumatoid arthritis, Crohn's disease	Chimeric IgG1κ	Binds soluble & bound TNF-α, blocks binding to target cell/Centocor
Xolair	Omalizumab	Allergies/asthma	Humanized	Binds IgE/Genentech
Zenapax	Daclizumab	Acute renal rejection, possibly MS & T-cell lymphoma	Humanized	Binds part of IL-2 receptor (CD25)/Roche Protein Design Labs
Rituxan	Rituximab	B-cell lymphoma NHL Perhaps MS	Chimeric IgG1κ	Binds CD20 on B-cells (therapeutic) Genentech/Centocor, J & J Biogen-IDEC
Zevalin	^{90}Y/^{111}In-Ibritumomab tiuxetan	B-cell lymphoma	Murine	Radiolabeled - binds CD20 on B-cells (therapeutic)
Bexxar	Tositumomab (+/− ^{131}I)	B-cell lymphoma	Murine IgG2a	Radiolabeled antibody binds CD20 on B-cells
Herceptin	Trastuzumab	Breast cancer	Humanized IgG1κ	Binds HER2 receptor (tyrosine kinase receptor) (therapeutic)/Genentech
Erbitux	Cetuximab	Breast cancer, non small cell lung cancer, metastatic colon cancer	Chimeric	Blocks HER1 EFGR
Mylotarg	Gemtuzumab ozogamicin	AML	Humanized bispecific conjugated with calicheamicin (anti-tumor antibiotic)	Binds CD33 on myeloid leukemia cells, and binds calicheamicin (potent antibiotic) (therapeutic) American Home Products
LymphoCide		B-cell leukemias		Binds CD20 on B-cells
Campath	Alemtuzumab	B-CLL Possibly transplant rejection MS	Humanized	Binds CD52 Millennium/ILEX
Oncolym	Lym-1	Lymphoma		Binds HLA-RD-encoded histocompatibility antigen
Vitaxin		Solid tumors	Humanized	Angiogenesis inhibitor. Binds vascular Integrin (alpha-v/beta-3)
Avastin	Bevacizumab	Metastatic colorectal cancers	Humanized	Blocks vascular endothelial growth factor (VEGF) receptor Genentech

Table 2.2. (*Continued*)

Trade Name	Generic Name	Application	Origin	Specifics
ReoPro	Abciximab	Post-angioplasty Anti-platelet	Chimeric Fab fragment	Inhibits platelet clumping by binding receptor for fibrinogen receptor II/III linking/Lilly Centocor
Campath	Alemtuzumab	B-cell chronic lymphocytic leukemia	Humanized	(therapeutic)
Avastin	Bevacizumab	Colorectal cancers (metastatic) Renal cell carcinoma		Blocks vascular endothelial growth factor (VEGF) receptor Inhibits angiogenesis
Simulect	Basiliximab	Organ rejection Liver transplants	Chimeric	IL-2Rα binding Novartis
Synagis	Palivizumab	RSV	Humanized	Anti-F glycoprotein Medimmune
Omnitarg (2C4)	Pertuzumab	Breast, other cancer	Humanized	Blocks HER-2 dimerization Genetech

Investigational Agents:

Trade Name	Generic Name	Application	Origin	Specifics
Erbitux	Cetuximab	Multiple solid tumors	Chimeric	Binds epidermal growth factor receptor (EGFR)
	H22xKi-4	Hodgkin's lymphoma	BsMab (2 x Fab') Murine/ humanized	CD30 (murine)/CD64 (humanized)
	Pexelizumab	Decreased myocardial damage	ScFv from humanized	Complement C5 Acute MI
	Edrecolomab Mab17-1A	Metastatic colorectal cancer	Murine IgG2a	EpCAM (a TAA) Centocor
Humira	Adalimumab	RA	Human	Anti-TNF Abbott
Omnitarg	Pertuzumab	Breast, other	Humanized	HER2 Dimerization blocker Genentech
	ABX-EGF	Metastatic renal cell carcinoma	Human	EGRF Abgenix
Raptiva	Efalizumumab	Severe plaque psoriasis	Humanized IgG1 Given SQ	CD11a (α-subunit of leukocyte function-associated antigen 1) (LFA-1) on T-cells
Bexxar	^{131}I-Tostitumomab	Follicular lymphoma	Murine IgG2a	CD20

(*Continued*)

Table 2.2. (*Continued*)

Trade Name	Generic Name	Application	Origin	Specifics
	Odulimomab	Protect against ischemia reperfusion injury after kidney transplant		LFA-1
	RhuMAB-E25	Asthma		IgE
Digibind	Digoxin immune Fab		Sheep IgG Fab from papain digest	Digoxin/digitoxin overdose
	Epratuzumab 90YDOTA-hLL2	NHL	Humanized IgG	CD22 (B-cells) Immunomedics
Oncolyn		NHL		HLADR 10 Perigrine Pharmaceuticals
	Pemtumomab	Ovarian cancer	Murine	90Y-labeled anti-human milk fat globulin 1 (MUC-1)
	Bivatuzumab	Head & neck squamous cell carcinoma	Humanized ^{186}Re-BIWA	
	ABX-EGF		Human IgG2 from Xenomouse®	EFGR Abgenix, Immunex, Amgen
	Afelimomab	Sepsis	Murine F(ab')$_2$	Anti-TNF-α
Tru-Scint AD	^{99m}Tc-Mab170	Ovarian cancer	Murine	For imaging ovarian cancer
Tysabri	Natalizumab	Crohn's disease	Humanized	Tx for Crohn's, MS
	MLN-02	Crohn's disease Ulcerative colitis	Humanized	Binds to the α4B$_7$ integrin
Enbrel	Etanercept	Rheumatoid arthritis inflammation	Fragment Dimeric fusion protein made with two extracellular portions of TNFR linked to human IgG1 FC	Anti-TNF Amgen, Wyeth

mAbs for Nuclear pharmacy:

Generic	Trade	Primary Uses
^{111}In – Capromab pendetide	ProstaScint	Monoclonal antibody for imaging prostate cancer
Tositumomab & Iodine I-131 Tositumomab	Bexxar	Treatment of non-Hodgkin's lymphoma

Table 2.2. (*Continued*)

Generic	Trade	Primary Uses
Tc-99m Arcitumomab	CEA-Scan	Monoclonal antibody for colorectal cancer
Tc-99m Fanolesomab	Tc-99m NeutroSpec	Monoclonal antibody for infectious imaging
Y-90 Ibritumom-ab Tiuxetan	Zevalin	Non-Hodgkin's lymphoma

can selectively target the malignant B cells when administered next. This gamma-emitting radioisotope allows for biodistribution assessment with a gamma camera. After acceptable biodistribution is determined, the second dose of the therapeutic, beta-emitting ^{90}Y-ibritumomab tiuxetan is administered.[24] A similar two-step dosing technique is used with ^{131}I-tositumomab, although it also can be used as a two-step monotherapy with positive results.[4,25] ^{90}Y-ibritumomab tiuxetan and ^{131}I-tositumomab will be discussed further in Chapter 11.

^{123}ImAb-14C5

^{123}I-mAb-14C5 is a newer radiolabeled monoclonal antibody developed specifically for radioimmunodetection of tumor growth and metastasis. ^{123}I emits a gamma photon that is detectable by nuclear medicine cameras. The cancer-associated antigen CA14C5 is thought to be involved in the construction and destruction of connective tissue and is highly expressed on many different tumors. Initial tests on mice show favorable biodistribution of the tracer with sufficient tumor uptake to provide acceptable imaging. The results prove promising for new approaches to radioimmunodetection and radioimmunotherapy.[26]

*Rituximab (Rituxan)

Rituximab is a chimeric monoclonal antibody for the treatment of NHL. It targets CD20.[27] Once bound to target cells, rituximab induces ADCC as well as complement-mediated cytotoxicity (CDC). Better results often are seen with adjunct therapy, either monoclonal antibodies with chemotherapy or with other monoclonal antibodies. For example, rituximab targets CD20 on malignant B cells and has been shown to be effective in many conditions in which B cells need to be selectively eliminated.[4,24,28,29] However,

it has been even more effective against these same conditions when used as adjunct therapy with the combination chemotherapy regimen of cyclophosphamide, doxorubicin, vincristine, and prednisone (CHOP), high-dose therapy, and other monoclonal antibodies.[4,24,28,30]

In addition to treatment of chronic lymphocytic leukemia (CLL), rituximab has several off-label uses in treating autoimmune diseases including rheumatoid arthritis, systemic lupus erythematosus (SLE), dermatomyositis, myasthenia gravis, refractory pemphigus vulgaris, and autoimmune hemolytic anemia.[31,32] The approved use of rituximab is for treatment of relapsed/refractory low-grade, or follicular, CD20-positive B-cell NHL.[33] But with the increased knowledge of the role B lymphocytes play in cancer and autoimmune diseases, there is great potential for expanded use of this antibody in treating disease.[31] One new area of use for rituximab is the treatment of multiple sclerosis (MS), with several clinical studies under way.[34] Rituximab will be discussed more completely in Chapter 11.

*Infliximab (Remicade)

Infliximab is a chimeric antibody recently approved by the FDA for treatment of rheumatoid arthritis when administered with methotrexate. Infliximab acts by binding to soluble and transmembrane tumor necrosis factor alpha (TNF-α), preventing it from binding to its receptors on activated macrophages.[7] Infliximab can also be used to treat Crohn's disease, an inflammatory bowel disorder. This may provide relief to patients with moderate to severe Crohn's disease.[7] Infliximab is also being used as a combined therapy in patients with myelodysplastic syndrome, an incurable bone-marrow disorder with no approved treatment. In this disease, TNF-α may play a role in initiating proinflammatory cytokines.[35]

*Basiliximab (Simulect) and *Daclizumab (Zenepax)

Several monoclonal antibodies are used to prevent graft-versus-host disease (GVHD) after transplantation. These antibodies include alemtuzumab, rituximab, basiliximab, and daclizumab.[36]

Basiliximab and daclizumab are used as immunosuppressive agents after acute organ rejection in adults recovering from renal transplantation.[37,38] Daclizumab is the humanized version of basiliximab, a chimeric antibody. They bind to the interleukin-2 alpha (IL-2α) receptor on the surface of activated T cells. IL-2 plays a significant role in the activation of alloreactive T cells. By binding to IL-2R, these antibodies inhibit the proliferation of antigen-activated T cells and prevent the generation of cytotoxic T cells. Daclizumab has been approved by the FDA for use in preventing acute kidney transplant rejection and is currently being evaluated for use in preventing acute rejection in other organs.[40] It is also being studied for the treatment of MS. For MS patients who cannot be controlled by conventional therapy, daclizumab is a good alternative. Larger studies are still needed to determine its benefit to the general MS population and to evaluate whether daclizumab can be effective as a stand-alone therapy.[39]

In a cost-comparison study of limited-dose daclizumab versus basiliximab, daclizumab was found to be both more effective and less costly than basiliximab. Yet basiliximab is still the primary antibody given in most cases of organ rejection.[41]

Abciximab

Abciximab is a chimeric antibody used to bind and block the platelet fibrinogen receptor II/III. This leads to a complete reduction of platelet aggregation and adhesion, promoting longer bleeding times and inhibiting platelet-induced thrombin generation. Better cardiovascular surgery is the final outcome.[7] Use of abciximab reduces the number of ischemic complications during cardiopulmonary bypass (CPB) surgery.[41] The antibody is administered during other cardiac surgeries, including coronary artery bypass grafting (CABG), to prevent coagulation.[42] Abciximab has the potential to reduce the number of single platelets and leukocytes lost in aggregates. It has been used to treat deep venous thrombosis, a rare condition with no clinical guidelines for treatment, and it achieved positive results when used in the treatment of arterial thrombosis.

Trastuzumab (Herceptin)

Trastuzumab is a humanized monoclonal antibody used to treat metastatic breast cancers. It consists of an antigen-binding fragment directed against the extracellular domain of the HER-2 receptor, which is overexpressed in breast cancer, spliced to the Fc fragment of human IgG. Because it is humanized, it has limited human-against-human antibody (HAHA) response and a heightened potential for recruiting immune effector cells. Its target is the extracellular domain of the HER-2 tyrosine kinase receptor. Recent studies have shown that when combined with pertuzumab (see following section), the two antibodies act synergistically against HER-2 breast cancer cells. The two antibodies target different regions of the HER-2 receptor; trastuzumab targets the HER-2 tyrosine kinase receptor, whereas pertuzumab sterically blocks the dimerization of HER-2 with other HER receptors.[43,44] Combined with chemotherapy, trastuzumab has improved the response rate and survival rate of women with breast cancer.[45] Trastuzumab will be more thoroughly discussed in Chapter 11.

Pertuzumab

Pertuzumab is a humanized monoclonal antibody developed as part of a new class of therapeutics known as HER dimerization inhibitors, used for the treatment of breast cancer. The role of HER-1, HER-2, and HER-3 in the development of many tumor types, such as breast, lung, prostate, and ovarian cancers, has been well documented.[43,46] Dimerization with other receptor proteins is essential for HER receptor activity and has a major role in survival and growth of most tumors.

*Bevacizumab (Avastin)

Bevacizumab is a humanized monoclonal antibody used to treat renal cell carcinoma (RCC), a malignancy that historically has been difficult to treat and very unresponsive to therapy. Bevacizumab blocks the vascular endothelial growth factor (VEGF) receptor. The most frequent cause of RCC is the inactivation of both VHL alleles, which act as tumor suppressor genes. This triggers a cascade of events beginning with a decrease in VHL protein, which normally functions to degrade hypoxia-inducible factor alpha (HIFα). Lack of degradation results in an accumulation of HIFα, which then translocates into the nucleus and associates with other HIF molecules. This leads to the induction of hypoxia-inducible genes, including VEGF. The increase in VEGF leads to an increase in vascular permeability, endothelial cell proliferation, and migration.[47]

Other cancers also are caused by an increase in VEGF. The progression of ovarian cancer is marked by an increase of VEGF, making this cancer a potential candidate for treatment with bevacizumab. Bevacizumab shows potential for treating other cancers that may involve an increase of VEGF, including colon, lung, and colorectal cancers.[48] Bevacizumab will be discussed more thoroughly in Chapter 11.

Alemtuzumab (Campath)

Alemtuzumab is a humanized monoclonal antibody used to treat B-cell chronic lymphocytic leukemia. It targets CD52, an overexpressed surface marker found on several different types of leukocytes including T cells. CD52 is a glycosylated protein linked to the cell membrane by a glycosylphosphatidylinositol (GPI) anchor. Alemtuzumab is directed against this surface protein.[36] Alemtuzumab exerts its cytotoxic effects through immunological mechanisms, such as CDC and ADCC. It also has been somewhat successful in treating MS. The drug has been found to eliminate the formation of new lesions and the inflammation associated with MS for at least 18 months. Trials with alemtuzumab show that it is tolerated reasonably well. One serious side effect observed, however, was the development of autoimmune thyroid disease (Graves disease). Despite its seriousness, Graves disease is relatively easy to manage.[49] In treating patients with CLL whose tumor cells are resistant to alemtuzumab alone, rituximab and alemtuzumab can be used together to obtain satisfactory results.[36]

Alemtuzumab is especially useful in treating CLL in patients who are unresponsive to other treatments. These patients often undergo stem cell transplantation as a last option. Unfortunately, these individuals have a low prognosis for survival because of GVHD. Alemtuzumab can induce remission of CLL even in patients with advanced CLL, leading to a better outcome after allogeneic transplantation. And treatment with alemtuzumab can lead to a reduced tumor mass in the blood and bone marrow which can, in turn, lead to improvement in all the affected organs.[50] Alemtuzumab will be discussed further in Chapter 11.

Palivizumab (Synagis)

Palivizumab is a humanized anti-F glycoprotein antibody that neutralizes respiratory syncytial virus (RSV) and prevents it from binding to cells.

While prophylactic treatment with palivizumab does not prevent RSV, it decreases the severity of the disease and reduces the rate of RSV hospitalization by 55% in high-risk children, including infants with chronic lung disease, premature infants, and infants with congenital heart disease. The high cost of this monoclonal antibody prevents its use in all children.[51]

Omalizumab (Xolair)

Omalizumab is a humanized anti-IgE antibody that was developed to relieve symptoms of asthma and allergic rhinitis. It binds to IgE in the same region of the antibody that binds to the IgE receptor on effector cells. This effectively blocks IgE from inducing degranulation, and reduces the concentration of free IgE in the plasma. Omalizumab is most often used as an add-on therapy to control the symptoms of asthma (especially in patients with asthma that is difficult to treat), and also in patients with poor lung function and those with a history of emergency treatment in the preceding year.[52] Omalizumab was humanized via CDR grafting from an anti-IgE antibody raised in mice onto a human IgG framework. It is the first anti-IgE agent to undergo clinical evaluation for the treatment of airway allergies. In many different trials, omalizumab demonstrated effective disease control and improved quality of life in asthma, allergic rhinitis, and other IgE-related allergic diseases.

Gemtuzumab ozogamicin (Mylotarg)

bsmAbs can have intrinsic binding sites to any two antigens, including a cytotoxic agent, eliminating the need for chemical conjugation to the cytotoxic agent. A specific example is gemtuzumab ozogamicin, a humanized bsmAb used for treatment of acute myeloid leukemia (AML). One arm of this antibody binds to the CD33 antigen expressed on myeloid leukemia cells, and the other is linked to calicheamicin, a potent antibiotic with an antitumor effect on the cell. Gemtuzumab ozogamicin will be discussed more thoroughly in Chapter 11.

[186]Re-BIWA4 (Bivatuzumab)

[186]Re-labeled BIWA4 is a humanized monoclonal antibody for treatment of head and neck squamous cell carcinoma (HNSCC).[19] BIWA4 targets v6-containing CD44, which is highly expressed and homogeneous on the outer cell surface of HNSCC. Prior studies with murine and chimeric

monoclonal antibody had proven promising for tumor targeting, but problems with HAMA and HACA were encountered. To eliminate these responses and possible allergic reactions, BIWA4 was created. It still displayed the superior tumor targeting of the murine and chimeric versions, and there was little HAHA response.[53]

90Y-DOTA-Epratuzumab

90Y-DOTA-epratuzumab, a humanized antibody targeting the CD22 antigen expressed on B cells, shows promise in treating NHL. In this treatment regimen, no predosing with an unlabeled antibody was needed, so the number of administrations was reduced. Because this is a humanized monoclonal antibody, the immunogenicity of the monoclonal antibody is low; therefore, multiple doses of lower radiation can be given repeatedly for successful tumor destruction.

ABX-EGF and Cetuximab (Erbutix)

Cetuximab is a chimeric monoclonal antibody with an anti–epidermal growth factor (EGF) receptor; ABX-EGF is fully human. Both are being studied for use in treating renal cancer. Predictably, cetuximab induced HACA in some patients, but there was neither hypersensitivity nor an anaphylactic reaction with ABX-EGF therapy. The preadministration of antihistamines and corticosteroids needed with cetuximab is apparently unnecessary when using ABX-EGF. HAHA was not detected, even after long-term treatment.[5] Cetuximab will be discussed further in Chapter 11.

H22xKi-4

H22xKi-4 is a bispecific molecule made from Fab′γ fragments derived from two separate monoclonal antibodies: a murine anti-CD30 monoclonal Ki-4 and a humanized anti-CD64 monoclonal H22. This novel monoclonal antibody (mAb) was studied as a potential treatment for refractory Hodgkin's lymphoma. The size of H22xKi-4, 104 kDa, allows quicker clearance and is believed to permit easier penetration into the malignant lymph nodes than rituximab and alemtuzumab, which are whole mAbs against lymphoma cells: NHL and B-cell chronic lymphocytic leukemia (B-CLL), respectively.[24,28,54]

MDX-210

Many bsmAbs are being tested in human clinical trials. Several of these target CD64, a CD antigen found on monocytes, macrophages, blood, and germinal-center dendritic cells. One of these bispecific antibodies is MDX-210.

2B1 and HRS-3/A9

Found on macrophages, NK cells, and neutrophils, CD16 is being studied as a target molecule. It may not be as attractive as CD64 because it is also found on neutrophils and is a soluble molecule, which may cause side effects including formation of immune complexes. 2B1 and HRS-3A9, two bsmAbs that use CD16 as the target molecule, are in clinical trials for the treatment of various cancers.

Other Bispecifics

bsmAbs are also undergoing extensive research for applications other than immunotherapy. Investigators in one study developed bispecific antibodies that inhibit the costimulatory pathways CD40-CD40L (on B cells and T cells, respectively) and CD80/86-CD28 (on B and T cells and CD3+ thymocytes, peripheral T cells, and plasma cells, respectively). They produced a bispecific anti-CD40/CD86 antibody that binds and inhibits CD40 and CD86 costimulatory molecules. Using products like these in medicine may help prevent allograft loss and autoimmunity.[55]

✳Etanercept (Enbrel)

Etanercept is an antibody fragment used to treat rheumatoid arthritis. It is made of a soluble, dimeric fusion protein. This protein consists of two copies of the extracellular ligand-binding portion of the TNF receptor linked to the constant portion of human IgG. It binds to TNF-α and blocks TNF-α's interaction with the cell surface receptors, preventing the cell from exerting its proinflammatory effect.[14] Etanercept is being used to treat patients with rheumatoid arthritis who have an inadequate response to other antirheumatic drugs, such as methotrexate and infliximab. It has also been effective in treating psoriatic arthritis and juvenile rheumatoid arthritis.[14]

Di-dgA-RFB4, RFB4(dsFv)-PE38 (BL22), Anti-Tac(Fv)-PE38 (LMB-2)

Many immunotoxins are in the midst of clinical testing. Di-dgA-RFB4, a ricin immunotoxin with two toxins attached to a single monoclonal antibody, targets CD22, a surface marker on B-cell malignancies. It is being investigated as a therapy against B-cell lymphoma and leukemia. Another product being investigated is RFB4(dsFv)-PE38 (BL22), a recombinant immunotoxin made from the monoclonal antibody's Fv domain-RFB4 fused with PE38, a *Pseudomonas* exotoxin (PE). BL22 is directed toward CD22, targeting leukemias and lymphomas displaying this surface antigen.[18]

A recombinant immunotoxin, anti-Tac(Fv)-PE38 (LMB-2), has shown great promise in a variety of different cancers.[19] It was previously believed that LMB-2 was only cytotoxic toward T-cell leukemic cells, but recent studies have shown that it is cytotoxic toward B-cell leukemic cells as well. Hairy cell leukemia, a B-cell neoplasm, is very sensitive to LMB-2. B-CLL, the most common type of leukemia in the western hemisphere, is also sensitive to the immunotoxins but to a lesser degree.[56] B-CLL cells can be further sensitized to LMB-2 by inducing the up-regulation of CD25 on the B-CLL cells (because LMB-2 is an anti-CD25 immunotoxin). This can be performed with the immunostimulatory DSP30, a phosphorothioate CpG-oligodeoxynucleotide.[57]

In recent studies, the side effects of LMB-2 limited the amount of immunotoxin that could be delivered to the patient. Side effects included nonspecific binding of the immunotoxin to normal tissues and human anti-PE antibodies. And the small molecular weight of the immunotoxin compared to other similar constructs gives it a short half-life in circulation, and makes it somewhat unstable and likely to distribute to tissue organs, specifically the liver and the kidney. This causes one of the major problems of LMB-2 therapy: liver damage.[58]

It was concluded that liver damage was caused by the production of TNF by Kupffer cells, and that treatment with indomethacin, an anti-inflammatory agent, inhibited the increase of TNF in the liver and protected the liver from damage.[59]

Crotalinae Polyvalent Immune Fab (CroFab)

Crotalinae polyvalent immune Fab is a sheep-derived antivenin consisting of highly purified ovine Fab fragments. Sheep are immunized with the venom of each of the four North American snakes: *Crotalus atrox, Crotalus adamanteus, Crotalus scutalatus,* and *Agkistrodon piscivorus.* All four antivenins are mixed together in the final product, which is capable of neutralizing the toxic effects of all North American Crotalidae venoms. The major objective of Crofab is to reduce invasive surgical procedures in the treatment of envenemation.[60]

Digoxin Immune Fab (Digibind)

Digoxin immune Fab is a papain-digested Fab fragment derived from specific antidigoxin antibodies produced by sheep. Digibind has been clinically proven successful in treating life-threatening or potentially life-threatening digoxin toxicity or overdose. The antigen is produced by conjugating digoxin, a hapten, to human albumin. Sheep are immunized with the conjugate to produce antibodies specific for the digoxin molecule. Digoxin immune Fab binds molecules of digoxin, keeping them from binding to their active sites.

Afelimomab

Afelimomab is an $F(ab')_2$ fragment of an anti-TNF murine mAb, which is being studied for efficacy and safety in patients with severe sepsis. Previous studies with other anti-TNF-α therapies failed to find a significant mortality benefit, yet treatment with afelimomab in studies revealed it may have a benefit. Its smaller size may contribute to quicker neutralization of TNF-α activity[61] (see Table 2.2).

SUMMARY

Monoclonal antibodies have advanced from murine origin to chimeric, to humanized, and to human antibodies. This progress has allowed a wider range of diagnostic and therapeutic applications as technology has progressed. Not only are the whole antibodies useful, but fragments (pieces) of the antibodies can have broad applications in medicine. Antibody and fragment technology is advancing quickly, so new products are being introduced at a rapid pace.

REFERENCES

1. Kohler G, Milstein C. Continuous cultures of fused cells secreting antibody of predefined specificity. *Nature.* 1975; 256:495–497.
2. Pavlou AK, Belsey MJ. The therapeutic antibodies market to 2008. *Eur J Pharm Biopharm.* 2005; 59(3):389–396.
3. Haruyama H, Ito S, Miyadai K, et al. Humanization of the mouse anti-Fas antibody HFE7A and crystal structure of the humanized HFE7A Fab fragment. *Biol Pharm Bull.* 2002; 25(12):1537–1545.
4. Stern M, Herrmann R. Overview of monoclonal antibodies in cancer therapy: present and promise. *Crit Rev Oncol Hematol.* 2005; 54(1):11–29.
5. Rowinsky EK, Schwartz GH, Gollob JA, et al. Safety, pharmacokinetics, and activity of ABX-EGF, a fully human anti-epidermal growth factor receptor monoclonal antibody in patients with metastatic

renal cell cancer. *J Clin Oncol.* 2004; 22(15): 3003–3015.

6. Green LL. Antibody engineering via genetic engineering of the mouse: XenoMouse strains are a vehicle for the facile generation of therapeutic human monoclonal antibodies. *J Immunol Methods.* 1999; 231(1–2):11–23.

7. Berger M, Shankar V, Vafai A. Therapeutic applications of monoclonal antibodies. *Am J Med Sci.* 2002; 324:14–30.

8. Funaro A, Horenstein AL, Santoro P, et al. Monoclonal antibodies and therapy of human cancers. *Biotechnol Adv.* 2000; 18(5):385–401.

9. Goldsby RA, Kindt TJ, Osborne BA, et al. *Immunology.* 5th ed. New York, NY: W.H. Freeman and Company; 2003.

10. van de Putte LB, Atkins C, Malaise M, et al. Efficacy and safety of adalimumab as monotherapy in patients with rheumatoid arthritis for whom previous disease modifying antirheumatic drug treatment has failed. *Ann Rheum Dis.* 2004; 63(5):508–516.

11. Vaquero C, Sack M, Chandler J, et al. Transient expression of a tumor-specific single-chain fragment and a chimeric antibody in tobacco leaves. *Proc Natl Acad Sci U S A.* 1999; 96:1128–1482.

12. Yau K, Lee H, Hall JC. Emerging trends in the synthesis and improvement of hapten-specific recombinant antibodies. *Biotechnol Adv.* 2003; 21:599–637.

13. Roque AC, Lowe CR, Taipa MA. Antibodies and genetically engineered related molecules: production and purification. *Biotechnol Prog.* 2004; 20:639–665.

14. Culy CR, Keating GM. Spotlight on etanercept in rheumatoid arthritis, psoriatic arthritis and juvenile rheumatoid arthritis. *Biodrugs.* 2003; 17:139–145.

15. Desogus A, Burioni R, Ingianni A, et al. Production and characterization of a human recombinant monoclonal Fab fragment specific for influenza A viruses. *Clin Diagn Lab Immunol.* 2003; 10(4):680–685.

16. Flanagan RJ, Jones AL. Fab antibody fragments: some applications in clinical toxicology [review]. *Drug Saf.* 2004; 27(14):1115–1133.

17. Barbas CF, Angray SK, Lerner RA, et al. Assembly of combinatorial antibody libraries on phage surfaces: the gene III site. *Proc Natl Acad Sci U S A.* 1991; 88:7978–7982.

18. Fitzgerald D, Kreitman R, Wilson W, et al. Recombinant immunotoxins for treating cancer. *Int J Med Microbiol.* 2004; 293:577–582.

19. Kreitman RJ. Immunotoxins in cancer therapy. *Curr Opin Immunol.* 1999; 5:570–578.

20. Sharkey R, Mcbride W, Karacay H, et al. A universal pretargeting system for cancer detection and therapy using bispecific antibody. *Cancer Res.* 2003; 63:354–363.

21. Cao Y, Lam L. Bispecific antibody conjugates in therapeutics. *Adv Drug Deliv Rev.* 2003; 55: 171–197.

22. Jung G, Ledbetter JA, Muller-Eberhard HJ. Induction of cytotoxicity in resting human T lymphocytes bound to tumor cells by antibody heteroconjugates. *Immunology.* 1987; 84:4611–4615.

23. van Laan S. Monoclonal antibodies. American Medical Association [online]. April 11, 2005 (Nomenclature 2005; [May 10, 2005]). Available at: http://www.ama-ssn.org/ama/pub/category/13280.html. Accessed 7/24/07 - keyword search: "monoclonal antibodies nomenclature." Go to www.ama-assn.org first, then search.

24. Fiola C. Monoclonal antibodies as anticancer agents. *US Pharm* 2003; 10(15). Available at: http://www.uspharmacist.com/index.asp?show=article&page=8_1147.htm. Accessed April 1, 2005.

25. Kaminski MS, Tuck M, Estes J, et al. ^{131}I-Tositumomab therapy as initial treatment for follicular lymphoma. *N Engl J Med.* 2005; 352(5):441–449.

26. Lahorte CM, Bacher K, Burvenich I, et al. Radiolabeling, biodistribution, and dosimetry of ^{123}I-mAb 14C5: a new mAb for radioimmunodetection of tumor growth and metastasis in vivo. *J Nucl Med.* 2004; 45(6):1065–1073.

27. Cerny T, Borisch B, Introna M, et al. Mechanisms of action of rituximab. *Anticancer Drugs.* 2002; 13(2):2301–2310.

28. Horwitz SM, Negrin RS, Blume KG, et al. Rituximab as adjuvant to high-dose therapy and autologous hematopoietic cell transplantation for aggressive Non-Hodgkin lymphoma. *Blood.* 2004; 103(3):777–783.

29. Zaja F, De Vita S, Mazzaro C, et al. Efficacy and safety of rituximab in type II mixed cryoglobulinemia. *Blood.* 2003; 101(10):3827–3834.

30. Usuda M, Fujimori K, Koyamada N, et al. Successful use of anti-CD20 monoclonal antibody (rituximab) for ABO-incompatible living-related liver transplantation. *Transplantation.* 2005; 79(1):12–16.

31. Chambers SA, Isenberg D. Anti-B cell therapy (rituximab) in the treatment of autoimmune diseases. *Lupus.* 2005; 14:210–214.

32. Bonduel M, Zelazko M, Figueroa C, et al. Successful treatment of autoimmune hemolytic anemia with rituximab in a child with severe combined immunodeficiency following nonidentical T-cell-depleted bone marrow transplantation. *Bone Marrow Transplant.* 2005; 35:819–821.

33. Saleh M. Monoclonal antibody therapy of non-Hodgkin's lymphoma: the rituximab story. *J Med Assoc Ga.* 2003; 92:39–46.

34. Rizvi SA, Bashir K. Other therapy options and future strategies for treating patients with multiple sclerosis. *Neurology.* 2004; 63:S47–S54.

35. Raza A, Candoni A, Khan U, et al. Remicade as TNF suppressor in patients with myelodysplastic syndromes. *Leuk Lymphoma.* 2004; 45:2099–2104.

36. Smolewski P, Szmigielska-Kaplon A, Cebula B, et al. Proapoptotic activity of alemtuzumab alone and in combination with rituximab or purine nucleoside

analogues in chronic lymphocytic leukemia cells. *Leuk Lymphoma*. 2005; 46:87–100.

37. Leonard PA, Woodside KJ, Gugliuzza KK, et al. Safe administration of a humanized murine antibody after anaphylaxis to a chimeric murine antibody. *Transplantation*. 2002; 74:1697–1700.

38. Baudouin V, Crusiaux A, Haddad E, et al. Anaphylactic shock caused by immunoglobulin E sensitization after retreatment with the chimeric anti-interleukin-2 receptor monoclonal antibody basiliximab. *Transplantation*. 2003; 76:459–469.

39. Panacek EA, Marshall JC, Albertson TE, et al. Efficacy and safety of the monoclonal anti-tumor necrosis factor antibody F(Ab')2 fragment afelimomab in patients with severe sepsis and elevated interleukin-6 levels. *Crit Care Med*. 2004; 32(11):2173–2182.

40. Waldmann TA, O'Shea J. The use of antibodies against the IL-2 receptor in transplantation. *Curr Opin Immunol*. 1998; 10:507–512.

41. Pham K, Kraft K, Thielke J, et al. Limited-dose daclizumab versus basiliximab: a comparison of cost and efficacy in preventing acute rejection. *Transplant Proc*. 2005; 37:899–902.

42. Straub A, Wendel HP, Azevedo R, et al. The GP IIb/IIIa inhibitor abciximab (ReoPro) decreases activation and interaction of platelets and leukocytes during in vitro cardiopulmonary bypass simulation. *Eur J CardioThorac Surg*. 2005; 27:617–621.

43. Bakker H, Bardor M, Molthoff JW, et al. Galactose-extended glycans of antibodies produced by transgenic plants. *Proc Natl Acad Sci U S A*. 2001; 98(5):2899–2904.

44. Nahta R, Hung MC, Esteva FJ. The HER-2-targeting antibodies trastuzumab and pertuzumab synergistically inhibit the survival of breast cancer cells. *Cancer Res*. 2004; 64(7):2343–2346.

45. Bussolati G, Montemurro F, Righi L, et al. A modified trastuzumab antibody for the immunohistochemical detection of HER-2 overexpression in breast cancer. *Br J Cancer*. 2005; 92:1261–1267.

46. Agus DB, Gordon MS, Taylor C, et al. Phase I clinical study of pertuzumab, a novel HER dimerization inhibitor, in patients with advanced cancer. *J Clin Oncol*. 2005; 23(11):2534–2543.

47. Rini BI, Halabi S, Taylor J, et al. Cancer and leukemia Group B 90206: A randomized phase III trial of interferon-alpha or interferon-alpha plus anti-vascular endothelial growth factor antibody (bevacizumab) in metastatic renal cell carcinoma. *Clin Cancer Res*. 2004; 10:2584–2586.

48. Alekshun T, Garrett C. Targeted therapies in the treatment of colorectal cancers. *Cancer Control*. 2005; 12:105–110.

49. Confavreux C, Vukusic S. Non-specific immunosuppressants in the treatment of multiple sclerosis. *Clin Neurol Neurosurg*. 2004; 106(3):263–269.

50. Harder S, Kirchmaier CM, Krzywanek HJ, et al. Pharmacokinetics and pharmacodynamic effects of a new antibody glycoprotein IIb/IIIa inhibitor (YM337) in healthy subjects. *Circulation*. 1999; 100:1175–1181.

51. Stevens TP, Hall CB. Controversies in palivizumab use. *Pediatr Infect Dis J*. 2004; 23:1051–1052.

52. Bousquet J, Wenzel S, Holgate S, et al. Predicting response to omalizumab, an anti-IgE antibody, in patients with allergic asthma. *Chest*. 2004; 125:1378–1386.

53. Borjesson PK, Postema EJ, Roos JC, et al. Phase I therapy study with [186]Re-labeled humanized monoclonal antibody BIWA4 (bivatuzumab) in patients with head and neck squamous cell carcinoma. *Clin Cancer Res*. 2003; 9(10 Pt 2):3961S-3972S.

54. Borchmann P, Schnell R, Fuss I, et al. Phase 1 trial of the novel bispecific molecule H22xKi-4 in patients with refractory Hodgkin lymphoma. *Blood*. 2002; 100(9):3101–3107.

55. Koenen H, Hartog M, Heerkens S, et al. A novel bispecific antihuman CD40/CD86 fusion protein with T-cell tolerizing potential. *Transplantation*. 2004; 78:1429–1438.

56. Robbins D, Margulies I, Stetler-Stevenson M, et al. Hairy cell leukemia, a B cell neoplasm that is particularly sensitive to the cytotoxic effects of Anti-Tac(Fv)PE38 (LMB-2). *Clin Cancer Res*. 2000; 6:693–700.

57. Decker T, Hipp S, Kreitman R, et al. Sensitization of B-cell chronic lymphocytic leukemia cells to recombinant immunotoxins by immunostimulatory phosphorothioate oligodeoxynucleotides. *Blood*. 2002; 99:1320–1326.

58. Onda M, Kreitman R, Vasmatzis G, et al. Reduction of the nonspecific animal toxicity of Anti-Tac(Fv)-PE38 by mutations in the framework regions of the Fv which lower the isoelectric point. *J Immunol*. 1999; 163:6072–6077.

59. Onda M, Willingham M, Wang Q, et al. Inhibition of TNF-α produced by kupffer cells protects against the nonspecific liver toxicity of immunotoxins anti-tac(Fv)-PE38, LMB-2. *J Immunol*. 2000; 176:7150–7156.

60. Drug Facts and Comparisons. Updated monthly. St. Louis, MO: Lippincott Williams & Wilkins; 2003:1499a.

61. Bielekova B, Richert N, Howard T, et al. Humanized anti-CD25 (daclizumab) inhibits disease activity in multiple sclerosis patients failing to respond to interferon beta. *Proc Natl Acad Sci U S A*. 2004; 101(23):8705–8708.

SELF-ASSESSMENT QUESTIONS

1. The original hybridoma technology, begun in 1975, produced which of the following monoclonal antibodies?

   A. Chimeric
   B. Humanized

C. Human
D. Murine

2. The human immune system often produces a response to the antibodies of question #1. This reaction has the acronym of:

   A. HAHA
   B. HAMA
   C. HACA
   D. HADA

3. Which monoclonal antibody type is *least* likely to cause an immune response in humans?

   A. Human
   B. Chimeric
   C. Humanized
   D. Murine

4. Chimeric antibodies contain approximately what percentage of their peptide sequence from murine origin?

   A. 100%
   B. 75%
   C. 33%
   D. 10%

5. What is sometimes an advantage of using mAb fragments instead of whole mAbs?

   A. Fragment production is much less time-consuming
   B. Fragments induce ADCC
   C. Fragments induce complement fixation
   D. Fragments contain about 75% human peptide sequence

6. Antibody fragments may be produced by inserting the V_H and V_L DNA into:

   A. Plasmids
   B. Bacterial chromosomal DNA
   C. Bacteriophage
   D. Both A and C are correct

7. Which fragment of the antibody is typically used for attachment of toxins?

   A. $F(ab')_2$
   B. Fv
   C. Fab
   D. Fc

8. Bispecific monoclonal antibodies:

   A. Have binding regions that can bind multiple targets due to their "loose" conformation
   B. Can be made to bind both arms of the mAb to the same target
   C. Have two different binding regions on the same mAb
   D. Have antibodies joined together to form quadromas

9. The best isotope to attach to a mAb for imaging purposes, based on its emission characteristics, is:

   A. ^{186}Re
   B. ^{90}Y
   C. ^{99m}Tc
   D. ^{212}Bi

10. The name "ibritumomab" indicates the antibody origin is from a:

    A. Mouse
    B. Human
    C. Rat
    D. Hamster

CHAPTER 3

Cytokines, Chemoattractants, and Adhesion Molecules

Arezoo Campbell

CHAPTER OUTLINE

Introduction
Learning objectives
Cytokines
    Cytokines needed for innate immune responses
    Cytokines mediating adaptive immunity
Chemokines
    C chemokines
    CC chemokines

CXC chemokines
CXXXC chemokines
Adhesion molecules
    Immunoglobulin superfamily
    Selectins
    Integrins
    Mucinlike vascular addressins
Summary
References
Self-assessment questions

INTRODUCTION

The primary purpose of the immune system is to protect the host from infections and environmental insults. Innate (or natural) immune responses are induced as an essential first line of defense; they are initiated by macrophages after they encounter antigens. Inflammation, an important process in innate immunity, recruits additional phagocytic cells to the site of infection. This allows the clearance of pathogens from the foci of infection, helps clear debris, and begins wound healing. In ancient times, Celsus described inflammation as redness (rubor), pain (dolor), swelling (tumor), and heat (calor), reflecting the vascular changes that accompany an inflammatory response.

In higher organisms, adaptive (or acquired) immune responses are activated if innate immunity fails to clear an infection. T and B lymphocytes are the mediators of adaptive immunity. Adhesion molecules and small secreted proteins known as cytokines and chemokines (**Figure 3.1**) are needed for both innate and adaptive immune responses. The first section of this chapter discusses the most common classes of cytokines, grouped according to their function in mediating innate or adaptive immune responses. The second part of the chapter explains the role of chemokines in recruiting other immunologically important cells. The last section covers the expression of adhesion molecules on the cell surface and how they mediate immune responses.

LEARNING OBJECTIVES

After completing this chapter, the reader should be able to:

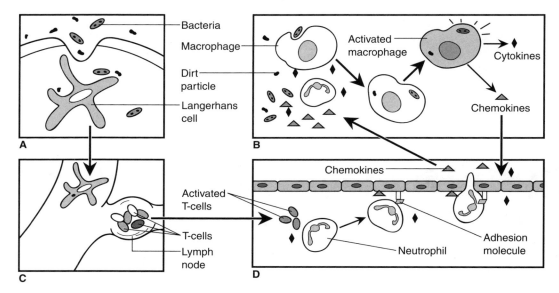

Figure 3.1. Orchestration of the inflammatory response by cytokines, chemokines, and adhesion molecules. Panel A: Disruption of the skin by minor cuts and burns leads to the entry of bacteria and dirt particles into the body. Panel B: Macrophages underlying the damaged tissue process the foreign material and pathogens and are activated. The activated macrophages secrete cytokines and chemokines to enhance the recruitment of additional phagocytes and other immune-competent cells. This initiates the inflammatory response. Panel C: Langerhans cells are specialized dendritic cells that lie in the dermis. When immature, they are highly phagocytic and will take up bacterial and dirt particles. Once activated, these cells travel to the closest lymph node and mature into antigen-presenting cells. Here, they interact with antigen-specific T cells, which then proliferate, mature into effector T cells, and enter the circulation. Panel D: The interaction of cell adhesion molecules expressed on leukocytes (in this case a neutrophil) with those expressed on the vascular endothelium of inflamed tissue causes extravasation of immune cells. The gradient of chemokines produced by activated macrophages directs the neutrophil into the area of damage.

1. Understand the purpose of the inflammatory response and the mediators that contribute to the underlying events.
2. Identify the cytokines mediating both the innate and the adaptive immune responses.
3. Describe the role of viral-induced cytokines.
4. Know the function of the major chemokines and characterize the four structure-based classes.
5. Describe the role of adhesion molecules in both innate and adaptive immune responses and categorize the four different classes of molecules based on their structural similarities.

CYTOKINES

Cytokines are secreted, biologically active proteins usually about 25 kDa in size and released by a variety of stimulated cells. Cytokines affect the behavior of cells that express the specific receptors that bind them. They use a rapid signaling system to activate specific gene expression in the cell nucleus. This signaling pathway includes the receptor-associated tyrosine kinases of the Janus kinase (JAKs) family; upon binding, phosphorylate signal transducers and activators of transcription (STATs). STAT proteins dimerize and translocate to the nucleus where they promote transcription of a variety of genes needed for the effector responses of the activated cell.[1] Several signal-transduction–attenuating proteins ensure appropriate and controlled responses to cytokines. These include the protein inhibitors of activated STATs (PIAS) and suppressors of cytokine signaling (SOCS). Deregulation in these signaling pathways can lead to a variety of hematologic malignancies.[2] Cytokines can be grouped according to their structural characteristics (**Table 3.1**) or their main immunological functions (**Table 3.2**). In the first part of the next section, the cytokines important for innate immune responses are discussed. The second part describes the cytokines involved in the adaptive immune responses. Although this distinction is being made, the innate and adaptive immune responses are highly interactive and dependent on each other.

Cytokines Needed for Innate Immune Responses

The main cytokines mediating innate immune responses—tumor necrosis factor-α (TNF-α),

✳ Table 3.1. Classification of the Major Cytokines Based on Structural Characteristics

Protein Family	Name of Cytokine	Cells Responsible for Production
TNF	TNF-α	Macrophages, NK cells, T cells
	TNF-β	T cells, B cells
Interferons	IFN-α	Dendritic cells
	IFN-β	Fibroblasts
	IFN-γ	T cells, NK cells
IL-10 related	IL-10	T cells, macrophages
	IL-29	T cells, NK cells
IL-12 related	IL-12	Macrophages, dendritic cells
	IL-23	Dendritic cells
Hematopoietins	IL-2	T cells
	IL-3	T cells, thymic epithelial cells
	IL-4	T cells, mast cells
	IL-6	T cells, macrophages, endothelial cells
	IL-7	Non–T cells
Miscellaneous	TGF-β	Monocytes, T cells
	IL-1	Macrophages, epithelial cells
	IL-25	T cells, mast cells

IFN = interferon; IL = interleukin; NK = natural killer; TGF = transforming growth factor; TNF = tumor necrosis factor.

✳ Table 3.2. Classification of the Major Cytokines Based on Effector Mechanisms

Function	Cytokine	Cause of Defect
Inflammation, acute phase protein production, and fever	TNF-α	Susceptibility to *Listeria*
	IL-1	Decreased IL-6 production
	IL-6	Decreased acute phase reaction
Anti-viral defense	IFN-α	Impaired anti-viral defenses
	IFN-β	
	IL-29	
B-cell proliferation	IL-7	Defective B-cell development
T-cell proliferation	IL-2	T-cell development defective (SCID)
	IL-7	
Th2 responses	IL-4	Impaired Th2 responses
	IL-25	
Th1 responses	IFN-γ	Impaired Th1 responses
	IL-12	
	IL-23	
Anti-inflammatory	IL-10	Uncontrolled inflammation
	TGF-β	
Hematopoiesis	IL-3	Bone marrow unresponsive to cytokines IL-5 and GM-CSF

GM-CSF = granulocyte-macrophage colony-stimulating factor; IFN = interferon; IL = interleukin; SCID = severe combined immunodeficiency; TGF = transforming growth factor; TNF = tumor necrosis factor.

interleukin-6 (IL-6), and IL-1β—are also known as proinflammatory cytokines. One pathway leading to production of these cytokines is activated by the interaction of pathogen-associated molecular patterns (PAMPs) with transmembrane toll-like receptors (TLRs). TLRs are part of an evolutionarily well-conserved signaling pathway that mediates innate immune responses in organisms as diverse as plants, insects, and mammals.[3] Once TLRs bind a specific ligand, a cascade of events causes the activation of the transcription factor NF-κB. This transcription factor is usually inactive in the cytoplasm because it is in a complex with an inhibitor protein (IκB). The IκB kinase (IKK) complex consists of IKKα, IKKβ, and NF-κB essential modifier (NEMO). IKK complex phosphorylates IκB, and allows its proteolytic degradation. NF-κB then translocates to the nucleus, binds to its consensus sequence in the promoter region of genes, and causes transcription of immune-related proteins.[4] Point mutations in the NEMO gene lead to X-linked ectodermal dysplasia and immunodeficiency characterized by recurrent infections. The dysplasia is caused by defects in ectodermal development, which depends on IKK activation through a receptor known as ectodysplasin A (a member of TNF receptor superfamily). The immunological dysfunction is manifold. One consequence of the lack of NF-κB activation is decreased production of TNF-α and IL-18. TNF-α is needed for amplification of immune responses, nitric oxide production, and phagocytic activation of macrophages harboring intracellular pathogens. Males with NEMO mutations will suffer from chronic mycobacterial infections. Viral infections are also common because natural killer (NK) cells are incapable of destroying viral-infected cells.[5]

One function of TNF-α, IL-1, and IL-6 is to cause fever; they are known as pyrogenic cytokines. Higher host temperature has many benefits. It defends host cells from the harmful effects of TNF-α, slows down the proliferation of pathogens, and promotes adaptive immunity, which responds more efficiently at higher temperatures. These three main proinflammatory cytokines also induce acute-phase protein secretion by hepatocytes. Acute-phase proteins include mannose-binding lectin, C-reactive protein, and pulmonary surfactant proteins (SP-A, SP-D). Their main function is opsonization of pathogens during the early, nonadaptive phases of immunity.[1]

Uncontrolled release of proinflammatory cytokines can have harmful consequences. This is clearly demonstrated by systemic secretion of TNF-α. The early function of this cytokine is to increase vascular permeability and adhesiveness of endothelial cells at the foci of infection. In the later phases of inflammation, TNF-α helps contain infections by occluding local blood vessels. However, this TNF-α–mediated clotting mechanism can be harmful if an infection spreads to the blood stream (sepsis). One consequence of a massive release of TNF-α by systemic tissues is clot formation in the small vessels of vital organs, leading to decreased perfusion and multiple organ failure. This condition, septic shock, has a high mortality rate.[6]

Interferons (IFNs) are antiviral cytokines, so named because they interfere with viral replication. IFN-α and IFN-β are considered type I interferons. They are monomeric, and activate a receptor complex composed of two subunits of interferon receptor (IFNAR) 1 and 2. The IFNAR uses the rapid JAK-STAT signaling pathway discussed earlier. When activated, IFN-sensitive genes are transcribed and the protein product of these genes mediates IFN-dependent immune responses.[7] Type I interferons have three main functions. First, they can stop replication of viruses by inhibiting the translation of proteins necessary for viral proliferation. Second, they can activate NK cells to release cytotoxic components onto the surface of viral-infected target cells. NK cells are part of the innate immune response and provide a fast-acting defense against viral infections; activated NK cells activate macrophages by producing IFN-γ. A third function of IFN-α and IFN-β is to enhance the production and expression of major histocompatibility (MHC) class I molecules on neighboring non-infected cells, making them less susceptible to destruction by NK cells.[1]

Although activation of NK cells controls viral replication, it does not clear the infection. Cytotoxic T cells (part of the adaptive immune response) are needed. IL-12 is produced early in infections and, similar to IFN-α and IFN-β, activates NK cells. Together with TNF-α, IL-12 causes NK cells to produce IFN-γ, which contains the infection until an adaptive immune response is mounted. Because type I interferons are such powerful modulators of the immune response, they are being used therapeutically in several human diseases. They have been shown to improve the degenerative autoimmune disease multiple sclerosis as well as hepatitis B and C viral infections.

Cytokines Mediating Adaptive Immunity

Many cytokines work in the vicinity in which they are released and require focal up-regulation of their receptors. Thus, clinical trials using systemic administration of cytokines are often disappointing.

The first part of this section reviews the essential cytokines responsible for B-cell and T-cell development. The second part focuses on the cytokines responsible for the effector function of B and T cells.

Development of lymphocytes. IL-7 is important for the development of both B cells and T cells in the central lymphoid tissues (bone marrow for B cells and thymus for T cells). The IL-7 receptor is expressed on early pro-B cells in the bone marrow; this cytokine, along with other factors secreted by stromal cells, is needed for the development of pro-B cells into pre-B cells. The IL-7 receptor is also important for development of T cells in the thymus, since a defect in the receptor greatly impedes this process. Once the lymphocytes are formed, they migrate to the peripheral lymphoid tissues where the secretion of chemokines and cytokines, along with interaction with adhesion molecules, direct them to specialized loci. The proinflammatory cytokine, TNF-α, also has a role in developing and maintaining the architecture of lymphoid tissue. Mutant mice lacking the TNF receptor (TNFR-I) develop spleens with an abnormal structure and missing follicular dendritic cells.[1]

Proliferation of activated T cells. IL-2 is a cytokine needed for division and differentiation of T cells. After transcription factor activation, the cytokine is produced when the T-cell receptor and coreceptor complexes receive signals. The costimulatory signals delivered by the cell surface protein, CD28, amplify the rate of transcription of IL-2 by stabilizing its mRNA and activating other transcription factors. The IL-2 receptor is expressed on T cells in a low-affinity conformation of γ and β chains. Upon activation of the T lymphocyte, the α chain is synthesized, and associates with γ and β chains. This is a high-affinity IL-2 receptor that strongly binds the IL-2 produced by the activated T cells, triggering cell division. The immunosuppressive drugs cyclosporin A and tacrolimus are potent inhibitors of T-cell activation and division because they disrupt the signals from T-cell receptors needed for IL-2 production.[6] These pharmaceutical agents are used for selective suppression of the immune response during tissue transplantation to inhibit graft rejection. Since the discovery of cyclosporine in the late 1970s, the clinical outcome of transplantation has dramatically improved.

Cytokines responsible for effector T-cell function. T cells can be divided in two groups, based on the coreceptor expressed. If they carry the CD8 coreceptor, they are called cytotoxic T (T$_C$) cells. If they carry the CD4 coreceptor, they are known as T-helper (Th) cells. The effector function of T cells is dependent on the type of cytokines they produce. Activated CD8 T cells mainly produce TNF-α, IFN-γ, and TNF-β. IFN-γ production directly inhibits viral replication and allows activation of macrophages. It also induces the up-regulation of MHC class I molecules on the infected cells, which are loaded with pathogen-associated antigens. TNF-α and TNF-β intensify macrophage activation while accelerating the death of some target cells through TNFR-I-mediated mechanisms (Table 3.2). These cytokines cooperate to allow cytotoxic T cells to confine the spread of infection caused by cytosolic pathogens.

CD4 T cells are subdivided based on the profile of cytokines they secrete; this determines their overall effector functions. Both the Th1 and Th2 subtypes of CD4 T cells derive from Th0 cells. The main role of Th1 cells is to activate macrophages. To accomplish this, the main cytokine produced is IFN-γ. Unlike the CD8 cells, which have preformed cytotoxic granules, Th1 cells have to synthesize the needed cytokines. Similar to CD8 cells, Th1 CD4 T cells also produce TNF-α and TNF-β, which not only work with IFN-γ to activate macrophages, but also mediate the migration of macrophages into the site of infection. IL-2 is also produced, allowing activated Th1 cells to proliferate. This subtype of CD4 cells is needed for defense against intravesicular pathogens, microorganisms that live in macrophages. These include mycobacteria responsible for tuberculosis or leprosy. Because they live in the vesicular system of macrophages, these pathogens cannot be reached by antibodies. Also, the MHC class I molecules cannot process and present peptides from these microorganisms. Therefore, cytotoxic T cells cannot kill infected macrophages. The function of the Th1 CD4 T cells becomes essential; they activate the macrophages to make them able to destroy the intravesicular microbes. Activated macrophages produce IL-12, which not only activates NK cells but also induces differentiation of the CD4 T cells to the Th1 lineage. This way, the macrophage itself can amplify the immune response to mycobacteria.[1]

The Th2 subset of CD4 T cells secretes IL-4, IL-5, IL-10, and IL-13, which work together to activate B cells. IL-5 also increases the production of eosinophils. The Th2 CD4 T cells are clinically important because they contribute to the development of allergic responses. IL-4, produced by Th2 cells, stimulates B cells to switch immunoglobulin isotypes and produce the antibody isotype IgE, which is responsible for most allergies. Once IgE is produced, activated eosinophils amplify the effects. The IL-4 and IL-10 produced by the Th2 CD4 T cells inhibit macrophage activation. Thus the cytokines produced by Th2 CD4 T cells inhibit the effects of the Th1 subset of CD4 T cells and vice-versa. A pharmacological intervention being studied for allergies involves using cytokines to promote Th1 responses to shift the antibody response away from IgE production.

Both Th1 and Th2 CD4 T cells are able to produce the cytokines IL-3 and granulocyte-macrophage colony-stimulating factor (GM-CSF). These two cytokines trigger production of macrophages and granulocytes from bone marrow by a process known as myelopoiesis. Clinical use of cytokines generally is limited because these molecules must be close to their target cells. However, IL-3 and GM-CSF can be effective therapeutically because they are able to act systemically. These two cytokines are used successfully to stimulate leukocyte production in patients who have undergone bone marrow transplantation.[1]

A subset of CD4 T cells known as regulatory, or suppressor, CD4 cells limit the function of activated T cells during an immune response, protecting healthy cells from indirect damage. T-regulatory cells differ from other CD4-positive cells by the abundance of CD25 on the cell membrane. They also have a distinct profile of cytokine secretion, which is mainly anti-inflammatory and consists of IL-4, IL-10, and transforming growth factor (TGF)-β. These cells are thought to help inhibit the pro-inflammatory responses that occur in such diseases as rheumatoid arthritis. When these cells fail, the common drug therapy includes immunosuppressive and anti-inflammatory medications. Treatment with antibodies against TNF-α has also been used to improve symptoms of rheumatoid arthritis.

CHEMOKINES

Chemokines are a large family of molecules with a pivotal role in the migration of leukocytes to an area of infection. Cells can produce chemokines to recruit leukocytes such as neutrophils and monocytes to the foci of infection or physical damage. Chemokines also play a role in lymphocyte development and migration, adaptive immune responses, and angiogenesis. All chemokines share similarities in their amino acid sequences, and function through G-coupled receptors composed of seven membrane-spanning domains. Chemokines generally are grouped according to their structure (**Table 3.3**). Two broad classes include the CC (contain two adjacent cysteines near the amino terminus) and the CXC (the two cysteines are separated by one amino acid) chemokines. There is also an XCL chemokine (lymphotactin) and a CX3CL chemokine (fractalkine).[6]

The varied expression of the chemokine receptor on different cell types determines if the cell will be recruited by a specific chemokine. Thus, CXCL8 guides the migration of neutrophils that express the CXC receptor (CXCR) specific for this chemokine while CCL2 promotes recruitment of monocytes that express the CC receptor (CCR).[1] The complement-derived fragments C3a, C4a, and C5a can also function in a chemokine-like way and enhance inflammation. C5a is the most potent fragment, and C4a is only weakly proinflammatory. The activity of C3a is intermediate.[6]

C Chemokines

The chemokines belonging to this class lack the first and third cysteines. So far two ligands for the XC receptor (XCR) have been identified. XCL1 is also known as lymphotactin; XCL2, the only other member of this class of chemokines, is known as lymphotactin-beta. XCL1 is glycosylated, which is important for its function as a chemokine. It is primarily chemoattractant and stimulatory for T cells. It has been proposed that lymphotactin can promote antitumor activity by enhancing CD8 T-cell mediated cytotoxicity.[8]

CC Chemokines

This class of chemokines is so named because of the presence of two adjacent cysteine residues in the amino-terminal region of the peptides without an intervening amino acid. To date, 27 members have been identified, and most are encoded on human chromosome 17. Ten CC receptors designated as CCR1-10 have been identified. These chemokines target a variety of immunologically competent cells including NK cells, T cells, monocytes, dendritic cells, and eosinophils.

Two CC chemokines, CCL19 (MIP-3β) and CCL21 (secondary lymphoid chemokines), are involved in the migration of T cells into the T zones of lymphoid organs. Both of these chemokines bind to the CCR7 receptor expressed on T cells. The chemokines are produced by endothelial cells of the high endothelial venules, stromal cells, and the interdigitating dendritic cells, which are all present at the T zones.[1] Another CC chemokine, CCL18, also called dendritic cell-chemokine (DC-CK), is produced by activated dendritic cells to attract naïve T cells; it is needed to activate antigen-specific clones of T-lymphocytes. CCL2, formerly known as macrophage chemoattractant protein (MCP), is produced by activated Th1 cells and is essential in migration of macrophages to the site of inflammation.

Table 3.3. Classification of Common Chemokines Based on Structural Similarities

Class	Examples	Main Function	Cells Capable of Production
CXXXC	CX3CL1 (Fractalkine)	Adhesion of leukocytes to endothelium	Monocytes, endothelium
CXC	CXCL1 (GROα)	Activates neutrophils	Monocytes
	CXCL7 (NAP-2)	Clot resorption	Platelets
	CXCL8 (IL-8)	Mobilizes neutrophils	Monocytes, macrophages Endothelial cells
	CXCL12 (SDF-1)	Lymphocyte homing	Stromal cells
CC	CCL2 (MCP-1)	Activates macrophages	Monocytes, macrophages
	CCL3 (MIP-1α)	Antiviral defense	Monocytes, T cells
	CCL4 (MIP-1β)	Competes with HIV-1	Monocytes, neutrophils, macrophages, endothelium
	CCL5 (RANTES)	Activates T cells	T cells, endothelium
	CCL11 (Eotaxin)	Allergic response	Endothelium, T cells Monocytes, epithelium
	CCL18 (DC-CK)	Activates naïve T cells	Dendritic cells
C	XCL1 (Lymphotactin)	Lymphocyte development	T cells

DC-CK = dendritic cell-chemokine; IL = interleukin; MCP = macrophage chemoattractant protein; SDF-1 = stromal cell–derived factor 1.

As noted earlier, Th2 cells produce IL-5, which stimulates production of eosinophils. The chemokines CCL5, CCL7, CCL11, and CCL13 bind to the CCR3 receptor expressed on eosinophils and allow the cells to migrate into tissues. CCL11, also known as eotaxin, has been shown to be especially important for eosinophil migration. Overactivated eosinophils can cause severe tissue damage, as seen in patients with high eosinophil counts (a condition known as hypereosinophilia). T-cell lymphomas that secrete IL-5 can predispose a patient to this disease. The highly reactive eosinophils cause damage to the endocardium of the heart and nerves, leading to heart failure and neuropathy.[1]

CXC Chemokines

These chemokines contain two cysteine residues separated by one amino acid in the N-terminus of the peptides. About 14 ligands have been identified, and they are mostly encoded on human chromosome 4. They bind to six CXC receptors designated as CXCR1-6. The first chemokine to be cloned, CXCL8, is also known as IL-8 because it was identified by a cytokine assay. Produced by activated macrophages, CXCL8 has two important functions. First, it changes the adhesive properties of leukocytes by changing the expression of cell surface molecules, allowing the cells to leave the general circulation and enter infected areas. Second, CXCL8 binds to proteoglycans in the extracellular matrix forming a concentration-based gradient. It also binds to proteoglycans on endothelial cells, and can direct the movement of leukocytes into foci of infection or tissue damage. Thus, the main function of CXCL8 is to recruit neutrophils from the systemic blood to infected areas.

While some chemokines recruit leukocytes from the periphery to sites of inflammation, others maintain the general homeostasis of lymphoid organs. CXCL12 and CXCL13 are in the second category. CXCL12 is also known as stromal cell–derived factor 1 (SDF-1); as its name implies, it is produced constitutively by the stromal cells of the bone marrow. It is thought that one of its functions is to ensure that B-cell precursors stay in the bone marrow. In mice lacking the gene to encode CXCL12, B cells fail to develop. CXCL13, produced by follicular dendritic cells, is an important cytokine for the migration of B cells into the follicular zones of the lymph nodes. Therefore, this cytokine is also known as B-lymphocyte chemokine (BLC). B cells express the CXCR5 receptor, which binds CXCL13 and directs the cells to the distinct follicular areas of lymphoid tissues.[6]

CXXXC Chemokines

The CX3CL1 chemokine, also known as fractalkine, is encoded on human chromosome 16. It binds the CX3R1 receptor and attracts both T cells and monocytes. It exists in both a soluble and an immobilized form, functioning both as a chemoattractant protein and as an adhesion molecule. The soluble form of CX3CL1 causes migration of NK cells, cytotoxic T cells, and macrophages; the membrane-bound form helps these cells enter inflamed tissue. Inappropriate expression of fractalkine is thought to be responsible for many clinical diseases including atherosclerosis, cardiovascular disease, and arthritis.[9]

ADHESION MOLECULES

Cell adhesion molecules play an important role in many kinds of immune responses. They allow the leukocytes to interact with the endothelial cells of the blood vessels, a crucial step to induce inflammation. They also regulate the homing of naïve T and B lymphocytes to secondary lymphoid tissue, where they interact with their specific antigens. Cell adhesion molecules also play a pivotal role in the interaction of T lymphocytes with antigen-presenting dendritic cells and the resulting activation of antigen-specific T cells.

Cell adhesion molecules can be grouped into four structural classes (**Table 3.4**). One is the immunoglobulin superfamily, which includes the intercellular adhesion molecules (ICAMs). Members of this family are needed for a variety of immune responses. They are present on activated endothelium at sites of infection or injury. They are also found on stromal cells of the bone marrow and are needed for the development of B cells. CD2 (also known as LFA-2), a member of the immunoglobulin superfamily, is present on T cells. Molecules belonging to another class, the selectins, are expressed on activated endothelial cells. These are glycoproteins with a lectin-like domain that interact with specific carbohydrate groups. The third class of adhesion molecules is the integrins, which are expressed on leukocytes. These interact with ICAM molecules expressed on activated endothelial cells to allow extravasation of leukocytes into sites of inflammation or naïve lymphocytes into secondary lymphoid tissues. The mucinlike vascular addressins, the fourth class of adhesion molecules, are expressed mainly by the endothelium, and bind to L-selectin.[6]

The nomenclature of cell adhesion proteins can be misleading. They were named randomly, based on the assay used to identify them, so their names do not reflect their function or their structural group. For instance, although LFA-1 is an integrin, LFA-2 is a member of the immunoglobulin superfamily. Pharmacology students new to the field of immunology must be careful not to confuse the terminology of the adhesion molecules with their actual structure and function.

Immunoglobulin Superfamily

This group includes the ICAMs. ICAM-1 is expressed by activated endothelial cells of the blood vessels, while ICAM-2 is expressed mainly in resting endothelium and dendritic cells. ICAM-3 is expressed on the T-cell surface. The ligand for ICAM molecules is usually LFA-1. ICAM-3 also interacts with high affinity to the lectin

Table 3.4. Structural Classes of the Main Adhesion Molecules

Class	Example	Ligands	Cells That Present Molecule	Main Function
Addressins	CD34	L-selectin	Endothelium	Initiate endothelial-leukocyte interactions
Immunoglobulin superfamily	LFA-2	LFA-3	T cells	Allow strong adhesion of immune cells
Integrins	LFA-1	ICAMs	Monocytes, macrophages, dendritic cells, T cells, neutrophils	Allow strong adhesion of immune cells
Selectins	L-selectin	CD34	Neutrophils, lymphocytes, monocytes, macrophages	Initiate leukocyte-endothelial interactions

ICAM = intercellular adhesion molecule.

dendritic cell–specific intercellular adhesion molecule 3–grabbing nonintegrin (DC-SIGN), which is present on activated dendritic cells. Platelet-endothelial cell adhesion molecule (PECAM) is expressed mainly by activated leukocytes and endothelial cell-to-cell junctions, and is essential for the extravasation of phagocytes into an area of injury. Interactions between the leukocytes and endothelial junctions involving PECAM allow the cells to move through the basement membrane. This process, known as *diapedesis*, also involves a series of enzymes that break down extracellular matrix proteins.[1]

Adhesion molecules may do more than activate immune cells and allow their migration. A new class of adhesion molecules known as the carcinoembryonic-antigen-related-adhesion molecule (CEACAM) family of proteins has been shown to help regulate cell proliferation in normal and cancer cells. They are differentially expressed on most human cells, including epithelial, endothelial, granulocytes, lymphocytes, and cells of myeloid origin, and consist of either long or short cytoplasmic tails. Depending on the activation state and cell types, the levels of the short and long isoforms of CEACAM can be varied. The long cytoplasmic domains of CEACAM1 seem to provide a predominantly coinhibitory function for T-cell proliferation and cytotoxic activity. In mice deficient in this adhesion molecule, stimulated T cells hyperproliferate and produce high levels of IL-2 and IFN-γ. Tumors that overexpress CAECAM1 have been shown to be highly aggressive, possibly due to the inhibition of T-cell–mediated killing of the cancer cells.[10]

Selectins

Selectins are membrane glycoproteins induced on activated endothelial cells. They bind oligosaccharides (sulfated sialyl-Lewis moieties) on the cell surface of circulating leukocytes, initiating the first interactions between the endothelium and immune-competent cells. Preformed P-selectins are present in granules called Weibel-Palade bodies. TNF-α, secreted by activated macrophages, causes the rapid externalization of P-selectin on endothelial cells and these adhesion molecules are expressed immediately. E-selectins synthesized in the endothelial cells in response to stress are expressed on the cells after a lag. After a few hours, E-selectin is the main adhesion molecule expressed on the vascular endothelium.[6]

L-selectin is expressed on naïve T cells, allowing them to recirculate through lymph nodes by entering high endothelial venules. Once they enter lymph nodes, they can interact with antigen-presenting cells carrying an MHC-peptide specific for the T-cell receptor. An activated T cell downregulates L-selectin on its membrane and instead expresses the integrin VLA-4. This adhesion molecule selectively interacts with VCAM-1, which is abundant on the endothelial cells of blood vessels in inflamed tissue.[1]

Integrins

Integrins are heterodimeric proteins expressed by the circulating leukocytes. They allow tight adhesion of the cells to activated endothelial cells expressing ICAMs. The main integrins are leukocyte functional antigen 1 (LFA-1) and complement receptor type 3 (CR3). In general, more LFA-1 is expressed by activated T cells compared to naïve T cells. Greater expression of LFA-1 increases the chance of interacting with ICAMs. Endothelium-bound chemokines change the conformational shape of integrins to an extended form that allows immediate arrest of leukocytes traveling under continuous-shear blood flow.[11]

Another example of how conformational change in LFA-1 binding to ICAMs allows tight binding between immune-competent cells is the interaction of mature dendritic cells with antigen-specific naïve T cells in secondary lymphoid tissue. When the T-cell receptor associates with a peptide-MHC complex on an antigen-presenting dendritic cell, it signals the LFA-1 to change shape so it can interact with ICAMs with higher affinity. This tight binding of the newly shaped LFA-1 to ICAMs on the dendritic cell allows the T cell to associate with the antigen-presenting cell for up to several days. During this time, costimulatory signals from members of the immunoglobulin superfamily (CD28 on T cells and B7 on professional antigen-presenting cells) allow activated T cells to proliferate and differentiate.[6] Once the response is no longer needed, there is a shift to express a different coreceptor, CTLA4 instead of CD28. This molecule dampens the activation of T cells, allowing regulation of proliferation.

The importance of integrins in phagocyte trafficking to infected tissue is demonstrated by the genetic defect leukocyte adhesion deficiency. Patients with this condition lack functional integrins on their phagocytes. These cells cannot be recruited to sites of inflammation so extracellular bacteria cannot be cleared. Children with this genetic defect have recurrent infections with capsulated bacteria, and wound healing is compromised.

Mucinlike Vascular Addressins

The vascular addressins, CD34 and glycosylation-dependent cell adhesion molecule 1 (GlyCAM-1), are expressed on the high endothelial venules. These addressins are important in initiating movement of naïve T cells into lymph nodes. CD34 and GlyCAM-1, which contain sulfated sialyl-Lewis moieties that interact with the L-selectin expressed on circulating naïve T cells, home these cells into the lymph nodes. GlyCAM-1 is expressed only on the high endothelial venules. Because it lacks transmembrane regions, it is not known how it attaches to the endothelial membrane. In contrast, CD34 has a transmembrane region and a form of it is found on other endothelial cells. But the glycosylated form is found only on high endothelial venule cells.

The mucosal addressin cell adhesion molecule-1 (MAdCAM-1) is expressed exclusively on mucosal endothelium. T cells, by binding to the MAdCAM-1 moieties, can be recruited to mucosal lymphoid tissue from distinct anatomical loci. When T cells are activated in the Peyer's patches (secondary lymphoid tissues on the gut epithelium), they are drained into the blood. These select T cells can enter all mucosal tissues by recognizing MAdCAM-1. Thus, initiation of the immune response by a few antigen-specific T cells in the gut can spread to all mucosal tissues.[6]

SUMMARY

The immune system has developed an intricate network of cytokines, chemokines, and adhesion molecules to fine-tune its response to different pathogens. Pathogens, on the other hand, have learned to manipulate this system to avoid elimination. For example, the vaccinia virus produces a soluble form of cytokine receptors that bind to the secreted forms of the molecules and render them ineffective. The Epstein-Barr virus, by inhibiting the expression of the adhesion molecule ICAM-1, prevents recruitment of immune-competent cells. Today our understanding of the interplay between cytokines, chemokines, and adhesion molecules in orchestrating an effective immune response is in its infancy. A better understanding of this system eventually will allow us to design selective therapeutic strategies. This will be especially important in diseases where immune responses, rather than being beneficial, have actually become destructive.

REFERENCES

1. Janeway CA, Travers P, Walport M, et al, eds. *Immunobiology*. 6th ed. New York, NY: Garland Science Publishing; 2005.
2. Valentino L, Pierre J. JAK/STAT signal transduction: regulators and implication in hematological malignancies. *Biochem Pharmacol*. 2006; 71:713–721.
3. Medzhitov R, Janeway CA. An ancient system of host defense. *Curr Opin Immunol*. 1998; 10:12–15.
4. Baeuerle PA, Henkel T. Function and activation of NF-κB in the immune system. *Ann Rev Immunol*. 1994; 12:141–179.
5. Rosen F, Ceha R. *Case Studies in Immunology, A Clinical Companion*. 4th ed. New York, NY: Garland Science Publishing; 2004.
6. Parham P. *The Immune System*. 2nd ed. New York, NY: Garland Science Publishing; 2005.
7. Brierley MM, Fish EN. Review: IFN-alpha/beta receptor interactions to biologic outcomes: understanding the circuitry. *J Interferon Cytokine Res*. 2002; 22:835–845.
8. Cao X, Zhang W, He L, et al. Lymphotactin gene-modified bone marrow dendritic cells act as more potent adjuvants for peptide delivery to induce specific antitumor immunity. *J Immunol*. 1998; 161:6238–6244.
9. Umehara H, Bloom ET, Okazaki T, et al. Fractalkine in vascular biology. *Arterioscle Thromb Casc Biol*. 2004; 24:34–40.
10. Gray-Owen SD, Blumberg RS. CEACAM1: contact-dependent control of immunity. *Nat Rev Immunol*. 2006; 6:433–446.
11. Shamri R, Grabovsky V, Gauguet JM, et al. Lymphocyte arrest requires instantaneous induction of an extended LFA-1 conformation mediated by endothelium-bound chemokines. *Nature Immunol*. 2005; 6:497–506.

SELF-ASSESSMENT QUESTIONS

1. The ancient definition of the inflammatory response consists of the following terms:

    A. Pain and redness
    B. Cold and heat
    C. Swelling and heat
    D. Both A and C
    E. None of the above

2. The cytokines responsible for proinflammatory responses are:

    A. TNF-α and TNF-β
    B. IFN-β and IFN-α
    C. IL-6, IL-1, and TNF-α
    D. IL-2, IL-4, and IL-5
    E. IL-4, IL-10, and TGF-β

3. What is the main event responsible for sepsis?

    A. Systemic release of TNF-α
    B. Activation of Type I interferons
    C. NK cell–mediated cytotoxicity

D. Systemic release of IL-5, which increases production of eosinophils
E. Massive release of IL-2 leading to uncontrolled T-cell proliferation

4. Which of the following are functions of type I interferons?

A. Macrophage activation and destruction of intravesicular microbes
B. Inhibition of viral replication and activation of NK cells
C. Initiation of acute phase reaction and opsonization of pathogens
D. B-cell activation and production of antibodies
E. Activation of B cells and NK cells

5. Th1 cells are different from Th2 cells based on:

A. Function
B. Main cytokines produced
C. Type of cells affected
D. All of the above
E. None of the above

6. The main anti-inflammatory cytokines are:

A. TNF-α and TNF-β
B. IFN-β and IFN-α
C. IL-6, IL-1, and TNF-α
D. IL-2, IL-4, and IL-5
E. IL-4, IL-10, and TGF-β

7. Cytokines produced by Th1 cells mainly affect:

A. Epithelial cells
B. B cells
C. NK cells
D. Macrophages
E. Neutrophils

8. Antibodies against TNF-α have been therapeutically successful in:

A. Lymphoma
B. Multiple sclerosis
C. Rheumatoid arthritis
D. Meningitis
E. All of the above

9. The structural classification of chemokines is based on the following:

A. Glycosylation
B. Lipid moieties
C. Cysteine residues
D. Alanine residues
E. Three-dimensional shape

10. Which of the following chemokines attracts leukocytes to sites of inflammation and directs them to the foci of infection by providing a concentration-based gradient?

A. CXCL8
B. CXCL12
C. CCL19
D. XCL1
E. All of the above

11. Which of the following is/are function(s) of adhesion molecules?

A. Interaction of antigen-presenting cells with T cells
B. Extravasation of neutrophils to sites of inflammation
C. Homing of B cells to secondary lymphoid tissues
D. Homing of naïve T cells to secondary lymphoid tissue
E. All of the above

12. Which of the following is an addressin?

A. CAECAM
B. PECAM
C. GlyCAM1
D. CXCL8
E. None of the above

Part II—Clinical Applications of Immunology

CHAPTER 4

Mechanisms of Hypersensitivity and Drug Allergy

Andrea K. Hubbard

CHAPTER OUTLINE

INTRODUCTION

Although allergic drug reactions account for only 6% to 10% of cases of adverse drug reactions, they are an important drug effect because of their unpredictability, their prevalence in certain risk groups, and their occurrence in response to commonly used medications (e.g., antibiotics). It is important to understand the immune mechanisms underlying these reactions and to acknowledge their role in normal immune defense. This chapter also highlights specific compounds that elicit immune-mediated adverse drug reactions and discusses possible treatment strategies.

Adverse drug reactions (ADRs) can be either type A (common, predictable, and occurring in any patient) or type B (uncommon, unpredictable, and occurring only in susceptible patients) (**Table 4.1**). Type A reactions account for about 80% of adverse drug reactions, are usually dose-dependent, and are produced by known pharmacologic actions of the drug. Type B reactions cause 6% to 10% of adverse reactions and are uncommon and usually unpredictable. These idiosyncratic reactions are generally unrelated to the pharmacologic actions of the drug and difficult to distinguish from an immune response. The immune responses in type B adverse reactions are collectively known as hypersensitivities.

Hypersensitivity reactions, first described in 1975 by Gell and Coombs,[1] have often been portrayed as events that can be either harmful or beneficial (**Figure 4.1**). These reactions evolved in response to immunogenic/pathogenic stimuli

Table 4.1. Adverse Drug Reactions

Type A	Type B
Common	Uncommon
Predictable	Usually unpredictable
Occurs in any patient	Occurs in few susceptible patients
Resembles pharmacologic activity of drug	Resembles immune response
Accounts for 80% of adverse drug reactions	Accounts for 6% to 10% of adverse drug reactions

to eliminate antigen without extensive damage to the host. They are broad strategies used by the body to combat classes of infectious agents.[2] Yet in some circumstances, these same reactions in response to foreign stimuli (or altered self) result in significant tissue damage or even death. Indeed, the word *anaphylaxis* means "protection again." These hypersensitivity reactions are classified by the immune effector mechanism responsible for cell, tissue, or organ damage.

This chapter describes the immunologic mechanisms underlying each of the four types of hypersensitivity (**Table 4.2**) and their role in drug allergy. Although cellular mechanisms differ among these hypersensitivities (**Figure 4.2,** page 66), they have several common elements: (1) These reactions are normal immune responses, often against pathogens, that have expanded to damage tissue. They are mechanistically identical to protective responses, differing only in the source and nature of the immunogen. (2) These reactions begin with a sensitization phase in which an immune response is initiated, then progress to a secondary immune response with antibody-isotype switching or sensitization of T lymphocytes. The sensitization phase is followed by an elicitation phase with the development of symptoms. (3) These reactions are not mutually exclusive; they can occur simultaneously or consecutively.

LEARNING OBJECTIVES

After completing this chapter, the reader should be able to:

1. Describe the immune mechanisms underlying each of the four hypersensitivity responses.
2. Understand the hapten hypothesis in the formation of immunogenic compounds.
3. Define the different pharmaceutical compounds that can lead to allergic adverse drug reactions.
4. Describe potential therapeutic strategies for treating drug-induced adverse reactions.

CELLULAR MECHANISMS UNDERLYING HYPERSENSITIVITIES

Type I Hypersensitivity

Similar to other immune responses, the immunoglobulin E (IgE)-mediated type I hypersensitivity reaction begins with immunogen (allergen) uptake by antigen-processing cells (APC), resulting in allergen processing and presentation to T helper cells. These T helper cells (Th2 cells)—with T-cell

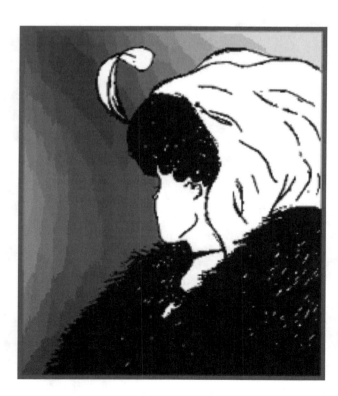

Figure 4.1. Hypersensitivities are often considered the double-edged sword as reflected by two images in one picture.

Table 4.2. The Double-Edged Sword of Hypersensitivities

Classifi- cation	Name	Initiation Time	Immunologic Mechanism	Destructive Immune Defense	Protective Immune Defense
Type I	IgE-mediated (immediate) type	2–30 min	Allergen cross-links mast-cell–bound IgE antibodies with release of vasoactive, lipid, and cytokine mediators	Systemic anaphylaxis Localized anaphylaxis: • rhinitis • asthma • hives • food allergies • eczema	Expulsion of parasites from the respiratory and gastrointestinal tracts
Type II	Antibody-mediated cytotoxic type	5–8 hr	IgG, IgM Ab specific for cell-surface or matrix antigens mediates cytotoxicity by complement or ADCC	Blood transfusion reactions Erythroblastosis fetalis Autoimmune hemolytic anemia	Elimination of extracellular microorganisms
Type III	Immune complex-mediated type	2–8 hr	Antigen-antibody (IgG, IgM) complexes deposited along basement membranes/joints with activation of complement and neutrophil influx	Localized Arthus reaction Generalized reactions: • serum sickness • glomerulonephritis • rheumatoid arthritis • systemic lupus erythematosus	Elimination of viral particles and/or toxins
Type IV	Cell-mediated (delayed) type	24–72 hr	Th1 lymphocytes specific for allergen activates macrophages and CTL mediates tissue damage	Contact dermatitis Tubercular reactions Graft rejection	Elimination of intracellular viral, parasitic, or bacterial microbes

Ab = antibody; ADCC = antibody-dependent cell cytotoxicity; CTL = cytotoxic T cells; Ig = immunoglobulin; Th1 = T helper 1.

receptors specific for individual epitopes within the allergen—undergo primary and secondary immune responses (upon reexposure to the same allergen). IgE antibody molecules predominate during the secondary immune response; the Fc portion of the antibody molecule interacts with high affinity to IgE receptors on connective tissue, mucosal mast cells, or circulating basophils. Mature mast cells reside close to epithelia, blood vessels, nerves, and in the airways and gastrointestinal (GI) tract near smooth muscle cells and mucus-producing glands.[3] Upon reexposure to allergen during the elicitation phase, the allergen interacts with and cross-links the mast-cell-bound IgE molecules. Cross-linking of receptor-bound IgE molecules with multivalent allergen activates mast cells or basophils and leads to (1) extracellular release of preformed mediators stored in the cells' cytoplasmic granules (e.g., histamine, major basic protein, cathepsin); (2) de novo synthesis of proinflammatory lipid mediators (e.g., prostaglandins, leukotrienes); and (3) synthesis and secretion of growth factors, cytokines, and chemokines (e.g., interleukins).[3–5] With the interaction of allergen with specific IgE bound to its high-affinity receptor (FcεRI) on the cell surface, there is aggregation of the receptors and initiation of intracellular signaling. Since this receptor lacks intrinsic tyrosine kinase activity, its cross-linking initiates activation of Src, Syk, and Tec families of protein tyrosine kinases. These early phosphorylation events lead to recruitment of adaptor molecules and activation of enzymes such as phospholipase Cγ, which regulates intracellular calcium release. It also activates protein kinase C (PKC) activity by hydrolyzing membrane phospholipids to soluble inositol triphosphate and membrane-bound diacylglycerol. The release of calcium from internal stores, along with PKC activation, leads to fusion

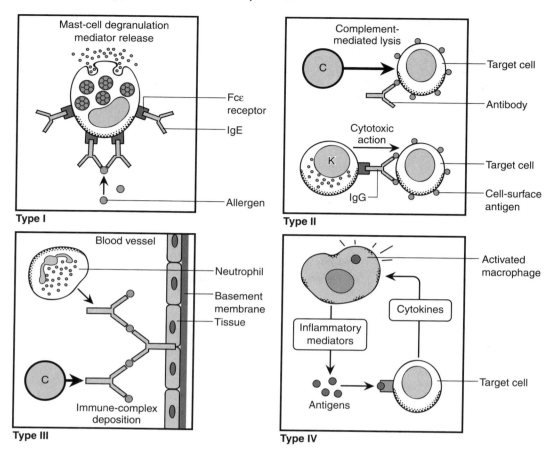

Figure 4.2. Summary of the immune mechanisms of the four hypersensitivities. (Adapted from Roitt I, Brostoff J, Male D, eds. *Immunology*. 6th ed. New York, NY: Mosby; 2001.)

of granules with the cell membrane and exocytosis of preformed mediators. Small guanosine triphosphates (GTPases) that regulate activation members of the mitogen-activated protein kinase (MAPK) family (extracellular signal-regulated kinase [ERK], Jun *N*-terminal kinase [JNK], and p38) are subsequently activated. These kinases help activate and regulate cytokine production and phospholipase A2 activity with resulting arachidonic acid metabolism. The release of preformed mediators begins a physiologic response (principally vasodilatation and smooth muscle contraction) within minutes of allergen exposure—immediate-type hypersensitivity. The route of allergen exposure and anatomic location of the mast cells results in both systemic and localized responses.[3]

Systemic responses often result from intravenous administration of allergen and release of mediators from mast cells in connective tissue. This potentially life-threatening response results in labored breathing and hypotension. Without pharmacologic intervention, bronchiole constriction and asphyxiation occur within 2 to 4 minutes

of allergen exposure. In susceptible individuals, this systemic anaphylaxis can be induced by bee, wasp, hornet, and ant stings; drugs (e.g., penicillin, insulin); plant pollens; molds; animal hair/dander; seafood; and nuts.

Localized responses are limited to specific organs and tissues. These can include allergic rhinitis in the conjunctiva and nasal tissue (watery exudation, sneezing, coughing), asthma (difficulty breathing, wheezing) in the lower airways, food allergies (vomiting, diarrhea), and atopic urticaria or hives (swollen eruptions in the skin).

Often a late-phase reaction (some 4 to 6 hours after allergen exposure) takes place, characterized by the infiltration of leukocytes (neutrophils, eosinophils, basophils monocytes, lymphocytes). Eosinophils in particular will bind both IgE and IgG molecules (via the Fc receptor) that have interacted with allergen; this releases a variety of mediators (e.g., major basic protein) to perpetuate this inflammatory response and tissue damage.

Most allergens are relatively small, highly soluble proteins that are inhaled in desiccated particles such as pollen grains or house dust mite feces. The soluble allergen elutes from the particle and diffuses into the mucosa with allergen exposure generally at very low doses. Host genetic factors—including the presence of atopy or high levels of circulating IgE antibodies—can play a role in the development of type I hypersensitivity.

Beneficial aspects of the immune mechanisms underlying type I hypersensitivity include the expulsion of parasites. On engagement of the mast-cell–bound IgE with the relevant allergen, mast cell degranulation and subsequent release of histamine (causing an immediate reaction), leukotrienes (more delayed symptoms), and other mediators occurs. This reaction is a strategy to prevent multicellular metazoan parasites from infecting respiratory and gastrointestinal systems. Mast cell degranulation contributes to vasodilatation and goblet cell hyperplasia with synthesis of mucin to increase viscosity and increase peristaltic and mucociliary movement to eliminate parasites.[2]

Type II Hypersensitivity

The mechanisms underlying this hypersensitivity with resulting tissue damage is antibody-mediated cell cytotoxicity. During the sensitization phase, IgM and IgG molecules are generated with specificity for and binding to the immunogen. Cell death is elicited by either complement activation or antibody-dependent cell cytotoxicity (ADCC) and killer cells.[4,5]

Physiologic responses from this hypersensitivity can include transfusion reactions, hemolytic disease of the newborn, drug-induced or idiopathic autoimmune hemolytic anemia, thrombocytopenia, or leukopenia. ABO blood group incompatibility and the resulting transfusion reactions are mediated by preexisting IgM antibodies and complement activation. During this reaction—often immediately following a mismatched transfusion—there is massive intravascular hemolysis of the transfused erythrocytes with the patient experiencing fever, chills, nausea, blood clotting, lower back pain, and hemoglobin in the urine. A more delayed transfusion reaction is often seen in response to Rh proteins or incompatibility between minor blood group proteins (such as Kidd, Kell, Duffy); it is usually mediated through IgG antibodies and complement. Symptoms can include fever, jaundice, and anemia. Hemolytic disease of the newborn (*erythroblastosis fetalis*) results from the reaction of an Rh-negative mother delivering an Rh-positive neonate. During delivery of the first Rh-positive neonate, fetal umbilical cord blood enters the mother's circulation resulting in anti-RH antibodies of the IgG isotype. During a second pregnancy with an Rh-positive child, these antibodies cross the placenta causing mild to severe anemia in the neonate with sometimes fatal outcomes. In addition, the conversion of hemoglobin to bilirubin can cause brain damage if the bilirubin accumulates in the brain of the neonate. This reaction may also be caused by IgG antibodies generated during ABO incompatibility, especially a type-O mother carrying an A- or B-type fetus.

Drug-induced hemolytic anemia can occur when certain antibiotics (e.g., penicillin) bind to the erythrocyte surface forming a hapten-self protein complex. The resulting IgM or IgG antibodies can then mediate damage. Idiopathic autoimmune hemolytic anemia has an unknown etiology and has been noted in Hashimotos thyroiditis, Goodpasture's syndrome, and myasthenia gravis.

The immune mechanisms underlying type II hypersensitivity defend the body against cellular pathogens such as extracellular bacteria. This reaction was designed to opsonize and eliminate small extracellular pathogens through leukocyte phagocytosis or through complement- or ADCC-mediated lysis.

Type III Hypersensitivity

Generation of immune complexes (the reaction of antibody with antigen) is critical in clearing soluble protein antigens (such as bacterial toxins) and terminating an immune response; however, large amounts of immune complexes generated in slight antigen excess can deposit along the basement member of capillaries in tissue and organs and cause significant damage. The pathogenicity of these immune complexes depends on their size. Large aggregates (antibody excess) are removed by phagocytes, whereas small aggregates (antigen excess) are not phlogogenic. In conditions of slight antigen excess, the complexes are large enough to activate complement, but not so large as to be phagocytosed.[4,5]

The type III reaction often begins with the introduction of immunogen into a host (or alteration of self into nonself) with preexisting IgG antibodies (in high concentration) following a secondary immune response. Formation of immune complexes near the site of administration elicits a localized Arthus reaction, whereas formation of complexes in the blood elicits deposition in blood vessel walls, synovial membranes of the joints, glomerular basement membranes of the kidney, and the choroid plexus of the brain. Deposition of these immune complexes activates complement, generating mediators (anaphylatoxins C3a, C5a) to cause localized mast cell degranulation and an increase in local vascular permeability. In response to C5a, neutrophils (PMNs) will accumulate at the site of immune complex deposition with resulting tissue damage from the extracellular release of lytic enzymes as these cells attempt to engulf the large complexes. Intradermal or subcutaneous administration of an immunogen into a sensitized host can lead to the formation and deposition of localized immune complexes (Arthus reaction) in 4 to 8 hours. Localized tissue and vascular damage follows as vasoactive mediators and PMNs are activated.

Intravenous administration of immunogen into a sensitized host can lead to the formation of circulating immune complexes. Within days to weeks of immunogen exposure and in the presence of slight antigen excess (often seen in recipients of antitoxins containing foreign serum), the host experiences fever, weakness, rash, edema, lymphadenopathy, arthritis, and sometimes glomerulonephritis.

This hypersensitivity reaction was designed to eliminate circulating viral particles or soluble protein antigens through the formation of antigen antibody complexes that can be effectively engulfed by the reticuloendothelial system. Elimination of virus by immune complexes during the viremic phase can prevent the virus from binding to and infecting host cells.

Type IV Hypersensitivity

Unlike the previous three types of hypersensitivity that rely on the formation of antibody (and thus Th2 lymphocytes) to mediate damage, type IV hypersensitivity relies on T lymphocytes (Th1, cytotoxic T cells [CTL]) and macrophages. With the introduction of immunogen into a host with a large population of previously sensitized T lymphocytes, an immune response occurs with the release of cytokines (e.g., interleukin [IL]-2 and interferon γ [IFNγ]) to attract and activate macrophages and lymphocytes. With activation, there is increased phagocytic activity and release of lytic enzymes into surrounding tissue by macrophages as well as cytotoxicity by CTL.[4,5] This reaction generally evolves 48 to 72 hours after immunogen exposure, giving rise to the name delayed-type hypersensitivity (in contrast to immediate type, or type I, which often takes only minutes to evidence physiologic symptoms).

Delayed-type hypersensitivity is manifested in granulomatous skin and pulmonary responses to mycobacteria and in the testing (by intradermal injection) for prior exposure to these pathogens. Contact dermatitis reactions from type IV hypersensitivity are also seen in certain individuals after exposure to metals (nickel), cosmetics (fragrances, hair dyes, preservatives), plants (poison ivy, poison oak), rubber, medications (bacitracin, penicillin, corticosteroids), resins, and some chemicals (e.g., formaldehyde). Most of these function as haptens (such as pentadecacatechol from poison ivy), forming covalent interactions with host proteins to compose the complete immunogen (described later in this chapter).

This reaction—designed in response to intracellular pathogens with the mobilization and activation of CTL and macrophages—eliminates infected host cells, preventing more microbial progeny and/or neoplastic cells.

HYPERSENSITIVITY RESPONSES TO PHARMACEUTICAL COMPOUNDS

Adverse drug reactions (ADRs) are defined by the World Health Organization as any noxious, unintended, and undesired effect of a drug that occurs at doses used for prevention, diagnosis, or treatment.[6] ADRs can increase the uncertainty of drug safety during development and create problems for patients who depend on these drugs. An allergic reaction to a drug can best be defined as an immune response to a drug or its metabolites that results in an adverse reaction.

Risk Groups

Most drug allergies occur after sensitization from previous drug exposure. Thus, drug allergies usually occur after second or subsequent exposure or after prolonged administration.[6] Drug-induced allergic reactions are known to account for only a small portion (6% to 10%[7]) of ADRs. The risk of an allergic reaction with potential fatality due to anaphylaxis for most drugs is 1% to 3%.[8] Risk factors for development of an allergic drug reaction can be associated with both the drug and the patient (**Table 4.3**). Characteristics of the drug, variations in metabolism, and drug exposure (dose, duration, frequency) can all influence development of drug allergy. Although sensitization may occur by any route of administration, topical administration presents the greatest risk and oral administration presents the least risk. A single prophylactic dose of a drug (such as an antibiotic) is less likely to sensitize an individual than high-dose prolonged parenteral therapy. Frequent courses of therapy are

Table 4.3. Factors That Increase Risk of Immune-Mediated Adverse Drug Reaction

- Prior exposure
- High dose, prolonged administration
- Administration by topical route
- Female gender
- HLA haplotype
- Parents with allergy
- Slow acetylator status

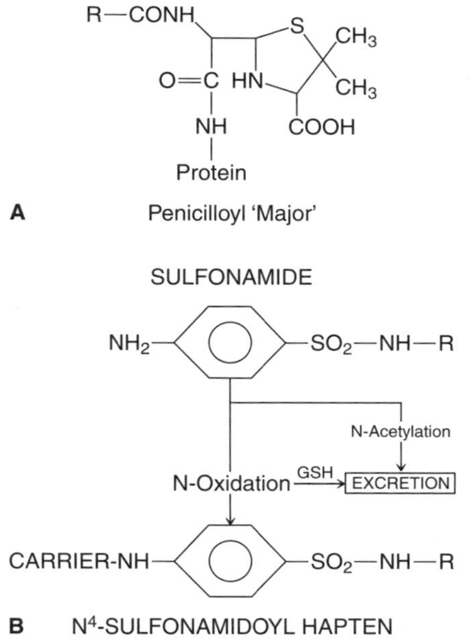

more likely to result in drug allergy than courses of therapy years apart. Certain patient populations are more at risk than others. Women have a 35% higher incidence of adverse cutaneous reactions and a 20-fold greater risk of anaphylaxis than men for compounds such as radiocontrast media. HLA haplotype (such as HLA-DR3) has been associated with specific drug allergies; children whose parents are allergic to an antibiotic have a 15-fold greater relative risk. In contrast, drug allergy is less common and less severe in infants and in the aged.

Hapten Hypothesis

The hapten hypothesis explains the origin of many drug-induced allergies.[9] Haptens are chemically reactive small compounds that bind to proteins or peptides through covalent bonds, modifying them (**Figure 4.3**). Some drugs such as penicillin can be directly chemically reactive (**Figure 4.4A**) because their molecular structure is unstable. Others such as sulfonamide must be metabolized or bioactivated to a reactive intermediate or metabolite (**Figure 4.4B**). Typically, this bioactivation occurs in hepatocytes via cytochrome P450 enzymes, although keratinocytes may also participate in

Figure 4.4. Metabolites from either penicillin (A) or sulfonamides (B) can become haptens.

bioactivation. These reactive intermediates or metabolites may bind to larger protein targets forming a complete immunogen that can elicit any of the hypersensitivity reactions. Another concept that may contribute to the initiation of these immune events has also been proposed.[10] Binding of hapten to self proteins may initiate cell damage or a "danger signal,"[11] which in turn could amplify the interaction of costimulatory molecules between APC and T cells. Should this coincide with the interaction of major histocompatibility complex (MHC) class II–bound immunogenic epitope with specific TCR on T cells, an immune response would follow.

Drugs Contributing to Type I Hypersensitivity

β *lactam antibiotics.* Antibiotics account for most drug-induced cutaneous allergic reactions as well as fatal anaphylaxis. β lactam drugs—especially penicillin—are common causes of drug-induced type I hypersensitivity and account for about 75% of fatal anaphylaxis in the United States each year.[12] Penicillins contain both a β lactam ring and a thiozolidine ring. Because of the instability of the β lactam ring, this structure readily opens and allows the carbonyl group to form amide linkages with amino groups of lysine residues on nearby proteins. The resulting immunogenic epitope is the penicilloyl moiety that

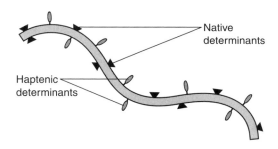

Figure 4.3. The formation of a hapten carrier complete immunogen. (Adapted from Mayer G, Microbiology and Immunology On-line, University of South Carolina School of Medicine. Available at: http://pathmicro.med.sc.edu/mayer/antigens2000.htm. Accessed May 2005.)

elicits IgE-mediated responses. In addition, the side-chain group that distinguishes the different penicillins may also elicit IgE-mediated responses. Thus, different penicillins may not only be cross-reactive through the shared β lactam ring, but also through similar side chain determinants.[13] Although penicillins and cephalosporins share a β lactam ring, clinically relevant cross-reactivity is uncommon. Rather, cephalosporins can induce distinct immune responses with IgE antibodies elicited against both side-chain moieties as well as against β lactam rings.[14] The frequency of an adverse reaction to penicillin in the general population is 0.7% to 10%. Manifestations of type I hypersensitivity are anaphylaxis, urticaria, angioedema, bronchospasm, laryngeal edema, hypotension, or arrhythmias. The remaining three types of penicillin allergies (types II, III, IV) usually occur after 72 hours with types II and III mediated by IgG or IgM antibodies. Type II hypersensitivity results in anemia and thrombocytopenia, type III hypersensitivity in immune complex disease, and type IV, contact dermatitis. In patients with a history of penicillin allergy, the frequency of allergic reactions to cephalosporin administration is only 5.6%.[14] Thus cephalosporins are well tolerated in 90% to 95% of patients with a type I allergy to penicillin. Since carbapenems and monobactams are also β lactam antibiotics, it is recommended that carbapenems not be used in patients with penicillin allergy, although monobactams can be administered to patients with type I allergy to penicillin.

Sulfonamides. These antimicrobial agents elicit drug-induced allergic responses as a cutaneous reaction (urticaria, erythroderma, fixed drug eruption, erythema multiforme) as well as an anaphylactic reaction in 2% to 4% of patients. Immediate type I hypersensitivity as well as type IV hypersensitivity (and specific T lymphocytes) are likely causes of these cutaneous reactions. Sulfonamides are metabolized in the liver by N-acetylation (yielding nontoxic metabolites) and by cytochrome P450 (yielding reactive hydroxylamines),[15] which then oxidize to nitroso species. These reactive nitroso metabolites are reduced by glutathione and excreted until the capacity for glutathione conjugation is exceeded. Then the hapten N,4 sulfonamidoyl may haptenate proteins forming immunogenic complexes. There is also some speculation of a potential cross-reactivity between sulfonamide nonantibiotics (such as furosemide) and sulfonamide antibiotics in allergic patients.[16]

Anticonvulsants. Phenytoin, phenobarbital, and carbamazepine are known to cause hyper-

sensitivity reactions characterized by fever, rash, lymphadenopathy, and varying degrees of internal organ involvement typically beginning several weeks into therapy. The aromatic anticonvulsants are metabolized in part by cytochrome P450 enzymes to reactive arene oxide metabolites, which may haptenate carrier proteins creating a complete immunogen. Cross-reactivity among the aromatic anticonvulsants may be as high as 75%, so alternatives should be considered.

Chemotherapy agents. The most common agents eliciting hypersensitivity reactions are the taxanes, platinum compounds, asparaginases, and epipodopyllotoxins. These reactions can range from mild cutaneous responses to anaphylaxis to death. It is suggested that both type I hypersensitivity reactions and direct mast cell degranulation (as with paclitaxel, docetaxel, etoposide, and teniposide) account for these reactions. Both cisplatin and carboplatin as well as asparaginase (a bacterial protease) commonly induce a typical type I hypersensitivity response.

Heparin. Heparin, a mucopolysaccharide of 6–20 kDa, can elicit several forms of type I hypersensitivity (urticaria, asthma, anaphylaxis) as well as type III IgG-mediated erythematous reactions.

Insulin and protamine. With the introduction of recombinant human insulin, allergic reactions to this drug have decreased dramatically. Rare local reactions at the injection site appear to be IgE-mediated. Protamine contained in insulin preparations to delay absorption has also been shown to induce IgE-mediated type I hypersensitivity reactions.

Radiocontrast media. Mild adverse reactions (e.g., vasodilation) to radiocontrast media during radiological procedures occur in about 3% of patients. Of more concern is the idiosyncratic anaphylactic reaction due to IgE-mediated events that can result in death (0.1% to 0.2%). It appears that both first-generation solutions (ionic, hyperosmolar) and second-generation solutions (nonionic, hypo- and iso-osmolar) can activate IgE antibodies and elicit an anaphylactic reaction. The response generally occurs 3 to 5 minutes after administration following a previous exposure.[17]

Drugs Contributing to Type II Hypersensitivity

Drug-induced cytopenia can affect erythrocytes, leukocytes, platelets, and probably hematopoietic precursor cells in the bone marrow. For unknown reasons, platelets are affected more than other cell types. Quinine, quinidine, and sulfonamides can cause acute, and sometimes severe and life-threatening, thrombocytopenia. In rare instances, penicillin can also elicit thrombocytopenia.[18]

Quinine-induced thrombocytopenia usually develops after 5 to 8 days of exposure or after a single exposure in a previously sensitized patient. Patients usually present with widespread petechial hemorrhages in the skin sometimes accompanied by urinary and gastrointestinal tract bleeding. After discontinuation of the drug, platelet counts usually return to normal in 3 to 5 days. IgG and/or IgM antibodies react with selected platelet membrane glycoproteins such as the fibrinogen receptor or von Willebrand factor receptor and only when the drug is present in soluble form.[18]

Thrombocytopenia has also been documented in patients receiving tirofiban, eptifibatide, or abciximab to prevent complications after coronary angioplasty. With the first two drugs, patients appear to have preexisting antibodies that recognize glycoproteins on platelets that participate in clotting. In patients receiving abciximab, IgG and IgM antibodies can recognize abciximab-coated platelets.[18]

Long-term high-dose therapy with other drugs has also been associated with immune hemolytic anemia. Quinidine and quinine can elicit drug-induced antibodies that (as immune complexes) bind to the erythrocyte and cause marked hemolytic anemia. Other drugs may cause a lower incidence of anemia presumably because the antidrug antibodies do not activate complement efficiently. Penicillin (or its metabolite) can adsorb to the erythrocyte membrane and elicit antibodies; methyldopa also elicits anti–red blood cell (RBC) antibodies that are not specific for the drug, but rather for the Rh or other intrinsic erythrocyte proteins.[19]

Halothane- and tienilic acid–induced hepatitis may also be the result of antibody-mediated cytotoxicity. Antibodies against the reactive intermediate of halothane bound to proteins are detected in patients with halothane hepatitis. In patients with tienilic acid–induced liver damage (tienilic acid is no longer on the market), antibodies against one of the cytochrome P450 isozymes are present.[10]

Drugs Contributing to Type III Hypersensitivity

It is estimated that up to 10% of cases of systemic lupus erythematosus (SLE) are drug induced[20] and that more than 40 drugs can cause it. Classes of these drugs include antiarrhythmics (procainamide), antihypertensives (hydralazine), antipsychotics, antibiotics, anticonvulsants, antithyroidals, anti-inflammatories, and diuretics

Table 4.4. Drugs Capable of Inducing Systemic Lupus Erythematosus

- Hydralazine
- Procainamide
- Isoniazid
- Methyldopa
- Chlorpromazine
- Quinidine
- Minocycline

(Adapted from Antonov C, Kazandjieva J, Etugov D, et al. Drug-induced lupus erythematosus. *Clin Dermatol.* 2004; 22(2):157–166.)

(**Table 4.4**).[19] The highest risk by far is in patients receiving procainamide or hydralazine with a 20% incidence for procainamide and a 5% to 8% risk for hydralazine.[21]

Patient factors such as specific HLA alleles (e.g., HLA-DR4, HLA-B47) may increase risk for this reaction; indeed the HLA-DR4 haplotype is present in 73% of patients with drug (hydralazine)-induced lupus. The slow acetylator status of a patient can also contribute to susceptibility to drug-induced lupus (see Table 4.4). Acetylation is involved in the metabolism of drugs such as hydralazine, procainamide, isoniazid, and sulfonamides. Slower acetylation (and thus slower elimination) of these drugs and enhanced formation of reactive metabolites is associated with increased risk. Unlike idiopathic SLE, which tends to present in patients in their 20s, older patients tend to present with drug-induced lupus more often since they are taking more medications. Finally, the probability of drug-induced SLE increases as the dose and duration of exposure increases.[19] In addition, other drugs such as procainamide, propylthiouracil, isonizid, hydralazine, quinidine, and chlorpromazine are readily oxidized to reactive species by activated leukocytes and thus may also generate haptens. Indeed, these reactive metabolites may bind to nucleoproteins and elicit antihistone antibodies. Other immune mechanisms underlying drug-induced lupus include disruption of T-cell maturation in the thymus by procainamide-hydroxylamine–reactive intermediates resulting in the loss of tolerance to chromatin.[22,23] DNA methylation inhibitors such as procainamide may also induce autoreactivity in Th2 cells.

The onset of symptoms of this adverse drug reaction can be slow or acute, although it is typically 1 to 2 months before a diagnosis is made. About half the patients have symptoms of fever, weight loss, and fatigue.[19] Arthralgia is present in about 90% of patients and myalgia in about 50%.

Other symptoms include pleurisy and pericarditis. Cutaneous manifestations especially from hydralazine include malar rash, alopecia, discoid lesions, and photosensitivity; severe anemia, leucopenia, or thrombocytopenia are unlikely. Antinuclear antibodies (e.g., antihistone antibodies) are present in about 90% of patients with drug-induced SLE compared to 50% in idiopathic SLE. There is also a high frequency of anti–single-stranded DNA antibodies in drug-induced SLE instead of anti–double-stranded DNA antibodies commonly found in idiopathic SLE.

Drugs Contributing to Type IV Hypersensitivity

Both topical and oral administration of drugs have the potential to elicit a type IV contact dermatitis (CD) response through the formation of reactive metabolites (**Table 4.5**). Drugs applied topically may be metabolized by keratinocytes with direct hapten-protein interactions responsible for CD following uptake and processing by resident Langerhans cells. Drugs administered orally may be metabolized by hepatocytes to reactive intermediates/metabolites, which can haptenate liver proteins and sensitize T cells (in draining lymphoid tissue) or may circulate and ultimately bind to cutaneous proteins.[24]

Personal care products have also been documented to cause contact dermatitis. These are typically from fragrances, chemicals, and preservatives found in deodorants, perfumes, skin care products, hair care products, ophthalmic products, and nail products.[25] In hospitals, many drugs have been documented to cause contact dermatitis, including penicillins, furosemide, prednisone, allopurinol, and carbamazepine.[26] Antiseptics also frequently cause contact dermatitis in patients undergoing surgery. Other compounds that can cause allergic sensitization include thimerosal (especially in patients previously exposed to tinctures), adhesive-coated pregelled foam disks, epoxy resins (as in pacemakers, catheters), cementing materials, topical medicaments, and rubber and metal components from hemodialysis apparatus.[27]

TREATMENT OF HYPERSENSITIVITIES

Drug-induced allergic reactions can be best predicted through skin testing. However, there are relatively few tests available to confirm the allergic status of a patient to a drug except the Pre-Pen, which detects penicillin-specific IgE antibodies. This test facilitates the use of penicillin without adverse reactions in 90% of patients with a previous history of penicillin allergy.[7] If the skin test is positive, the simplest approach is to avoid the drug and use an alternate compound. Otherwise, a graded challenge with the implicated drug could be performed if the reaction is not life threatening. Finally, desensitization could also be considered. Penicillin and other drug allergies can often be treated by desensitization orally or intravenously. Once the starting dose has been determined, drug doses are doubled every 15 minutes with vital signs monitored throughout. Corticosteroids can also be administered if symptoms are severe, and epinephrine is commonly prescribed to treat systemic anaphylactic reactions. Indeed, physicians sometimes tell patients who have had an anaphylactic reaction to carry an epinephrine syringe designed for self-administration (Ana-Kit®, EpiPen®, or EpiPen Jr.® for children)—particularly if the allergen that causes the reaction is difficult to avoid.

Table 4.5. Drugs and Respective Reactive Metabolites That Can Elicit Contact Dermatitis

Drug	Metabolite
Abacavir	Aldehyde
Carbamazepine	Arene oxide Iminoquinone
Hydralazine	Phthalazinone
Phenytoin	Arene oxide Quinone
Lamotrigine	Arene oxide
Procainamide	Nitroso
Sulfamethoxazole	Nitroso
Trimethoprim	Iminoquinone methide

(Adapted from Naisbitt DJ. Drug hypersensitivity reactions in skin: understanding mechanisms and the development of diagnostic and predictive tests. *Toxicology*. 2004; 194(3):179–196.)

SUMMARY

Immune-mediated reactions account for 6% to 10% of adverse reactions to drugs and are classified as type B reactions—uncommon, unpredictable, and rarely occurring. Hypersensitivity reactions (normal immune responses with potential to damage cells and tissue) typically are responsible for these adverse reactions. In general, drugs or their metabolites form covalent interactions with self proteins to become complete immunogens and elicit deleterious responses. In addition, certain risk groups may be more susceptible to immune-mediated adverse drug reactions. Of the four types of hypersensitivities discussed, immediate type—mediated by IgE antibodies and mast cell degranulation—has the greatest potential for causing death through anaphylaxis. Antibiotics appear to be the class of drug with the greatest risk for fatality. Health care workers prescribing and dispensing these medications must be vigilant in recognizing risk groups and the potential for immune-mediated adverse drug reactions.

REFERENCES

1. Gell PGH, Coombs RRA. The classification of allergic reactions underlying disease. In: Coombs RRA, Gell PGH, eds. *Clinical Aspects of Immunology.* Philadelphia, PA: Blackwell Sciences; 1963:217–237.
2. Rajan TV. The Gell-Coombs classification of hypersensitivity reactions: a re-interpretation. *Trends Immunol.* 2003; 24(7):376–379.
3. Galli SJ, Kalesnikoff J, Grimbaldeston MA, et al. Mast cells as "tunable" effector and immunoregulatory cells: recent advances. *Annu Rev Immunol.* 2005; 23:749–786.
4. Kuby J. *Immunology.* 2nd ed. New York, NY: WH Freeman & Co; 1991.
5. Roitt I, Brostoff J, Male D, eds. *Immunology.* 6th ed. New York, NY: Mosby; 2001.
6. World Health Organization. *International Drug Monitoring: The Role of the Hospital.* Geneva, Switzerland: WHO; 1966.
7. Borda IT, Slone D, Jick H. Assessment of adverse reactions within a drug surveillance program. *JAMA.* 1968; 205(9):645–647.
8. deShazo RD, Kemp SF. Allergic reactions to drugs and biologic agents. *JAMA.* 1997; 278(22):1895–1906.
9. Naisbitt DJ, Williams DP, Pirmohamed M, et al. Reactive metabolites and their role in drug reactions. *Curr Opin Allergy Clin Immunol.* 2001; 1(4):317–325.
10. Uetrecht J. Role of drug metabolism for breaking tolerance and the localization of drug hypersensitivity. *Toxicology.* 2005; 209(2):113–118.
11. Matzinger P. Tolerance, danger, and the extended family. *Annu Rev Immunol.* 1994; 12:991–1045.
12. Joint Task Force on Practice Parameters; American Academy of Allergy, Asthma, and Immunology; American College of Allergy, Asthma, and Immunology; and the Joint Council of Allergy, Asthma, and Immunology. The diagnosis and management of anaphylaxis. *J Allergy Clin Immunol.* 1998; 101(6 Pt 2):S465–528.
13. Gruchalla RS. Drug allergy. *J Allergy Clin Immunol.* 2003; 111(2 Suppl):S548–559.
14. Salkind AR, Cuddy PG, Foxworth JW. The rational clinical examination. Is this patient allergic to penicillin? An evidence-based analysis of the likelihood of penicillin allergy. *JAMA.* 2001; 285(19):2498–2505.
15. Cribb AE, Spielberg SP. Hepatic microsomal metabolism of sulfamethoxazole to the hydroxylamine. *Drug Metab Dispos.* 1990; 18(5):784–787.
16. Sicherer SH, Leung DY. Advances in allergic skin disease, anaphylaxis, and hypersensitivity reactions to foods, drugs, and insect stings. *J Allergy Clin Immunol.* 2004; 114(1):118–124.
17. Brown V, Brandner B, Brook J, et al. Cardiac arrest after administration of Omnipaque radiocontrast medium during endoluminal repair of abdominal aortic aneurysm. *Br J Anaesth.* 2002; 88(1):133–135.
18. Aster RH. Drug-induced immune cytopenias. *Toxicology.* 2005; 209(2):149–153.
19. Rubin RL. Drug-induced lupus. *Toxicology.* 2005; 209(2):135–147.
20. Hess E. Drug-related lupus. *N Engl J Med.* 1988; 318(22):1460–1462.
21. Antonov D, Kazandjieva J, Etugov D, et al. Drug-induced lupus erythematosus. *Clin Dermatol.* 2004; 22(2):157–166.
22. Kretz-Rommel A, Rubin RL. Disruption of positive selection of thymocytes causes autoimmunity. *Nat Med.* 2000; 6(3):298–305.
23. Datta SK. Positive selection for autoimmunity. *Nat Med.* 2000; 6(3):259–261.
24. Naisbitt DJ. Drug hypersensitivity reactions in skin: understanding mechanisms and the development of diagnostic and predictive tests. *Toxicology.* 2004; 194(3):179–196.
25. Orton DI, Wilkinson JD. Cosmetic allergy: incidence, diagnosis, and management. *Am J Clin Dermatol.* 2004; 5(5):327–337.
26. Rademaker M, Oakley A, Duffill MB. Cutaneous adverse drug reactions in a hospital setting. *N Z Med J.* 1995; 108(999):165–166.
27. Ancona A, Arevalo A, Macotela E. Contact dermatitis in hospital patients. *Dermatol Clin.* 1990; 8(1):95–105.

SELF-ASSESSMENT QUESTIONS

1. Type B adverse drug reactions share which of the following characteristics?

   A. Uncommon
   B. Unpredictable
   C. Resembles an immune response
   D. All of the above

2. IgE-mediated Type I hypersensitivity is responsible for which of the following physiologic outcomes?

   A. Anaphylaxis
   B. Hemolytic anemia
   C. Arthritis
   D. Pulmonary granulomas

3. Which of the following mediators released from mast cells is/are responsible for the immediate effects of type I hypersensitivity?

   A. Growth factors
   B. Preformed mediators
   C. IgE molecules
   D. Allergens

4. The reaction that often occurs 4 to 6 hours after *allergen* exposure is known as:

   A. Delayed hypersensitivity
   B. Immune complex disease
   C. Late-phase reaction
   D. Atopy

5. The beneficial aspect of type I hypersensitivity is:

   A. Elimination of toxins
   B. Expulsion of parasites
   C. Elimination of cancer cells
   D. All of the above

6. Drug-induced adverse reactions in which type II hypersensitivity can participate would include:

   A. Serum sickness
   B. Arthus response
   C. Hemolytic anemia/leukopenia
   D. Asthma

7. The beneficial response of type II hypersensitivity is:

   A. Elimination of extracellular bacteria
   B. Elimination of soluble toxins
   C. Expulsion of parasites
   D. Vasodilation and smooth muscle contraction

8. Deposition of immune complexes in the synovial membranes of joints from a type III hypersensitivity response would elicit:

   A. Arthritis
   B. Vasculitis
   C. Pneumonitis
   D. Glomerulonephritis

9. Localized skin and vascular damage from immune complex deposition occurring within 4 to 8 hours is known as:

   A. Rhinitis
   B. Granulomatous disease
   C. Arthus reaction
   D. Serum sickness

10. Which of the following cell type(s) participates in type IV hypersensitivity?

    A. Eosinophils
    B. Th1 lymphocytes
    C. Macrophages
    D. Both B and C

11. A form of type IV hypersensitivity known as contact dermatitis can be elicited by:

    A. Metals
    B. Perfumes
    C. Plant proteins
    D. All of the above

12. The beneficial response of type IV hypersensitivity is:

    A. Expulsion of parasites
    B. Elimination of cells infected with intracellular pathogens
    C. Elimination of extracellular bacteria
    D. Neutralization of toxins

13. Which route of drug administration presents the greatest risk for the development of an allergic drug reaction?

    A. Intramuscular
    B. Oral
    C. Topical
    D. Inhalation

14. Which of the drugs below must be metabolized or enzymatically bioactivated to form a hapten?

    A. Sulfonamide
    B. Halothane
    C. Penicillin
    D. Both A and B

15. In patients with an allergy to penicillin, what is the frequency of allergic reactions to cephalosporins?

    A. Greater than 70%
    B. Less than 10%
    C. Never
    D. Always 100%

16. Quinine can induce which of the following physiologic outcomes?

    A. Thrombocytopenia
    B. Anemia
    C. Pneumonitis
    D. Both A and B

17. Which of the following increase the risk for developing drug-induced type III hypersensitivity?

    A. HLA haplotypes
    B. Slow acetylator status
    C. Increased dose and duration of administration
    D. All of the above

18. Drugs that elicit type IV hypersensitivity may be administered topically or orally and may be metabolized by:

    A. Hepatocytes
    B. Keratinocytes
    C. Thymocytes
    D. Both A and B

19. Physicians will often advise individuals who have had an anaphylactic response to carry a syringe for self-administration that contains:

    A. Epinephrine
    B. Histamine
    C. Penicillin
    D. Corticosteroids

20. Which class of drugs presents the greatest potential for eliciting death by anaphylaxis?

    A. Antibiotics
    B. Antiarrhythmics
    C. Cancer chemotherapeutics agents
    D. Skin-care products

CHAPTER 5

Inflammatory Diseases and Autoimmunity

Stephen O'Barr

LEARNING OBJECTIVES

After completing this chapter, the reader should
be able to:

1. Explain the pathogenesis and treatment of
acute inflammatory states.
2. Describe prevention and treatment strategies
for anaphylaxis.
3. Compare and discriminate between the con-
tribution of CD4$^+$ T cells, MHC, and non-HLA
associations in the induction and pathogenesis
of autoimmune diseases.
4. Develop reasoned therapeutic regimens for
autoimmune diseases based on known genetic
and molecular pathogenesis.
5. Illustrate the mechanism of action of various
immunotherapies, and describe how these
MOAs alter disease state pathologies.

6. Generate novel applications for experimental immunotherapy.

PHARMACOLOGIC THERAPIES OF ACUTE INFLAMMATION

Antihistamines

Antihistamines act as inverse agonists that bind to H_1 or H_2 histamine receptors in the treatment of perennial and seasonal allergic rhinitis, allergic conjunctivitis, and chronic urticaria.

Unfortunately, because histamine is only one mediator in the pathogenesis of these reactions, blocking histamine receptors only partially alleviates symptoms. The H_1 histamine receptor is predominantly involved in allergic reactions, and H_1 antagonists are therefore used for these conditions. The second-generation H_1 antagonists, such as loratadine (Claritin®), desloratadine (Clarinex®), and fexofenadine (Allegra®), cause minimal sedation—a major advantage compared with many older antihistamines (e.g., diphenhydramine). H_2-receptor antagonists, such as cimetidine (Tagamet®), have no effect on type I human immunoglobulin E (IgE)-mediated allergic responses. For patients refractory to standard H_1-receptor antihistamines, though, the addition of an H_2-receptor antihistamine may be beneficial. H_2 receptors are present in cutaneous vasculature, and the combination of H_1-receptor and H_2-receptor antihistamines has been most effective in certain urticarial syndromes.

Some H_1-receptor antagonists may also improve allergic symptoms through mechanisms unrelated to their histamine-blocking effects. The second-generation antihistamines azelastine (Astelin) and cetirizine (Zyrtec) inhibit production of leukotrienes; loratadine can reduce the release of histamine and prostaglandin D2 (PGD_2). More work is needed to define the mechanisms of action of antihistamines; however, it is likely that many antihistamine drugs have multiple mechanisms of action beyond histamine antagonism (**Table 5.1**).

Sympathomimetic Agents

Sympathetic nervous stimulation is useful to counteract some manifestations of mast cell degranulation. For example, stimulation of β_2-adrenergic

Table 5.1. Acute Inflammation Therapies

Generic Name (Brand Name)	MOA	Indications and Usage	Adult Dose, Route	Adult Frequency
Loratadine (Claritin®)	H_1-receptor antagonist	Seasonal allergic rhinitis, perennial allergic rhinitis, chronic idiopathic urticaria	10 mg, PO	24 hr
Desloratadine (Clarinex®)	H_1-receptor antagonist	Seasonal allergic rhinitis, perennial allergic rhinitis, chronic idiopathic urticaria	5 mg, PO	24 hr
Fexofenadine (Allegra®)	H_1-receptor antagonist	Seasonal allergic rhinitis, chronic idiopathic urticaria	60 mg or 180 mg, PO	12 hr or 24 hr
Azelastine (Astelin®)	H_1-receptor antagonist	Seasonal allergic rhinitis, vasomotor rhinitis	1–2 sprays per nostril	12 hr
Cetirizine (Zyrtec®)	H_1-receptor antagonist	Seasonal allergic rhinitis, perennial allergic rhinitis, chronic idiopathic urticaria	5 mg or 10 mg, PO	24 hr
Zileuton (Zyflo®)	5-lipoxygenase inhibitor	Chronic asthma	600 mg, PO	6 hr
Zafirlukast (Accolate®)	Leukotriene receptor antagonist, LTD4 and LTE4	Prophylaxis and chronic treatment of asthma	20 mg, PO	12 hr
Montelukast (Singulair®)	Leukotriene receptor antagonist, CysLT1	Prophylaxis and chronic asthma, seasonal allergic rhinitis, perennial allergic rhinitis	10 mg, PO	24 hr

receptors leads to bronchodilation, promoted by cyclic adenosine monophosphate (cAMP), and may reverse some or all of the bronchoconstricting effects of allergen-induced asthma. α_1-Agonists, such as phenylephrine, constrict mucosal vasculature and are used predominantly as nasal decongestants. For systemic anaphylaxis, epinephrine is the preferred sympathomimetic agent because of its potent α- and β-adrenergic receptor-stimulating effects.

Antiallergy Agents

Antiallergy drugs are classified as noncorticosteroidal anti-inflammatory agents that can modify the acute and chronic tissue responses associated with type I reactions. Cromolyn sodium, the prototype drug in this class, can inhibit mast cell degranulation and prevent the clinical symptoms that follow antigen exposure. Cromolyn sodium can also modulate the effector functions of neutrophils and eosinophils, both of which may have active roles in many allergic reactions. Likewise, nedocromil sodium exhibits anti-inflammatory properties by modulating cellular components of inflammation, including eosinophils, neutrophils, macrophages, and mast cells.

Corticosteroids

Many allergic conditions, such as asthma and allergic rhinitis, include chronic inflammation. Corticosteroids do not relieve the acute allergic symptoms that follow allergen exposure, but they help suppress the inflammatory response seen in late-phase and chronic allergic reactions.

The mechanisms of action of corticosteroids are still unclear. It has been observed that steroids do not prevent mediator release from mast cells and that (among their many functions) they inhibit the actions of leukocytes, decrease edema by reducing vascular leakage, and prevent the influx of inflammatory cells into the area of mast cell degranulation. Corticosteroids can also increase the quantity of β-adrenergic receptors on tissues, enhancing the efficacy of β-agonists.

Corticosteroids can be given systemically or topically. Topical corticosteroids have proven effective for diseases such as asthma and hay fever. The use of inhaled and intranasal corticosteroids has circumvented many side effects of systemic administration.

Leukotriene Antagonists

Because leukotrienes have a major role in type I hypersensitivity reactions, drugs that inhibit their synthesis or block their actions have been synthesized. Many drugs that inhibit the formation of leukotrienes by blocking the action of 5-lipoxygenase have been studied in allergic conditions. Clinical trials have shown that leukotriene receptor antagonists or synthesis inhibitors decrease bronchoconstriction in exercise-induced asthma, improve baseline pulmonary function, decrease symptoms, and decrease the need for β-agonist use in moderate to severe asthmatic individuals. These agents have also been demonstrated to have clinical efficacy in allergic rhinitis. Leukotriene B4 (LTB_4) and leukotriene D4 (LTD_4) antagonists have received the most study.

Two new agents that block the effects of leukotrienes are currently approved for clinical use. Zileuton (Zyflo®), a 5-lipoxygenase inhibitor, is indicated for treatment of chronic asthma. Zafirlukast (Acolate®) and montelukast (Singulair®) are leukotriene receptor antagonists (LTRAs) indicated for chronic asthma. All have been shown to reduce the need for other medications to control the symptoms of asthma. More study is needed to determine the therapeutic role of leukotriene antagonists and synthesis inhibitors in allergic inflammatory diseases.

IMMUNOTHERAPY

Prevention and Treatment of Anaphylaxis

Anaphylaxis is usually an extreme type I allergic response most commonly triggered by medicines, food, latex, and other environmental allergens, and also by insect and plant toxins. It leads to systemic release of histamine, leukotriene C4, prostaglandin D2, and trypase. Rapid systemic release of histamine causes bronchoconstriction, mucosal edema, vasodilation, and decreased effective plasma volume, leading to system shock.

Currently the only prevention of anaphylaxis is avoidance of the trigger. When the trigger is not avoided, the primary treatment for anaphylaxis is self-injected epinephrine (EpiPen®). Epinephrine is a sympathomimetic catecholamine that acts on both α and β adrenergic receptors and, when injected subcutaneously, has a rapid onset and short duration of action. The strong vasoconstrictor action of epinephrine through its effect on α adrenergic receptors acts quickly to counter vasodilation and increased vascular permeability, which can lead to loss of intravascular fluid volume and hypotension during anaphylactic reactions. Epinephrine binding to β receptors on bronchial smooth muscle causes relaxation, which alleviates wheezing and dyspnea. Patient counseling should include recognition of symptoms and proper self-administration. Patients who are also prescribed antihistamines, leukotriene receptor antagonists, or steroids as disease state modifiers should be counseled that these medications do not replace epinephrine treatment during acute attacks.

Hyposensitization

Immunotherapy, also known as hyposensitization or desensitization, is an effective adjunct therapy for patients with seasonal allergic rhinitis, allergic asthma, or insect venom hypersensitivity. Immunotherapy consists of injecting allergens subcutaneously, or introducing them orally, in increasing doses over a prolonged period. Many controlled trials using immunotherapy have been carried out in patients with allergic rhinitis or asthma. Most studies demonstrate clinical improvement in 60% to 90% of patients. Allergy immunotherapy results in reduction, not complete elimination, of symptoms. The selection of allergens for injection is based on positive skin test results, clinical history, and sometimes a radioallergosorbent test (RAST) when the other methods of diagnosis are inconclusive.

Immunotherapy is used mainly in patients whose symptoms are not adequately controlled by pharmacologic means or avoidance of the offending antigens. Immunotherapy usually begins with weekly injections of low concentrations of appropriate allergens. The amount of allergen administered is increased weekly until a maintenance dose is achieved. Under certain circumstances, rush immunotherapy has been used to achieve maintenance dose within a few days. This form of therapy has been shown to result in a more rapid IgG response. Therapy then continues with monthly injections. Duration of treatment is different for each patient; therapy should be discontinued if symptoms do not improve after 2 or 3 years. The usual recommended length of treatment is 3 to 5 years, although some patients may require longer treatment. There is always a risk of inducing an anaphylactic reaction with each injection. Because of this potentially severe risk, for a disease such as allergic rhinitis a combination of a second-generation antihistamine plus a topical corticosteroid may be the preferred therapy. Immunotherapy should be used only after appropriate pharmacotherapy fails to improve symptoms satisfactorily.

The mechanisms by which hyposensitization reduces allergic symptoms are not clearly established. Skin test reactivity to the offending antigens decreases after a successful course of immunotherapy. Antigen-specific serum IgE levels diminish with a concomitant rise in antigen-specific serum IgG levels. This IgG is thought to be a "blocking antibody" competing with mast cell–bound IgE for binding to the allergen. Immunotherapy has also been shown to induce regulatory T lymphocytes (Treg), which suppress production of antigen-specific IgE, and increase class switching to non-IgE isoforms.

Omalizumab

Omalizumab (Xolair®) is a recombinant DNA-derived humanized IgG1 monoclonal antibody that selectively binds to IgE on the same Fc site as FcεR1. This prevents the binding of IgE to the high-affinity IgE receptor (FεR1) on the surface of mast cells and basophils. It has also been reported that basophil FcεR1 expression levels decrease after omalizumab treatment. A reduction in surface-bound IgE on FcεR1-bearing cells limits release of mediators of the allergic response, and has demonstrated effectiveness in treating patients with persistent asthma. Omalizumab is the first in a new class of biologicals aimed at preventing sensitization to an allergen and can be used in patients who are inadequately controlled with appropriate combination therapy. Once dosing is determined by calculating patient weight and IgE serum level, omalizumab is injected subcutaneously every 2 or 4 weeks.

INDUCTION OF AUTOIMMUNITY (CD4⁺, T CELL, MHC, AND TCR)

Role of CD4⁺ T Cells and Th1/Th2 Balance

Autoimmunity occurs when T cells that escape clonal deletion in the thymus are no longer regulated by Treg cells in the periphery. In most autoimmune disease, there is an immunological balance between T helper cells (Th1 and Th2), accompanied by corresponding cytokine profiles. Generally speaking, disease states that favor Th1 proliferation tend to induce cellular-mediated processes, while Th2-mediated disease states lean toward humoral processes. While some disease states show prominence in either Th1 or Th2 activation (as determined by cytokine profiles), many diseases present with mixed Th1 and Th2 pathologies. In rheumatoid arthritis, for example, autoantibodies appear in all stages of the disease and although this disease is mainly a Th1-driven condition, the Th2 response is robust early in the disease process (**Figure 5.1**).

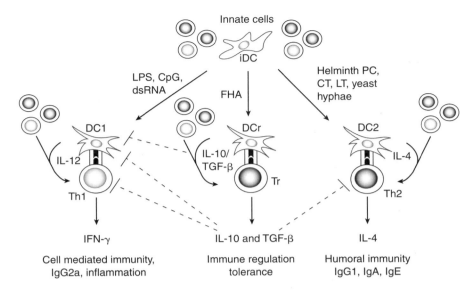

Figure 5.1. Role of CD4$^+$ T cells and Th1/Th2 balance. Proposed model for CD4$^+$ T-cell differentiation and function in immunity to infection. Certain pathogen-derived immunomodulatory molecules bind to dendritic cells (DCs) or other innate cells, including macrophages, and stimulate maturation of immature DCs (iDCs) into DC1 and DC2, which direct the differentiation of Th1 and Th2 cells, respectively. Other pathogen-derived molecules might activate maturation of iDCs into DCs, which direct the induction of regulatory T (Tr) cells (designated DCr). The function of Tr cells is to suppress Th1 and, in certain cases, Th2 responses, by the release of anti-inflammatory cytokines or contact-dependent mechanisms, acting directly on the T cell or the antigen-presenting cell (APC). Abbreviations: CT = cholera toxin; FHA = filamentous haemagglutinin; IFN = interferon; IL = interleukin; LPS = lipopolysaccharide; LT = labile enterotoxin; TGF = transforming growth factor. (Reproduced, with permission, from McGuirk P, Mills KH. Pathogen-specific regulatory T cells provoke a shift in the Th1/Th2 paradigm in immunity to infectious diseases. *Trends Immunol.* 2002; 23(9):450–455.)

Association with the MHC

The genetic influence of autoimmunity is complex and involves many genes. One of the most well studied genetic associations in autoimmunity includes autoreactive T-cell recognition of either foreign- or self-antigenic peptides presented by the major histocompatibility complex (MHC). The entire HLA region contains more than 250 gene loci and together HLA-I and HLA-II genes have been associated with over 100 different diseases. HLA association varies with disease; diseases such as insulin-dependent diabetes mellitus (IDDM) and multiple sclerosis (MS) correlate with both HLA-I and HLA-II alleles, while others, such as ankylosing spondylitis (AS), have an almost absolute association with one allele (HLA-B27).[1]

Non-HLA Genetic Association

There are more than 30 identified non-HLA genes associated with autoimmune disease. Most of these contribute directly or indirectly to antigen presentation and include genes encoding processing proteins (TAP2), cytokines (TNF, IL1, IL18, IL10, IFNG), cytokine receptors (IL4R,

IL6R), interleukin 1 receptor antagonist (IL1RN), cell surface proteins, cytotoxic T-lymphocyte-associated protein 4 (CTLA4), cellular maintenance, nitric oxide synthase 3 (NOS3), apoptotic proteins, B-cell CLL/lymphoma 2 (BCL2), programmed cell death 1 (PDCD1), signal transduction proteins, protein tyrosine phosphatase, non-receptor type 22 (PTPN22), and TNF receptor–associated factor 2 (TRAF2). As with MHC, there is both positive and negative regulation depending on the polymorphism.[2]

CHRONIC INFLAMMATION—ORGAN-SPECIFIC AUTOIMMUNE DISEASES MEDIATED BY DIRECT CELLULAR DAMAGE

Hashimoto's Thyroiditis

Hashimoto's thyroiditis (HT), also known as goitrous autoimmune thyroiditis, is an autoimmune disease caused by lymphocyte infiltration into the thyroid gland, leading to tissue destruction and hypothyroidism. Patients with HT have positive antibodies to thyroglobulin or thyroperoxidase, or both, in their blood. Although only 2% of the general population presents clinically with the disease, it is the most common cause of thyroid disease in the pediatric population and the most common cause of acquired hypothyroidism with or without goiter. The clinical course is variable, and spontaneous remission may occur in adolescence.

Autoimmune Hemolytic Anemia

Autoimmune hemolytic anemia is a group of type II hypersensitivity diseases—paroxysmal nocturnal hemoglobinuria, immune complex-mediated autoimmune disease, cold-induced immune hemolytic anemia—that lead to direct or indirect destruction of red blood cells. IgG or IgM autoantibodies bind to Rh blood group antigens (mainly Band 3, an ion transporter) on the red blood cell surface, activating the classical complement pathway. This results in direct C5b-9 (membrane attack complex [MAC]) cellular lysis. Alternatively, IgG1, IgG2, or IgG3 antibody and C3b-coated red blood cells can be opsonized by macrophages in the spleen and liver by FcRγ and CD35 (CR1), leading to indirect destruction of red blood cells. Current therapies include down-regulation of FcRγ expression with prednisone and dexamethasone and high-dose intravenous immunoglobulin therapy; in severe cases, a splenectomy may be considered. Future therapies showing promise include treatment with eculizumab (Soliris™), a humanized chimeric antibody that binds specifically to C5, inhibiting its cleavage into C5a and C5b, and preventing the formation of MAC.[3]

Goodpasture's Syndrome

Goodpasture's syndrome is an antiglomerular basement membrane disease in which autoantibodies bind to two dominate epitopes (E_A and E_B) of the α3 chain of type IV collagen (α3[IV]), causing rapidly progressive glomerulonephritis and pulmonary hemorrhage. Presented in young men in their 20s and women older than 60, there is a common increased susceptibility restricted to MHC, HLA-DRB1*1501 and DRB1*1502 alleles. Conversely, HLA-DR7 and DR1 have been shown to be protective. Renal injury in Goodpasture's syndrome includes complement-mediated damage after autoantibody binds to α3(IV); protease activation, which leads to filtration disruption; proteinuria; and glomerular epithelial crescent formation. Subsequent CD4+ and CD8+ T-cell activation induces macrophage and neutrophil migration into the kidney, where cytokine release (interleukin [IL]-12 and interferon [IFN]-γ) mediates further damage, leading to interstitial nephritis and ultimate fibrosis.

Once autoantibodies to α3(IV) have been detected by the antiglomerular basement membrane assay, patients are treated with plasmapheresis along with oral prednisone and cyclophosphamide. In cases of kidney failure, dialysis or kidney transplantation may be warranted. Future therapies may include blockage of T-cell activation, immune modulation with IL-4 or IL-10, or inhibition of macrophage migration.[4]

Insulin-Dependent Diabetes Mellitus

Insulin-dependent diabetes mellitus (IDDM), also known as type I diabetes, is a B- and T-cell-mediated autoimmune disease that results in destruction of the insulin-producing β-cells located in the islets of Langerhans within the pancreas. Destruction of β cells leads to glucose urea, a clinical sign of the disease.

Eighty percent of IDDM patients are positive for autoantibodies against glutamic acid decarboxylase (GAD), though other β-cell-specific proteins may also be autoantibody targets. The T-cell component of IDDM is highlighted by the fact that about 95% of all patients have either the HLA-DRB1*03, HLA-DQB1*0201, HLA-DRB1*04, or HLA-DQB1*0302 haplotype. It is postulated that because MHC-II alleles cannot effectively present GAD-like peptides to T cells in the thymus, autoreactive T cells are allowed to migrate to the periphery. Another theory is that peripheral CD4+ CD25+ Treg cells, which normally regulate pancreatic β-cell destruction of cytotoxic T lymphocytes (CTLs) and Th1 cells, have become depleted in patients with IDDM. More recently, attention has focused on the hypothesis that the loss of β cells is initiated by inappropriate induction of apoptosis through the Fas-Fas Ligand (FasL) mechanism. Because treatment for IDDM consists of rapid-acting, regular- or short-acting, intermediate-acting, and long-acting insulin, immunotherapy for IDDM is not a current clinical option. Fortunately, several clinical trials and animal experiments are under way to investigate the clinical benefit of cytokine therapy in IDDM patients. Most exciting is the potential treatment of patients with IFN-α, which increases levels of IL-4 and IL-10, both of which attenuate Th1 activity.

DISEASE MEDIATED BY STIMULATING OR BLOCKING AUTOANTIBODIES

Graves' Disease

Graves' disease occurs when autoantibodies, binding to the thyroid-stimulating hormone receptor (TSH-R), cause a chronic release of thyroid hormones from thyroid follicles. Hyperthyroid patients may present with an enlarged thyroid and bulging eyes (exophthalmos), along with insomnia, heat intolerance, tachycardia, weight loss, and irritability. Treatment options are limited to antithyroid medication, radiotherapy, or surgery, none of which alter the immune response. Patients who undergo antithyroid therapy must maintain lifelong thyroid hormone replacement therapy (L-thyroxine).

Because therapy only addresses thyroid hormone production, researchers are interested in therapeutically reintroducing immunological tolerance to TSH-R reactive cells or modifying the intrathyroidal autoimmune process. Several TSH-R autoantigens that accelerate both autoantibody production and autoreactive T-cell proliferation have been identified; however, reintroducing immunological tolerance using modified autoantigens is difficult because of the commonly slow initiation of the autoimmune response in Graves' disease.

Another approach being studied is modification of the intrathyroidal autoimmune process by regulating proliferation of Treg and Th1/Th2 populations of T cells. Cytokine profiles reveal that, while both Th1 and Th2 T cells are activated in Graves' disease, Th2 cells predominate, as expected by the production of autoantibodies. Cytokine therapy to increase Treg populations or deviate the Th2 response to a Th1 response, or both, are thought to hold promise in altering the immunopathology.[5]

Myasthenia Gravis

Myasthenia gravis (MG) is an autoimmune disease characterized by a fluctuating pathological weakness with remissions and exacerbations involving one or several skeletal muscle groups. It is caused mainly by antibodies to the α-subunit of the acetylcholine receptor (AChR) at the postsynaptic site of the neuromuscular junction. Apart from directly blocking AChR ligand binding, both AChR-specific and non-AChR autoantibodies of the IgG1 and IgG3 subclasses initiate complement-mediated focal muscle membrane damage, further accelerating the degradation of AChR.

First-line pharmacotherapy for MG is acetylcholinesterase inhibitors, which promote enhanced binding of acetylcholine to the diminished number of AChRs on the myasthenic muscle cell membrane, causing contractility improvement. In the 15% of MG patients who co-present with thyoma, or those with early-onset MG who do not respond well to acetylcholinesterase inhibitors, thymectomy is a treatment option. Second-line agents include immunosuppressive drugs, including corticosteroids, azathioprine, cyclophosphamide, cyclosporine, and methotrexate; all have undesired side effects. Other immunosuppressive agents that have shown some favorable effect in MG are tacrolimus and rituximab.

SYSTEMIC AUTOIMMUNE DISEASES

Systemic Lupus Erythematosus

Systemic lupus erythematosus (SLE), a chronic, type III hypersensitivity autoimmune inflammatory disease involving multiple organ systems, is caused by tissue damage resulting from antibody- and complement-fixing immune complex deposition. Autoantibodies, specific for both apoptotic and necrotic cell debris, cause inflammation in skin, joints, kidneys, and nervous system.

SLE predominates in the female population (9:1 ratio to males) between the child-bearing ages of 20 to 40. Genetic predisposition to the disease includes HLA-DR2, HLA-DR3; complement components C4, C2, C1q, and C1r/s; and polymorphisms in IL-10, CTLA-4, myelin basic protein (MBP), BCL-2, and Fcγ-R. Apart from genetic predispositions, environmental factors also appear needed to initiate the disease process in some patients at risk.

Treatment for SLE can include nonsteroidal anti-inflammatory drugs (NSAIDS), anti-malarials such as hydroxychloroquine sulfate (Plaquenil®), corticosteroids, and immunosuppressants such as cyclophosphamide (Cytoxan®, Neosar®), methotrexate (Rheumatrex® dose pack), and azathioprine (Imuran).

Multiple Sclerosis

Multiple sclerosis (MS) is a T-cell-mediated autoimmune disease against self-myelin or self-oligodendrocytic antigens in the white matter of both the brain and the spinal cord. It causes plaques to be formed on the myelin sheath of nerve cells, resulting in demyelination. Although the brain is normally immune privileged, in MS, effector cells enter the central nervous system (CNS), where they recognize as self-antigen the MBP, myelin oligodendrocyte glycoprotein (MOG), and proteolipid protein (PLP). Locally released IFN-γ and tumor necrosis factor (TNF)-α stimulate macrophage and microglia cells to attack the MBP or the myelin protein, respectively. Additionally, the release of chemotactic factors results in recruitment of macrophages and B cells, which when combined with autoantibodies and complement, increases CNS damage.

CTL cells induce production of lytic granules and activate apoptotic responses initiated by peptide:MHCI and Fas:FasL interaction. CTL release of IFN-γ activates macrophages and local microglia effector cells leading to more demyelination and tissue damage. IFN-γ production diverts the T-cell response to Th1, thus increasing CNS damage.

Multiple forms of IFN-β are used to reduce the number and severity of relapses in relapsing-remitting MS (RRMS): subcutaneous (SC) IFN beta-1β (Betaseron®); intramuscular (IM) IFN beta-1α (Avonex®); and SC IFN beta-1α (Rebif®). Although the mechanisms of action of these drugs are unknown, it is possible that their effects in MS may result from their immunomodulating properties, including their ability to augment Treg functions. These drugs inhibit T-cell migration across the blood-brain barrier and decrease the production IFN-γ, while at the same time increasing IL-10 levels.

Mitoxantrone (MX; Novantrone®) belongs to a class of antitumor antibiotics, and has been approved by the Food and Drug Administration (FDA) for treatments of MS. Mitoxantrone inhibits DNA repair and synthesis in dividing and nondividing cells through inhibition of DNA topoisomerase II. MX down-regulates CD4 Th1 T cells, inhibits demyelination activity performed by macrophages, inhibits T cell activation, reduces proliferation of B and T cells, and decreases antibody production. It is administered intravenously, dosed at 12 mg/m^2 every 3 months.

Copaxone (Glatiremer acetate [GA]), a synthetic polypeptide, shows marked inhibition of effector T cells, and reduced inflammation, demyelination, and axonal damage. It is administered once daily as 20 mg, subcutaneously.

One of the most widely used classes of drugs for treatment of MS includes glucocorticoids. Prednisone, a member of the glucocorticoid class, is administered initially 60–80 mg orally once a day; the dosage is tapered over the next 7 days.

Rheumatoid Arthritis

Rheumatoid arthritis (RA) is an inflammatory, autoimmune, often chronic disease that targets the synovial tissues of many joints. The disease often affects the wrist and finger joints, and sometimes affects the joints of the neck, shoulders, elbows, hips, knees, ankles, and feet. Inflamed joints are typically distributed symmetrically. In RA, inflammation of the synovium occurs, causing warmth, redness, swelling, and pain. White blood cells in the synovium eventually invade and destroy the cartilage and bone within the joint. The surrounding muscles, ligaments, and tendons that support and stabilize the joint become weak and lose function.

Susceptibility to RA has been linked to several genetic factors. Studies have shown that a large number of RA patients express HLA-DRB1 subtypes. Although there are numerous subtypes, patients with HLA-DRB1*0401, *0404, *0405, or *0408 expression have a greater risk of developing RA. Analysis of the amino acid sequences of HLA-DRB1 alleles identified a conserved sequence, glutamine-lysine-arginine-alanine-alanine (QKRAA), located on the third hypervariable region, which may serve as an epitope for RA-specific T-cell receptors (TCRs). It is clear, however, that more than one gene is involved in determining whether a person will develop the disease and how severe the disease will become. Agents in the environment (such as viruses and bacteria) are thought to trigger the disease in people who are more susceptible to RA. In addition, some studies suggest that hormonal factors may play a role.

The synovial joints of RA patients have a large number of CD4$^+$ T cells, indicating that the pathogenesis of RA is mediated by CD4$^+$ T-cell responses. CD4$^+$ T cells interact with macrophage-like type A synoviocytes that have acquired self-antigens on their MHC-II; this interaction initiates ongoing destruction of synovial tissue by causing secretion of proinflammatory cytokines, such as IL-1, IL-6, IL-12, IL-15, IL-17, and TNF-α.

The pleiotropic effects of proinflammatory cytokines include T-cell and macrophage activation and nitric oxide synthase, cyclooxygenase-2 (COX-2), and C-reactive protein production. Cytokines can also recruit neutrophils, basophils, and T cells to the synovial joints, causing inflammation and tissue damage. IL-12 activates natural killer (NK) cells and induces IFN-γ production as well as the differentiation of CD4$^+$ T cells into Th1 cells, which further enhance the pathogenesis of the disease.

Even though effector T cells and B cells play a large role in the pathology of RA, cells of the innate immune system appear to have a pivotal role as well. The synovial joints of RA patients have a high concentration of activated macrophages and fibroblasts. Macrophages in RA patients show signs of overproduction of proinflammatory cytokines and an overexpression of MHC-II molecules. Macrophage-produced IL-1 and TNF-α induce fibroblasts and chondrocytes to secrete cytokines, prostaglandins, and proteases, which erode and destroy bone and cartilage. Neutrophils, recruited to the joint by IL-8, release oxygen-derived free radicals that damage the joint by depolymerizing hyaluronic acid and inactivating protease inhibitors. Matrix metalloproteinases (MMPs) destroy bone and cartilage by degrading proteins that make up the intracellular matrix of these tissues. Working through separate pathways, both innate and adaptive immune responses intensify the effects of one another, shortening the time period of tissue damage.

Pharmacological treatment of RA includes NSAIDs, disease-modifying anti-rheumatologic drugs (DMARDs), and glucocorticoids. NSAIDs provide relief from pain and stiffness in the early stages of disease. In general, NSAIDs block prostaglandin synthesis pathways by inhibiting either the cyclooxygenase I (COX-1) or cyclooxygenase II (COX-2) isoenzymes. The two classes of NSAIDs are selective COX-2 inhibitors and nonselective COX inhibitors. COX-2 inhibitors bind only to the COX-2 isoenzyme, while nonselective COX inhibitors can bind to both COX-1 and COX-2. Highly selective COX-2 inhibitors are 10 to 20 times more selective for COX-2 than for COX-1. The advantage of selective COX-2 inhibitors is that they minimize some adverse effects commonly associated with COX-1 inhibitors. The only selective COX-2 inhibitor currently on the market is celecoxib (Celebrex®), since rofecoxib (Vioxx®) and valdecoxib (Bextra®) have been voluntarily withdrawn from the market because of unfavorable overall risk-versus-benefit profiles.

Some common nonselective COX inhibitors include ibuprofen (Motrin®) and naproxen (Naprosyn®). NSAIDs mainly offer symptomatic relief by reducing inflammation and pain to preserve the function of the joint, but they have little effect on slowing down the progression of bone and cartilage destruction.

Glucocorticoids are used in 60% to 70% of RA patients because of their immunosuppressive and anti-inflammatory properties. Prednisone (Meticorten®) is a glucocorticoid commonly used to treat RA.

DMARDs are used to retard or stop the progression of RA. These medications relieve pain, reduce swelling of the joints, and slow down joint damage. In comparison to NSAIDs, DMARDs are slow acting and may take weeks to months before their therapeutic effects are noticeable. DMARDs are either nonbiologic or biologic, and each has its own mechanism of action.

Nonbiologic DMARDs. Methotrexate (Rheumatrex®) is an antimetabolite that irreversibly binds to dihydrofolic acid reductase, inhibiting the formation of reduced folates, and thymidylate synthetase. It is considered the DMARD of choice for treating of RA, being used at low dosages in up to 60% of RA patients. Patients usually notice a decrease in the rate of appearance of new erosions. Leflunomide (Arava®), another antimetabolite that inhibits dihydroorotate dehydrogenase and thus pyrimidine synthesis, is a nonbiologic DMARD and is available in dosages of 10-, 20-, or 100-mg tablets.

Biologic DMARDs. Etanercept (Enbrel®), infliximab (Remicade®), and adalimumab (Humira®) all belong to a subclass of biologic DMARDs, sometimes called "anti-TNF" antibodies, which inhibit TNF from binding to its receptor (described in detail later in this chapter). Infliximab is on-label to be used in combination with methotrexate as a first-line regimen to treat patients with moderate to severe RA. Anakinra (Kineret®), another biologic DMARD, is an interleukin-1 receptor antagonist (IL-1Ra).

A new class of biologic DMARDs has been approved for treatment of RA by the FDA. The first in this class is abatacept (Orencia®; CTLA4-Ig), which works upstream of TNF release by blocking B7:CD28 interactions and T cell activation.

Since many patients do not respond adequately to therapy using a single drug from one of the above classes, combination therapy is becoming more common. Combination DMARD therapy decreases inflammation and slows down joint destruction with tolerable toxic effects.

TREATMENT OF AUTOIMMUNE DISEASES

Glucocorticoids

Glucocorticoids decrease the symptomatology of inflammation by affecting leukocyte function and suppressing cytokines, chemokines, and other inflammatory mediators. After administration of glucocorticoid, the concentration of neutrophils increases while the population of eosinophils, basophiles, monocytes, and T and B cells decreases. The increased levels of blood neutrophils results from increased production of neutrophils in the bone marrow. However, the migration of B and T cells through the blood to the site of inflammation causes their decrease in the blood at the same time. The lymphocytes, monocytes, eosinophils, and basophils move to the secondary lymphoid tissues, accounting for their reduced concentration in the blood. Glucocorticoids reduce inflammation caused by cytokines (IL-1, IL-3, IL-4, IL-5, TNF-α, IL-8, and granulocyte-macrophage colony-stimulating factor [GM-CSF]), and they also prevent the movement of nuclear factor κB (NFκB)—the major factor in transcribing inflammatory genes—into the nucleus. Finally, these drugs inhibit the function of tissue macrophages, other antigen-presenting cells (APCs), and leukocytes, thus inhibiting the release of inflammatory cytokines TNF-α, IFN-γ, IL-1, and IL-12.

As immunosuppressive drugs, glucocorticoids inhibit macrophages and other APCs from releasing IL-1, TNF-α, and MMPs. IL-12 and IFN-γ are also reduced, limiting the induction of Th1 cell activity. Glucocorticoids decrease inflammation by reducing the expression of COX-2 isoenzyme, limiting the production of prostaglandins and leukotrienes.

Antimetabolites

Methotrexate (Rheumatrex®) is used to treat severe psoriasis and adult RA. It inhibits dihydrofolic acid reductase, an enzyme used in the synthesis of purine nucleotides and thymidylate, thereby interfering with DNA synthesis, repair, and cellular replication. Two reports describe in vitro methotrexate inhibition of DNA precursor uptake by stimulated mononuclear cells, and another describes partial correction by methotrexate of spleen cell hyporesponsiveness and suppressed IL-2 production in animal polyarthritis. Other laboratories, however, have been unable to demonstrate similar effects. Clarification of methotrexate's effect on immune activity and its relation to rheumatoid immunopathogenesis await further studies. In RA, methotrexate is given at 7.5 mg once weekly, much lower than the dose for neoplastic diseases.

Leflunomide (Arava®) is indicated in adults for the treatment of active RA. It is a pyrimidine synthesis inhibitor, and induces its antiproliferative activity by inhibiting dihydroorotate dehydrogenase. It decreases ribonucleotide synthesis and arrests stimulated cells in the G1 phase of cell growth. Ultimately, leflonomide inhibits T-cell proliferation and production of autoantibodies by B cells. Secondary effects include up-regulation of IL-10 receptors, down-regulation of type A IL-8 receptors, and decreased activation of NFκB. For RA, it is recommended that leflonomide therapy be initiated with a loading dose of one 100-mg tablet per day for 3 days, then maintained at 20 mg/day. Concomitant treatment with other DMARDs is not contraindicated.

IMMUNOTHERAPY

Anti-TNF (Infliximab, Etanercept, Adalimumab, Abatacept)

Infliximab (Remicade®) is a chimeric IgG1κ monoclonal antibody composed of human constant and murine variable regions. Infliximab neutralizes the biological activity of TNF-α by binding with high affinity to the soluble and transmembrane forms of TNF-α, and inhibits binding of TNF-α with its receptors. Infliximab does not neutralize TNF-β (lymphotoxin α), a related cytokine that uses the same receptors as TNF-α.

By blocking TNF-α, infliximab reduces levels of proinflammatory cytokines such as IL-1 and IL-6; decreases leukocyte migration by decreasing endothelial layer permeability and expression of adhesion molecules by endothelial cells and leukocytes; attenuates neutrophil and eosinophil functional activity; lowers acute phase reactant levels and other liver proteins; and decreases tissue-degrading enzymes produced by synoviocytes and chondrocytes. Cells expressing transmembrane TNF-α bound by infliximab can be lysed by complement or by antibody-dependent cell-mediated cytotoxicity (ADCC).

Infliximab is indicated for use in moderately to severely active RA, Crohn's disease, and AS. In RA it is on-label to be used in combination with methotrexate as a first-line regimen.

Anti-IL-1 (Anakinra)

Anakinra (Kineret®) is a recombinant, nonglycosylated form of the human IL-1Ra. Unlike native human IL-1Ra, anakinra has the addition of a single methionine residue at its amino terminus.

IL-1Ra is expressed on a wide variety of tissues and organs, and when bound by IL-1, mediates various physiologic responses, including inflammatory and immunological responses. IL-1 can produce several systemic changes, including cartilage degradation through induction of the rapid loss of proteoglycans, as well as stimulation of bone reabsorption. The levels of the naturally occurring IL-1Ra in synovium and synovial fluid obtained from RA patients are not sufficient to compete with the elevated amount of locally produced IL-1.

Anakinra is indicated for the reduction in signs and symptoms of moderately to severely active RA, in patients 18 or older who have failed one or more DMARDs.

Anti-CD2 (Alefacept)

Alefacept (AMEVIVE®) is an immunosuppressive dimeric fusion protein consisting of the extracellular CD2-binding portion of the human leukocyte function antigen-3 (LFA-3) linked to the Fc (hinge, CH2 and CH3 domains) portion of human IgG1. It interferes with lymphocyte activation by specifically binding to the lymphocyte antigen CD2, and inhibiting LFA-3/CD2 interaction. Activation of T lymphocytes involving the interaction between LFA-3 on APCs and CD2 on T lymphocytes plays a role in the pathophysiology of chronic plaque psoriasis. The majority of T lymphocytes in psoriatic lesions are of the memory effector phenotype, characterized by the presence of the CD45RO marker 1, express activation markers (e.g., CD25, CD69), and release inflammatory cytokines, such as interferon γ.

Alefacept also causes a reduction in subsets of $CD2^+$ T lymphocytes (primarily $CD45RO^+$), presumably by bridging between CD2 on target lymphocytes and immunoglobulin Fc receptors on cytotoxic cells, such as NK cells. Total counts of circulating $CD4^+$ and $CD8^+$ T lymphocytes are also reduced by alefacept treatment. Since CD2 is also expressed at low levels on the surface of NK cells and certain bone marrow B lymphocytes, the potential exists for alefacept to affect the activation and numbers of cells other than T lymphocytes.

Alefacept is indicated for the treatment of adult patients with moderate to severe chronic plaque psoriasis, who are candidates for systemic therapy or phototherapy.

Natalizumab (Anti-α4 integrin)

Natalizumab (Tysabri®) is a recombinant humanized IgG4 monoclonal antibody containing human framework regions and the complementarity-determining regions of a murine antibody. It binds to the α4-subunit of α4β1 and α4β7 integrins expressed on the surface of all leukocytes except neutrophils, and inhibits the α4-mediated adhesion of leukocytes to their counterreceptor(s). The receptors for the α4 family of integrins include vascular cell adhesion molecule-1 (VCAM-1) and mucosal addressin cell adhesion molecule-1

(MadCAM-1). Disruption of these molecular interactions prevents transmigration of leukocytes across the endothelium into inflamed parenchymal tissue. In vitro, anti-α4-integrin antibodies block α4-mediated cell binding to ligands, such as osteopontin, and block an alternatively spliced domain of fibronectin connecting segment-1 (CS-1). In vivo, natalizumab may further act to inhibit the interaction of α4-expressing leukocytes with their ligand(s) in the extracellular matrix and on parenchymal cells, inhibiting further recruitment and inflammatory activity of activated immune cells.

The specific mechanism(s) by which natalizumab exerts its effects in MS have not been fully defined. MS-specific leukocyte migration across the blood-brain barrier involves interaction between adhesion molecules on inflammatory cells and their counter-receptors, which are present on endothelial cells of the vessel wall. The clinical effect of natalizumab in MS may be secondary to the blockade of the molecular interaction of α4β1-integrin (expressed by inflammatory cells) with VCAM-1 (present on vascular endothelial cells) and CS-1 and osteopontin (expressed by parenchymal cells in the brain).

Natalizumab is indicated for the treatment of patients with relapsing forms of MS to reduce the frequency of clinical exacerbations. Although pulled from the market after only 3 months because of increased incidence of progressive multifocal leukoencephalopathy, the drug was reintroduced into the market in June 2006 after establishment of a risk-minimization program with mandatory patient registration and periodic follow-up.

Glatiramer Acetate (Copaxone®)

Glatiramer acetate (Copaxone®), formerly known as copolymer-1, consists of the acetate salts of synthetic polypeptides. It contains four naturally occurring amino acids, and is chemically identified as L-glutamic acid polymer—with L-alanine, L-lysine, and L-tyrosine-acetate (salt).

How glatiramer acetate exerts its effects in patients with MS is not fully understood. It is thought to act by modifying immune processes currently believed to be responsible for MS pathogenesis. This hypothesis is supported by studies that explored the pathogenesis of experimental allergic encephalomyelitis (EAE), a condition induced in several animal species through immunization against central nervous system-derived material containing myelin. (This condition is often used as an experimental animal model of MS.) Studies in animals and in vitro systems suggest that on administration of glatiramir-acetate, glatiramer acetate-specific suppressor T cells are induced and activated in the periphery.

Glatiramer acetate is indicated for reduction of the frequency of relapses in patients with RRMS, and is administered 20 mg per day injected subcutaneously.

Type I Interferons (IFN-β1a, IFN-β1b)

Interferon β-1b (Betaseron®) is a purified, sterile, lyophilized protein produced by recombinant DNA techniques from a genetically engineered plasmid containing the gene for human interferon beta$_{ser17}$. The native gene was obtained from human fibroblasts and altered in a way that substitutes serine for the cysteine residue found at position 17. It does not include the carbohydrate side chains found in the natural material.

The mechanism of action of IFN-β1b in patients with MS is unknown. IFN-β1b receptor binding induces the expression of proteins responsible for the pleiotropic bioactivities of IFN-β1b. A number of these proteins (including neopterin, β2–microglobulin, MxA protein, and IL-10) have been measured in blood fractions from both patients and healthy volunteers treated with IFN-β1b. Immunomodulatory effects of IFN-β1b include enhancement of suppressor T-cell activity, reduction of proinflammatory cytokine production, the down-regulation of antigen presentation, and the inhibition of lymphocyte trafficking into the CNS. It is not known which of these immunomodulatory effects are responsible for the clinical improvement seen in IFN-β1b treatment MS patients.

IFN-β1b is indicated for treatment of relapsing forms of MS to reduce the frequency of clinical exacerbations and is administered subcutaneously every other day at a dose of 0.25 mg.

IFN-β1a (Rebif® and Avonex®) is produced by recombinant DNA technology from a genetically engineered plasmid carrying the human interferon beta gene. The amino acid sequence of IFN-β1a is identical to that of natural fibroblast-derived human interferon β. Natural IFN-β and IFN-β1a are both glycosylated, with each containing a single N-linked complex carbohydrate moiety.

The binding of IFN-β to its receptors initiates a complex cascade of intracellular events leading to the expression of numerous IFN-induced gene products and markers, including 2′, 5′-oligoadenylate synthetase, β2-microglobulin, and neopterin. Although many of the affected genes have been identified, specific IFN-induced protein profiles and cellular mechanisms by which IFN-β1a exerts its clinical effects in MS have not been fully defined.

IFN-β1a is indicated for the treatment of patients with relapsing forms of MS to decrease the frequency of clinical exacerbations and delay the accumulation of physical disability. Rebif® is administered subcutaneously 3 times a week at a dosage between 22 and 44 μg, whereas Avonex® is administered IM once a week at a dosage of 30 μg.

Efalizumab (Anti-LFA-1)

Efalizumab (Raptiva®) is an immunosuppressive recombinant humanized IgG1 kappa isotype monoclonal antibody that binds to human CD11a (LFA-1a). Efalizumab inhibits binding of LFA-1 to intercellular adhesion molecule-1 (ICAM-1), thereby inhibiting the adhesion of leukocytes to other cell types. Interaction between LFA-1 and ICAM-1 contributes to the initiation and maintenance of multiple processes, including activation of T lymphocytes, adhesion of T lymphocytes to endothelial cells, and migration of T lymphocytes to sites of inflammation including psoriatic skin. Lymphocyte activation and trafficking to skin play a role in the pathophysiology of chronic plaque psoriasis. In psoriatic skin, ICAM-1 cell surface expression is upregulated on endothelium and keratinocytes. CD11a is also expressed on the surface of B lymphocytes, monocytes, neutrophils, NK cells, and other leukocytes. So the potential exists for efalizumab to affect the activation, adhesion, migration, and numbers of cells other than T lymphocytes.

Efalizumab is indicated for treatment of adult patients (18 years or older) with chronic moderate to severe plaque psoriasis who are candidates for systemic therapy or phototherapy. Treatment is initiated with a single 0.7-mg/kg subcutaneous conditioning dose followed by weekly subcutaneous doses of 1 mg/kg (maximum single dose not to exceed 200 mg).

EXPERIMENTAL THERAPEUTIC APPROACHES

Interactions between TCR and MHC are involved in both stimulatory and inhibitory functions. Thus, cutting-edge therapies are being developed to reduce or enhance T-cell-mediated responses in a wide variety of disease states.

T-Cell Vaccination

With advances in identifying autoantigens and tumor-specific or tumor-associated antigens, novel therapeutic approaches can manipulate the cellular response of the immune system to target autoimmune and oncological diseases.

Autoimmunity. In autoimmunity, therapy is aimed at increasing populations of antigen-specific Treg cells. Phase II clinical trials show promise in treating nonresponder relapsing-remitting MS patients with whole autologous attenuated myelin-stimulated T cells. After three vaccinations, patient relapse rates decreased by almost 50%, and patients showed significant improvements in both neurologic and pathologic outcomes with no noted adverse events. Previous studies showed the improved clinical outcomes corresponded closely with a decrease in myelin-reactive T-cell populations. This same strategy may also be used in other autoimmune diseases such as RA, in which known T-cell antigens have been identified.[6,7]

Cancer. Cancer vaccine strategies aim to generate an immune-mediated, antitumor-associated antigen response that leads to the complete destruction of cancerous tissue. Some tumors induce anti-inflammatory responses and many tumor-specific T-cell populations are peripherally anergized or deleted due to lack of expression of costimulatory molecules; the primary objective of cancer-specific T-cell vaccines is to enhance activation of tumor-specific CTLs through ex vivo adoptive immunotherapy. Alternatively, APC therapy (autologous dendritic cells) can be used to enhance T-cell activation in vivo.[8]

Altered Peptide Ligand Immunotherapy

Treatment with pathogenic peptide sequences, which have been altered by one or more amino acid substitutions at key MHC or TCR contact points, produces both agonistic and antagonistic effects on T-cell activation. At low doses, antagonistic peptides have been shown to render autoreactive T cells (usually Th1 cells) anergic to later stimulation by native antigen, with higher doses inducing complete selective clonal deletion via activation-induced apoptotic cell death. The proposed mechanism is through Th2 activation and release of IL-10. Conversely, agonistic peptides have been shown to stimulate Treg cells in autoimmune models; and in cancer models, they stimulate activation of CTLs and enhance tumor destruction (**Table 5.2**).

In humans, experimental recombinant peptide therapy has been used to treat RA, psoriasis vulgaris, and MS, all with modest results. Although the majority of patients showed measurable immunological response to the peptide, fewer than 40% showed any degree of favorable clinical benefit. The greatest clinical benefit occurred mainly in patients with robust T-cell responses, which indicated a positive correlation between T-cell activation and disease state pathology. In animal

Table 5.2. Comparative Table of Monoclonal Antibody Therapies (Generic/Brand, Structure/Isotype/Species, Antigen, On-Label Approval)

Generic Name (Brand Name)	Structure	Species	Antigen	Indications and Usage	Dose, Route	Frequency
Omalizumab (Xolair)	IgG1κ monoclonal antibody	All mouse with human CDRs	Human IgE	Moderate to severe persistent asthma	150–375 mg, SC	Every 2 or 4 weeks
Infliximab (Remicade)	IgG1κ monoclonal antibody	Human constant and murine variable regions	Human TNF-α	Moderately to severely active rheumatoid arthritis Moderately to severely active Crohn's disease Active ankylosing spondylitis Active arthritis in patients with psoriatic arthritis Moderately to severely active ulcerative colitis	3 mg/kg, IV	Two and 6 weeks after the first infusion, then every 8 weeks thereafter

(Continued)

Table 5.2 (*Continued*)

Generic Name (Brand Name)	Structure	Species	Antigen	Indications and Usage	Dose, Route	Frequency
Etanercept (Enbrel)	IgG1-TNF-R fusion protein	All human CH2/CH3 Fc region fused to the extracellular ligand-binding portion of the human 75 kDa (P75) TNF-R	Human TNF-α	Moderately to severely active rheumatoid arthritis Moderately to severely active polyarticular-course juvenile rheumatoid arthritis in patients who have had an inadequate response to one or more DMARDs Ankylosing spondylitis Chronic moderate to severe plaque psoriasis	50 mg, SC	Weekly
Adalimumab (Humira)	IgG1κ monoclonal antibody	Human	Human TNF-α	Moderately to severely active rheumatoid arthritis	40 mg, SC	Every other week
Abatacept (Orencia)	IgG1-fusion protein	Extracellular domain of human CTLA-4 linked to modified Fc (hinge, CH2, and CH3 domains)	Human CD80 (B7-1), CD86 (B7-2)	Moderately to severely active rheumatoid arthritis	500 mg–1.0 g; 30-min intravenous infusion	Two and 4 weeks after the first infusion, then every 4 weeks thereafter
Anakinra (Kineret)	Recombinant, IL-1Ra with the addition of a single methionine residue at its amino terminus	Human	Interleukin-1 type I receptor (IL-1RI)	Moderately to severely active rheumatoid arthritis	100 mg by subcutaneous injection	Daily
Alefacept (AMEVIVE)	IgG1 fusion protein	Extracellular CD2-binding portion of human LFA-3 linked to human Fc (hinge, CH2 and CH3 domains)	Human CD2 (LFA-2)	Moderate to severe chronic plaque psoriasis	7.5- or 15-mg IV bolus	Once weekly for 12 weeks
Natalizumab (Tysabri)	IgG4κ monoclonal antibody	All mouse with human CDRs	Human α4-integrin	Relapsing forms of multiple sclerosis	300-mg IV infusion	Every 4 weeks

CDR = complement-determining region; CTLA-4 = cytotoxic T-lymphocyte-associated protein 4; DMARDs = disease-modifying anti-rheumatologic drugs; Ig = immunoglobulin; IL = interleukin; IV = intravenous; SC = subcutaneous; TNF = tumor necrosis factor.

models, peptide therapy has been used in models of breast cancer and experimental autoimmune anterior uveitis, both with significant efficacy in altering T-cell profiles and improving clinical outcomes[9] (**Figure 5.2**).

There is only one T-cell-modifying peptide currently on the market: glatiramer acetate (Copaxone®), described above. Composed of four amino acids found in myelin, glatiramer acetate has been shown to bind both MHC and TCR, inducing IL-4, IL-10, and transforming growth factor (TGF) β-1 release from Th2/Treg cells and thus decreasing Th1/CTL cell activation in MS patients.[10]

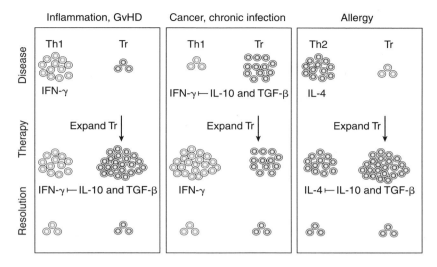

Figure 5.2. Experimental therapeutic approaches: T-cell regulation. Possible disease therapies based on regulatory T (Tr)-cell manipulation in vivo. In a healthy individual, Tr cells maintain homeostasis and prevent inflammation at mucosal surfaces, including the gut and lungs, but permit Th1 and cytotoxic T-lymphocyte (CTL) responses to control infection and tumors. However, imbalances in regulatory and effector arms of the immune response are apparent in certain disease states. Tr cells might be expanded in chronic infection and possibly cancer, resulting in suppressed Th1 responses. By contrast, overactive Th1 responses contribute to the pathology in autoimmune diseases, infection-induced inflammation, graft-versus-host disease (GVHD), and graft rejection, whereas Th2 cells mediate allergy. So strategies that can inhibit or expand Tr cells in vivo might offer therapeutic potential for treatment of these diseases. Abbreviations: IFN = interferon; IL = interleukin; TGF = transforming growth factor. (Reproduced, with permission, from McGuirk P, Mills KH. Pathogen-specific regulatory T cells provoke a shift in the Th1/Th2 paradigm in immunity to infectious diseases. *Trends Immunol.* 2002; 23(9):450–455.)

REFERENCES

1. Shiina T, Inoko H, Kulski JK. An update of the HLA genomic region, locus information and disease associations: 2004. *Tissue Antigens.* 2004; 64(6):631–649.
2. Serrano NC, Millan P, Paez MC. Non-HLA associations with autoimmune diseases. *Autoimmun Rev.* 2006; 5(3):209–214.
3. Rosse WF, Hillmen P, Schreiber AD. Immune-mediated hemolytic anemia. *Hematology Am Soc Hematol Educ Program.* 2004:48–62.
4. Hudson BG, Tryggvason K, Sundaramoorthy M, et al. Alport's syndrome, Goodpasture's syndrome, and type IV collagen. *N Engl J Med.* 2003; 348(25):2543–2556.
5. Weetman AP. Cellular immune responses in autoimmune thyroid disease. *Clin Endocrinol (Oxf).* 2004; 61(4):405–413.
6. Achiron A, Lavie G, Kishner I, et al. T cell vaccination in multiple sclerosis relapsing-remitting nonresponders patients. *Clin Immunol.* 2004; 113(2):155–160.
7. Lee E, Sinha AA. T cell targeted immunotherapy for autoimmune disease. *Autoimmunity.* 2005; 38(8):577–596.
8. Dermime S, Gilham DE, Shaw DM, et al. Vaccine and antibody-directed T cell tumour immunotherapy. *Biochim Biophys Acta.* 2004; 1704(1):11–35.
9. Vandenbark AA, Morgan E, Bartholomew R, et al. TCR peptide therapy in human autoimmune diseases. *Neurochem Res.* 2001; 26(6):713–730.
10. Arnon R, Aharoni R. Mechanism of action of glatiramer acetate in multiple sclerosis and its potential for the development of new applications. *Proc Natl Acad Sci U S A.* 2004; 101(Suppl 2):14593–14598.

SELF-ASSESSMENT QUESTIONS

1. All of the following are true of second-generation H_1 antagonists *except*:

   A   Cause minimal sedation
   B.   Are ineffective in patients with Type I hypersensitivity
   C.   May also improve allergic symptoms independent of binding to the H_1-receptor
   D.   In the case of loratadine, reduces PGD2 release

E. All of the above are true of second-generation H$_1$ antagonists

2. Which of the following is the only proven effective *prevention* for anaphylaxis?

A. Prophylactic treatment with epinephrine (EpiPen®)
B. Hyposensitization immunotherapy
C. Subcutaneous injection of omalizumab (Xolair®) every 2 to 4 weeks
D. Avoidance of the trigger
E. None of the above are proven effective preventions for anaphylaxis

For questions 3–6 concerning induction of autoimmunity, use the following (use each answer only once):

A. Th1 CD4$^+$ T cells
B. Th2 CD4$^+$ T cells
C. MHC genes
D. Non-HLA genes

3. Is most closely linked to ankylosing spondylitis.

4. Predominant populations of these cells lean toward humoral processes.

5. Associated with diseases with prevalence of cytokine gene polymorphisms.

6. Predominant populations of these cells tend to induce cellular-mediated processes.

7. It has been shown that attenuation of Th1 CD4$^+$ T cell activity in IDDM shows potential therapeutic benefit. Which of the following treatment(s) could theoretically assist in Th1 CD4$^+$ T-cell attenuation? Mark all that apply.

A. Increased IL-10 levels
B. Increased IL-4 levels
C. IFN-α cytokine therapy
D. Glatiramer acetate (Copaxone®) peptide therapy
E. None of the above would be a potential regimen for IDDM

8. Fill in the missing information in the following chart:

Generic Name (Brand Name)	Structure	Species	Antigen	Indications and Usage	Dose, Route	Frequency
Omalizumab (_____)	IgG1κ monoclonal antibody	All mouse with human CDRs	_____ _____	Moderate to severe persistent asthma	150–375 mg, SC	Every 2 or 4 weeks
_____ (Enbrel)	_____ _____ _____	All human CH2/CH3 Fc region fused to the extracellular ligand-binding portion of the human 75 kDA (P75) TNF-R	Human TNF-α	Moderately to severely active rheumatoid arthritis Moderately to severely active polyarticular-course juvenile rheumatoid arthritis in patients who have had an inadequate response to one or more DMARDs Ankylosing spondylitis Chronic moderate to severe plaque psoriasis	50 mg, SC	Weekly

(Continued)

Generic Name (Brand Name)	Structure	Species	Antigen	Indications and Usage	Dose, Route	Frequency
Abatacept (_____)	IgG1-fusion protein	Extracellular domain of human CTLA-4 linked to modified Fc (hinge, CH2, and CH3 domains)	_____ _____	Moderately to severely active rheumatoid arthritis	500 mg–1.0 g; 30-minute intravenous infusion	Two and 4 weeks after the first infusion, then every 4 weeks thereafter
Anakinra (Kineret)	Recombinant, IL-1Ra with the addition of a single methionine residue at its amino terminus	Human	_____ _____	_____ _____	100 mg by subcutaneous injection	Daily
_____ (AMEVIVE)	IgG1 fusion protein	Extracellular CD2-binding portion of human LFA-3 linked to human Fc (hinge, CH2 and CH3 domains)	Human CD2 (LFA-2)	_____ _____	7.5- or 15-mg IV bolus	Once weekly for 12 weeks
Natalizumab (Tysabri)	IgG4κ monoclonal antibody	_____ _____	Human α4-integrin	Relapsing forms of multiple sclerosis	300-mg IV infusion	_____ _____

CHAPTER 6

Common Infectious Diseases and Immunization

Gail Goodman Snitkoff

CHAPTER OUTLINE

INTRODUCTION

The immune system has developed diverse mechanisms to deal with infections caused by pathogens. As part of the adaptive immune response, these mechanisms include antibodies, effector CD4$^+$ T cells, and cytotoxic T cells. While each component of specific immunity is designed to provide protection and recovery from diseases based in different cellular and extracellular compartments, they all develop immunological memory and provide long-term protection from reinfection. This protection is stimulated naturally by infection with a particular pathogen; protection from reinfection with the same pathogen has been recognized for centuries. This recognition led to investigation of ways to artificially produce immunity against disease. Today, the widespread use of vaccines has led to the global eradication of smallpox, elimination of polio in the United States, and dramatic reductions in the incidence of other infectious diseases.

Pharmacists can play a major role in the field of immunization, including educating patients about vaccines as prophylaxis for disease along with the need for accurate timing of vaccine administration, and recommending passive and/or active immunization for the treatment of diseases. This can help prevent outbreaks of diseases that are primarily due to failure to vaccinate children at recommended ages (although some outbreaks may be attributed to waning of the immunity provided by vaccines). Passive immunization and therapeutic intervention with intramuscular and intravenous immune globulins continue to be expanding fields in medicine.

This chapter is designed to highlight how the body protects itself from various infectious pathogens. It also identifies the achievements of early investigations into active immunization, followed by a discussion of both biotechnological and traditional approaches to modern vaccine development. Finally, the principles of immunotherapy are presented, with a focus on the use of immune globulins for imparting passive immunity. For additional information, the following resources may be useful:

- Janeway CA, Travers P, Walport M, et al. *Immunobiology*. 6th ed. London: Garland Science; 2004.
- Plotkin SA, Orenstein WA. *Vaccines*. 4th ed. Philadelphia, PA: WB Saunders; 2004.

LEARNING OBJECTIVES

After completing this chapter, the reader should be able to:

1. Describe the different types of immune responses used to clear infections caused by different types of microorganisms.
2. Describe risk factors associated with active immunization.
3. Describe development of traditional vaccines.
4. Discuss biotechnological production methods of modern vaccines.
5. Describe potential advantages and disadvantages of simultaneous administration of vaccines.
6. Discuss therapeutic applications of intramuscular immune globulins.
7. Discuss considerations in the use of intravenous immune globulins.

IMMUNE RESPONSE TO INFECTIOUS DISEASES

As human beings, we are at constant risk of infection because we live in an environment full of microorganisms. We are not constantly ill because we have evolved strategies to protect ourselves from infectious diseases. These host strategies include barriers to infection, inflammation, and acquired immunity.

Barriers—such as skin, mucous membranes, fatty acids, and the low pH of the stomach—prevent viable pathogens from entering our bodies and establishing an infection. When these barriers are breached, the inflammatory response, involving the cells and chemicals of innate immunity, is often enough to stop the infection and prevent disease. But when innate defense mechanisms are insufficient, the infectious agent is carried to

the local lymphoid tissue and a specific immune response is initiated. The type of immune response is based on the pathogenic microorganism and type of infection.

Different types of specific immunity, including antibodies (Ab), effector CD4+ T cells (Th1 and Th2), and cytotoxic T cells (CTLs), are produced by the host's immune system in response to different types of microorganisms. Abs provide protection by neutralizing the ability of a pathogen or toxin to bind to the host cell, and by increasing phagocytosis of the bacteria (opsonization) and activation of complement (**Figure 6.1**). Th1 cells produce and secrete cytokines that recruit macrophages to the site of infection and activate macrophages for increased intracellular killing (**Figure 6.2**). CTLs are able to specifically recognize and kill pathogens that reproduce in the cytoplasm of host cells via induction of apoptosis and release of lytic molecules (**Figure 6.3**).

Viral Infections

Viruses are obligate intracellular parasites that reproduce in the host cells. Over 400 different viruses can cause disease in humans, ranging from acute disease to persistent infections. Some viruses, such as retroviruses, papillomaviruses, adenoviruses, and hepadnaviruses, are able to integrate into the host genome; others, especially herpesviruses, are able to establish latency in the host. Because of the wide variety of viruses and types of infections, the host's immune system has devised a number of different mechanisms—both innate and adaptive—for defending against viral infections.

Innate immune responses to viral infections are initiated by macrophages binding to pathogen-associated molecular patterns (PAMPs) on the virion and activation of the macrophage's Toll receptors. These receptors activate signaling pathways to stimulate production of inflammatory cytokines leading to activation of primarily cell-mediated immune responses. In addition to stimulating specific immune responses, macrophages produce interferon γ (IFN-γ, immune interferon), and the virally infected cells produce IFN-α and IFN-β. Interferons can affect cell function throughout the body. The effects of IFNs on cells of the immune system include activation of natural killer (NK) cells to hold the viral infection in check until acquired immunity is established; stimulation of antigen presentation and costimulator (B7) expression by antigen presenting cells; and enhancement of CD4+Th1 responses. The effect of IFNs on other cells is to

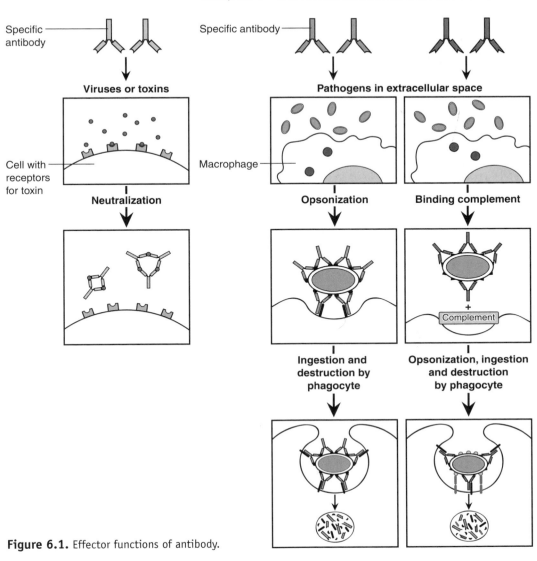

Figure 6.1. Effector functions of antibody.

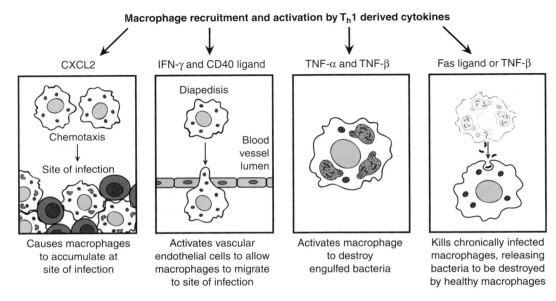

Figure 6.2. Effector functions of T-helper cells.

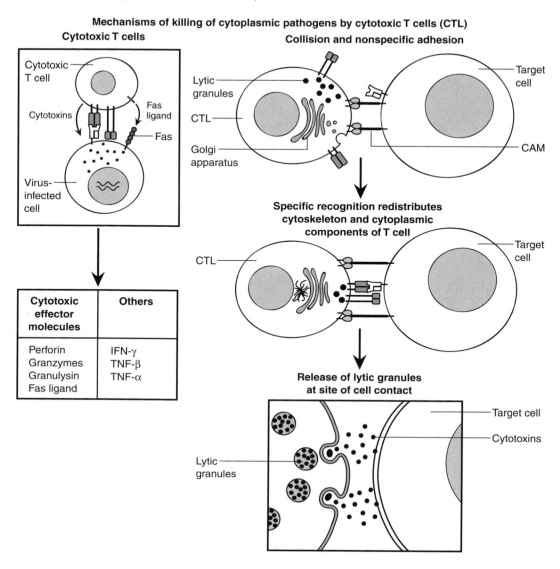

Figure 6.3. Effector functions of cytotoxic T cells.

inhibit viral infection in susceptible cells. Viral infection is inhibited by decreasing cellular receptors for the virions; reducing virus entry into the host cell; inhibiting transcription of viral genes; and inhibiting production of viral DNA and RNA genomes. IFNs and NK cell activation are able to reduce the viral load until the adaptive immune response is activated 4 to 5 days after infection.

In the host, viruses are found both intracellularly and extracellularly. Infectious virions are present in extracellular fluids, and viruses reproduce inside host cells. So the host's adaptive immune system interacts with the virus as both exogenous antigen (antigen from outside the cell) and endogenous antigen (antigen from inside

the cell). Two different processing and presentation pathways exist; these lead to different types of immune responses, depending on where the antigen is found. Exogenous antigen stimulates production of Abs, while endogenous antigen stimulates development of cell-mediated immunity. Antigens (such as viruses) that reproduce in the cytoplasm of the host cell activate CD8+ T cells to become CTL.

During an infection, CD4+ Th2 cells stimulate B cells to produce Ab directed against viral proteins and glycoproteins. Virus-specific Abs are able to recognize viral antigens on either extracellular virions or on infected host cells. When an Ab recognizes extracellular viral antigen, it can neutralize the virus and stimulate increased phagocytosis of the opsonized (Ab-coated) virion. Ab recognition of viral antigen on the surface of an infected host cell can lead to antibody-dependent cell-mediated cytotoxicity (ADCC) by NK cells. However, Abs cannot recognize a cell in which the virus is replicating. To eliminate virus from an infected host cell, cell-mediated immunity is required.

Development of cell-mediated immunity, including activation of CD4+ Th1 cells and CTLs, is needed to clear the viral infection. Th1 cells are needed for the activation of CD8+ T cells into CTLs. They do this by secreting interleukin (IL)-2, which in conjunction with antigen binding by the CD8+ T cells, results in activation of the T cells to CTLs. In addition, Th1 cells can stimulate macrophages to increase antigen presentation and expression of costimulator molecules, which, in turn, can directly activate the resting CD8+ T cells. CTLs are the optimum mechanism for clearing viral infections; they can recognize cells in which the virus is growing by recognizing viral peptides presented on the cell's class I major histocompatibility complex (MHC) molecules. This allows the specific immune response to recognize an infected cell early in the replication of the virus and to eliminate that cell.

The CTLs can eliminate a virally infected host cell by inducing apoptosis through a variety of mechanisms: release of perforin, expression of FAS ligand (FasL), and expression of tumor necrosis factor (TNF)-related apoptosis-inducing ligand (TRAIL). Perforin, a protein related to the C9 component of complement, creates holes in the plasma membrane of an infected cell. These holes allow granzymes access to the cytoplasm of the cell, inducing apoptosis. Expression of FasL by the CTL allows the CTL to bind to Fas (CD95) on the virus-infected host cell and also stimulates apoptosis. CTLs expressing TRAIL are able to bind DR4, DR5, which stimulate programmed cell death in these cells.[1,2] CTLs are able not only to induce apoptosis in infected cells, but also to release IFN-γ upon binding to class I MHC molecules. IFN-γ not only reduces viral replication, but is also important in clearing infections caused by viruses such as herpes simplex.[3]

Thus, for viral infections, both cell-mediated and humoral immunity are needed to clear the infection, and each of these arms of acquired immunity works at different sites during the infection.

Bacterial Infections

Most bacteria live in a commensal or symbiotic relationship with humans. Indeed, while humans have 10^{12} of their own cells, each of us is colonized with about 10^{14} bacteria. Although pathogenic bacteria are relatively rare—less than 1% of all bacterial species can cause disease—they are quite varied. In an individual, pathogenic bacteria can replicate either extracellularly or intracellularly; the site of growth is dependent on the bacterial species and growth requirements. The variety of bacterial pathogens and their sites of growth require the host's immune system to be able to respond to infections no matter where the bacteria are growing. Initial host defenses against all bacteria include barriers, antibacterial products (lactoferrin, lactoperoxidase, defensins, mucin, lysozyme), and mechanical clearing by cilia and peristalsis. If these defenses fail, innate defenses and inflammation are activated before activation of specific responses.

Upon entry into the host, bacteria activate inflammation by interactions with the complement system and with phagocytic cells (macrophages, neutrophils). These phagocytes recognize bacteria through PAMP receptors that recognize microbial products including glycolipids, lipoproteins, and flagella. These receptors (in cooperation with Toll receptors) activate the phagocytic cells. Other receptors recognize bacterial polysaccharides, glycolipids, lipopolysaccharides, and lipoarabinomannans, and aid in the phagocytosis of the bacteria. Following bacterial ingestion, the phagosome is acidified and fuses with a lysosome. The resulting phagolysosome contains not only typical lysosomal enzymes, but also an array of highly reactive toxic oxygen and nitrogen intermediates. For pathogenic bacteria to survive, they must be able to circumvent the host's immune response.

During an infection, extracellular bacteria are able to survive by evading or inhibiting phagocytosis, and intracellular bacteria survive within phagocytes by using one of several different strategies. Intracellular survival strategies include inhibiting acidification of the phagosome; decreasing or neutralizing the production of toxic intermediates; preventing fusion of the phagosome and lysosome; or escaping the phagosome and replicating in the cytoplasm of the cell. So bacteria that cause disease may be found growing extracellularly, in a phagosome, or in the cytoplasm of the cell. Because of the diverse sites of bacterial growth, a variety of host immune responses are needed.

Extracellular organisms that are common causes of disease are listed in **Table 6.1.** Diseases caused by these organisms are due to growth and avoidance of phagocytosis at the site of infection,

Table 6.1. Extracellular Organisms Responsible for Common Infections or Diseases

Bordetella pertussis	Neisseria meningitidis
Clostridium sp.	Pseudomonas aeruginosa
Corynebacterium diphtheria	Staphylococcus aureus
Escherichia coli gram (-) bacilli	Streptococcus agalctiae
Haemophilus ducreyi	Streptococcus pneumoniae gram (+)
Haemophilus influenzae (type b and nontypeable)	Streptococcus pyogenes
Helicobacter pylori	Treponema pallidum
Neisseria gonorrhoeae	Vibrio sp.

or to the effects of exotoxins and endotoxins produced by the organism. Since the bacteria and their toxins are extracellular, host defense mechanisms must be able to recognize the bacteria and their components as they occur naturally. Specific recognition of these organisms and toxins is the purview of Abs. In the case of extracellular pathogens, Ab functions to protect the host and clear the infection by three mechanisms: neutralization, complement activation, and opsonization (Figure 6.1).

Ab-mediated neutralization of toxins and bacterial infection prevents the protein or bacteria from binding to receptors on host cells. Without binding, toxins cannot affect cell function, and bacteria cannot attach to and colonize a site. Thus Abs can prevent toxin-mediated disease and decrease the presence of bacteria at a site.

In addition, Abs can activate complement by binding C1qrs to the Fc portion of immunoglobulin (Ig)M and IgG. Complement components are able to increase inflammation at the site of infection, and opsonize and lyse the bacteria. Opsonization occurs because activation of the complement system leads to deposition of complement proteins C3b and C4b on the surface of the bacteria. Phagocytic cells have receptors for these proteins, so C3b and C4b on the surface of bacteria act as handles for phagocytes to bind, enhancing phagocytosis. Finally, Ab itself is able to act as an opsonin. Receptors on phagocytic cells for the Fc portion (FcγR) of IgG function to increase the ability of these cells to bind and ingest Ab-coated bacteria. Since extracellular bacteria survive by evading or inhibiting phagocytosis, these Ab functions are vitally important for enabling the phagocytic cells to ingest and kill extracellular bacteria.

Bacteria that can survive in host cells are listed in **Table 6.2.** These organisms survive by inhibiting phagosome function or by escaping the phagosome to replicate in the cytoplasm of the cell. Because these organisms are growing inside host cells, Abs are unable to recognize, bind, and clear them. Cell-mediated immunity is needed for clearance, recovery, and protection from infection with intracellular bacteria. The type of effector T-cell response developed is also dependent on the intracellular site of bacterial growth, with antigens from cytosolic pathogens activating CD8+ T cells and antigens from vesicular or phagosomal pathogens activating

Table 6.2. Intracellular Organisms Responsible for Human Disease

Chlamydia pneumoniae

Chlamydia tracomatis

Legionella pneumoniae

Listeria monocytogenes

Mycobacterium avium/intracellulare

Mycobacterium tuberculosis, leprae

Rickettsia sp.

Salmonella enterica serovar typhi

CD4⁺ T cells. With the exception of chlamydia and rickettsia, these bacteria are not obligate intracellular pathogens and their entry into the host cell is generally by conventional uptake by a phagocytic cell (usually a macrophage). Once in the macrophage, the bacteria have unique survival strategies.

Bacteria (e.g., mycobacteria) are able to replicate inside the macrophage, so macrophage actions alone are ineffective in clearing the infection. However, because the bacteria are ingested via Toll-like receptors, the macrophages are activated and release many different cytokines. The pathogen's location within the cell stimulates the expression of IL-12, a cytokine that preferentially activates Th1 cells. For intracellular bacteria, activation of acquired immunity may lead to rapid clearance of the infection or containment of the infection at specific sites.

For bacteria that replicate in vesicles, activation of Th1 cells and development of granulomas are primary mechanisms for recovery or containment of the infection. Granulomas are used to wall off infections caused by these bacteria, *Mycobacterium tuberculosis* being the archetypal organism. Granuloma formation and maintenance are dependent on IFN-γ, TNF-α, and lymphotoxin-α3 secreted by Th1 cells. The granuloma is surrounded by effector T cells; it contains mature macrophages, multinucleated giant cells, epithelioid cells, and new monocyte arrivals, along with host cells and dead and dying bacteria. The bacteria are killed by macrophages that are preferentially activated by IFN-γ and TNF-α, cytokines that increase the activation of macrophages, and the production and secretion of toxic radicals. This makes bacterial killing outside the macrophage possible. The granuloma center is often described as caseous, because of its resemblance to cottage cheese. Although granulomas protect the host by containing the infection, they can also lead to loss of function in the tissues where they develop. As long as the host's immune system is intact, cellular immunity is an effective mechanism for containing infections caused by intracellular bacteria.

For cytosolic bacteria, whose antigens are presented by class I MHC molecules, activation of CD8⁺ T cells is important for clearing the infection. Indeed, for listeria, the role of effector CTLs has been amply demonstrated. CTLs kill the bacterially infected cells the same way they destroy cells with a viral infection.

In summary, because bacteria can grow both intracellularly and extracellularly, acquired host defense mechanisms for recovery from, and protec-tion against, these organisms include Abs as well as cell-mediated immunity.

Protozoan Infections

Protozoan diseases (malaria, schistosomiasis, leishmaniasis) cause significant morbidity and mortality in tropical and developing countries. But these diseases are not restricted to the tropics; protozoa such as giardia, toxoplasma, and cryptosporidia have been responsible for disease outbreaks in the United States in recent years. With increased numbers of immunocompromised people living in developed countries, protozoan infections are likely to increase. Most of these parasites are designed to survive initial host immune responses and to produce chronic infection, allowing transmission to others. For some protozoans, the infection is latent, with little or no reproduction of the parasite; this allows the organism to hide from the host's immune response, thus preventing clearance of the organism.

Immune responses to protozoan infections are complex and not fully understood. While both Ab- and cell-mediated mechanisms can be effective in containing protozoan infections, it has been observed that there is a strong polarization of the CD4⁺ T-cell response between Th1 and Th2 phenotypes for many of these organisms. This results in immune responses being skewed toward either cell-mediated immunity or Ab production. It is generally true that intracellular protozoans stimulate Th1 responses, while helminths (parasitic worms, see below) stimulate Th2 responses that lead to the production of IgE, eosinophilia, and mastocytosis.

With entry of protozoa into the host, innate immune responses (including inflammation) are activated. Phagocytic cells and humoral components (such as complement) are often initiating factors, and NK cells and γδ T cells are also activated early in infection. Activation of these cells is important for containing the infection until adaptive immunity is established.

For diseases such as malaria, which can be found both intracellularly and extracellularly, Ab is important for neutralizing the organism's ability to enter either the erythrocytes or hepatocytes. Ab also acts as an opsonin, increasing phagocytosis. Once the protozoa have entered the host cells, cell-mediated immunity is required for clearance and protection. Both T cytotoxic (Tc or CTL) and Th1 cells are activated by intracellular protozoan infections. Th1 cells secrete a number of different cytokines responsible for activation of other T cells and macrophages. It is likely that IFN-γ is important for activating macrophages to increased production of toxic radicals and enhanced intracellular killing, while CTL induces apoptosis in infected host cells.

Intestinal protozoans such as giardia stimulate both humoral and cell-mediated immunity. Experimental models have identified IgA and mast cells as being important to controlling the infection[4,5]; however, the exact mechanisms of recovery and protection in people are still unknown.

Many other protozoans elicit a similar spectrum of immune responses, and it is generally accepted that cell-mediated immune responses are required for protection and recovery from protozoan infections. For diseases like malaria, it is likely that both Ab- and cell-mediated immunity provide some degree of protection. However, this protection is often short-lived and time away from an area of endemic infection results in waning immunity and susceptibility to reinfection.[6]

Diseases Caused by Parasitic Worms

Parasitic worms colonize a variety of niches in the human body. They can be found not only in the gastrointestinal tract, but also in blood, lymphatics, and other deep tissues. The worms gain access to these areas by crossing epithelial barriers. Helminths come in a variety of sizes, and many are multicellular. The size of these pathogens can be problematic, as most parasitic worms are too large to be ingested by phagocytic cells; thus Ab is the major specific host defense mechanism available to recognize and defend against infection. While much still needs to be understood about immune responses to helminths, a strong Th2 response appears to be important in protection from and clearance of parasitic worms, especially those that colonize the gut.

Innate immune response cells participating in host protection include mast cells and eosinophils. Full activation of these responses is dependent on an adaptive Th2 response leading to production of IgE and IgA. IgE mediates mast cell activation by binding to high-affinity receptors on these cells. Once antigen has bound IgE, the mast cell degranulates, releasing mediators including histamine and heparin that are toxic to the parasites. The activated mast cells also secrete cytokines and chemokines to activate inflammation and recruit additional cells to the site of infection, and leukotrienes to stimulate mucous production and smooth muscle contraction.

Ab may also be important in removing tissue and lymphatic helminthes through ADCC. Finally,

Th2-derived cytokines, such as IL-3, IL-4, IL-5, and IL-9, further activate mast cells and eosinophils.

Taken together, host defense mechanisms against helminths are skewed toward Ab production and cytokines to expel the worms from both the gut and deep tissues. Thus, mechanisms of humoral immunity are clearly important for clearance of parasitic worms.

In summary, pathogens grow at many different sites within the host. The type of pathogen and the site at which it replicates determine the type of immune response needed for clearance and protection. A summary of the types of responses generated to different organisms is shown in **Figure 6.4.**

EMERGING INFECTIOUS DISEASES

In 1992, the Institute of Medicine released a report outlining the problem of emerging infectious disease. Emerging diseases are defined as "diseases whose incidence in humans has increased within the past two decades or threatens to increase in the near future.[7]" In the past 30 years, a number of new diseases have been identified. These include hemorrhagic viruses like Marburg (1967) and Ebola (1973); Legionnaire's disease and *Legionella pneumophila* (1976); acquired immune deficiency syndrome (AIDS) (1981) and the human immunodeficiency virus (1984); hantavirus (1993); *Escherichia coli* 0157:H7 (1996); the outbreak of "bird flu" (H5N1) in Hong Kong (1997); West Nile encephalitis in the New York City area (1999); and severe acute respiratory syndrome (SARS) in Asia (2003). Some of these diseases occur sporadically in isolated outbreaks, coming and going without scientists ever identifying the reservoir or vector (e.g., Ebola and Marburg viruses in Africa). Others, like *E. coli* 0157:H7, are related to food and food preparation and also occur sporadically. AIDS has emerged and become pandemic in less than 30 years, devastating large portions of Africa and Asia. Diseases like "bird flu" and SARS are currently contained, but remain a concern because of their potential to cause pandemic disease.

Other diseases considered to be "emerging diseases" are recognized human pathogens, such as *Mycobacterium tuberculosis* and *Staphylococcus aureus*, which have evolved multiple drug resistance. Diseases caused by these organisms are increasingly difficult to treat and are spreading across the world.

The Institute of Medicine also identified demographic and environmental conditions that favor spread of emerging diseases (**Table 6.3**). Recognizing this threat, the Centers for Disease

Immune responses to different types of infectious agents

Type of Agent	Effector mechanism		
	Antibody	T_h1 cells	CTL
Viruses 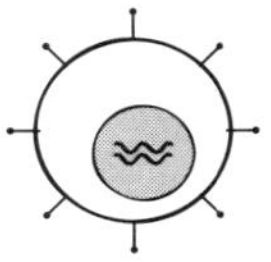	IgG Neutralization of virions extracellularly ADCC infected cells		Induction of apoptosis in infected cells
Extracellular bacteria 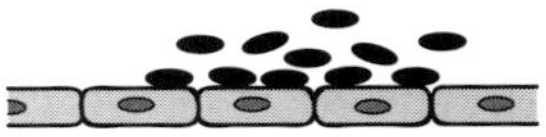	IgM, IgG Neutralization Opsonization Complement activation		
Intracellular bacteria 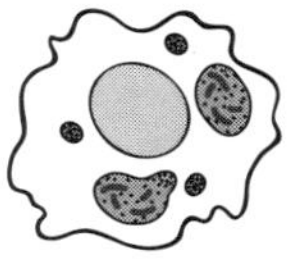	IgG +/-	Macrophage activation Granuloma formation	Apoptosis of cells with cystolic bacteria
Protozoans 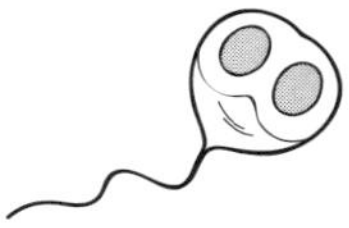	IgG Neutralization Opsonization Complement activation	Macrophage activation	
Parasitic worms 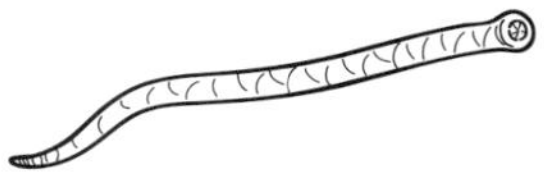	IgE Mast cell activation		

Figure 6.4. Immunologic effector functions based on type of pathogen.

Control and Prevention (CDC) has adopted emergency management plans that include surveillance to rapidly identify new disease threats. By partnering with public health officials in the United States and beyond, scientists and physicians can develop strategies for responding to newly emerging pathogens. Early response allows basic research into the identification of new drugs and agents, such as vaccines, to combat the diseases and protect the public.[7]

Table 6.3. Conditions That Contribute to the Emergence of New Infectious Disease

Increased population growth

Increased international travel

Changes in human behavior

Humans entering, living in, and modifying wilderness habitats and encountering new infectious agents and disease vectors

Development of drug resistance in pathogens that were previously treatable

Increased transport of animal and food products

Changes in food processing

PREVENTION AND TREATMENT OF INFECTIOUS DISEASES

One of the most important mechanisms for preventing infectious disease is hygiene. The advent of clean water supplies brought a rapid decrease in deaths from infectious illness. Although in most developed countries clean water is considered the norm, clean water is a luxury and a public health goal yet to be achieved in many areas. Beyond clean water, food supplies need to be secure from pathogenic microorganisms. Indeed, recent outbreaks of hepatitis A, *Salmonella agona* and *E. coli* 0157:H7 have been linked to contaminated and prepared foods. Personal hygiene and avoidance of risky behaviors are also important for preventing disease.

Many diseases are not directly preventable by monitoring our food and water or by changing our behavior. They may be spread by aerosols or droplets, or by vectors we cannot totally avoid, so treatment is often necessary. In many cases, diseases caused by pathogenic bacteria can be treated with antibiotics, greatly reducing the morbidity and mortality previously associated with them. Some viral diseases—in particular those caused by HIV, herpes viruses (including herpes simplex virus, cytomegalovirus, and varicella-zoster virus) and influenza viruses—can be treated with synthetic agents that block specific pathways in the virus life cycle. Infections with hepatitis B and C viruses are treatable with recombinant interferons. Fungal and protozoan infections are often difficult to treat because of the similarity of these organisms' metabolic pathways to those of human cells. Although many diseases can be treated with specific antimicrobials, there are many pathogens for which we have not found an appropriate drug therapy, and some infectious agents have developed drug resistance. Development of new antimicrobials continues to be an important area of biomedical research.

One mechanism for prevention is the generation of artificial immunity. Immunization is the induction of a specific immune response to a killed or weakened pathogen. While immunization against smallpox has been practiced in some form for hundreds of years, immunization has succeeded in reducing the burden of many infectious diseases in the last century. One of the greatest achievements of vaccination was the worldwide elimination of smallpox in 1979. Another infectious disease, polio, is on the verge of being eliminated, with pockets remaining only in Africa and the Indian subcontinent. The incidence of many other diseases has also been reduced in this country through the use of vaccines. Most of these vaccines are discussed in greater detail below.

ACTIVE AND PASSIVE IMMUNIZATION

Active Immunization

Specific active immunity may be acquired naturally, through exposure to infectious agents, or it may be induced by immunization with inactivated (killed) or attenuated live organisms or toxoids. As described in Chapter 1, the body's first contact with an organism (i.e., an antigen) stimulates immunologic memory, allowing the body to effectively prevent later infection by the same organism. Because we develop complete and long-lasting immunity to many pathogens, we rarely suffer twice from the same disease. Active immunization (vaccination) takes advantage of this process by exposing the body to a relatively harmless form of the pathogen to stimulate the body's defenses and induce immunologic memory against subsequent exposure to the antigen.

Active immunization traditionally uses either attenuated live microorganisms or inactivated microbial products and some synthetic peptides. For some diseases, such as poliomyelitis, both approaches have been used.

Generally, live vaccines induce an immunologic response closely resembling natural infection. The organisms in attenuated live vaccines replicate in the host until halted by the immunologic response to the vaccine. This multiplication of organisms allows live vaccines to produce greater antigenic loads than can be achieved with inactive vaccines, even though the amount of antigen initially administered with inactivated vaccines is generally greater. An inactivated vaccine may contain killed whole organisms (e.g., pertussis), inactivated bacterial toxins (toxoids), extracts of capsular material (e.g., *H. influenzae* type b), or other components (e.g., hepatitis B surface antigen) (**Table 6.4**).

The relative merits of inactivated vaccines have been debated. The controversy focuses on their relative immunogenicity, safety, ease of production, distribution, administration, stability, and cost.

Attenuated live vaccines. Attenuated organisms are live pathogens whose virulence and ability to replicate in the host have been significantly reduced so they do not cause disease in healthy individuals. The first systematically attenuated vaccine was produced by Louis Pasteur for chicken cholera. To develop a safe vaccine, the pathogenicity of an organism must be reduced substantially, but for the vaccine to be effective, the organism must retain sufficient

Table 6.4. Characteristics of Vaccines

Attenuated live vaccines
Diminished pathogenicity
Both cell-mediated and humoral immunity
Longer lasting antibody protection
Ability to revert to pathogenic variant

Killed, inactivated vaccines
Nonreplicating and noninfectious
Need for multiple, booster administrations
Primarily humoral response
May be composed of whole organisms or subunits

pathogenicity to infect the host. Organisms have been attenuated by species adaptation (smallpox), tissue adaptation (measles, mumps, rubella), and temperature-selected mutants (influenza). Such organisms, although unable to reproduce in numbers adequate to result in disease, cause a subclinical infection sufficient to stimulate both cellular and humoral responses. Because these organisms reproduce the same way as the pathogens, the host's immune response to an attenuated vaccine will mirror the immune response generated by a natural infection.

The use of cowpox virus (vaccinia) to prevent smallpox (caused by the variola virus) is an example of a relatively nonpathogenic virus used to stimulate immunity to a closely related pathogen. More commonly, however, attenuated live vaccines have been produced by adaptation of virulent viruses to unnatural host cells, or temperatures. Examples include the attenuation of Sabin poliovirus strain; measles, mumps, and rubella vaccines through growth in diploid cell lines; and cold-adapted influenza and poliovirus. The success of attenuation through adaptation depends on characteristics of the organisms involved, types of culture media and conditions, and the number of passages through laboratory culture.

The infection caused by an ideally attenuated organism should provoke an immune response that mimics the response to the natural infection as closely as possible while producing little or no illness. The live virus should not be teratogenic, abortogenic, or oncogenic, and it should be unable to establish a latent infection. The organism's ability to disseminate throughout a population should be minimal. And the attenuated organism must be genetically stable and incapable of reverting to a pathogenic form.

The genetic stability of attenuated strains is an important concern. Even a minimal level of reversion, such as producing one case of disease per 100,000 vaccinated subjects, is unacceptable

if that case provides a focus of outbreak. The attenuated oral polio vaccine provides an example of genetic reversion to pathogenicity. In the United States, about one in 2.4 million individuals receiving the live vaccine developed polio as a result of genetic reversion. Since the last known case of wild-type polio occurred in the United States in 1979 and polio is considered to have been eradicated in the western hemisphere, the risk of vaccine-derived polio led to the discontinuation of its use in the United States in 2000.[8] (http://www.cdc.gov/nip/ed/vpd2004/vpd04polio-script.pdf). The killed injectable vaccine is still used, however. Even in areas where polio is endemic (Central and West Africa and the Indian subcontinent), the risks of vaccine-derived polio have caused the World Health Organization (WHO) to recommend discontinuation of the use of the attenuated oral polio vaccine as soon as feasible after certification of eradication to prevent vaccine-acquired polio.[9]

Killed/inactivated vaccines. Inactivated, or killed, vaccines do not replicate, and are generally less efficient in inducing an immune response than attenuated vaccines. The antigenic mass needed for an inactivated vaccine to generate a protective immune response is often many times greater than that for attenuated live vaccines. Differences in vaccine production procedures, cost, and administration created by the larger dose size may be considerable. Because there is no replication of the bacteria or virus, inactivated vaccines need multiple doses to achieve protective levels of immunity and primarily a humoral response is stimulated. Usually, two or three doses of inactivated vaccine must be given to stimulate the primary and secondary responses needed to produce long-lasting immunity. Furthermore, inactivated vaccines prepared from infected cell or tissue cultures may contain large amounts of extraneous material, increasing the possibility of adverse reactions. Because inactivated vaccines do not replicate within the host, they cannot revert to a pathogenic variant and cause clinical disease.

The classic approaches to producing inactivated vaccines use biochemical purification and biophysical inactivation, such as physical inactivation of whole viruses (e.g., intramuscular influenza vaccine, polio, hepatitis A) or bacteria (e.g., *Vibrio cholerae*). Because of the wide variety of antigens, inactivated whole cell vaccines can stimulate strong protective immune responses and are therefore highly effective vaccines. Indeed, some of the most promising vaccines for diseases like malaria include inactivated whole pathogens.[10]

Purified macromolecules as vaccines.
Macromolecules such as proteins and polysaccharides can act as immunogens. Use of macromolecules as vaccines is dependent on identification of protective epitopes in these moieties. Historically, identification of protective epitopes has relied on genetics, biochemistry, and immunology to pinpoint sites that stimulated the production of protective Abs. The revolution in genomics has meant that viral and bacterial sequences can be searched for proteins homologous to others that stimulate protective immune responses. And previously unrecognized proteins can be identified and tested for their ability to induce protective immune responses. Because organisms do not have to be cultured to identify important proteins and epitopes, this technology will allow scientists to design vaccines for medically significant organisms we cannot successfully cultivate in vitro.[11,12]

Polysaccharide vaccines. Many important pathogenic bacteria have capsules able to inhibit phagocytosis of bacteria and protect the microorganisms from innate host defenses (e.g., *Streptococcus pneumoniae, Haemophilus influenzae, Neisseria meningitidis*). The polysaccharides that form these capsules are antigenically important because Abs specific for these polysaccharides act as an opsonin, facilitating phagocytosis and providing protective immunity. Gram-negative bacteria also contain antigenic lipopolysaccharides. Polysaccharides, and the polysaccharide portion of lipopolysaccharides, can be isolated from the bacteria or purified from the culture medium; they are made up of hundreds of repeats of primarily monosaccharide and phosphate. The repeats are unique for each bacterial species and subtype, and have been used for immunologic identification of bacteria.

Because of their structure, polysaccharides and lipopolysaccharides are T-independent antigens; primarily, the B-1 subset of B cells is activated. While vaccines made from pure polysaccharides of *H. influenzae, N. meningitidis,* and *S. pneumoniae* are immunogenic in adults and older children, children under 2 do not develop any immune response to naturally occurring polysaccharides, placing them at increased risk of infections with these organisms.

To counter these problems, polysaccharides have been conjugated to proteins, changing the polysaccharide into a T-dependent antigen. T-dependent Ags are able to induce production of IgG and immunologic memory in all age groups. For children under 2 years, conjugate polysaccharide vaccines are used to develop protective immunity and immunologic memory. Four conjugate vaccines for *H. influenzae* serotype "b" have been

developed and licensed for use in children, as has a conjugate pneumococcal vaccine.

Toxoid vaccines. Bacterial toxins are proteins responsible for pathogenesis in infections such as tetanus and diphtheria. In the early 1900s it was demonstrated that Abs to toxins could prevent disease. A toxoid is a chemically inactivated toxin with the same three-dimensional structure as the active toxin; when used as an immunogen, it stimulates production of neutralizing Ab. Unfortunately, chemical inactivation has potential problems, including structural changes that result in the loss of epitopes important for eliciting protective immunity, and incomplete inactivation could result in reversion to a biologically active toxin.

The problems inherent in chemical inactivation are being addressed by genetic inactivation of the toxin. Genetic inactivation involves the production of two or more mutations in the toxin gene, because multiple mutations decrease the likelihood of reversion to wild-type toxin. These genetically mutated toxins are able to stimulate protective immunity to the naturally occurring toxin without the risks of incomplete inactivation or loss of important epitopes. This technique has been successful in the development of pertussis and diphtheria toxoids.

Recombinant-antigen vaccines. Recombinant DNA (rDNA) technology has been used to engineer both subunit and attenuated viral and bacterial vaccines. Attenuation by recombination, achieved by introducing multiple mutations or deleting important proteins, results in the production of organisms with low reversion rates. Attenuated herpes simplex vaccines have been tested in animals, but are not currently in clinical trials, and an attenuated cholera vaccine is being tested.[13] rDNA technology has excelled in the development of protein subunit vaccines.

Proteins from rDNA technology have been expressed in a wide variety of hosts, including bacteria, yeast, mammalian cells, mammals, and plants. The most successful use of recombinant technology for vaccine production is the expression of hepatitis B surface antigen (HBsAg) in the *Saccharomyces cerevisiae* yeast. Expression of HBsAg in this vector resulted in the formation of highly immunogenic particles containing this Ag. These particles resemble the immunogenic Dane particles, which had been purified from human plasma. In addition, recombinant HBsAg lack the potential pathogenicity of plasma-derived vaccines. Interestingly, expression of HBsAg in a bacterial system does not result in particle formation and is of decreased immunogenicity. Proteins from human papillomavirus (HPV) have also been expressed and are approved for use in humans. The now-withdrawn vaccine for Lyme disease was produced by expressing outer-surface protein A of *Borrelia burgdorferi* in *E. coli*. The vaccine was withdrawn because of vaccine-induced arthritis.

Recombinant-vector vaccines. Immunization with a live vaccine is advantageous because there is generally a greater immune response when antigens are produced within the host. The development of live vectors carrying unrelated genes is being investigated. These vectors, which include both viruses and bacteria, can deliver a variety of foreign proteins. Because the antigens are presented in the context of a live infection, they stimulate the production of broad-based immunity. Currently, there are no licensed vaccines using this technology, although vaccinia, herpes simplex virus, and adenoviruses have been engineered as live-vector vaccines. The only recombinant viral vector that has been clinically tested is a vaccinia vector expressing glycoprotein 160 (gp160) from the human immunodeficiency virus. Unfortunately, it was poorly immunogenic for gp160 in phase I clinical trials.

Recombinant bacterial vectors have been designed to deliver foreign antigens to the gastrointestinal mucosa following oral delivery. Bacteria used for oral immunization include *Salmonella typhi*, *Listeria monocytogenes*, *Vibrio cholerae*, and *Shigella flexneri*. Bacille Calmette-Guérin has also been modified to present foreign proteins and has been tested in mice for immunogenicity, using several delivery routes. It has been observed that many of the genetically engineered bacteria either retain too much virulence or lose the ability to replicate in the gut, significantly decreasing the immunogenicity of the foreign antigens.[13]

DNA vaccines. DNA vaccines are nonreplicating vaccines that deliver the genetic information for the vaccine antigen directly into the cell. They are derived from plasmid technology, in which a cell is transformed through the uptake of a plasmid to express a particular antigen. The DNA can be injected as naked DNA, or it can be incorporated into microparticles that enhance the uptake of the vaccine by the cell.

DNA vaccines work by stimulating transcription and translation of the vaccine antigen by the transformed host cell. In the transformed cell, protein may be expressed on the cell surface, as secreted protein, peptides associated with class I MHC molecules, or both. These different routes of antigen presentation result in stimulation of both Ab production and cell-mediated immunity. The transformed cell also can express multiple copies of the vaccine antigen, which amplifies both the amount of antigen and the immune response.

DNA vaccines have been demonstrated to be effective in many animal models.

While the immune response to vaccination with naked DNA is not robust, facilitating uptake of DNA or including adjuvants in the vaccine has the potential to significantly increase immune responses. Immunogenicity of DNA vaccines can be enhanced through use of a "gene gun," microemulsions, and microparticles made from lipids, lipospermines, and poly lactide co-glycide (PLG). All of these mechanisms have been used to increase the delivery of DNA into the cell and promote immune responses.[14,15]

Safety issues still to be resolved with DNA vaccines include possible production of anti-DNA Abs and integration of DNA into the host cell genome. Initial results suggest these are not clinical problems and that DNA vaccines have an excellent safety record.

While both Ab- and cell-mediated immunity are seen following vaccination with DNA vaccines, the production of vaccine antigen in the cytoplasm of the host cell makes this technology especially good for the elicitation of CTL.

Synthetic peptide vaccines. In an immune response to naturally occurring antigens, neither Abs nor T-cell receptors recognize the entire macromolecule; rather they bind to a portion of the antigen called an epitope. In the case of Abs (B-cell epitopes), the epitope may be linear (successive amino acids or monosaccharides) or conformational (formed by bringing together distant amino acids in the three-dimensional folding of a protein). For T cells, the epitopes are always linear and are peptides 7–30 amino acids in length. Shorter peptides are able to bind class I MHC molecules, while longer peptides can bind class II MHC molecules.

Technology exists to identify B-cell and T-cell epitopes. If an important B-cell epitope is conformationally determined, the full macromolecule is usually needed for immunogenicity. There is a report, however, that a conformational epitope has been maintained in a synthesized peptide vaccine.[16] Linear epitopes of fewer than 20 amino acids have been successfully produced for use as vaccines. For T-cell epitopes, it is also possible to synthesize epitopes that interact with an MHC molecule and a T-cell receptor.

Peptides encoding B-cell epitopes are often poorly immunogenic, so their immunogenicity must be increased before they can be used as a vaccine. Much of the work on epitope-derived vaccines has been directed toward development of a malaria vaccine. This work has demonstrated that increasing the immunogenicity of the peptides makes production of synthetic epitope-derived vaccines feasible. It has been shown that immunogenicity can be enhanced by chemically conjugating the peptide to an immunogenic carrier protein such as tetanus toxoid; genetically fusing it to a carrier protein, creating aggregates of the peptide; or producing a complex containing multiple antigenic peptides.[10,16]

Epitopes recognized by CTL are also poorly immunogenic. To stimulate immunity to these peptides, the CTL epitope must be presented with an epitope or protein that can activate a T-helper cell.

Thus peptide vaccines need to overcome immunogenicity hurdles to become clinically effective. Many of these hurdles may be overcome by using multiple epitopes, appropriate adjuvants, and better delivery vehicles.

Multivalent subunit vaccines. Multivalent vaccines are vaccines that contain more than one purified antigen. With a single injection, multivalent vaccines stimulate an immune response to a number of different antigens and induce immunity to more than one disease.

A multivalent subunit vaccine can be composed of either multiple proteins or peptides. If proteins are used, they may be toxoids or viral surface proteins. An example of a widely used, toxoid-based multivalent subunit vaccine is the diphtheria/tetanus vaccine; it includes two purified toxoids and stimulates immunity to each with one injection. Multivalent subunit vaccines may also be composed of peptide subunits rather than whole proteins. Many different peptides can be combined into a single vaccine, although when using peptides, problems with immunogenicity and inclusion of the appropriate epitopes remain.

While multivalent vaccines offer a mechanism for developing broad-based immunity, when designing them it is important to ensure that inclusion of one subunit does not suppress the immune response to a second subunit. This and a similar phenomenon known as "original antigenic sin" have been demonstrated with both Ab and T-cell immunity. When they occur, the immune response to one antigen inhibits the response to a second or newer Ag, leaving the individual unprotected to the second antigen.

Multivalent subunit vaccines hold great promise for simplifying vaccine administration, but the vaccines will need to be carefully constructed to assure appropriate immune responses.

Adjuvants. Adjuvants enhance the immune response to vaccines. Even though adjuvants have been used for more than 80 years, the mechanisms by which they enhance immune responses are not fully understood. It was originally believed that adjuvants, such as oil-in-water emulsions and aluminum salts, acted primarily as deposition agents to extend the time an antigen remained at the site of injection. But this explanation is insufficient to explain all the effects of adjuvants. Today it is believed that adjuvants work by affecting antigen delivery and presentation, inducing immunologically important cytokines, and affecting antigen-presenting cells. Not all adjuvants are effective with all antigens, nor do all adjuvants have the same effects on the immune response. For example, aluminum salts can increase vaccine antigen uptake by antigen-presenting cells and generate high-tittered antiserum, but they do not stimulate cell-mediated immunity. Adjuvants fall into a number of different classes (**Table 6.5**), of which only three—aluminum salts, MF59 (a microfluidized emulsion), and monophosphoryl-lipid A (a detoxified lipid A)—are either licensed or have received significant clinical evaluation.

Historically and today, aluminum salts are the major adjuvant used in human vaccines. Three aluminum salts are used: crystalline aluminum oxyhydroxide, amorphous aluminum hydroxyphosphate, and alum, a phosphate precipitate of aluminum potassium sulfate. The mechanism by which aluminum salts potentiate immune

Table 6.5. Types of Adjuvants

Type of Adjuvant	Example
Mineral Salt	Aluminum hydroxide/phosphate (alum)
Microbial	Muramyl dipeptide (MDP) Bacterial exotoxins Monophosphoryl lipid A (MPL) Bacterial DNA
Particulate	Biodegradable polymer microspheres Immune-stimulating complexes Liposomes
Oil-emulsions and surfactant-based adjuvants	Freund's incomplete adjuvant Microfluidized emulsions (MF59) Saponins
Synthetic	MDP derivatives Non-ionic block copolymers Synthetic polynucleotides
Cytokines	IL-2, IL-12, GM-CSF, IFN-γ

(Adapted from Plotkin SA, Orenstein WA. *Vaccines.* 4th ed. Philadelphia, PA: WB Saunders; 2004:Ch. 6.)

responses to adsorbed antigens is still not known, but the possible mechanisms include (1) acting as a deposition agent, keeping the antigen at the injection site for slow release; (2) induction of an inflammatory response at the site of immunization; and (3) conversion of soluble antigen to a particulate antigen. Antigen retention at the injection site results in slow movement of the antigen to the draining lymph nodes, and stimulation of the immune response over an extended time—mimicking the presence of antigen during an infection. Since inflammatory responses are the initial responses in an infection (leading to stimulation of acquired immunity), if aluminum salts were to stimulate inflammation they would attract macrophages. The macrophages would ingest the antigen, carry it to a draining lymph node, and initiate a specific immune response. Finally, conversion of the antigen from a soluble to particulate form would help retain antigen at the injection site and increase phagocytosis and presentation of the vaccine antigen.

Oil-in-water emulsions can also lead to increased antigen uptake and presentation. But in the absence of bacterial components, most of these emulsions do not appear to significantly increase macrophage activation. Also, adjuvants, such as incomplete Freund's adjuvant, have been associated with adverse effects. One oil-in-water emulsion approved for use in humans is MF59. MF59 is a microfluidized emulsion of squalene and two surfactants. It is as safe as aluminum salt adjuvants but is more potent, stimulating increased Ab production.

Many structural components of microorganisms are themselves antigenic and may be suitable adjuvants, because microbial products bind to phagocytes through PAMP and Toll receptors. The binding activates the inflammatory pathway including cytokine production and release, which can upregulate immune responses. Unfortunately bacterial products are often toxic and have significant adverse effects in animal models including fever, adjuvant arthritis, and uveitis, precluding their use in humans. There are two bacterial products with little toxicity: monophosphoryl lipid A and muramyl dipeptide.

Monophosphoryl lipid A is derived from a heptoseless mutant of *Salmonella minnesota*. The lipopolysaccharide structure has been modified to remove a phosphate and a fatty acid. It is much less toxic than the parent lipopolysaccharide and is able to activate macrophages without the potential toxic effects of other bacterial components. It can enhance not only Ab production, but also Th1 responses, leading to increased cell-mediated immunity to the vaccine antigen.[17]

Another bacterial-derived adjuvant with reduced toxicity is muramyl dipeptide (MDP), a mycobacterial peptide. Unlike other mycobacterial components, the adjuvant properties of MDP are present when administered either parenterally or orally in water-in-oil emulsions, but it is rapidly excreted in the urine when given in an aqueous solution.[17] MDP is not currently licensed for use in any country.

Liposomes, particles composed of vaccine antigens within a phospholipid bilayer, and other particulate adjuvants have the potential to release antigen into the cytoplasm of antigen-presenting cells. Presentation of antigens from the cytoplasm of cells would result in activation of CTL rather than Ab or T-helper cells—an advantage for development of immunity to viral antigens. Two virosomal vaccines (viral membrane glycoproteins incorporated into liposomes) have been licensed: Inflexal for influenza and Epaxal for hepatitis A.[17]

Vaccine boosting and schedules. The Advisory Committee on Immunization Practices (ACIP) regularly reviews and recommends immunization schedules for children and adolescents to ensure the schedule is current with changes in vaccine formulations and reflects revised recommendations for the use of licensed vaccines. These recommendations are approved by ACIP, the American Academy of Family Physicians, and the American Academy of Pediatrics and published by the CDC; recommendations for 2006 are presented in **Table 6.6.**[18] A new addition to these recommendations is that of yearly influenza immunization for individuals aged 6 months to 18 years.

Vaccine recommendations for adults are made by the ACIP, American College of Obstetricians and Gynecologists, and the American Academy of Family Physicians; their 2004–2005 recommendations are shown in **Table 6.7.**[19]

Recommendations for vaccinations change regularly; the most current recommendations are available from the CDC.

Risks and benefits of vaccines. The purpose of vaccination is to establish an immune response with memory cells adequate to provide immunity upon renewed contact with the antigen, but the first contact with the antigen (during vaccination) should not be harmful to the patient. The goal in developing a vaccine is to modify the pathogenic effect of the organism without losing its antigenicity.

Risk of complications from vaccine administration must be balanced against the risk of contracting the disease. For diseases that have been eradicated (such as smallpox), the risk of untoward effects from vaccination outweighs the possible benefits. In the developed world, the risk of vaccine-induced paralysis with the attenuated polio

Table 6.6. Immunization Schedule for Children

DEPARTMENT OF HEALTH AND HUMAN SERVICES • CENTERS FOR DISEASE CONTROL AND PREVENTION

Recommended Immunization Schedule for Persons Aged 0–6 Years—UNITED STATES • 2007

Vaccine ▼ Age ►	Birth	1 month	2 months	4 months	6 months	12 months	15 months	18 months	19–23 months	2–3 years	4–6 years
Hepatitis B[1]	HepB	HepB		see footnote 1	HepB				HepB Series		
Rotavirus[2]			Rota	Rota	Rota						
Diphtheria, Tetanus, Pertussis[3]			DTaP	DTaP	DTaP		DTaP				DTaP
Haemophilus influenzae type b[4]			Hib	Hib	Hib[4]	Hib		Hib			
Pneumococcal[5]			PCV	PCV	PCV	PCV				PCV / PPV	
Inactivated Poliovirus			IPV	IPV	IPV						IPV
Influenza[6]					Influenza (Yearly)						
Measles, Mumps, Rubella[7]						MMR					MMR
Varicella[8]						Varicella					Varicella
Hepatitis A[9]						HepA (2 doses)				HepA Series	
Meningococcal[10]										MPSV4	

Legend:
- Range of recommended ages
- Catch-up immunization
- Certain high-risk groups

This schedule indicates the recommended ages for routine administration of currently licensed childhood vaccines, as of December 1, 2006, for children aged 0–6 years. Additional information is available at http://www.cdc.gov/nip/recs/child-schedule.htm. Any dose not administered at the recommended age should be administered at any subsequent visit, when indicated and feasible. Additional vaccines may be licensed and recommended during the year. Licensed combination vaccines may be used whenever any components of the combination are indicated and other components of the vaccine are not contraindicated and if approved by the Food and Drug Administration for that dose of the series. Providers should consult the respective Advisory Committee on Immunization Practices statement for detailed recommendations. Clinically significant adverse events that follow immunization should be reported to the Vaccine Adverse Event Reporting System (VAERS). Guidance about how to obtain and complete a VAERS form is available at http://www.vaers. hhs.gov or by telephone, 800-822-7967.

1. Hepatitis B vaccine (HepB). *(Minimum age: birth)*

At birth:
- Administer monovalent HepB to all newborns before hospital discharge.
- If mother is hepatitis surface antigen (HBsAg)-positive, administer HepB and 0.5 mL of hepatitis B immune globulin (HBIG) within 12 hours of birth.
- If mother's HBsAg status is unknown, administer HepB within 12 hours of birth. Determine the HBsAg status as soon as possible and if HBsAg-positive, administer HBIG (no later than age 1 week).
- If mother is HBsAg-negative, the birth dose can only be delayed with physician's order and mother's negative HBsAg laboratory report documented in the infant's medical record.

After the birth dose:
- The HepB series should be completed with either monovalent HepB or a combination vaccine containing HepB. The second dose should be administered at age 1–2 months. The final dose should be administered at age ≥24 weeks. Infants born to HBsAg-positive mothers should be tested for HBsAg and antibody to HBsAg after completion of ≥3 doses of a licensed HepB series, at age 9–18 months (generally at the next well-child visit).

4-month dose:
- It is permissible to administer 4 doses of HepB when combination vaccines are administered after the birth dose. If monovalent HepB is used for doses after the birth dose, a dose at age 4 months is not needed.

2. Rotavirus vaccine (Rota). *(Minimum age: 6 weeks)*
- Administer the first dose at age 6–12 weeks. Do not start the series later than age 12 weeks.
- Administer the final dose in the series by age 32 weeks. Do not administer a dose later than age 32 weeks.
- Data on safety and efficacy outside of these age ranges are insufficient.

3. Diphtheria and tetanus toxoids and acellular pertussis vaccine (DTaP). *(Minimum age: 6 weeks)*
- The fourth dose of DTaP may be administered as early as age 12 months, provided 6 months have elapsed since the third dose.
- Administer the final dose in the series at age 4–6 years.

4. Haemophilus influenzae type b conjugate vaccine (Hib). *(Minimum age: 6 weeks)*
- If PRP-OMP (PedvaxHIB® or ComVax® [Merck]) is administered at ages 2 and 4 months, a dose at age 6 months is not required.
- TriHiBit® (DTaP/Hib) combination products should not be used for primary immunization but can be used as boosters following any Hib vaccine in children aged ≥12 months.

5. Pneumococcal vaccine. *(Minimum age: 6 weeks for pneumococcal conjugate vaccine [PCV]; 2 years for pneumococcal polysaccharide vaccine [PPV])*
- Administer PCV at ages 24–59 months in certain high-risk groups. Administer PPV to children aged ≥2 years in certain high-risk groups. See *MMWR* 2000;49(No. RR-9):1–35.

6. Influenza vaccine. *(Minimum age: 6 months for trivalent inactivated influenza vaccine [TIV]; 5 years for live, attenuated influenza vaccine [LAIV])*
- All children aged 6–59 months and close contacts of all children aged 0–59 months are recommended to receive influenza vaccine.
- Influenza vaccine is recommended annually for children aged ≥59 months with certain risk factors, health-care workers, and other persons (including household members) in close contact with persons in groups at high risk. See *MMWR* 2006;55(No. RR-10):1–41.
- For healthy persons aged 5–49 years, LAIV may be used as an alternative to TIV.
- Children receiving TIV should receive 0.25 mL if aged 6–35 months or 0.5 mL if aged ≥3 years.
- Children aged <9 years who are receiving influenza vaccine for the first time should receive 2 doses (separated by ≥4 weeks for TIV and ≥6 weeks for LAIV).

7. Measles, mumps, and rubella vaccine (MMR). *(Minimum age: 12 months)*
- Administer the second dose of MMR at age 4–6 years. MMR may be administered before age 4–6 years, provided ≥4 weeks have elapsed since the first dose and both doses are administered at age ≥12 months.

8. Varicella vaccine. *(Minimum age: 12 months)*
- Administer the second dose of varicella vaccine at age 4–6 years. Varicella vaccine may be administered before age 4–6 years, provided that ≥3 months have elapsed since the first dose and both doses are administered at age ≥12 months. If second dose was administered ≥28 days following the first dose, the second dose does not need to be repeated.

9. Hepatitis A vaccine (HepA). *(Minimum age: 12 months)*
- HepA is recommended for all children aged 1 year (i.e., aged 12–23 months). The 2 doses in the series should be administered at least 6 months apart.
- Children not fully vaccinated by age 2 years can be vaccinated at subsequent visits.
- HepA is recommended for certain other groups of children, including in areas where vaccination programs target older children. See *MMWR* 2006;55(No. RR-7):1–23.

10. Meningococcal polysaccharide vaccine (MPSV4). *(Minimum age: 2 years)*
- Administer MPSV4 to children aged 2–10 years with terminal complement deficiencies or anatomic or functional asplenia and certain other high-risk groups. See *MMWR* 2005;54(No. RR-7):1–21.

The Recommended Immunization Schedules for Persons Aged 0–18 Years are approved by the Advisory Committee on Immunization Practices (http://www.cdc.gov/nip/acip), the American Academy of Pediatrics (http://www.aap.org), and the American Academy of Family Physicians (http://www.aafp.org).

SAFER • HEALTHIER • PEOPLE™

CS103164

Table 6.6. *(Continued)*

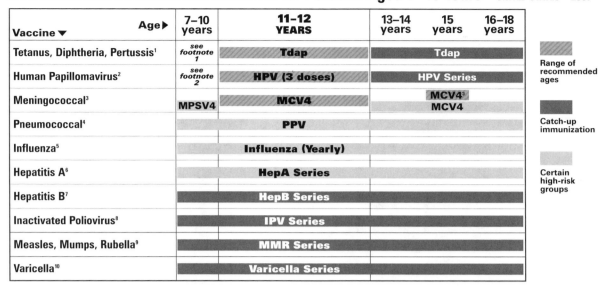

DEPARTMENT OF HEALTH AND HUMAN SERVICES • CENTERS FOR DISEASE CONTROL AND PREVENTION

Recommended Immunization Schedule for Persons Aged 7–18 Years—UNITED STATES • 2007

Vaccine ▼ Age▶	7–10 years	11–12 YEARS	13–14 years	15 years	16–18 years
Tetanus, Diphtheria, Pertussis[1]	see footnote 1	Tdap	Tdap		
Human Papillomavirus[2]	see footnote 2	HPV (3 doses)	HPV Series		
Meningococcal[3]	MPSV4	MCV4	MCV4[3] / MCV4		
Pneumococcal[4]	PPV				
Influenza[5]	Influenza (Yearly)				
Hepatitis A[6]	HepA Series				
Hepatitis B[7]	HepB Series				
Inactivated Poliovirus[8]	IPV Series				
Measles, Mumps, Rubella[9]	MMR Series				
Varicella[10]	Varicella Series				

Range of recommended ages
Catch-up immunization
Certain high-risk groups

This schedule indicates the recommended ages for routine administration of currently licensed childhood vaccines, as of December 1, 2006, for children aged 7–18 years. Additional information is available at **http://www.cdc.gov/nip/recs/child-schedule.htm.** Any dose not administered at the recommended age should be administered at any subsequent visit, when indicated and feasible. Additional vaccines may be licensed and recommended during the year. Licensed combination vaccines may be used whenever any components of the combination are indicated and other components of the vaccine are not contraindicated and if approved by the Food and Drug Administration for that dose of the series. Providers should consult the respective Advisory Committee on Immunization Practices statement for detailed recommendations. Clinically significant adverse events that follow immunization should be reported to the Vaccine Adverse Event Reporting System (VAERS). Guidance about how to obtain and complete a VAERS form is available at **http://www.vaers.hhs.gov** or by telephone, **800-822-7967.**

1. Tetanus and diphtheria toxoids and acellular pertussis vaccine (Tdap).
(Minimum age: 10 years for BOOSTRIX® and 11 years for ADACEL™)
- Administer at age 11–12 years for those who have completed the recommended childhood DTP/DTaP vaccination series and have not received a tetanus and diphtheria toxoids vaccine (Td) booster dose.
- Adolescents aged 13–18 years who missed the 11–12 year Td/Tdap booster dose should also receive a single dose of Tdap if they have completed the recommended childhood DTP/DTaP vaccination series.

2. Human papillomavirus vaccine (HPV). *(Minimum age: 9 years)*
- Administer the first dose of the HPV vaccine series to females at age 11–12 years.
- Administer the second dose 2 months after the first dose and the third dose 6 months after the first dose.
- Administer the HPV vaccine series to females at age 13–18 years if not previously vaccinated.

3. Meningococcal vaccine. *(Minimum age: 11 years for meningococcal conjugate vaccine [MCV4]; 2 years for meningococcal polysaccharide vaccine [MPSV4])*
- Administer MCV4 at age 11–12 years and to previously unvaccinated adolescents at high school entry (at approximately age 15 years).
- Administer MCV4 to previously unvaccinated college freshmen living in dormitories; MPSV4 is an acceptable alternative.
- Vaccination against invasive meningococcal disease is recommended for children and adolescents aged ≥2 years with terminal complement deficiencies or anatomic or functional asplenia and certain other high-risk groups. See *MMWR* 2005;54(No. RR-7):1–21. Use MPSV4 for children aged 2–10 years and MCV4 or MPSV4 for older children.

4. Pneumococcal polysaccharide vaccine (PPV). *(Minimum age: 2 years)*
- Administer for certain high-risk groups. See *MMWR* 1997;46(No. RR-8):1–24, and *MMWR* 2000;49(No. RR-9):1–35.

5. Influenza vaccine. *(Minimum age: 6 months for trivalent inactivated influenza vaccine [TIV]; 5 years for live, attenuated influenza vaccine [LAIV])*
- Influenza vaccine is recommended annually for persons with certain risk factors, health-care workers, and other persons (including household members) in close contact with persons in groups at high risk. See *MMWR* 2006;55 (No. RR-10):1–41.
- For healthy persons aged 5–49 years, LAIV may be used as an alternative to TIV.
- Children aged <9 years who are receiving influenza vaccine for the first time should receive 2 doses (separated by ≥4 weeks for TIV and ≥6 weeks for LAIV).

6. Hepatitis A vaccine (HepA). *(Minimum age: 12 months)*
- The 2 doses in the series should be administered at least 6 months apart.
- HepA is recommended for certain other groups of children, including in areas where vaccination programs target older children. See *MMWR* 2006;55 (No. RR-7):1–23.

7. Hepatitis B vaccine (HepB). *(Minimum age: birth)*
- Administer the 3-dose series to those who were not previously vaccinated.
- A 2-dose series of Recombivax HB® is licensed for children aged 11–15 years.

8. Inactivated poliovirus vaccine (IPV). *(Minimum age: 6 weeks)*
- For children who received an all-IPV or all-oral poliovirus (OPV) series, a fourth dose is not necessary if the third dose was administered at age ≥4 years.
- If both OPV and IPV were administered as part of a series, a total of 4 doses should be administered, regardless of the child's current age.

9. Measles, mumps, and rubella vaccine (MMR). *(Minimum age: 12 months)*
- If not previously vaccinated, administer 2 doses of MMR during any visit, with ≥4 weeks between the doses.

10. Varicella vaccine. *(Minimum age: 12 months)*
- Administer 2 doses of varicella vaccine to persons without evidence of immunity.
- Administer 2 doses of varicella vaccine to persons aged <13 years at least 3 months apart. Do not repeat the second dose, if administered ≥28 days after the first dose.
- Administer 2 doses of varicella vaccine to persons aged ≥13 years at least 4 weeks apart.

The Recommended Immunization Schedules for Persons Aged 0–18 Years are approved by the Advisory Committee on Immunization Practices (http://www.cdc.gov/nip/acip), the American Academy of Pediatrics (http://www.aap.org), and the American Academy of Family Physicians (http://www.aafp.org).

SAFER • HEALTHIER • PEOPLE™

CS100131

Table 6.7. Immunization Schedule for Adults

Recommended Adult Immunization Schedule, by Vaccine and Age Group
UNITED STATES • OCTOBER 2006–SEPTEMBER 2007

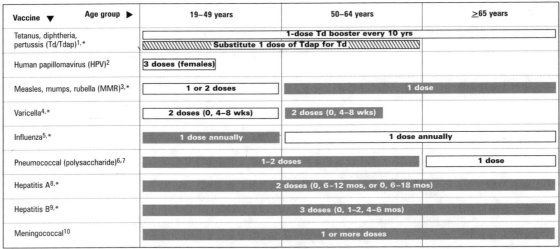

Vaccine ▼ / Age group ▶	19–49 years	50–64 years	≥65 years
Tetanus, diphtheria, pertussis (Td/Tdap)[1],*	1-dose Td booster every 10 yrs / Substitute 1 dose of Tdap for Td		
Human papillomavirus (HPV)[2]	3 doses (females)		
Measles, mumps, rubella (MMR)[3],*	1 or 2 doses	1 dose	
Varicella[4],*	2 doses (0, 4–8 wks)	2 doses (0, 4–8 wks)	
Influenza[5],*	1 dose annually	1 dose annually	
Pneumococcal (polysaccharide)[6,7]	1–2 doses		1 dose
Hepatitis A[8],*	2 doses (0, 6–12 mos, or 0, 6–18 mos)		
Hepatitis B[9],*	3 doses (0, 1–2, 4–6 mos)		
Meningococcal[10]	1 or more doses		

*Covered by the Vaccine Injury Compensation Program. NOTE: These recommendations must be read with the footnotes (see reverse).

☐ For all persons in this category who meet the age requirements and who lack evidence of immunity (e.g., lack documentation of vaccination or have no evidence of prior infection)

▨ Recommended if some other risk factor is present (e.g., on the basis of medical, occupational, lifestyle, or other indications)

This schedule indicates the recommended age groups and medical indications for routine administration of currently licensed vaccines for persons aged ≥19 years, as of October 1, 2006. Licensed combination vaccines may be used whenever any components of the combination are indicated and when the vaccine's other components are not contraindicated. For detailed recommendations on all vaccines, including those used primarily for travelers or that are issued during the year, consult the manufacturers' package inserts and the complete statements from the Advisory Committee on Immunization Practices (www.cdc.gov/nip/publications/acip-list.htm).

Report all clinically significant postvaccination reactions to the Vaccine Adverse Event Reporting System (VAERS). Reporting forms and instructions on filing a VAERS report are available at www.vaers.hhs.gov or by telephone, 800-822-7967.

Information on how to file a Vaccine Injury Compensation Program claim is available at www.hrsa.gov/vaccinecompensation or by telephone, 800-338-2382. To file a claim for vaccine injury, contact the U.S. Court of Federal Claims, 717 Madison Place, N.W., Washington, D.C. 20005; telephone, 202-357-6400.

Additional information about the vaccines in this schedule and contraindications for vaccination is also available at www.cdc.gov/nip or from the CDC-INFO Contact Center at 800-CDC-INFO (800-232-4636) in English and Spanish, 24 hours a day, 7 days a week.

Recommended Adult Immunization Schedule, by Vaccine and Medical and Other Indications
UNITED STATES • OCTOBER 2006–SEPTEMBER 2007

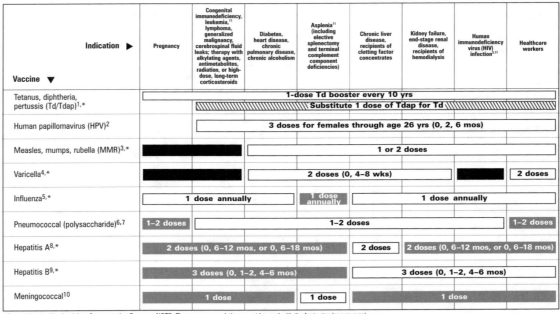

Vaccine ▼ / Indication ▶	Pregnancy	Congenital immunodeficiency, leukemia,[11] lymphoma, generalized malignancy, cerebrospinal fluid leaks; therapy with alkylating agents, antimetabolites, radiation, or high-dose, long-term corticosteroids	Diabetes, heart disease, chronic pulmonary disease, chronic alcoholism	Asplenia[11] (including elective splenectomy and terminal complement component deficiencies)	Chronic liver disease, recipients of clotting factor concentrates	Kidney failure, end-stage renal disease, recipients of hemodialysis	Human immunodeficiency virus (HIV) infection[3,11]	Healthcare workers
Tetanus, diphtheria, pertussis (Td/Tdap)[1],*	1-dose Td booster every 10 yrs / Substitute 1 dose of Tdap for Td							
Human papillomavirus (HPV)[2]	3 doses for females through age 26 yrs (0, 2, 6 mos)							
Measles, mumps, rubella (MMR)[3],*	(contraindicated)		1 or 2 doses					
Varicella[4],*	(contraindicated)		2 doses (0, 4–8 wks)			(contraindicated)	2 doses	
Influenza[5],*	1 dose annually		1 dose annually	1 dose annually				
Pneumococcal (polysaccharide)[6,7]	1–2 doses	1–2 doses						1–2 doses
Hepatitis A[8],*	2 doses (0, 6–12 mos, or 0, 6–18 mos)			2 doses	2 doses (0, 6–12 mos, or 0, 6–18 mos)			
Hepatitis B[9],*	3 doses (0, 1–2, 4–6 mos)			3 doses (0, 1–2, 4–6 mos)				
Meningococcal[10]	1 dose		1 dose	1 dose				

*Covered by the Vaccine Injury Compensation Program. NOTE: These recommendations must be read with the footnotes (see reverse).

☐ For all persons in this category who meet the age requirements and who lack evidence of immunity (e.g., lack documentation of vaccination or have no evidence of prior infection)

▨ Recommended if some other risk factor is present (e.g., on the basis of medical, occupational, lifestyle, or other indications)

■ Contraindicated

Approved by
the Advisory Committee on Immunization Practices,
the American College of Obstetricians and Gynecologists,
the American Academy of Family Physicians,
and the American College of Physicians

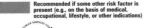

DEPARTMENT OF HEALTH AND HUMAN SERVICES
CENTERS FOR DISEASE CONTROL AND PREVENTION

Table 6.7. (*Continued*)

Footnotes
Recommended Adult Immunization Schedule • UNITED STATES, OCTOBER 2006–SEPTEMBER 2007

1. **Tetanus, diphtheria, and acellular pertussis (Td/Tdap) vaccination.** Adults with uncertain histories of a complete primary vaccination series with diphtheria and tetanus toxoid–containing vaccines should begin or complete a primary vaccination series. A primary series for adults is 3 doses; administer the first 2 doses at least 4 weeks apart and the third dose 6–12 months after the second. Administer a booster dose to adults who have completed a primary series and if the last vaccination was received ≥10 years previously. Tdap or tetanus and diphtheria (Td) vaccine may be used; Tdap should replace a single dose of Td for adults aged <65 years who have not previously received a dose of Tdap (either in the primary series, as a booster, or for wound management). Only one of two Tdap products (Adacel® [sanofi pasteur]) is licensed for use in adults. If the person is pregnant and received the last Td vaccination ≥10 years previously, administer Td during the second or third trimester; if the person received the last Td vaccination in <10 years, administer Tdap during the immediate postpartum period. A one-time administration of 1 dose of Tdap with an interval as short as 2 years from a previous Td vaccination is recommended for postpartum women, close contacts of infants aged <12 months, and all healthcare workers with direct patient contact. In certain situations, Td can be deferred during pregnancy and Tdap substituted in the immediate postpartum period, or Tdap can be given instead of Td to a pregnant woman after an informed discussion with the woman (see www.cdc.gov/nip/publications/acip-list.htm). Consult the ACIP statement for recommendations for administering Td as prophylaxis in wound management (www.cdc.gov/mmwr/preview/mmwrhtml/00041645.htm).

2. **Human papillomavirus (HPV) vaccination.** HPV vaccination is recommended for all women aged ≤26 years who have not completed the vaccine series. Ideally, vaccine should be administered before potential exposure to HPV through sexual activity; however, women who are sexually active should still be vaccinated. Sexually active women who have not been infected with any of the HPV vaccine types receive the full benefit of the vaccination. Vaccination is less beneficial for women who have already been infected with one or more of the four HPV vaccine types. A complete series consists of 3 doses. The second dose should be administered 2 months after the first dose; the third dose should be administered 6 months after the first dose. Vaccination is not recommended during pregnancy. If a woman is found to be pregnant after initiating the vaccination series, the remainder of the 3-dose regimen should be delayed until after completion of the pregnancy.

3. **Measles, mumps, rubella (MMR) vaccination.** *Measles component:* adults born before 1957 can be considered immune to measles. Adults born during or after 1957 should receive ≥1 dose of MMR unless they have a medical contraindication, documentation of ≥1 dose, history of measles based on healthcare provider diagnosis, or laboratory evidence of immunity. A second dose of MMR is recommended for adults who 1) have been recently exposed to measles or in an outbreak setting; 2) have been previously vaccinated with killed measles vaccine; 3) have been vaccinated with an unknown type of measles vaccine during 1963–1967; 4) are students in postsecondary educational institutions; 5) work in ahealthcare facility; or 6) plan to travel internationally. Withhold MMR or other measles-containing vaccines from HIV-infected persons with severe immunosuppression.

   Mumps component: adults born before 1957 can generally be considered immune to mumps. Adults born during or after 1957 should receive 1 dose of MMR unless they have a medical contraindication, history of mumps based on healthcare provider diagnosis, or laboratory evidence of immunity. A second dose of MMR is recommended for adults who 1) are in an age group that is affected during a mumps outbreak; 2) are students in postsecondary educational institutions; 3) work in a healthcare facility; or 4) plan to travel internationally. For unvaccinated healthcare workers born before 1957 who do not have other evidence of mumps immunity, consider giving 1 dose on a routine basis and strongly consider giving a second dose during an outbreak. *Rubella component:* administer 1 dose of MMR vaccine to women whose rubella vaccination history is unreliable or who lack laboratory evidence of immunity. For women of childbearing age, regardless of birth year, routinely determine rubella immunity and counsel women regarding congenital rubella syndrome. Do not vaccinate women who are pregnant or who might become pregnant within 4 weeks of receiving vaccine. Women who do not have evidence of immunity should receive MMR vaccine upon completion or termination of pregnancy and before discharge from the healthcare facility.

4. **Varicella vaccination.** All adults without evidence of immunity to varicella should receive 2 doses of varicella vaccine. Special consideration should be given to those who 1) have close contact with persons at high risk for severe disease (e.g., healthcare workers and family contacts of immunocompromised persons) or 2) are at high risk for exposure or transmission (e.g., teachers of young children; child care employees; residents and staff members of institutional settings, including correctional institutions; college students; military personnel; adolescents and adults living in households with children; nonpregnant women of childbearing age; and international travelers). Evidence of immunity to varicella in adults includes any of the following: 1) documentation of 2 doses of varicella vaccine at least 4 weeks apart; 2) U.S.-born before 1980 (although for healthcare workers and pregnant women, birth before 1980 should not be considered evidence of immunity); 3) history of varicella based on diagnosis or verification of varicella by a healthcare provider (for a patient reporting a history of or presenting with an atypical case, a mild case, or both, healthcare providers should seek either an epidemiologic link with a typical varicella case or evidence of laboratory confirmation, if it was performed at the time of acute disease); 4) history of herpes zoster based on healthcare provider diagnosis; or 5) laboratory evidence of immunity or laboratory confirmation of disease. Do not vaccinate women who are pregnant or might become pregnant within 4 weeks of receiving the vaccine. Assess pregnant women for evidence of varicella immunity. Women who do not have evidence of immunity should receive dose 1 of varicella vaccine upon completion or termination of pregnancy and before discharge from the healthcare facility. Dose 2 should be administered 4–8 weeks after dose 1.

5. **Influenza vaccination.** *Medical indications:* chronic disorders of the cardiovascular or pulmonary systems, including asthma; chronic metabolic diseases, including diabetes mellitus, renal dysfunction, hemoglobinopathies, or immunosuppression (including immunosuppression caused by medications or HIV); any condition that compromises respiratory function or the handling of respiratory secretions or that can increase the risk of aspiration (e.g., cognitive dysfunction, spinal cord injury, or seizure disorder or other neuromuscular disorder); and pregnancy during the influenza season. No data exist on the risk for severe or complicated influenza disease among persons with asplenia; however, influenza is a risk factor for secondary bacterial infections that can cause severe disease among persons with asplenia. *Occupational indications:* healthcare workers and employees of long-term–care and assisted living facilities. *Other indications:* residents of nursing homes and other long-term–care and assisted living facilities; persons likely to transmit influenza to persons at high risk (e.g., in-home household contacts and caregivers of children aged 0–59 months, or persons of all ages with high-risk conditions); and anyone who would like to be vaccinated. Healthy, nonpregnant persons aged 5–49 years without high-risk medical conditions who are not contacts of severely immunocompromised persons in special care units can receive either intranasally administered influenza vaccine (FluMist®) or inactivated vaccine. Other persons should receive the inactivated vaccine.

6. **Pneumococcal polysaccharide vaccination.** *Medical indications:* chronic disorders of the pulmonary system (excluding asthma); cardiovascular diseases; diabetes mellitus; chronic liver diseases, including liver disease as a result of alcohol abuse (e.g., cirrhosis); chronic renal failure or nephrotic syndrome; functional or anatomic asplenia (e.g., sickle cell disease or splenectomy [if elective splenectomy is planned, vaccinate at least 2 weeks before surgery]); immunosuppressive conditions (e.g., congenital immunodeficiency, HIV infection [vaccinate as close to diagnosis as possible when CD4 cell counts are highest], leukemia, lymphoma, multiple myeloma, Hodgkin disease, generalized malignancy, or organ or bone marrow transplantation); chemotherapy with alkylating agents, antimetabolites, or high-dose, long-term corticosteroids; and cochlear implants. *Other indications:* Alaska Natives and certain American Indian populations and residents of nursing homes or other long-term–care facilities.

7. **Revaccination with pneumococcal polysaccharide vaccine.** One-time revaccination after 5 years for persons with chronic renal failure or nephrotic syndrome; functional or anatomic asplenia (e.g., sickle cell disease or splenectomy); immunosuppressive conditions (e.g., congenital immunodeficiency, HIV infection, leukemia, lymphoma, multiple myeloma, Hodgkin disease, generalized malignancy, or organ or bone marrow transplantation); or chemotherapy with alkylating agents, antimetabolites, or high-dose, long-term corticosteroids. For persons aged ≥65 years, one-time revaccination if they were vaccinated ≥5 years previously and were aged <65 years at the time of primary vaccination.

8. **Hepatitis A vaccination.** *Medical indications:* persons with chronic liver disease and persons who receive clotting factor concentrates. *Behavioral indications:* men who have sex with men and persons who use illegal drugs. *Occupational indications:* persons working with hepatitis A virus (HAV)–infected primates or with HAV in a research laboratory setting. *Other indications:* persons traveling to or working in countries that have high or intermediate endemicity of hepatitis A (a list of countries is available at www.cdc.gov/travel/diseases.htm) and any person who would like to obtain immunity. Current vaccines should be administered in a 2-dose schedule at either 0 and 6–12 months, or 0 and 6–18 months. If the combined hepatitis A and hepatitis B vaccine is used, administer 3 doses at 0, 1, and 6 months.

9. **Hepatitis B vaccination.** *Medical indications:* persons with end-stage renal disease, including patients receiving hemodialysis; persons seeking evaluation or treatment for a sexually transmitted disease (STD); persons with HIV infection; persons with chronic liver disease; and persons who receive clotting factor concentrates. *Occupational indications:* healthcare workers and public-safety workers who are exposed to blood or other potentially infectious body fluids. *Behavioral indications:* sexually active persons who are not in a long-term, mutually monogamous relationship (i.e., persons with >1 sex partner during the previous 6 months); current or recent injection-drug users; and men who have sex with men. *Other indications:* household contacts and sex partners of persons with chronic hepatitis B virus (HBV) infection; clients and staff members of institutions for persons with developmental disabilities; all clients of STD clinics; international travelers to countries with high or intermediate prevalence of chronic HBV infection (a list of countries is available at www.cdc.gov/travel/diseases.htm); and any adult seeking protection from HBV infection. Settings where hepatitis B vaccination is recommended for all adults: STD treatment facilities; HIV testing and treatment facilities; facilities providing drug-abuse treatment and prevention services; healthcare settings providing services for injection-drug users or men who have sex with men; correctional facilities; end-stage renal disease programs and facilities for chronic hemodialysis patients; and institutions and nonresidential daycare facilities for persons with developmental disabilities. *Special formulation indications:* for adult patients receiving hemodialysis and other immunocompromised adults, 1 dose of 40 μg/mL (Recombivax HB®) or 2 doses of 20 μg/mL (Engerix-B®).

10. **Meningococcal vaccination.** *Medical indications:* adults with anatomic or functional asplenia, or terminal complement component deficiencies. *Other indications:* first-year college students living in dormitories; microbiologists who are routinely exposed to isolates of *Neisseria meningitidis*; military recruits; and persons who travel to or live in countries in which meningococcal disease is hyperendemic or epidemic (e.g., the "meningitis belt" of sub-Saharan Africa during the dry season [December–June]), particularly if their contact with local populations will be prolonged. Vaccination is required by the government of Saudi Arabia for all travelers to Mecca during the annual Hajj. Meningococcal conjugate vaccine is preferred for adults with any of the preceding indications who are aged ≤55 years, although meningococcal polysaccharide vaccine (MPSV4) is an acceptable alternative. Revaccination after 5 years might be indicated for adults previously vaccinated with MPSV4 who remain at high risk for infection (e.g., persons residing in areas in which disease is epidemic).

11. **Selected conditions for which *Haemophilus influenzae* type b (Hib) vaccine may be used.** Hib conjugate vaccines are licensed for children aged 6 weeks–71 months. No efficacy data are available on which to base a recommendation concerning use of Hib vaccine for older children and adults with the chronic conditions associated with an increased risk for Hib disease. However, studies suggest good immunogenicity in patients who have sickle cell disease, leukemia, or HIV infection or who have had splenectomies; administering vaccine to these patients is not contraindicated.

Use of trade names and commercial sources is for identification only and does not imply endorsement by the U.S. Department of Health and Human Services.

vaccine is greater than the risk of contracting the disease naturally, so only the killed vaccine is used in those countries. In contrast, the documented benefits of vaccines against other diseases, such as measles, far outweigh the small percentage of postvaccination complications. Factors in assessing risks and benefits of vaccination include the risk of infection, the consequences of natural unmodified illness, the availability of a safe and effective vaccine, and the duration of vaccine effect. Even today, certain vaccines still carry real, if rare, risks to the recipient. Measles and rabies vaccines have been associated with postvaccination complications such as encephalitis, which has resulted in permanent brain damage. The rate of postvaccination encephalitis with the measles vaccine is about one case per million vaccinations. This small incidence rate is only one fifth to one tenth the rate of encephalitis following natural measles. Since the introduction of measles vaccine, the rate of postmeasles encephalitis has dropped tenfold; the potential benefit from measles vaccination far outweighs the small risk of postvaccination encephalitis. The information documented in historical reports and postmarketing surveillance data provides the basis for making decisions about the risk-to-benefit relationship for currently used vaccines.

Another risk is the potential for the vaccine to elicit an allergic response. Allergenicity usually results from the method of production, as in the use of chicken embryo culture media. When such methods are used to produce a vaccine, complete purification may not be possible, and trace contaminants (e.g., egg protein) may persist in the final product; this is true for some influenza vaccines. The use of human diploid cell lines as viral hosts, a method developed in the 1980s, has limited the risk of allergenicity.

Clearly, immunization is a vital component of pediatric and adult health care. Even so, immunization is underutilized, although it is one of the most cost-effective measures available for preserving and protecting health. Incidence rates of vaccine-preventable diseases in the United States have decreased dramatically since the mid-1950s, primarily because of the widespread public acceptance and availability of effective vaccines. But the perception of a change in the risk-to-benefit relationship between disease and vaccine may lead to a resurgence of vaccine-preventable diseases. An example of this is whooping cough, caused by *Bordetella pertussis*.

Pertussis may present as a severe illness characterized by prolonged coughing spells lasting several weeks to months. In children and infants, these bouts can lead to difficulty eating, drinking, and breathing. The coughing is often ended by vomiting, so dehydration is common. The disease has a mortality rate of 0.1% to 1%; it can lead to brain damage, seizures, and mental retardation. Following introduction of a pertussis vaccine in the 1940s, the incidence of disease dropped sharply (**Figure 6.5**). But the rate of infection has risen consistently since the 1980s; vaccine coverage has decreased because of bad publicity about the whole-cell vaccine and an increasing refusal to vaccinate because of religious or philosophical beliefs (Figure 6.5). Recent studies

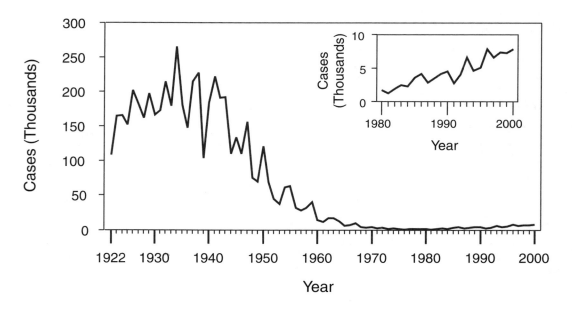

Figure 6.5. Decrease in incidence of pertussis in the United States following the introduction of a pertussis vaccine.

of children diagnosed with pertussis demonstrated that 65% of patients had not received the recommended schedule of immunizations and 39% had not received any pertussis vaccine at all. Also, 12% of the diagnosed pertussis cases are in individuals older than 15 and may reflect waning immunity. The increased incidence of disease is of concern for the entire community. Based on experience in other countries, it is expected that in the absence of vaccination, the rate of pertussis infections and associated morbidity and mortality would increase 10- to 100-fold.[20]

Other considerations for immunization include socioeconomic factors. In early 1995, the Food and Drug Administration (FDA) approved the live attenuated varicella vaccine for use in individuals older than 1 year who had not had varicella. Varicella-zoster virus (VZV) causes varicella (chickenpox), the primary infection, and zoster (shingles), a secondary infection caused by reactivation of the latent VZV. Varicella is generally a mild, self-limiting, but highly contagious childhood disease that, in most cases, provides lifelong immunity to varicella. Almost 4 million cases of varicella occur in the United States each year, with a mortality rate estimated at 1.4 deaths per 100,000 cases in children and 30.9 deaths per 100,000 cases in adults. Varicella also has a major socioeconomic impact. Because of the contagiousness of the disease, a child generally misses 7–10 days of school, and the parents generally lose several days of work. The estimated annual health care costs for varicella infections reach $399 million. In 1994, a cost-benefit analysis estimated the routine use of varicella vaccine would cost $384 million annually—a net savings from routine vaccination of $15 million. The major controversy with this vaccine is not about its efficacy for childhood varicella, but long-term protection against both varicella and zoster. It should be noted that the potential costs associated with lack of long-term protection were not included in the cost-savings analysis for the vaccine.

Although studies document the efficacy of the vaccine against varicella, it is unclear how this will affect the epidemiology of VZV infection. Will the incidence of zoster in middle age decrease because of a lower latency infection rate associated with the attenuated virus, or will waning immunity place older individuals at risk of VZV infection when the risks associated with varicella are higher? Are the estimated cost savings associated with routine pediatric vaccination still valid if the epidemiology of VZV infection changes? Are the risks associated with these unknowns worth the socioeconomic benefits? These questions will only be answered with continued surveillance of

varicella vaccine recipients. Pharmacists should be aware of the benefits and risks associated with the vaccine, so they can advise patients, parents, and other health care providers.

Companies that develop and produce vaccines carefully weigh all known risks associated with vaccination to minimize adverse effects on patients. Even so, some adverse events occur in such a small percentage of patients that the incidence and severity of the effect may be unknown until mass production and vaccination are under way.

The 1976 nationwide "swine flu" immunization program was a classic example of this problem. A careful retrospective monitoring program revealed a fivefold increase in development of Guillain-Barré syndrome after vaccination over its incidence in unvaccinated controls. The rarity of this complication made it impossible to detect it prior to widespread administration, illustrating the difficulty of predicting all the risks of immunization. This experience underscores the need for extensive post-licensure and post-marketing surveillance to identify unexpected adverse events.

Vaccine initiative. In response to the resurgence of childhood diseases, the Childhood Immunization Initiative (CII) was implemented in 1993. The goals that CII intended to accomplish by 1996 were to (1) eliminate indigenous cases of diphtheria, *Haemophilus influenzae* infection, measles, polio, rubella, and tetanus; (2) increase vaccination coverage of 2-year-old children to at least 90%; and (3) establish a system that maintains and further improves vaccination coverage levels. This initiative also attempts to increase knowledge of vaccines and reduce vaccination costs to parents or guardians through the "Vaccines for Children" program. In effect since October 1994, this program provides free vaccinations to children not covered by health insurance. The most recent update from the national immunization survey indicates that in January to June 2004, 80% to 95% of children in the United States were appropriately vaccinated.[21] It also indicated there were still areas where vaccination coverage was suboptimal and that completion of vaccination series is more difficult to achieve than the goals for individual vaccines. Proven strategies for increasing vaccine coverage still need to be implemented in these areas.

Pharmacists can assist in meeting the goals of CII by encouraging parents to comply with vaccination recommendations from the CDC. They can also educate other health care workers about different vaccine products and administration schedules. But it is also the responsibility of pharmacists and physicians to advise the patient or patient's guardian about the risks of immunization, and it is the responsibility of all health care providers to use (i.e., store, dose, and administer) the vaccines appropriately. Pharmacists should advocate and ensure compliance with patient safety measures. The pharmacist can act as an advocate for immunization not only in infants and children, but also in adults and special populations. The goals of CII are attainable, but unless universal immunization is implemented, eradication of vaccine-preventable diseases will not be achievable.

Specific vaccines. A number of vaccines are available in the United States for immunization against specific pathogens. Some of these vaccines are available as single vaccines and others as multivalent subunit vaccines. Some vaccines, such as the tetanus toxoid vaccine, are available in different configurations. Historical and epidemiologic information for each disease and vaccine is summarized below; **Table 6.8** summarizes additional information on the vaccines. For additional information on dosage and scheduling, please see ImmunoFacts.[22]

Anthrax. Anthrax is a zoonotic infection caused by *Bacillus anthracis*. The most common form of anthrax in humans is cutaneous anthrax or infection of the skin; other forms of the disease are gastrointestinal and inhalation anthrax. The cutaneous disease is seen primarily in people working with animal skins contaminated with anthrax spores. While it is unusual to contract the disease naturally, anthrax is important because of its po-

tential as a bioterrorism agent. One example of this potential danger occurred in the Soviet Union in 1979, when an accidental release of anthrax spores from a biological weapons laboratory attracted the world's attention. Because of anthrax's potential as a biological weapon, American troops engaged in the 1991 Gulf War were immunized against anthrax. There is no evidence it was used during that war, although Iraqi officials did acknowledge filling missile heads with anthrax spores. Following the terrorist attacks of September 11, 2001, 18 people in the United States were infected with weaponized anthrax distributed through the mail. Of those, 11 cases were of inhalation anthrax; five resulted in death.

Anthrax vaccine is a cell-free culture filtrate consisting of a protein called protective antigen (PA). PA is one part of a three-part toxin; the others are lethal factor and edema factor. Abs directed toward PA neutralize the ability of the anthrax toxin to bind to host cells, thus inhibiting the functions of lethal factor and edema factor. The vaccine has been shown to protect against cutaneous infection in people and against aerosolized spores in monkeys and rabbits. Experiments with aerosolized spores mimicked the likely form of exposure in the event of a terrorist attack. For greatest efficacy, multiple doses of the vaccine are needed.

Diphtheria/tetanus/pertussis. Diphtheria, tetanus, and pertussis are clinically distinct diseases that have been recognized for centuries. Diphtheria

Table 6.8. Characteristics and Recommendations for Common Vaccines[a]

Disease	Type of Vaccine	Adjuvant	Indications	Route
Anthrax	Subunit containing PA (protective antigen). Strain avirulent, nonencapsulated, nonproteolytic V770-NP1-R	Aluminum hydroxide	Based on exposure to *B. anthracis*	SC[b]
Diphtheria, tetanus, pertussis	Subunits, inactivated diphtheria and tetanus toxoids. Available with or without acellular pertussis vaccine (pertussis toxoid, filamentous hemagglutinin, pertactin, fimbriae).[c] See text for strains	Aluminum phosphate[c]/Aluminum hydroxide	Induction of active immunity in children without added pertussis used in adults as booster immunizations	IM
Haemophilus influenzae b	Conjugate vaccine, *H. influenzae* oligosaccharide and polyribosyl-ribitol-phosphate conjugated to tetanus toxoid or diphtheria CRM$_{197}$ protein or meningococcal protein conjugate	None None Aluminum hydroxide	Induction of active immunity to *H. influenzae* type b. Especially important for children less than 24 months of age, those in day care, of low socioeconomic status, blacks, Native Americans, and individuals with asplenia, sickle-cell disease, and Ab deficiency syndromes	

Table 6.8. (Continued)

Disease	Type of Vaccine	Adjuvant	Indications	Route
Hepatitis A[d]	Inactivated lysed whole virus Strain CR326F' Strain HM-175	Aluminum hydroxy-phosphate sulfate[c] Aluminum hydroxide	Induction of active immunity to hepatitis A virus. Recommended for children and adults in selected states and at those high risk for disease. High-risk individuals include travelers, military personnel, people living in areas of high endemicity of hepatitis A, people with chronic liver disease, people engaging in high-risk sexual activity, food handlers, and people exposed to hepatitis A through household contacts	IM
Hepatitis B	Subunit, purified hepatitis B surface antigen (HBsAg) Lipoprotein complex is expressed in and purified from *Saccharomyces cerevisiae* Strain Hepatitis B adw_2 Strain Hepatitis B adw	Aluminum hydroxide[c] Aluminum hydroxyphosphate sulfate	Induction of active immunity in persons of all ages. Prevention of hepatitis B prevents liver cancer	IM
Human papilloma-virus	Subunit, purified L1 capsid proteins Quadrivalent contains proteins from types 6, 11, 16, and 18	Aluminum hydroxyl-phosphate sulfate	Induction of active immunity in females 9–26 years old	
Influenza Traditional	Inactivated viral subunits. Subvirion or purified surface protein antigens. Trivalent contains 2 influenza A and 1 influenza B serotype; serotypes revised annually	None	Induction of active immunity against influenza. Recommended for annual immunization in children up to 18 years old and adults over 50. Also recommended for at-risk individuals 19–49. At-risk individuals include those with chronic cardiac or pulmonary disease, diabetes mellitus, renal dysfunction, hemoglobinopathies, immunosuppression, pregnant women, and health care professionals	IM
Live	Live, cold attenuated. Trivalent (for composition see above)	None	Induction of activity immunity against influenza in healthy individuals 5–49 years old	Intranasal
MMR	Combination vaccine contains live attenuated whole viruses of measles, mumps, and rubella Strain Measles: Moraten Strain Mumps: Jeryl Lynn (B level) Strain Rubella: Wistar Institute RA27/3	None	Induction of immunity against measles, mumps, and rubella simultaneously. Preferred immunizing agent for children and adults	SC

(Continued)

Table 6.8. (*Continued*)

Disease	Type of Vaccine	Adjuvant	Indications	Route
Meningococcal	Subunit, capsular polysaccharide fragments, strains A-1, C-11, 6306Y, W-135-308	None	Induction of active immunity to specific serotypes of *Neisseria meningitidis* in specific persons at risk, including college freshmen, military recruits, those with anatomic or functional asplenia, as adjunct to prophylactic chemotherapy for those exposed to *Neisseria meningitidis*, and immunosuppressed individuals	SC
	Subunit, capsular polysaccharide fragments, strains A, C, Y, W-135 individually conjugated to diphtheria toxin	None	Induction of active immunity to specific serotypes of *Neisseria meningitidis* in individuals over 11 years of age	SC
Pneumococcal 7-Valent	Subunit, capsular polysaccharide fragments of 7 distinct *S. pneumoniae* serotypes (4, 6B, 9V, 14,18C, 19F,23F) conjugated to diphtheria CRM_{197} protein	Aluminum phosphate	Induction of active immunity in infants against the serotypes of *S. pneumoniae* that cause 80% of invasive disease in children less than 5 years. Also for children at increased risk, including blacks, Native Americans and Alaskans, children with sickle-cell disease, immunosuppression, HIV, or chronic diseases	IM
23-Valent	Subunity, capsular polysaccharide fragments of 23 distinct *S. pneumoniae* serotypes (1, 2, 3, 4, 5, 8, 9, 12, 14, 17, 19, 20, 22, 23, 26, 34, 43, 51, 54, 56, 57, 68, 70)	None	Induction of active immunity against serotypes of *S. pneumoniae* that cause invasive disease in older children and adults Children: as an adjunct to the 7-valent vaccine for children older than 23 months of age with sickle-cell disease, asplenia, immunosuppression, HIV, or chronic disease Adults: all adults 65 or older, individuals at increased risk for pneumococcal disease because of chronic cardiac, pulmonary, hepatic, or renal disease; diabetes, alcoholism, cirrhosis, chronic cerebrospinal fluid leaks	SC/IM
Polio	Inactivated, killed, whole Virus, serotypes 1, 2, and 3 Strains; serotype 1–Mahoney Serotype 2–MEF-1 Serotype 3–Saukett	None	Induction of active immunity against serotypes 1, 2, and 3 of polio and prevention of poliomyelitis. Recommended for infants older than 2 months of age. Also recommended for household contacts of immunosuppressed individuals, adults traveling to areas where polio is endemic, and those with incomplete immunizations	SC/IM

Table 6.8. (*Continued*)

Disease	Type of Vaccine	Adjuvant	Indications	Route
Rabies	Inactivated/killed whole virus Strains: PM-1503-3M CVS Flury LEP-C 25	None Aluminum phosphate[c]	Induction of active immunity against rabies before or after exposure to the virus Preexposure: individuals who are at high risk of exposure because of occupation (i.e., veterinarians, some laboratory workers, animal handlers, forest rangers) Postexposure: following a bite from an unprovoked animal	IM
Smallpox	Live, attenuated virus vaccina Strain NYCBOH	None	Induction of activate immunity against smallpox and vaccinia in individuals with potential exposure to the virus, including laboratory workers, military personnel, health care professionals, and selected public health and community workers	Percutaneous with bifurneedle
Typhoid				
Typhoid Vi	Subunit, bacterial polysaccharide strain Ty-2	None	Induction of active immunity against typhoid fever in specific populations, including travelers to endemic areas, individuals with prolonged contact with a known typhoid carrier, and laboratory personnel who work with *Salmonella typhi*	IM
Oral	Live, attenuated bacteria plus non-viable cells strain Ty21a	None	Induction of active immunity against typhoid fever in specific populations, including travelers to endemic areas, individuals with prolonged contact with a known typhoid carrier, and laboratory personnel who work with *Salmonella typhi*	Oral
Varicella	Live, attenuated whole virus Oka/Merck strain	None	Induction of active immunity against infections caused by varicella-zoster virus, especially chicken pox. The vaccine is currently recommended for children older than 1 year of age and at-risk adults. These include individuals without a history of disease or immunization who work with young children, in institutional settings such as colleges, or military barracks, nonpregnant women, and travelers	SC
Yellow fever	Live attenuated whole virus 17D-204	None	Induction of active immunity against yellow fever. Vaccine is recommended for individuals 9 months of age and older living or traveling to areas where yellow fever is endemic	SC

[a] Derived from information in ImmunoFacts.[22]
[b] SC = subcutaneous; IM = intramuscular.
[c] Depending on manufacturer.
[d] May be combined with hepatitis B vaccine.

and pertussis are both communicable diseases; tetanus is not communicable. For all these organisms, disease pathogenesis is from the exotoxins produced. Diphtheria and pertussis are common illnesses that caused severe epidemics. In the early part of the twentieth century, each organism was responsible for significant morbidity and mortality. It is not uncommon today for both diphtheria and pertussis to have mortality rates of 5% to 15% in unvaccinated individuals. WHO estimates more than 400,000 deaths per year due to pertussis. Tetanus, while not common, is striking in its ability to kill previously healthy individuals following a traumatic injury.

Immunization to diphtheria was begun in the early 1900s using a combination of toxin and horse-derived antitoxin. Although this was able to provide protection, it was not without adverse reactions. In the early 1920s it was discovered that formalin and heat treatment of diphtheria toxin destroyed its toxicity, but not its antigenicity. These findings led to the development of diphtheria toxoid, which is the current vaccine formulation.

Pertussis vaccine was first developed from whole cells in the early 1900s, following laboratory culture of the organism. This whole-cell vaccine was initially difficult to standardize, but a greater problem was its adverse reaction profile. In most cases the reactions were minor, but occasional serious reactions occurred. The reactions were generally self-limited, but widespread negative publicity led to decreasing immunization rates in many countries. In the 1980s and 1990s, better identification of important protective antigens within the bacteria led to development of an acellular vaccine containing predominantly pertussis toxin and filamentous hemagglutinin derived from bacterial cultures. Today, although whole-cell vaccines for pertussis are still used in certain countries, only the acellular pertussis vaccine is licensed in the United States.

As with diphtheria, tetanus toxin was isolated in the early part of the twentieth century and by the 1920s was being produced by formaldehyde treatment. As early as 1927, tetanus toxoid was combined with diphtheria toxoid without a loss of immunogenicity in either. Tetanus toxoid did not come into common use in the United States until World War II, when the military began using it to prevent tetanus associated with wounds.

In 1948, diphtheria, pertussis, and tetanus vaccines were combined and shown to be highly effective. The trivalent vaccine, containing the acellular pertussis vaccine, is the preferred agent for immunizing children and the combination of diphtheria and tetanus toxoids is preferred for adult immunization.

Haemophilus influenzae type b. *Haemophilus influenzae* type b (Hib) is the major cause of meningitis in children under 5. In the United States it was estimated that there were 12,000 cases of meningitis and 1000 deaths caused by Hib each year in the 1980s. Protection against this organism is based on the presence of anticapsular Abs. Unfortunately, children in this age group have trouble developing Abs to polysaccharide antigens, and purified polysaccharides are not antigenic for this age group. Development of conjugate vaccines led to effective immunization protocols against Hib.

Conjugate vaccines use an immunogenic protein cross-linked to the polyribosyl-ribitol-phosphate (PRP), the major antigenic polysaccharide of Hib. The PRP has been successfully conjugated to a recombinant diphtheria toxoid (CRM_{197}), meningococcal outer membrane protein, and tetanus toxoid. Since 1991, the use of these vaccines has led to a greater than 90% decrease in incidence of Hib meningitis in children.

Hepatitis A. Hepatitis A is a viral disease transmitted person-to-person by the fecal-oral route. Infections with hepatitis A virus (HAV) are sporadic in the United States with about 30,000 cases reported annually. In other parts of the world, HAV is endemic with 80% to 90% of the population having been infected by the age of 18. In most individuals, HAV causes an acute infection with complete recovery and lifelong protective immunity for most patients. In patients with underlying chronic liver disease, however, the infection can become fulminant and lead to death.

Two HAV vaccines are licensed in the United States; both contain inactivated lysed whole hepatitis A virus and HAV antigen. There are no reference standards for comparison of the antigens present in each vaccine. However, studies have shown that both preparations provide 95% to 97% protection against infection with the virus. This vaccine is currently recommended for all children 1 year and older.

Hepatitis B. Hepatitis B is an infectious disease transmitted by blood, blood products, and sexual contact. Because of the chronic nature of hepatitis B, individuals who develop the disease are at increased risk for developing cirrhosis and cancer of the liver. It is estimated that more than 1 million people in the United States have this chronic infection. Other countries, particularly those in Southeast Asia and other tropical areas, have rates of infection six to 25 times higher than the United States. The high rates of infection and chronic nature of HBV infection, along with its lasting effects, make

HBV a significant cause of morbidity and mortality worldwide. These factors have led to aggressive immunization programs whose aim is to decrease the rates of infection throughout the world.

Hepatitis B vaccine was originally manufactured from serum-derived, heat-inactivated hepatitis B surface antigen (HBsAg). The heat-inactivated material was particulate and highly immunogenic. But because it was derived from infectious material, the risks associated with the initial vaccine included developing hepatitis B. In the mid-1980s, rDNA technology allowed for the expression of HBsAg from *Saccharomyces cerevisiae*. The recombinant HBsAg formed particles identical to the serum-derived material, but was totally noninfectious. The availability of a safe, effective vaccine for hepatitis B led to the recommendation of universal immunization in 1991.

Human papillomavirus. The human papillomavirus (HPV) family of viruses is responsible for warts, including genital warts; it is the most common sexually transmitted disease in the United States. While common warts rarely progress to cancer, four types of HPV (6, 11, 16, and 18) are responsible for most of squamous-cell cervical cancer and cervical adenocarcinoma. HPV is also responsible for 35% to 50% of vulvar and vaginal cancers. Current therapy for these cancers has depended on routine screening for early detection of lesions and early intervention. The recent development of vaccine for the prevention of infection by HPV types associated with cancer will shift the focus to prevention of the disease entirely.

The HPV vaccine is a quadrivalent preparation that includes the major capsid protein (L1) of HPV types 6, 11, 16, and 18. These proteins are produced by rDNA technology in *Saccharomyces cerevisiae* using individual fermentation tanks. Production of the L1 protein results in self-assembly of noninfectious viruslike particles (VLP) released following disruption of the yeast cells. The four different VLP are then combined to form the quadrivalent vaccine. Studies demonstrated that use of the vaccine resulted in the production of neutralizing Abs to the different types of HPV contained in the vaccine, thus preventing nearly 100% of infections and precancerous lesions. In June 2006, the FDA approved the use of the vaccine for females 9–26 years of age.

Influenza. The influenza virus is responsible for respiratory disease occurring in epidemic and pandemic form. From 1918 to 1920, pandemic influenza killed more people than were killed in combat during World War I. Since that time, influenza has caused seasonal epidemics and occasional pandemics. Influenza is generally a self-limiting disease, but because it is spread easily, it contributes significantly to loss of work and school time. In addition, both the initial infection and secondary bacterial infections are responsible for increased hospitalizations and deaths each year.

Influenza viruses occur as A, B, and C groups, with A and B being responsible for most of the human disease. All these viruses undergo gradual or significant antigenic change over time (antigenic drift and antigenic shift) due to point mutations in the viral surface proteins (hemagglutinin and neuraminidase). Because of these changes in the surface antigens, recovering from an influenza infection does not provide lifelong immunity to reinfection. The presence of Abs to the old surface proteins causes the new antigens to predominate in the population. The changes in viral surface antigens provide a challenge to the public health departments and vaccine manufacturers, as new formulations are needed each year.

Global surveillance during influenza season (winter in both hemispheres) allows for identification of the viral strains likely to be present during the next outbreak. In the northern hemisphere, strain selection occurs by the end of March. This gives manufacturers time to produce a new vaccine for release during the summer, and immunization begins in September or October. Because of the antigenic changes in the virus and the corresponding changes in the vaccine, yearly immunization is required.

The influenza vaccine is available as an injectable preparation or nasal spray. The injection is an inactivated vaccine made up of viral subunits or purified surface proteins and is recommended for use in all age groups. Contrary to popular belief, the inactivated influenza vaccine does not cause influenza. It does, however, stimulate the production of protective Ab to the virus.

The intranasal vaccine is a live, cold-adapted vaccine. This virus can replicate well at 25°C, but not at 37°C. The cold-adaptation means that the virus will replicate well in the nasal mucous of an individual, but not in the lower respiratory tract. Thus, intranasal immunization with the cold-adapted vaccine results in a localized infection and this infection results in the production of both systemic and localized Ab- and cell-mediated immunity. The local production of Ab means that there are significant levels of IgA on the nasal mucosa that may inhibit entry of infectious virus into the cells. As discussed earlier, cell-mediated immunity, especially CTL, is important for recovery from a viral infection. The intranasal vaccine, because it is a live vaccine, will stimulate CTL—something the killed, subvirion injectable influenza vaccine does not do. Currently, the intranasal vaccine is only licensed for healthy individuals between the ages of 5 and 49.

MMR. Measles, mumps, and rubella are common childhood diseases. In developed countries, these diseases are usually self-limiting, although measles and mumps have potentially serious complications. Rubella is unique in that it poses little danger for the infected individual, but can cause congenital rubella syndrome (CRS) in children whose pregnant mothers have contracted the disease. Measles is an infectious disease that causes a recognizable and distinguishing rash. There is little mortality associated with measles in developed countries, but in developing countries, mortality rates range between 2% and 5%. Measles deaths are usually due to complications of the disease, which vary based on age. The most common complication in children is pneumonia; in adults, encephalitis is the primary complication. Following measles virus infection, subacute sclerosing panencephalitis (SSPE) is a late complication for a small percentage of children. Occurring 2–10 years after the initial measles infection, SSPE is a progressive degenerative disease that is fatal. Since the introduction of measles vaccine and immunization protocols, the rate of SSPE has decreased 90%.

Mumps, a disease initially described by Hippocrates, is characterized by painful swelling of the parotid glands. In young children, mumps may appear as a respiratory infection without the parotitis; in adults, inapparent infections are common. Major complications of mumps include inflammation of the testicles in adolescent boys with a decrease or loss of fertility; oophoritis in young women and increased rates of miscarriage in pregnant women; meningoencephalitis; and deafness.

Rubella infection is characterized by a mild rash in most individuals, child or adult. In a pregnant patient, the virus is transmitted to the fetus and causes CRS, a disastrous syndrome affecting all organs. At birth, congenitally infected infants are found to have a constellation of defects such as cataracts, glaucoma, cochlear deafness, patent ductus arteriosus, mental retardation, autism, hepatosplenomegaly, and diabetes. The damage caused by the viral infection may continue after birth. An immunization initiative was begun to prevent CRS.

The combination measles, mumps, and rubella vaccine is composed of live attenuated viruses that are able to elicit both Ab- and cell-mediated immunity following immunization. In studies comparing the efficacy of individual vaccines to the combination vaccine, no suppression of any immune response to the combination was found when compared to administration of the vaccines individually. The combination vaccine makes it easier to achieve vaccination goals since patients do not need to return to the physician for additional immunizations. Because this is an attenuated vaccine, immunity to the viruses appears to wane following immunization. A booster immunization is recommended to induce lifelong immunity.

Meningococcal. Meningococcal disease is a relatively rare but serious disease among children and young adults. The disease no longer occurs in epidemic form in the United States, but rather in sporadic outbreaks with about 3000 cases reported each year. Important characteristics of this disease are its rapid onset and high mortality rate (15%) even with appropriate antibiotic treatment. Characteristic clinical signs include fever, rash, and meningitis, often resulting in hospitalization less than 24 hours after the initial symptoms. Among patients who recover, 10% to 20% have lasting complications, including cognitive deficits, seizures, and limb loss. In the United States, close contact among young adults is a risk factor for the disease, with college freshmen and military recruits at highest risk. To reduce this risk, immunization is recommended for all children 11–12 years of age and others under specific circumstances (see Tables 6.7 and 6.8).

The current meningococcal vaccine contains capsular polysaccharide fragments from four common strains for *Neisseria meningitidis.* Because the vaccine does not contain protein, it is unable to stimulate T-cell immunity or significant memory responses. However, sufficient levels of immunity are produced to protect the populations most at risk. A conjugate vaccine, containing a polysaccharide from the four most common strains of *N. meningitidis* cross-linked to either diphtheria toxoid CRM[197], was licensed in 2005 and is recommended for all age groups although the polysaccharide vaccine may be substituted in some age groups.

Pneumococcal. Streptococcus pneumoniae is the causative agent of pneumonia and meningitis; more than 90 different serotypes of the bacterium have been identified. *S. pneumoniae* is the leading cause of meningitis in children between the ages of 1 and 5 and adults older than 19, so effective vaccine strategies were needed. The age differences among the individuals most at risk required different strategies for vaccine development. Small children do not mount effective immune responses to polysaccharides and would not respond to the available adult vaccine. In addition, different strains of *S. pneumoniae* cause the disease for the different age groups. Today, two different pneumococcal vaccines are on the market, targeted to the two different groups. Since inclusion of antigens from 90 different serotypes is impractical, only the most common disease-causing organisms were included.

The pneumococcal conjugate vaccine was licensed in 2000 and contains capsular polysaccharides from seven different strains of *S. pneumoniae* conjugated to diphtheria toxoid CRM[197]. The vaccine is recommended for use in all children 2–23 months old and for some older children. The seven strains included in the vaccine are responsible for almost 90% of pneumococcal disease seen in American and Canadian children under 5. Conjugating the polysaccharide to a toxoid converts the T-independent polysaccharide to a T-dependent antigen and stimulates both Ab production and memory responses in children. One shortcoming of this vaccine is that diseases caused by other serotypes may arise.

In adults, protection from both pneumonia and meningitis is important. The 23 serotypes of *S. pneumoniae* responsible for more than 80% of adult pneumococcal disease are included in a vaccine composed of capsular polysaccharide fragments. This vaccine is able to stimulate Ab production toward the organisms included in the vaccine. Studies show the effectiveness of adult immunization ranges from 45% to 80%, possibly because of invasive diseases from serotypes of the bacteria not included in the vaccine. Because polysaccharides are T-independent Ags, this vaccine is intended primarily for adults, but may be used in high-risk children older than 2. In addition, reimmunization may be recommended depending on age at initial immunization.

Polio. Polio, a viral illness that results in paralysis, has been eradicated from much of the world through intensive immunization programs. While no indigenous cases of polio have been identified in the United States in more than 20 years, polio vaccination is still recommended. In the United States, both inactivated and attenuated polio vaccines had been available. In 1999 the use of oral polio vaccine was limited to exceptional circumstances because the risk of developing paralytic poliomyelitis from the attenuated vaccine was greater than the risk of contracting wild-type polio.

The current polio vaccine is an inactivated whole virus vaccine of enhanced potency, containing virus particles from the three serotypes known to cause disease. Administration of the vaccine results in production of neutralizing Abs but not development of cell-mediated immunity.

Rabies. Rabies is a zoonotic infection caused by the bite of a rabid animal. Because rabies is endemic in the fox, skunk, and raccoon populations of the United States, humans may come in contact with a rabid animal and therefore be at risk for infection. Currently the rabies vaccine is limited to specific populations and special circumstances. The vaccination may be administered preexposure to laboratory workers, animal control officers, veterinarians, and forest rangers who, by virtue of their occupations, are at greater risk for contact with rabid animals. Postexposure vaccination is warranted for individuals who have been bitten by an animal with known or suspected rabies. In cases where exposure to rabies is likely (i.e., unprovoked bites from bats or wild animals), both rabies immune globulin (RIG) and active vaccination are indicated. The RIG is injected into the skin around the wound or, if there is no obvious wound, into the buttock or thigh muscles with the goal of neutralizing any infectious virus before it becomes established in the individual. The active vaccine is then given as a series of five injections into the arm muscle. The immunizations take place over a period of 28 days.

Smallpox. Smallpox was the first disease for which active vaccination was attempted. Reports suggest that methods for actively stimulating immunity against smallpox were developed in India about 1000 years ago. This practice, called variolation, spread throughout Asia and the Middle East, and was introduced to England and the rest of Europe in the 1700s. Because of the risks associated with variolation, the practice was not readily adopted. In 1796, Edward Jenner demonstrated that material from a cowpox lesion could be used to immunize against smallpox—the beginning of modern vaccination therapy and the beginning of the eradication of smallpox.

In 1980, WHO declared that smallpox had been eradicated throughout the world. At that time, wild-type smallpox virus was believed to be confined to two freezers, one in the United States and the other in the Soviet Union. We now know the Soviet Union continued to culture smallpox as part of its biological weapons program. Because of this, there is a possibility that weaponized smallpox survives in parts of the former Soviet Union, or has been carried to other countries by scientists who worked with the virus. So the specter of smallpox reappearing as a biological weapon exists today.

It is important that a vaccine continue to be available today. Vaccinia vaccine is a live attenuated vaccine that induces immunity to vaccinia and related viruses, including smallpox, monkeypox, and cowpox. Following the September 11, 2001, terrorist attacks, there have been efforts to increase the amount of vaccinia vaccine available in case of a terrorist attack that releases smallpox. Studies have shown that immunity can be induced with one fourth the usual immunizing dose if needed. All doses are given percutaneously.

Typhoid. Typhoid fever, caused by *Salmonella typhi,* is a disease of the reticuloendothelial system, the lymphoid system, and the gallbladder, characterized by fever, malaise, abdominal discomfort, and headache. The disease is spread through the fecal-oral route, and—although rare in the United States—is endemic in areas of Latin America, Asia, and Africa. Use of the vaccine is limited to specific populations of individuals, including travelers to endemic areas, laboratory personnel who work with *S. typhi,* and those who have close contact with typhoid carriers.

Two vaccines are currently available for immunization against typhoid fever. One is a subunit vaccine composed of purified polysaccharide from the outer member of *S. typhi,* and the other is a live attenuated vaccine. The polysaccharide vaccine is delivered as an intramuscular injection; the live attenuated vaccine is given orally. The live attenuated vaccine stimulates not only systemic immunity, but also local immunity in the gastrointestinal tract.

Varicella. Varicella-zoster virus (VZV) is the virus responsible for the diseases recognized as chickenpox and shingles. Infections with VZV have only rare complications in children, but may be associated with more significant morbidity and mortality in unimmunized adults. As discussed earlier, concomitant socioeconomic factors with chickenpox often affect school and work productivity. Following the initial infection, VZV becomes latent in the host's dorsal route and trigeminal ganglia. For most individuals, latency is lifelong; however, if host immunity wanes, the virus may become reactivated causing a painful vesicular rash recognized as shingles. Shingles is more frequently seen in adults over 50 and may be complicated by long-lasting post-herpetic neuralgia. The neuralgia may cause either constant or stabbing pain for as long as 6 months after the lesions have healed.

The varicella virus vaccine is a live attenuated vaccine that stimulates an immune response in children 1 year or older. It can be used in adults who have no record of having had chickenpox and who have not been immunized. The vaccine is highly effective, inducing immunity in more than 95% of immunized children, and providing additional socioeconomic benefits.

Since shingles is caused by waning immunity to varicella, recent studies have been undertaken to examine the effects of the vaccine on the development of shingles. A large-scale study showed that the varicella vaccine is able to decrease the inci-

dence of shingles in the elderly by 50%. In those who developed shingles, the severity of symptoms was significantly decreased.

Yellow fever. Yellow fever, a disease that killed more than 4000 people in Philadelphia in 1793, is reemerging in the southern United States and Central and South America. Its reemergence is the result of a resurgence of the mosquito that spreads the virus, believed to be due to global warming.

Although a live attenuated vaccine for yellow fever was developed in 1953, the currently available vaccine was licensed in 1978. It is used in special circumstances, primarily for those traveling to areas where yellow fever is endemic.

Passive Immunization

In active immunization, a patient receives a relatively harmless antigenic form of an organism to stimulate production of an endogenous immune response and impart memory to the host's immune system. In contrast, passive immunization protects a susceptible individual by directly administering exogenous replacement or supplemental immunoglobulins obtained from an immune donor. An individual may acquire specific passive immunity by either natural or induced means. An example of natural passive immunity is the Abs newborns receive from their mothers either across the placenta or in breast milk; an example of induced passive immunity is that imparted by the administration of exogenous animal or human immune globulins.

It was first recognized in the late 1800s that certain diseases (e.g., diphtheria and tetanus) are caused by specific toxins secreted by organisms. Soon after, researchers discovered that animals that survived exposure to these toxins had Abs in their serum and that these Abs were the source of this immunity. Serum containing these Abs came to be known as antitoxins. Passive transfer of immunoglobulins is currently used for much more than protection from infectious diseases or toxins. Immunoglobulins can also be used to supplement a patient's own immune response in cases of agammaglobulinemia or immunodeficiency due to disease or chemotherapy.

Intramuscular immune globulins. Humoral immunity can be transferred from a sensitized person to a nonsensitized person through Abs. The source of Ab for induced passive immunization may be immune globulin in serum from immunized animals (heterologous), or it may be antigen-specific or nonspecific pooled human immune globulin (homologous). **Tables 6.9 and 6.10** list the animal antisera and human immune

Table 6.9. Currently Available Animal Antisera for Passive Immunization

Disease	Product	Source
Black widow spider bite	Antivenin	Equine
Botulism	Botulism antitoxin	Equine
Diphtheria	Diphtheria antitoxin	Equine
Snakebite	Antivenin polyvalent; Antivenin polyvalent Fab fragment	Equine Ovine
Tetanus	Tetanus antitoxin	Human

globulin products, respectively, currently available for passive immunization.

Passive immunization often involves injection of a specific immunoglobulin that targets a specific antigen. This process is referred to as seroprophylaxis or serotherapy. Serotherapy provides only temporary protection against an antigen because it does not promote formation of protective antibodies by the recipient. Normal body catabolism and the rapid depletion of antibody as it combines with antigen contribute to the short duration of protection of exogenous immunoglobulin (21–28 days).

Immunoglobulins for serotherapy are derived from either animal or human sources. Although antitoxins derived from active immunization of animals (e.g., horses and rabbits) will neutralize the same toxins in humans, they are less desirable than those from human sources; the human immune system recognizes the foreign proteins and produces Ab in response. Use of animal antisera frequently causes serum sickness or anaphylactic reactions, so human immunoglobulin should be used whenever possible.

Animal sera may be given in life-threatening situations when human sources are not available. However, patients must be carefully assessed by the pharmacist or other health care provider for preexisting hypersensitivity to animal sera and

Table 6.10. Immune Globulins Available for Passive Immunization

Disease	Product
Cytomegalovirus	Cytomegalovirus immune globulin IV (CMV-IVIG)
Hepatitis A	Immune globulin IM
Hepatitis B	Hepatitis B immune globulin (HBIG) IM
Hypogammaglobulinemia	Immune globulin IM, immune globulin IV
Measles	Immune globulin IM (not available in the U.S.)
Mumps	Immune globulin IM (not available in the U.S.)
Pertussis	Immune globulin IM (not available in the U.S.)
Pseudomonas	Immune globulin IM (not available in the U.S.)
Rabies	Rabies immune globulin IM
Respiratory syncytial virus	Immune globulin IV, humanized monoclonal IgG IM
Rh isoimmunization	$Rh_o(D)$ immune globulin IM
Rubella	Immune globulin IM
Staphylococcus aureus & *Streptococcus pyogenes*	Immune globulin IM (not available in the U.S.)
Varicella-zoster	Varicella-zoster immune globulin (VZIG) IM
Vaccinia	Vaccinia immune globulin IM

IM = intramuscular; IV = intravenous.

possible type I hypersensitivity reactions. A history of atopy or hypersensitivity greatly increases the likelihood of such a reaction. This history, along with concomitant skin testing, is critical to patient safety.

Although serotherapy may provide immediate protection to a naive or specific antibody-free patient and has a variety of theoretical uses, the number of current clinical uses is limited. Its primary use is as prophylaxis in patients exposed to diseases such as hepatitis and rabies. It is especially useful when the anticipated incubation period of the disease is shorter than the onset of protection with standard vaccination techniques (7–10 days). The effectiveness of passive immunization depends on prompt administration of the Abs, which must be given early in the incubation period to avoid the clinical illness. For instance, diphtheria antitoxin should be given within 1 hour of symptom onset to prevent any irreversible damage. The effectiveness of the antitoxin rapidly decreases as the period between the onset of symptoms and administration increases.

The current uses of intramuscular immune globulins (IMIGs) outlined here include their use in treating established toxin-induced illnesses and in prophylaxis of viral infections.

IMIGs in toxin-induced diseases. The role of IMIGs in treating toxin-induced diseases is primarily limited to antitoxins and antivenins used to prevent onset of disease in exposed patients. Toxin-induced diseases that can be treated with IMIGs include botulism, diphtheria, tetanus, and black widow spider or snake bites. All IMIGs for this use are derived from horse or sheep sera (see Table 6.9).

IMIGs in prophylaxis of viral infections. WHO currently recommends using IMIGs only for patients exposed to hepatitis A, hepatitis B, varicella-zoster, measles, rubella, or rabies. This use of IMIGs is much more common than their use for toxin-induced diseases. IMIGs are useful for the prophylaxis of viral infections because they can decrease the severity or modify the effects of the diseases. Some of these immune globulins are antigen-specific and are derived from the serum of convalescent patients with very high circulating levels of Ab to that particular pathogen, while other human IMIG is nonspecific (see Table 6.10). Nonspecific IMIGs can be used for infections such as hepatitis A, measles, and rubella. The two specific types of IMIGs highlighted in this section are HBIG and VZIG.

Hepatitis B immune globulin. HBIG is the agent of choice in postexposure prophylaxis against hepatitis B. Active immunization with HBV vaccine is the most effective preventative tool for all individuals and is recommended by the CDC for children and adolescents. For accidentally exposed unvaccinated individuals and newborns whose mothers are HBsAg positive, administration of HBIG provides high levels of anti-HBV antibody immediately. HBIG should be administered intramuscularly as soon as possible, preferably within 24 hours of exposure, to people who have come in contact with blood from a patient with hepatitis B or other materials contaminated with HBV virus. Prompt serotherapy will provide protection until vaccination can induce active immunity to the exposed individual.

The ACIP of the CDC recommends a combination of active (HBV vaccine) and passive (HBIG, human) immunization for postexposure and prevention of HBV infection.

Varicella-zoster immune globulin. VZIG is prepared from the plasma of adults who have high titers of anti-VZV antibodies. In contrast to HBIG, the use of VZIG is directed toward high-risk patients, especially neonates whose mothers were infected with varicella just before delivery, and immunocompromised children and adults who have been exposed to VZV. Despite VZIG administration, one third to one half of immunocompromised people exposed to VZV will develop clinical disease, but VZIG makes the clinical course of the disease less severe. When used appropriately, VZIG significantly decreases the expected severity of chickenpox, significantly decreases mortality, and decreases the incidence of encephalitis and pneumonia to less than 25% of the expected rate for those not receiving treatment.

Palivizumab. Palivizumab is the first monoclonal Ab licensed for the treatment of an infectious disease. Palivizumab is a humanized monoclonal Ab containing 95% human protein and 5% mouse protein; the large human component in this protein decreases the immunogenicity of the antibody. Intramuscular administration of the Ab provides protection from serious respiratory syncytial virus infection (RSV) in premature infants and infants with chronic lung disease. Studies show that palivizumab can reduce hospitalization from RSV bronchiolitis by more than 50%.[23]

Intravenous immune globulins. Immune globulin suitable for intravenous use is an important development in passive immunization in the past 25 years. Before the mid-1970s, no immune globulin products could be given intravenously because they caused IgG aggregate formation, complement activation, and anaphylactic reactions. Aggregate formation was linked to the method of production. Reformulation has eliminated these problems,

Table 6.11. Intravenous Immune Globulin (IVIG) Products Licensed in the United States

Product	Manufacturer	Formulation
Carimune NF	ZLB Behring	Lyophilized powder
Flebogamma	Instituto Grifols	Solution
Gamimune N	Bayer	Liquid in 10% maltose
Gammagard S/D	Baxter Healthcare Corporation	Lyophilized powder*
Gammar-PIV	ZLB Behring	Lyophilized powder
Gamunex	Bayer	Solution
Iveegam EN	Baxter Healthcare Corporation	Lyophilized powder
Panglobulin	American Red Cross Blood Services/Swiss	Lyophilized powder
Polygam S/D	American Red Cross Blood Services/Hyland	Lyophilized powder*
Venoglobulin-S	Grifols Biologicals	Solution*

*Solvent/detergent in manufacturing process.

and now intravenous immune globulin (IVIG) products are available in the United States.

IVIGs are derived from IgG isolated from pooled human serum. Although it contains primarily IgG, other Ab classes (IgE, IgM, and IgA) and other serum proteins may be present in trace amounts. The larger the donor pool, the wider the spectrum of antigens recognized by the IgG contained in the serum. In fact, WHO recommends that all IVIG products be derived from pools of at least 1000 donors.

The intravenous route for administering immune globulins has many advantages over the intramuscular route. The greatest advantage is that IVIGs can be given in much larger doses than IMIGs. Other advantages include an immediate rise in blood levels, greater bioavailability, easy and relatively painless administration, fewer severe adverse reactions, and a half-life more closely resembling that of endogenous IgG. All plasma donor units must be free of HIV, hepatitis C virus (HCV), and HBsAg. All IVIG products should contain not less than 90% of their immunoglobulin content as gamma globulin (as recommended by WHO). **Table 6.11** lists the currently licensed IVIG products available in the United States. Normal serum contains four subclasses of IgG (IgG1, IgG2, IgG3, and IgG4), each with its own unique structure and function; these should be present in roughly the same ratios in IVIG products. WHO has recognized a "reference plasma" as a guideline for subclass distribution. The percentage of each subclass in currently available IVIG products, compared with the WHO reference,

is presented in **Table 6.12.** Use of IVIG is not without side effects; although generally mild (e.g., chills, nausea, abdominal pain), they are observed in about 1% to 10% of patients. These adverse reactions can often be avoided by premedicating the patient or by slowing the rate of infusion.

IVIG is the treatment of choice for primary immunodeficiencies, such as hypogammaglobulinemia, because it exerts its therapeutic action through replacement of Abs. The presence of impaired antibody responses is associated with an increased risk of infection and a beneficial response to IVIG. Diseases characterized as "secondary" or "acquired" immunodeficiencies vastly outnumber primary immunodeficiencies. IVIG has been approved for treatment of both primary and secondary immunodeficiency and shows efficacy for the treatment of a number of other immunologically mediated disorders (**Table 6.13**).

IVIG has also been studied extensively in the treatment of antibody-dependent autoimmune diseases, including immune thrombocytopenia, Kawasaki disease, and myasthenia gravis. The exact mechanism of action in treating these diseases is unclear. Suggested mechanisms include saturation of Fc receptors on platelets; producing antibody-coated cells that are less susceptible to Fc-mediated phagocytosis and destruction; and down-regulation of Ab production through inhibitory Fc receptors on B cells. Although several mechanisms may actually be involved, IVIG is clinically effective in ameliorating Ab-dependent autoimmune diseases.

Table 6.12. Percentage of IgG Subclasses in Licensed IVIG Products

Product	IgG1 (%)	IgG2 (%)	IgG3 (%)	IgG4 (%)
WHO reference plasma	60–70	23–29	4–8	2–6
Carimune NF	61	30	7	3
Flebogamma	70	25	3.1	1.9
Gamimune N	59	29	6	5
Gammagard S/D	69	22	4	5
Gammar-PIV	69	23	6	2
Gammunex	65	26	5.6	2.6
Iveegam	64	30	4	1.5
Panglobulin	61	30	7	3
Polygam S/D	57	30	8	5
Venoglobulin-S	66	25	6	3

WHO = World Health Organization.

Table 6.13. Potential and FDA-Approved Indications for IVIGs

Primary immunodeficiencies

Substitution therapy for agammaglobulinemia, hypogammaglobulinemia due to a number of primary immunodeficiency states[a]

Secondary (acquired) immunodeficiencies

Malignancies associated with antibody deficiency
    Chronic lymphocytic leukemia (CLL),[a] multiple myeloma

Bacterial infections
    Pseudomonas, group B streptococcus

Bone marrow transplant patients[a]

Viral infections
    Cytomegalovirus (CMV), herpes simplex

Kidney/heart/transplant patients

High-risk premature infants/neonates

AIDS patients, primarily children[a]

Burn patients

Guillain-Barré syndrome

Chronic inflammatory demyelinating polyneuropathy

Thrombocytopenias
    Immune thrombocytopenia purpura (ITP)[a]
    Neonatal alloimmune thrombocytopenia
    Posttransfusion purpura

Other autoimmune disorders
    Collagen vascular diseases
    Myasthenia gravis
    Kawasaki disease[a]
    Autoimmune neutropenia and hemolytic anemia

[a]FDA-approved indications.

The effectiveness of IVIG in other secondary (acquired) immunodeficiencies is thought to be caused by both its immunomodulatory effect and its ability to replace specific antibodies. The infectious complications—bacterial, viral, and fungal—that often accompany secondary immunodeficiencies can be devastating, especially in transplant patients, cancer patients, and premature infants.

In conclusion, each IgG subclass plays an important role in the immune system. Clinical deficiency of a subclass may manifest itself as disease, most commonly as a chronic respiratory infection. IVIG products, with adequate subclass representation, can normalize the plasma of patients with subclass deficiency.

SUMMARY

The body is able to respond to many different types of organisms. These responses are unique for each organism and the type of immune response—Ab, Th1 cell-mediated, or CTL—is determined by the type of pathogen and site of replication. Specific immune responses not only clear the infection, but also provide long-term immunity, protecting the host from developing the same disease a second time.

Protection from disease can also arise without a primary infection, through active or passive immunization. Active immunization exposes the immune system to a relatively harmless form of an antigen to stimulate the body's defenses against a specific disease. Passive immunization facilitates the antigen-antibody response by administering exogenous immunoglobulin from an immune donor to an unprotected individual.

Active immunization uses vaccines composed of live attenuated pathogens, inactivated organisms, or subunits of the organism (protein or polysaccharide). Active immunization can provide long-lasting protection if appropriate protocols are followed. Most vaccines, even live attenuated ones, require multiple administrations because a single dose does not usually provide permanent protection.

Biotechnological methods of producing vaccine subunits include cloning antigenic viral peptides (e.g., hepatitis B and HPV vaccines) or creating synthetic antigenic peptides (e.g., influenza and malaria vaccines) to produce large amounts of a critical antigen. Recombinant technology is used to produce attenuated vaccines that are genetically altered to a nonpathogenic state. Through recombinant DNA technology, vaccinia viruses can be altered to express the antigenic peptides of a variety of pathogens, thus functioning as a carrier organism. Adjuvants are also being studied to discover if there are ways they can enhance immunogenicity.

Although active immunization has had significant beneficial public health outcomes, it is not without risks. For example, when a live attenuated vaccine is used, there is a risk that the patient will develop the disease rather than only an immune response. Also, allergic reactions can be caused by residual antigens present in the culture media. The risk of vaccination must be assessed within the context of the disease and the relative risk of adverse or long-term effects.

Passive immunization can be transmitted through animal or human sera. Passive immunization provides more immediate protection than active immunization, but its protection is only temporary. Animal sera may produce a higher incidence of serum sickness than human products. Intramuscular immune globulin vaccines are used to treat toxin-induced illnesses and to prevent viral infections. Intravenous immune globulin vaccines are used for many therapeutic purposes, such as agammaglobulinemias and immunodeficiencies. Antigen-specific immune globulins can prevent disease, but their use is limited by high cost and restricted supply.

Pharmacists have an important role in the implementation of immunization programs. With knowledge of the products available and the recommendations for their use, pharmacists can actively assist in the goal of the elimination of vaccine-preventable diseases.

REFERENCES

1. Bharhani MS, Grewal JS, Pilgrim MJ, et al. Reovirus serotype 1/strain Lang-stimulated activation of antigen-specific T lymphocytes in Peyer's patches and distal gut-mucosal sites: activation status and cytotoxic mechanisms. *J Immunol*. 2005; 174:3580–3589.
2. Musgrave BL, Watson CL, Hoskin DW. CD2-CD48 interactions promote cytotoxic T lymphocyte induction and function: anti-CD2 and anti-CD48 antibodies impair cytokine synthesis, proliferation, target recognition/adhesion, and cytotoxicity. *J Interferon Cytokine Res*. 2003; 23:67–81.
3. Ellermann-Eriksen S. Macrophages and cytokines in the early defense against herpes simplex virus. *Virol J*. 2005; 2:59. Available at: http://www.pubmedcentral.gov/articlerender.fcgi?tool=pmcentrez&artid=1215526. Accessed June 5, 2006.
4. Velazquez C, Beltran M, Ontiveros N, et al. *Giardia lamblia* infection induces different secretory and

systemic antibody responses in mice. *Parasite Immunol.* 2005; 27:351–356.

5. Faubert G. Immune response to *Giardia duodenalis*. *Clin Microbiol Rev.* 2000; 13:35–54.

6. Centers for Disease Control and Prevention (CDC). Frequently asked questions about malaria. Available at: http://www.cdc.gov/malaria/faq. htm. Accessed June 12, 2006.

7. Centers for Disease Control and Prevention (CDC). Preventing emerging infectious diseases. A strategy for the 21st century. Centers for Disease Control and Prevention. 1998. Available at: http://www.cdc.gov/mmwr/preview/mmwrhtml/00054779.htm. Accessed June 14, 2005.

8. CDC Pink Book on Vaccines. www.cdc.gov. vaccines/pubs/pinkbook/downloads/polio.pdf. Accessed August 31, 2007.

9. Bompart F. Vaccination strategies for the last stages of global polio eradication. *Indian Ped.* 2005; 42:163–169.

10. Moorthy VS, Good MF, Hill AV. Malaria vaccine developments. *Lancet.* 2004; 363:150–156.

11. Scarselli M, Guiliani MM, Adu-Bobie J, et al. The impact of genomics on vaccine design. *Trends Biotechnol.* 2005; 23(2):84–91.

12. Capecchi B, Serruto D, Adu-Bobie J, et al. The genome revolution in vaccine design [review]. *Curr Issues Mol Biol.* 2004; 6(1):17–28.

13. Plotkin SA, Orenstein WA. *Vaccines.* 4th ed. Philadelphia, PA: WB Saunders; 2004:1193.

14. Ulmer JB. Enhancement of vaccine potency through improved delivery. *Expert Opin Biol Ther.* 2004; 4:1045–1053.

15. O'Hagen DT, Rappuoli R. Novel approaches to vaccine delivery. *Pharmacutical Res.* 2004; 21:1519–1530.

16. Haro I, Gomara MJ. Design of synthetic peptidic constructs for the vaccine development against viral infections. *Curr Protein Pept Sci.* 2004; 5:425–433.

17. McGeary RP, Olive C, Toth I. Lipid and carbohydrate based adjuvant/carriers in immunology. *J Pept Sci.* 2003; 9:405–418.

18. Centers for Disease Control and Prevention (CDC). Recommended childhood and adolescent immunization schedules. Available at: http://www.cdc.gov/mmwr/preview/mmwrhtml/mm5451-Immunizationa1.htm. Accessed June 13, 2006.

19. Centers for Disease Control and Prevention (CDC). Recommended Adult Immunization Schedule by Vaccine and Age Group. Available at: http://www.cdc.gov/mmwr/pdf/wk/mm5540-Immunization.pdf. Accessed August 30, 2007.

20. Centers for Disease Control and Prevention (CDC). Pertussis—United States, 1997–2000. *MMWR Morb Mortal Wkly Rep.* 2002; 51(4):73–76.

21. Centers for Disease Control and Prevention (CDC). National, state, and urban area vaccination coverage among children aged 19–35 months—United States. 2004. *MMWR Morb Mortal Wkly Rep.* 2005; 54(29):717–721. Available at: http://www.cdc.gov/mmwr/preview/mmwrhtml/mm5429a1.htm. Accessed June 13, 2006.

22. Grabenstein JD. *ImmunoFacts 2006: Vaccines and Immunologic Drugs.* Philadelphia, PA: Lippincott, Williams and Wilkins; 2005.

23. The IMpact-RSV Study Group. Palivizumab, a humanized respiratory syncytial virus monoclonal antibody, reduces hospitalization from respiratory syncytial virus infection in high-risk infants. *Pediatrics.* 1998; 102:531–537.

SELF-ASSESSMENT QUESTIONS

1. Adaptive immune responses necessary to clear pathogens, such as intracellular and extracellular bacteria and viruses, include:

   A. Antibody
   B. Th2 T cells
   C. Cytotoxic T-effector cells
   D. A and C
   E. All of the above

2. Innate immune responses responsible for holding viral infections in check until the development of adaptive immunity include:

   A. Interferons
   B Interleukins
   C. Natural killer cells
   D. A and C
   E. All of the above

3. Cytotoxic T-effector cells eliminate virally infected cells by:

   A. Antibody and complement
   B. Secretion of IFN-α and IFN-β
   C. Releasing perforin
   D. Activating macrophages

4. Activation of an innate response to pathogens involves binding to pathogen-associated molecular pattern (PAMP) receptors on the macrophage surface. These receptors are linked to signaling pathways within the cell and recognize _____ on the pathogens.

   A. Lipoproteins
   B. Polysaccharides
   C. Lipopolysaccharides
   D. Lipoarabinomannans
   E. All of the above

5. Parasitic worms are generally too large to be ingested by host cells; therefore, the main defense against these organisms is antibody.

The classes of antibody most important for host defense are:

A. IgA
B. IgG
C. IgE
D. A and C
E. All of the above

6. Immunization may be defined as the induction of a specific immune response to a killed or weakened pathogen, or component of a pathogen.

A. True
B. False

7. For a live pathogen to be used for active immunization, it should be:

A. Attenuated (weakened)
B. Genetically stable and unable to revert to a pathogenic form
C. Unable to establish a latent infection
D. All of the above

8. Advantages of inactivated (killed) vaccines compared to attenuated vaccines include the following:

A. They require less antigen in the immunization than an attenuated vaccine
B. They contain large amounts of extraneous material
C. They cannot replicate within the host and cause disease
D. All of the above

9. The *Haemophilus influenzae* serotype b vaccine (Hib) is a conjugate vaccine. This means that:

A. It contains both polysaccharide and protein
B. It is a T-independent antigen
C. It is able to stimulate immune responses in children
D. A and C
E. All of the above

10. For a toxoid vaccine to be effective, it must:

A. Be structurally identical to the toxin
B. Be completely inactivated

C. Both A and B
D. Neither A nor B

11. Recombinant DNA technology is used to produce vaccines from both bacteria and viruses. Examples of recombinant DNA technology include:

A. Tetanus vaccine
B. Hepatitis B vaccine
C. Measles vaccine
D. Hib vaccine

12. Adjuvants are used to increase immune response. Classes of adjuvants can include:

A. Mineral salts
B. Bacterial products
C. Particulate
D. Synthetic compounds
E. All of the above

13. Passive immunization provides the patient with preformed antibody. Passive immunization is used to treat patients who have been exposed to:

A. Toxins and venoms
B. Hepatitis A
C. Cytomegalovirus
D. Rh incompatibility
E. All of the above

14. Intravenous immunoglobulins (IVIG) are used to treat patients:

A. With primary agammaglobulinemias
B. Who have undergone bone marrow transplants
C. Diagnosed with thrombocytopenias
D. A and C
E. All of the above

15. Multivalent vaccines are unable to induce immunity to more than one disease.

A. True
B. False

CHAPTER 7

Immunology of HIV Infection and AIDS

Christopher W. James, Beulah Perdue Sabundayo

CHAPTER OUTLINE

Introduction
Learning objectives
Etiology/epidemiology
Viral replicative cycle
Immunopathogenesis
Transmission and prevention
   Sexual exposure
   Parenteral exposure
   Perinatal exposure
Natural history, diagnosis, and stages
HIV testing
   Standard testing
   Alternative testing
   Quantitation of HIV RNA
   Resistance testing

Opportunistic infections
   Pneumocystis jiroveci pneumonia
   Cryptococcal meningitis
   Toxoplasmosis
   Mycobacterium avium complex and *mycobacterium tuberculosis*
   Candidiasis
   Herpsesvirus/cytomegalovirus
Neoplasms
   Kaposi's sarcoma
   Non-Hodgkin's lymphoma
Summary
References
Self-assessment questions

INTRODUCTION

Since its recognition in 1981, acquired immune deficiency syndrome (AIDS) has affected a substantial portion of the U.S. population. As of December 2004, almost 920,000 cases of AIDS had been reported in the United States alone and over 500,000 AIDS patients have died.[1] By the end of 2003, an estimated 1,039,000 to 1,185,000 people were living with human immunodeficiency virus (HIV) infection in the United States.[2] The World Health Organization (WHO) estimates that, as of 2005, more than 40 million adults were infected with HIV worldwide, with over 95% of new infections occurring in developing countries.[3]

As accessible members of the health care profession, pharmacists can play an important role in educating their communities and patients about HIV infection. In practice, pharmacists may be asked to advise individuals about high-risk behaviors, risk-reduction strategies, and the appropriateness of HIV testing. Pharmacists may serve in a different capacity by advising AIDS patients about adverse drug reactions, drug interactions, and the potential of investigational treatment strategies. This chapter highlights the immunologic aspects of HIV infection and discusses its etiology, pathogenesis, transmission, prevention, and clinical manifestations. With such a background, pharmacists should be able to provide sound counsel, not only to HIV-infected patients, but also to the communities in which they live.

LEARNING OBJECTIVES

After completing this chapter, the reader should be able to:

1. Describe the pathogenesis of HIV infection.
2. Discuss the modes of transmission of HIV.
3. Identify the stages of the viral replicative cycle that have potential for antiviral attack.
4. Describe various methodologies of testing for HIV infection.
5. Identify opportunistic infections associated with HIV infection.

ETIOLOGY/EPIDEMIOLOGY

HIV was first isolated in 1983 by groups in the United States and France, and shortly thereafter was identified as the cause of AIDS.[4,5] The virus is believed to have been present for several decades in localized areas of central Africa and has since spread extensively throughout both developed and undeveloped countries.

HIV type 1 (HIV-1), a lentivirus belonging to a group of nontransforming cytopathic retroviruses, is the predominant type of HIV in the United States.[6] It is very closely related to a simian immunodeficiency virus (SIV) that causes a form of simian AIDS with encephalitis.[7] HIV type 2 (HIV-2), relatively uncommon in the United States, was isolated in 1986 in West African AIDS patients, and was found to cause an immunodeficiency syndrome similar to AIDS.[8] Isolates of HIV-2 appear more closely related, both antigenically and genetically, to SIV than to HIV-1.[7,9] There is cross-reactivity between the core proteins of HIV-1 and HIV-2, but the envelope glycoproteins are not cross-reactive.[7,9] Though HIV-1 and HIV-2 are transmitted by similar modes, HIV-2 appears to develop and advance more slowly than HIV-1. The first case of HIV-2 infection in the United States was documented in 1987; the virus continues to have a presence, although it is uncommon.[10,11]

The impact of the AIDS epidemic is partially reflected by the increase in adult mortality. Between 1993 and 1995, HIV became a leading cause of death among people 25–44 years old.[1] With the advent of more effective treatment, AIDS dropped to the sixth leading cause of death in this age group by 2001.[1]

More than 43,000 AIDS cases were reported to the Centers for Disease Control and Prevention (CDC) in 2004, with some 18,000 AIDS-related

deaths. Today, more than 400,000 people are estimated to be living with AIDS in the United States. Although the death rate from HIV and AIDS continues to decline due to better therapies (a 3% decrease in 1999–2003), the rate of diagnoses continues to increase (an estimated 4% during the same period). The proportion of cases occurring among women, racial and ethnic minorities, and by heterosexual transmission increased from 1993 to 2004 (**Table 7.1**). The largest decline in HIV cases is among perinatal transmission. Between 1992 and 1997, perinatally acquired AIDS cases declined 66% in the United States.[1]

Table 7.1. Characteristics of Reported AIDS Cases in the United States—1993 and 2004[1]

Characteristic	1993, %	2004, %
Sex		
Male	84	73
Female	16	27
Race/Ethnicity		
White	45	30
Black, non-Hispanic	36	49
Hispanic/Latino(a)	18	19
Asian/Pacific Islander, American Indian/ Alaska Native	<1	2
HIV Exposure		
Male-to-male sexual (MSM) contact	47	42
Injection drug use (IDU)	28	22
MSM/IDU	6	5
High-risk heterosexual contact	9	31
Other/not identified*	10	1

*Other/not identified includes hemophilia, blood transfusion, perinatal, and risk not identified or reported.

Source: Adapted from Centers for Disease Control and Prevention (CDC). *HIV/AIDS surveillance report, 2004.* Vol. 16. Atlanta, GA: U.S. Department of Health and Human Services, Centers for Disease Control and Prevention; 2005:1–46. Available at http://www.cdc.gov/hiv/stats/hasrlink.htm. Accessed May 3, 2006. Centers for Disease Control and Prevention [CDC]. *HIV/AIDS Surveillance Report.* Year-end Edition. Atlanta, GA: U.S. Department of Health and Human Services, Centers for Disease Control and Prevention; 1996:1–39.

VIRAL REPLICATIVE CYCLE

As shown in **Figure 7.1**, infection with HIV begins when the envelope glycoprotein of HIV, gp120, attaches to a CD4+ T lymphocyte or other type of cell (e.g., monocytes and macrophages, eosinophils, microglial cells, and dendritic cells).[12] The life cycle of the virus is complete with budding and maturation, at which point the virus can infect other cells through the same process.[13,14]

Three steps are needed for HIV to enter cells: attachment, co-receptor binding, and HIV fusion. The HIV-1 envelope contains surface glycoproteins (gp120) and transmembrane glycoproteins (gp41). The initial attachment between virus and cell is the coupling of the viral gp120 subunit to the CD4+ T cell. Coupling causes a conformational change in gp120, allowing interaction with the chemokine co-receptors CCR5 or CXCR4. The conformational change exposes the crucial gp41 fusion peptide, bringing the cell and viral membranes close, allowing fusion and ultimately viral entry.[15,16]

CCR5 is preferentially transmitted from person to person so it is more commonly encountered than CXCR4 early in the course of HIV-1 infection. Individuals who do not express CCR5 receptors on their lymphocyte cell surfaces (CCR5 gene deletion) are resistant to HIV-1 infection. CCR5 gene deletion occurs in approximately 10% to 20% of Caucasians, particularly those of Northern European descent, and has not been found to occur in African or Asian populations. Only about 1% of Caucasians are homozygous for this deletion. Heterozygous individuals are more commonly found and are frequently associated with long-term nonprogression of the disease.[17]

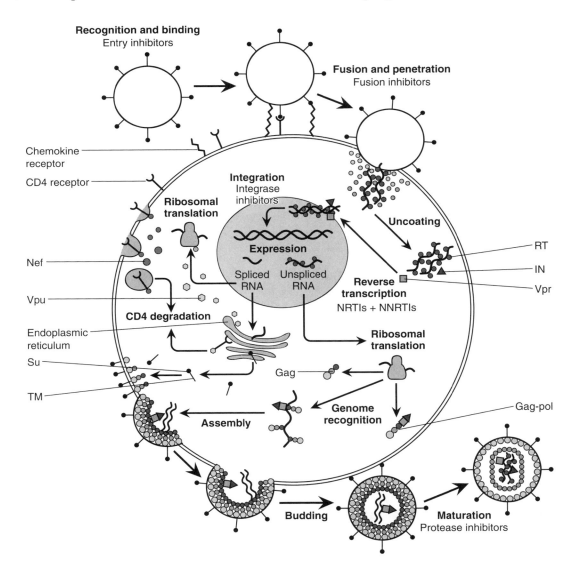

Figure 7.1. HIV life cycle and targets for therapy.

Post fusion, viral genomic RNA and the enzyme reverse transcriptase are released into the cytoplasm of the cell once the viral envelope uncoats. Genomic RNA is then transcribed by viral reverse transcriptase to double-stranded proviral DNA with LTR (long terminal repeats) regions at each end. Proviral DNA either remains accumulated in the cytoplasm in linear or circularized form (latent state) or moves into the cell's nucleus (facilitated by the HIV proteins vpr and matrix [MA]) and integrates into the host's chromosomal DNA with the help of the viral enzyme integrase. Restricted gene expression also allows integrated provirus to remain latent for many years until the cell is activated.[17-19] These latent reservoirs make eradication of HIV-1 unlikely with today's therapies.

When the infected cell becomes activated, the provirus—with the help of host RNA polymerase—is transcribed into viral genomic RNA and messenger RNA (mRNA) through the process of transcription. The mRNA is used for synthesis of HIV gag and gag-pol polyproteins (gp120, gp41) and six regulatory proteins (vif, vpr, vpu, tat, rev, and nef). The newly formed mRNA is then transported to the cytoplasm. Translation of mRNA results in formation of viral proteins, ENV gp 160 (contains gp 120 and gp41), GAG p55 (contains MA, CA, and NC), and GAG-POL p160 (contains MA, CA, PR, RT, and INT). Viral proteins, enzymes, and genomic RNA are assembled, forming an immature viral particle that buds off from the cell and acquires a lipid coat carrying the gp120 and gp41 proteins. Viral enzyme protease cuts the viral particle into smaller pieces. The final step, maturation, is responsible for the catalytic conversion of a capsid precursor protein to the mature capsid form, resulting in infectious particles.[17-19]

With viral replication and release, the CD4$^+$ T cell is usually killed. This cytopathic effect may result from accumulation of large amounts of unintegrated DNA, the presence of high levels of viral RNA and aberrant RNA in the cytoplasm, or the weakening of the cellular membrane during budding of the mature virion.[20] In addition, cell-to-cell fusion and syncytia formation result in cytolysis of both infected and uninfected cells. These mechanisms may contribute to the disproportionate quantitative deficiency in CD4$^+$ T cells relative to the number of cells actually infected.[18] An inappropriate induction of apoptosis (programmed cell death) in CD4$^+$ T cells may also play a role in CD4$^+$ T-cell depletion.[21]

IMMUNOPATHOGENESIS

Primary HIV infection is associated with very active replication of the virus, resulting in high levels of plasma viremia and dissemination of the virus to lymphatic tissue and latent reservoirs. As a result, the circulating population of CD4$^+$ T cells transiently declines (**Figure 7.2**). Within the first few weeks to months, both cellular and humoral responses are observed.[22]

An understanding of HIV dynamics has emerged by studying the effects of potent inhibitors

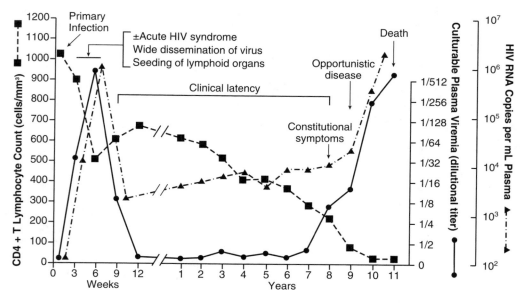

Figure 7.2. Natural history of untreated HIV infection. (Source: Bartlett JG, Gallant JE. *2005–2006 Medical Management of HIV Infection*. Baltimore, MD: Johns Hopkins Medicine Health Publishing Business Group; 2005.)

of viral replication on viral load, as measured by sensitive assays for HIV RNA. The life span of plasma virus is short. Free HIV particles have a half-life of approximately 1.5–4.5 minutes, producing about 50–500 billion viral particles per day in an untreated person. HIV has a reproductive rate of about 10, meaning that virus from 1 cell is able to infect 10 new cells. Infected active CD4$^+$ T cells have a half-life of about 1.1–1.5 days, while HIV-infected macrophages have a half-life of about 14 days and latently infected memory T cells have a half-life of up to 43.9 months. Although potent antiretroviral drugs may decrease plasma viremia by an average of 98.5% to 99%, eradication would still require current antiretroviral therapy to be administered for more than 60 years.[23–27] The majority of circulating virus must therefore be the result of newly infected cells, not chronically or latently infected cells. The observation that CD4$^+$ T-cell counts increase following initiation of antiretrovirals is consistent with a continuous and brisk recruitment of CD4$^+$ T cells into a rapidly cleared virus-expressing pool. It is likely the decline in CD4$^+$ T cells over time reflects destruction, not lack of production. There is a progressive diminution over time in the number of circulating CD4$^+$ T cells at a modal rate of about 30–50 cells/mL over 6 months.[28] This unrelenting cycle of new infection, viral replication, and rapid cell death may be the key dynamic driving HIV pathogenesis.[23,24]

Normally, when an infectious pathogen is encountered, the immune response triggers both humoral and cellular factors, the pathogen is eliminated, and the immune system restores itself to its resting state. Because HIV is persistently replicating, the normal return to quiescence does not occur, so the immune system enters a state of chronic activation.[22]

The immune system's primary antigen-presenting cells are dendritic cells (DC), macrophages, and B cells. Specific immune responses, induced by DC, are needed for primary antigen-specific immune reactions. Some viruses can infect DC. B and T lymphocytes are controlled by DC. Once exposed to antigen, DC expresses these antigens on the cell surface and, in the presence of interleukin-12 (IL-12), initiates T-cell activation. DC-SIGN, a type of lectin, is expressed on submucosal and intradermal DC; it has been postulated as a mechanism by which HIV is transmitted to T cells.[17]

Lymphoid tissue is the primary site of HIV-1 viral replications throughout the entire course of disease. Plasma viremia is extremely high following primary HIV-1 infection, but declines without antiretroviral therapy in response to an HIV-1-specific cytotoxic T-cell (CTL) response. Follicular DC (FDC) trap HIV virions in lymphoid tissue, leading to accumulation of virus in the lymph nodes. The lymph nodes are closely populated by CD4$^+$ T cells, FDC, antigen-presenting cells, and pro-inflammatory cytokines (such as IL-1, IL-6, and tumor necrosis factor alpha [TNFα]). Infection or vaccination can increase HIV-1 replication and induce antigen activation of CD4$^+$ T cells. In contrast, antiretroviral therapy decreases the number of actively infected CD4$^+$ T cells in lymphatic tissue. The pool of latently infected cells is not affected and remains ready to be activated once antiretroviral therapy is discontinued. Over the usual course of HIV-1 disease, viral replication increases and the total number of CD4$^+$ T cells declines. Disease progression leads to destruction of lymphatic architecture that leads to a lost viral trapping ability.[17,29]

Genetic polymorphisms have either a negative or positive impact on the course of HIV disease. Individual human leukocyte antigen (HLA) patterns determine an HIV-specific response, with CD$^+$ T cells dependent on HLA class II molecules and CD8$^+$ T cells dependent on HLA class I molecules.[17]

Less is known about HLA class II alleles. HLA class II antigens have been associated with a long-term non-progressive HIV disease state as a result of an HIV-1-specific CD4$^+$ T-cell response.[17] More is known about CD8$^+$ T-cell response to HLA class I molecules. Being homozygous for HLA-Bw4 is thought to be protective against infection with HIV, whereas being heterozygous is associated with a slower disease progression once infected. A slower disease progression is associated with HLA types B14, B27, B51, B57, and C8, whereas faster disease progression is seen with HLA types A23, B37, and B49. Discordant heterosexual couples appear to have a protective effect if they have "mismatched" HLA class I types.[17]

Virus-specific cytotoxic T lymphocytes play a critical role in recognition, control, and elimination of infected cells. They do not, however, appear to protect against superinfection. During the first stages of primary HIV infection, CTLs are thought to play a major role in initial control of plasma viraemia. In addition, patients who undergo planned structured treatment interruptions from antiretroviral therapy show strong CTL responses. Recently, CTL "escape" mutations have been described in stable chronic infection that leads to a rapid decline in CD4$^+$ T-cell counts. The mechanism for CTL escape has not been explained.[17,29]

CD4$^+$ T cells may be differentiated into T-helper1 (T$_H$1) or T$_H$2 cells. CD4$^+$ T cells that differentiate into T$_H$1 produce interferon γ (IFNγ) and IL-2 that are needed for CTL, natural killer (NK) cells, and macrophages, which produce the immune system's effector functions. T_H2 CD4$^+$ T cells primarily produce IL-4, IL-5, IL-6, and IL-10 that are needed to produce a humoral response.[17]

The body's HIV-1-specific humoral immune response is not well understood. Previous studies substantiate that neutralizing antibodies to HIV-1 do exist, although their role in protection from infection and progression of disease is unclear. HIV-1-infected persons develop neutralizing antibodies to their initial virus later in the disease course; but new resistant virus has already developed by the time these antibodies are developed, and the viruses can escape. Slow disease progressors have high titers of anti-p24 antibodies, persistent neutralizing antibodies, and do not have antibody against gp120 epitopes. It is unknown if these events are protective or a response to the virus by the healthy immune system.[17,29]

TRANSMISSION AND PREVENTION

HIV transmission occurs primarily by sexual or blood exposures, as well as mother-to-child transmission. It is usually preventable. Infection occurs when mucous membranes or breaks in the skin come in contact with infected blood, semen, vaginal secretions, amniotic fluid, or cerebrospinal fluid. Transmission by organ donation has also been reported. Education on appropriate condom use, safe needle practices, needle exchange programs, postexposure prophylaxis, and treatment of HIV-infected pregnant women dramatically decreases transmission rates. Transmission depends on the concentration of virus and the extent or type of exposure.[30,31]

Sexual Exposure

The risk of transmission varies depending on the type of sexual exposure. The rates from receptive anal intercourse are greatest at 0.1% to 3.0%.[32] Receptive vaginal intercourse rates are 0.1% to 0.2%; cases of receptive oral sex are possible, though very rare.[32] The risk of transmission during sex is associated with viral load, type of body fluid, and presence of genital ulcer disease or inflammation (such as concurrence of other sexually transmitted disease). Exposures to blood during sex, such as sex during menses or traumatic sex, may increase risk as well.[30,33,34]

Nonoccupational postexposure prophylaxis (PEP) for sexual exposures is primarily unproven

to work. As with occupational PEP, optimal outcomes should occur if treatment is started within first 2 hours and certainly within 24 hours of exposure, as efficacy diminishes after this time.[35,36] Given the paucity of data for choice of therapies, most clinicians draw from the occupational PEP guidelines for treatment recommendations and use dual NRTI or triple-drug regimens including a protease inhibitor. However, the most effective way to prevent sexual transmission continues to be appropriate condom use.[30]

Parenteral Exposure

The risk of transmission depends on the type of parenteral exposure. The rate of transmission from an infected blood transfusion is over 90%.[37-41] In the United States, antibody testing of blood donations began in March 1985 for HIV-1 and in June 1992 for HIV-2. Since then, the risk of transmission of HIV from receiving infected blood has decreased dramatically. In August 1995, the U.S. Food and Drug Administration (FDA) recommended further screening using the HIV-1 p24 antigen test that should detect cases in the "window period" before seroconversion.[42]

Today, injection drug use and occupational exposures are the most common routes of parenteral exposure. Single occupational exposures have a transmission risk of 0.4%[43] and injection drug use, 0.67%.[44,45] Increased risk depends on higher viral load, depth of the puncture wound, visible blood on the instrument, or entry into a vein or artery. Deep injuries have a 15-fold increased risk of transmission, visible blood on the instrument increases risk 6.2 times, entry into a vein or artery increases risk 4.3-fold, and if the source patient dies within 2 months of exposure, then the risk is 5.6 times greater.[46,47]

The CDC has published guidelines for evaluation and treatment of occupational exposures.[48] Occupational PEP with zidovudine has an 81% efficacy rate (48% to 94%).[49] Therapy should ideally begin within the first 2 hours and certainly within 24 hours. The type of exposure and circumstances of the source patient determine the recommendation for treatment, either dual NRTI or triple therapy with a protease inhibitor. Confounding factors for appropriate therapy include delayed presentation (>24 hours), pregnancy, unknown source patient, viral resistance in the source patient, and toxicity of PEP leading to nonadherence or early discontinuation of the course.[30,48]

Transmission by injection drug use can be reduced or prevented by appropriate needle use, including education on sharing of needles, needle exchange programs, dispensing of clean needles and supplies, and education on how to clean needles appropriately.[30,45]

Perinatal Exposure

Mother-to-child HIV infection transmission rates are 25% to 35% when the mother goes untreated during pregnancy.[50,51] Widespread use of zidovudine, as after the PACTG 076 trial, lowered transmission rates to below 4%.[50] The use of highly active antiretroviral therapy (HAART) is now common practice for HIV-infected pregnant women and has lowered rates even further.[52] Women who do not receive prenatal treatment may receive zidovudine during delivery or perhaps single-dose nevirapine. The concern for single-dose nevirapine is the development of resistance, which effectively renders the class of NNRTIs useless for future treatment.[51] Postpartum, newborn babies should receive zidovudine for their first 6 weeks to further lower the risk of transmission.[50,51]

NATURAL HISTORY, DIAGNOSIS, AND STAGES

The course of infection varies from person to person. The estimated median time from infection to the development of AIDS is about 10–12 years without antiretroviral therapy (Figure 7.2). However, an estimated 10% of those with new infections will progress to AIDS in 2–3 years. Another 5% will remain asymptomatic with stable CD4+ T-cell counts for at least 7 years, resulting in a long-term nonprogressive infection.[53,54]

Because of the nonspecific viral syndrome that occurs after HIV infection, most cases of acute HIV transmission go undiagnosed. Anywhere from 40% to 90% of those with newly acquired HIV infection will experience an acute viral syndrome characterized by fever and rash among other complaints (Table 7.2).[55–61] This syndrome generally lasts about 2 weeks, but can range from a few days to more than 10 weeks. Plasma HIV RNA can be detected 4–20 days after infection, and occurs about 3–4 days before p24 antigen is detectable.[54,62] So the best way to diagnose acute cases is through plasma viremia testing. Positive viremia of less than 3000 copies/mL is generally considered a false positive since true seroconversion syndromes usually result in much higher viremia.[59,63] HIV antibodies take longer to form, becoming detectable in the blood 1–3 months after infection, with few taking as long as 6 months. Diagnosis of established infection is generally by two different antibody tests, enzyme-linked immunosorbent assay (ELISA) and Western blot. ELISA antibodies can be detectable in the blood about 1–2 weeks after detectable viremia, and the Western blot will begin to develop positive bands about 2 weeks after detectable viremia.[64–66] These tests are described in more detail later. Criteria for the diagnosis of AIDS are detailed in Table 7.3.

Table 7.2. Symptoms Associated with Acute HIV Infection Seroconversion

Sign or Symptom	Frequency, %
Fever	80–90
Fatigue	70–90
Rash	40–80
Adenopathy	40–70
Pharyngitis	50–70
Myalgias/arthralgias	50–70
Headache	32–70
Nausea/vomiting	30–60
Night sweats	50
Oral ulcers	10–20

Source: Adapted from Kahn JO, Walker BD. Acute human immunodeficiency virus type 1 infection. *N Engl J Med*. 1998; 339:33–39.

Table 7.3. 1993 Centers for Disease Control and Prevention HIV/AIDS Classification System

CD4 Cell Categories	Clinical Categories		
	A Asymptomatic, or PGL or Acute HIV Infection	B Symptomatic (Not A or C)	C AIDS Indicator Condition*
500 cells/mm³ (≥29%)	A1	B1	C1
200–499 cells/mm³ (14%–28%)	A2	B2	C2
<200 cells/mm³ (<14%)	A3	B3	C3

Shaded areas indicate AIDS diagnosis.

PGL = persistent generalized lymphadenopathy

Source: Adapted from Appendix: Revised surveillance case definition for HIV infection. *MMWR Morb Mortal Wkly Rep.* December 10, 1999/48(RR13):29–31.

*AIDS-indicator conditions:

- Recurrent bacterial pneumonia
- Invasive cervical carcinoma, confirmed by biopsy
- Candidiasis of the bronchi, trachea, or lungs
- Esophageal candidiasis
- Cryptococcosis, extrapulmonary
- Coccidioidomycosis, chronic intestinal (>1 month duration)
- Cryptosporidiosis, chronic intestinal (>1 month duration)
- Cytomegalovirus disease (other than liver, spleen, or nodes)
- Cytomegalovirus retinitis (with loss of vision)
- HIV encephalopathy
- Herpes simplex: chronic ulcers (>1 month duration) or bronchitis, pneumonitis, or esophagitis
- Histoplasmosis, disseminated or extrapulmonary
- Isosporiasis, chronic intestinal (>1 month duration)
- Kaposi's sarcoma
- Lymphoma, Burkitt's (or equivalent term)
- Lymphoma, immunoblastic (or equivalent term)
- Lymphoma, primary in brain
- *Mycobacterium avium* complex or *Mycobacterium kansasii,* disseminated or extrapulmonary
- *Mycobacterium tuberculosis,* pulmonary, disseminated, or extrapulmonary
- *Pneumocystis carinii* pneumonia
- Progressive multifocal leukoencephalopathy
- Salmonella septicemia, recurrent
- Toxoplasmosis of brain
- Wasting syndrome (weight loss >10% of baseline body weight, associated with either chronic diarrhea or fever)

HIV TESTING

Serologic tests for antibodies to HIV are the mainstay of diagnosis of HIV infection in adults and children older than 18 months. Seroconversion occurs, on average, 6 weeks after initial HIV infection, with 95% of individuals seroconverting within 6 months.[67] An individual infected with HIV may have a negative test for antibodies during this period.

Currently available antibody tests are generally inadequate for diagnosing infection in infants born to HIV-seropositive mothers. Almost all infants will passively acquire maternal antibodies in utero. Maternal antibodies may persist up to 15–18 months, and serologic antibody tests will detect these passively acquired antibodies. True HIV infection of the infant cannot be serologically detected until maternal antibodies have cleared. Therefore, these tests lack the specificity needed for detection of infection in infants younger than 18 months.[68]

This section briefly summarizes the serologic tests currently available for detection of antibodies to HIV and other diagnostic tests that may become useful in diagnosing HIV infection.

Standard Testing

Enzyme-linked immunosorbent assay. ELISA was first licensed by the FDA in 1985, primarily for screening blood and plasma products. Testing by ELISA is now the most useful screening tool for HIV infection, and many commercially available ELISA kits are licensed by the FDA. Evolution of ELISA testing has resulted in improved sensitivity for the detection of rare HIV subtypes and HIV-2. In testing patients with chronic HIV infection, ELISAs have a sensitivity and specificity of greater than 99.9%.[69–71]

A "window period" of low sensitivity—the time between initial infection and the production of antibodies—has been noted with ELISA.[72] Seroconversion generally occurs within 6 weeks, and false-negative results may occur during this window period. An individual is still considered infectious at this time despite the absence of antibodies to HIV. Fourth-generation assays detect both HIV-1 antibodies and p24 antigen, increasing sensitivity and the ability to detect patients with acute HIV infection.[73,74] Hypogammaglobulinemic children of HIV-seropositive mothers also may have false-negative ELISA results because their immune systems cannot produce antibodies to HIV.[64,75]

Serum samples deemed positive by ELISA must be tested again in duplicate. Only samples tested by ELISA that are repeatedly reactive are considered positive. A positive ELISA is not sufficient to make the diagnosis of HIV infection, especially in low-prevalence populations; it must be followed by a confirmatory test. A diagnosis of HIV infection is made when an individual has repeatedly tested positive with ELISA and has a positive confirmatory test.

Western blot. The Western blot is the most commonly used confirmatory test, though some laboratories have used a radio-immunoprecipitation assay (RIPA) or indirect immunofluorescence assay (IFA).[76,77] Controversy exists among various groups as to the interpretation of a positive Western blot.[78] The CDC and the Association of State and Territorial Public Health Laboratory Directors suggest that a positive test should be defined by the presence of at least two of the following HIV protein bands: p24, gp41, or gp120/160.[79] A negative test is the absence of all bands. An indeterminate result is one in which at least one band is present, but the additional band(s) needed for a positive test are not. Indeterminate results can be seen in recently infected individuals with incomplete serologic response and in patients with advanced disease.[78] An indeterminate result in patients whose physical examination and medical history are highly suggestive of HIV infection should be repeated by a second Western blot in 6 months, which will likely yield a positive result. Conversely, repeat testing of an indeterminate result in individuals at low risk for infection will generally yield the same banding pattern as the previous indeterminate results. Such individuals are rarely, if ever, truly infected with HIV.[79] Indeterminate Western blot results may also be associated with conditions that produce cross-reacting nonspecific antibodies, including autoimmune diseases, collagen-vascular disease, lymphoma, multiple sclerosis, and recent immunizations.

Alternative Testing

p24 antigen assay. The detection of p24 antigen, one of the HIV core proteins, in the serum of an HIV-infected person is an indicator of active viral replication. Serum p24 antigen can be detected during two different phases of HIV infection: immediately after HIV infection but before the development of antibodies to HIV, and in the late stages of illness.[80–82] The p24 antigen assay is, at present, primarily used as a research tool. One of the major disadvantages of this assay is that it cannot detect p24 antigen in the presence of high titers of HIV-specific antibodies because of the formation of antibody-antigen complexes.[67] This assay is valuable in detecting HIV infection during the "window period" before people develop antibodies to HIV and in hypogammaglobulinemic children.[67,83] The assay for p24 antigen also has been used to monitor the progression of disease and the effect of antiviral therapy in patients with advanced disease.[84,85]

Less than 30% of HIV-infected patients have detectable p24 antigen at any given point in the infection, using the standard assay.[86] To increase its sensitivity, the assay was recently modified by using an "acid-dissociated method" in which p24 antibody-antigen complexes dissociate, allowing more p24 antigen to be detected by the ELISA. With this modified method, over 50% of HIV-infected patients have detectable p24 antigen.[86,87]

Polymerase chain reaction. Polymerase chain reaction (PCR) is a method for amplifying the viral DNA a million times or more to increase the probability of detection.[69] This method offers several advantages over other diagnostic tests, including its potential use in detecting virus in infants younger than 18 months. PCR is not affected by the presence of maternal antibodies.[88] The assay can be completed in 1 day, making it less labor-intensive than an HIV culture.

Because PCR detects viral genetic material, not antibodies, infection with HIV can be detected earlier. Early detection may have favorable prognostic implications because antiretroviral therapy and other medical interventions may be initiated earlier in the course of infection. PCR may also be used to (1) resolve the infection status of individuals with an indeterminate Western blot, (2) directly detect and quantify HIV DNA and RNA from cells of infected people, and (3) define the patterns of transmission and evolution of the virus through the population.[89] The sensitivity of PCR can vary with the course of HIV illness, and it may be less sensitive during asymptomatic periods and highly sensitive in patients with AIDS.[90]

Home testing kits. Today, only one over-the-counter home HIV testing kit is commercially available: Home Access Express™ by Home Access Health Corporation.[91] This kit allows people to be tested and counseled about their test results in the privacy of their own homes. The user provides a drop of blood on blot paper and sends it to an FDA-licensed laboratory (per instructions on the box) where both the ELISA and IFA are performed. After a specified period of time, the user calls for the result and receives appropriate counseling. The entire process is anonymous. The manufacturer received 174,316 home sample collection tests in the first year of availability, with 97% of those tested calling for their results. Less than 1% of the tests were positive for HIV.[92] About half of those testing positive for HIV had not been previously tested,[92] so home testing expands access to testing in populations at risk for HIV infection.

Rapid testing. Three FDA-approved rapid HIV antibody screening tests are available: OraQuick® Advance Rapid HIV-1/2 Antibody Test (OraSure Technologies, Inc), Uni-Gold™ Recombigen® HIV (Trinity Biotech), and Reveal G-2™ Rapid HIV-1 Antibody Test (MedMira, Inc).[93] These enzyme immunoassay (EIA) tests are categorized by Clinical Laboratory Improvement Amendments (CLIA) as waived or moderate complexity. The sensitivity and specificity of rapid assays range from 99.3% to 100%.[94] Results are available in 10–20 minutes, which is particularly helpful when rapid information is needed for occupational exposures or patients who may not return for their test results.[95] All positive results should be confirmed by standard antibody testing.[95] The OraQuick Advance product is the only rapid assay to detect HIV-2.[94] It is also the only assay able to perform testing on oral fluid; it is not approved for testing on serum.[94] In December 2005, public health officials in San Francisco, New York, and Los Angeles reported high rates of false-positive results when using oral fluids with the OraQuick Advance assay.[94] Although similar problems were not encountered at other sites using the same assay, it is the subject of ongoing investigation by OraSure Technologies and several government agencies.

Saliva and urine tests. Assays for detecting HIV antibodies in saliva have been studied. Earlier studies of these assays demonstrated a specificity and sensitivity ranging from 93% to 100% and from 98.7% to 100%, respectively.[96] In December 1994, the FDA approved the first saliva-based collection kit for HIV-antibody screening, OraSure HIV-1 test (Epitope; Beaverton, Oregon).[91,97] The sensitivity and specificity were 99.9% when compared to ELISA assays of the serum and clinical diagnosis.[98] Individuals repeatedly testing positive by this test should undergo standard testing methods. Assays for detecting antibodies in urine have also been studied.[99–102] EIA and Western blot urine testing is available from Calypte Biomedical Corporation. The reported sensitivity and specificity compared to standard serologic testing is 99% and 94%, respectively.[101,102] Potential advantages of these tests are ease of collection, lower cost, and the detection of HIV infection in places where technical skills may be lacking.

Quantitation of HIV RNA

The ability to quantitate the amount of HIV in the blood aids in monitoring disease progression, as well as in evaluating the response to antiretroviral therapy. A more rapid progression to AIDS has been observed in patients with a high viral load at the time of seroconversion ($>10^5$ copies/mL) compared with patients with lower viral loads.[103] Viral load testing is part of the standard-of-care management for HIV infection.

Several methods are available for quantitating viral load: reverse transcriptase-coupled polymerase chain reaction (RT-PCR), nucleic acid sequence-based amplification (NASBA), and branched DNA signal amplification (bDNA).[104–106] Sensitivity and specificity is comparable between methodologies, though some variability does exist when assessing low-level viremia.[107–109] Current RT-PCR and bDNA techniques are able to detect HIV-1 viremia as low as 50 copies/mL.

Resistance Testing

Antiretroviral resistance testing has become an essential adjunctive measure in the care of HIV-infected patients. Guidelines address the proper use of genotypic and phenotypic assays in the investigation of antiretroviral drug resistance.[63,110] Genotypic assays consist of gene sequencing to detect mutations that confer antiretroviral resistance, while phenotypic assays assess individual drug susceptibility to plasma virus.[110] U.S. Department of Health and Human Services guidelines recommend that resistance assays be conducted in patients who have not responded to antiretroviral therapy or have suboptimal suppression of HIV RNA after initiating antiretroviral therapy.[63]

OPPORTUNISTIC INFECTIONS

Because of the profound, irreversible immunodeficiency in AIDS patients, opportunistic infections are generally less responsive to conventional therapy and frequently recur when therapy is discontinued. Opportunistic infections are the leading cause of death in patients with AIDS, so lifelong suppressive therapy is often required for many of these infections. However, antiretroviral therapy and chemoprophylaxis for opportunistic infections have dramatically decreased the morbidity and mortality of HIV/AIDS.[111,112] Coinciding with the widespread availability of HAART, the overall incidence of opportunistic infections decreased more than 50% from 1992 to 1997.[113] Current guidelines for prophylaxis of opportunistic infections indicate it is safe to discontinue primary and secondary chemoprophylaxis for certain infections with immune reconstitution secondary to antiretroviral therapy.[111] Discontinuation of chemoprophylaxis for opportunistic infections should be considered case-by-case.[114]

Pneumocystis Jiroveci Pneumonia

Pneumocystis jiroveci (formerly known as *Pneumocystis carinii*) pneumonia occurs in up to 80% of AIDS patients not receiving primary prophylaxis;

it is the initial opportunistic infection in about 60% of AIDS patients.[115,116] The rate of occurrence in individuals with a CD4+ T-cell count below 200 cells/mm^3 is about 8% and 18% after 6 months and 1 year, respectively.[117]

As with other infections, *Pneumocystis* pneumonia (PCP) may represent reactivation of latent infection.[118] The presentation of PCP in HIV-infected patients is a more subtle, indolent process than that observed in patients whose immunodeficiencies are not caused by HIV. In one study, the median duration of symptoms at the time of diagnosis was 28 days in AIDS patients, compared with 5 days in patients whose immunodeficiencies are not caused by HIV.[119] Clinical manifestations of PCP include fever, shortness of breath, and nonproductive cough, with only subtle changes on chest radiography. Definitive diagnosis is made by identification of the organism in the sputum, by bronchoscopy with bronchoalveolar lavage, or by biopsy.[120,121] The treatment of choice for PCP is trimethoprim/sulfamethoxazole (TMP/SMX) for 21 days.[111,122]

Although 80% of patients survive their initial hospitalization, 60% relapse within 1 year without prophylaxis.[117,123] Medications including trimethoprim/sulfamethoxazole, dapsone, atovaquone, and aerosolized pentamidine can prevent the development of PCP, thus improving survival in people with HIV disease. Current guidelines recommend starting PCP prophylaxis in patients with a CD4+ T-cell count of less than 200 cells/mm^3.[111] TMP/SMX is also the treatment of choice for prophylaxis of PCP based on both clinical efficacy and cost effectiveness. A meta-analysis of randomized trials demonstrated superior efficacy of TMP/SMX compared with dapsone and aerosolized pentamidine for PCP prophylaxis.[124] In addition, TMP/SMX and high-dose dapsone (100 mg/day) demonstrate superior efficacy over aerosolized pentamidine in patients with CD4+ T-cell counts less than 100 cells/mm^3.[125] TMP-SMX is also effective in preventing toxoplasmosis and bacterial infections.[111,126]

Cryptococcal Meningitis

Cryptococcal meningitis occurs in about 5% to 10% of HIV-infected patients. In addition to the central nervous system, cryptococcal infection can occur in the lungs, skin, genitourinary tract, bone marrow, and blood.[127–129] Manifestations of cryptococcal meningitis may be subtle. Fever and headache are the most common symptoms; meningismus, photophobia, mental status changes, and seizures occur less frequently.[127–129] Time from onset of symptoms to diagnosis ranges from a day to 4 months, with a mean of 31 days.[129] Diagnosis is made by detecting yeast cells by India ink stain and culture or the presence of cryptococcal antigen in the cerebrospinal fluid (CSF).[127–129] Cryptococcal antigen can also be detected in the serum, although even with therapy, cryptococcal antigen titers may remain elevated. Patients who present with altered mental status, high cryptococcal antigen titers in the CSF (>1:1024), and low white-cell count in the CSF (<20 cells/mm^3) are at increased risk of death.[130] Initial treatment for cryptococcal meningitis includes amphotericin B, combined with flucytosine to decrease risk of relapse, for 2 weeks.[111,131,132] This is followed by consolidation treatment with fluconazole for 8 weeks and secondary prophylaxis. Once acute therapy is completed, suppressive therapy is always indicated, unless immune reconstitution occurs secondary to antiretroviral therapy.[111] Secondary prophylaxis may be discontinued in patients who remain asymptomatic and have adequate immune reconstitution (CD4$^+$ T-cell count >100–200 cells/mm^3) for 6 months.[111]

Toxoplasmosis

Toxoplasmosis is the most common cause of focal encephalitis in patients with AIDS.[133] Symptoms include fever, confusion, hemispheric signs (such as hemiparesis and aphasia), meningeal signs, coma, and seizures. The most useful tool in diagnosing toxoplasmosis has been the computerized tomography scan, which reveals multiple low-density lesions or ring-enhancing lesions.[133,134] Serology has proven of limited value. Definitive diagnosis requires demonstration of tachyzoites in brain tissue obtained through biopsy, though brain biopsy is generally reserved for patients who fail to respond to empiric therapy.

Empiric therapy with sulfadiazine, pyrimethamine, and leucovorin may be considered in patients with positive serology and a clinical and radiologic profile suggestive of toxoplasmosis.[135,136] In patients with a sulfonamide allergy, clindamycin may be used in place of sulfadiazine.[135,136] An initial response is usually observed after 2 weeks of therapy.[133,134] As with many of the opportunistic infections, relapse is common when treatment is stopped. Secondary prophylaxis may be safely discontinued in patients who have successfully completed initial therapy and maintain a sustained increase in CD4$^+$ T-cell count (>200 cells/mm^3 for 6 months) secondary to antiretroviral therapy.[111] Primary prophylaxis is not recommended, but many patients receive protective efficacy from TMP/SMX for PCP prophylaxis as discussed above.[126]

Mycobacterium Avium Complex and Mycobacterium Tuberculosis

Mycobacterium avium complex (MAC) and *Mycobacterium tuberculosis* infection occur frequently in AIDS patients, often as disseminated disease.[137] Before the AIDS epidemic, MAC infection was a rare condition seen only occasionally in patients with chronic pulmonary disease. Diagnosis of MAC infection is usually made in the late stages of HIV illness, and the presence of MAC has been documented in as many as 53% of AIDS patients at autopsy.[137–139] Manifestations of MAC infection range from asymptomatic to a constellation of nonspecific findings including diarrhea, abdominal pain, malabsorption, persistent fevers, anemia, and weight loss.[137–139] Quantitative blood cultures and cultures of bone marrow, lymph node, and liver biopsies may be used in the diagnosis of disseminated infection. Positive cultures from respiratory secretions, urine, and stool also have been reported to precede disseminated infection.[137] Initial treatment for disseminated MAC infection should consist of at least two antimycobacterial drugs, including a macrolide antibiotic and ethambutol.[111,140] Primary prophylaxis is recommended with azithromycin or clarithromycin for HIV-infected patients with CD4$^+$ T-cell counts less than 50 cells/mm^3; discontinuation of primary and secondary prophylaxis may be considered in patients with adequate immune reconstitution secondary to antiretroviral therapy.[111]

Tuberculosis is prevalent among individuals infected with HIV, particularly those living in endemic areas.[137,141] Tuberculosis typically precedes development of other AIDS-defining opportunistic infections. As in the general population, tuberculosis usually represents reactivation of latent infection acquired earlier in life, although reinfection has also been observed. Disseminated, extrapulmonary disease is encountered frequently, representing 67% of tuberculosis seen in patients with AIDS.[137,140] Clinical manifestations depend on the site involved. As with MAC, diagnosis is made with the finding of *M tuberculosis* in the affected tissues or secretions. Standard therapy for tuberculosis is effective in HIV infection, although directly observed therapy is strongly recommended given the severity of disease in immunocompromised individuals.[111]

Candidiasis

Candidiasis, often presenting as oral thrush and/or esophagitis, is the most common fungal infection in HIV-infected patients.[142] Unexplained oral or vaginal candidiasis in individuals at risk for HIV infection may indicate impending progression of HIV infection. Without antiretroviral therapy, about 60% of patients will develop an opportunistic infection or Kaposi's sarcoma (KS) within a median of 3 months after the diagnosis of oral candidiasis.[143] Topical therapy with clotrimazole or nystatin may be used for oropharyngeal candidiasis, but systemic therapy with azole antifungals is needed for esophagitis.[111] Relapses following antifungal therapy are common in the absence of antiretroviral therapy.

Herpesvirus/Cytomegalovirus

Infections with herpesviruses, such as herpes simplex and cytomegalovirus (CMV), are frequently encountered in HIV-infected individuals. Mucocutaneous herpes simplex (oral, genital, or perianal) can be painful, and patients may experience frequent relapses.[144] Like other herpesviruses, CMV can cause persistent infection, with viral shedding in a number of body sites.[145,146] Viremia occurs in about half of AIDS patients, and more than 90% show tissue evidence of CMV at autopsy.[144] Retinitis is the most common manifestation of CMV infection and is a leading cause of blindness in patients with AIDS.[147,148] Treatment options for CMV retinitis include oral valganciclovir, intravenous ganciclovir, ganciclovir ocular implants, cidofovir, and foscarnet.[147-154] Other clinical syndromes seen with CMV include colitis, esophagitis, encephalitis, adrenalitis, pneumonitis, sclerosing cholangitis, and hepatitis. Relapse rates are high, especially with CMV retinitis, so long-term suppressive therapy is often necessary.[145,146,155,156] Secondary prophylaxis for CMV may be discontinued in patients with immune reconstitution secondary to antiretroviral therapy; these decisions should be made in consultation with an ophthalmologist.[111]

NEOPLASMS

Severe cellular suppression and polyclonal B-cell activation may contribute to the development of cancers in patients with AIDS. Although both KS and non-Hodgkin's lymphoma (NHL) are relatively rare outside the HIV setting, these tumors occur more frequently and often present atypically in patients with AIDS.

Kaposi's Sarcoma

KS was one of the first described clinical manifestations of AIDS.[157,158] It occurs in about 12% of patients diagnosed with AIDS, with the highest prevalence among homosexual men (19%) and homosexual male injection drug users (15%).[158] KS is more likely to occur in white men than in black men and rarely occurs in women or children infected with HIV.[159] Although the incidence of KS in HIV-infected patients declined from 22% in 1985 to 8% in 1993, a significant number of cases are still reported each year, and this cancer continues to be a major cause of morbidity in HIV patients.[159] The presence of herpes-like DNA sequences has been detected in the KS lesions of both HIV-infected and non-HIV-infected individuals. This and other epidemiologic data suggest that AIDS-related KS may have an infectious etiology.[160]

Before the AIDS epidemic, KS was a rare tumor occurring predominantly among middle-aged men of Eastern European or Mediterranean extraction. The clinical presentation of KS in AIDS patients is very diverse and differs from the classic, localized presentation. In HIV-infected patients, KS tends to involve the skin, especially the head, neck, and trunk; lymph nodes; mucous membranes; and the entire gastrointestinal tract.[161] More than 50% of patients have visceral lesions, particularly in the gastrointestinal tract, at the time of initial presentation.[162] The rate of progression varies among patients. Most patients with KS have rapid, progressive disease with multiple organ involvement, particularly the gastrointestinal tract and pulmonary parenchyma. A small percentage experiences a slow and indolent process similar to that seen in the classic form. Patients with cutaneous KS and no history of opportunistic infections or symptomatic HIV infection have the most favorable prognosis. Patients with gastrointestinal KS have a slightly reduced survival rate, and those with pulmonary KS have the worst prognosis.[162]

Antiretroviral therapy is an integral part of the management of KS.[163] Treatment of KS is individualized based on the location and severity of disease and may include local therapy, radiation therapy, interferon-alpha, or cytotoxic chemotherapy.[164]

Non-Hodgkin's Lymphoma

NHL occurs in about 5% to 10% of AIDS patients.[165] It has been reported in homosexual men, male and female injection drug users, and hemophiliacs.[165-167] Although the reason for the increased incidence of aggressive lymphomas in AIDS patients is unclear, the presence of Epstein-Barr virus, which results in polyclonal B-cell proliferation, may have a permissive effect.[161] AIDS-related lymphomas differ from lymphomas in other populations because they occur in a younger population, are often disseminated, are predominantly high- or intermediate-grade B-cell type, and generally follow a rapidly progressive clinical course.[168,169] More than 70% of these patients have involvement of extranodal sites, especially the brain, bone marrow, and bowel.[170] Primary lymphoma of the brain in patients with AIDS carries a poor prognosis and is associated with advanced disease and CD4$^+$ T-cell count below 50 cells/mm^3.[165] Treatment of patients with AIDS-related NHL is associated with a complete response rate of about 50% and high relapse and mortality rates.[171,172] Decisions about aggressive chemotherapy are made case-by-case.

SUMMARY

The acquired immunodeficiency syndrome is clearly a disease of both national and global consequence. The long incubation period of the virus and the growing number of people infected with HIV ensure that AIDS will continue to have a major impact on our health care system for years to come. Infections from opportunistic pathogens are commonly seen in HIV/AIDS and may be the presenting symptoms in newly diagnosed individuals. In addition to a working knowledge of antiretroviral therapy, it is important for pharmacists to be aware of the appropriate modalities for the treatment and prophylaxis of opportunistic infections.

REFERENCES

1. Centers for Disease Control and Prevention (CDC). *HIV/AIDS surveillance report, 2004.* Vol. 16. Atlanta, GA: US Department of Health and Human Services, Centers for Disease Control and Prevention; 2005:1–46. Available at: http://www.cdc.gov/hiv/stats/hasrlink.htm. Accessed May 3, 2006.
2. Glynn M, Rhodes P. Estimated HIV prevalence in the United States at the end of 2003. Paper presented at: National HIV Prevention Conference; June 12–15, 2005; Atlanta, GA. Abstract 595.
3. WHO HIV/AIDS programme. Available at: http://www.who.int/hiv/en. Accessed May 3, 2006.
4. Gallo RC, Salahuddin SZ, Popovic M, et al. Frequent detection and isolation of cytopathic retroviruses (HTLV III) from patients with AIDS and at risk for AIDS. *Science.* 1984; 224:500–503.
5. Barre-Sinoussi F, Chermann JC, Rey F, et al. Isolation of a T-lymphotropic retrovirus from a patient at risk for the acquired immune deficiency syndrome (AIDS). *Science.* 1983; 220:868–871.
6. Clavel F, Guetard D, Brun-Vezinet F, et al. Isolation of a new human retrovirus from West African patients with AIDS. *Science.* 1986; 233:343–346.
7. Franchini G, Gurgo C, Guo H-G, et al. Sequence of simian immunodeficiency virus and its relationship to the human immunodeficiency viruses. *Nature.* 1987; 238:539–543.
8. Clavel F, Mansinho K, Chamaret S, et al. Human immunodeficiency virus type 2 infection associated with AIDS in West Africa. *N Engl J Med.* 1987; 316:1180–1185.
9. Kanki PJ, Barin F, M'Boup S, et al. New human T-lymphotropic retrovirus related to simian T-lymphotropic virus type III (STLV-III$_{AGM}$). *Science.* 1986; 232:238–243.
10. Armstrong W, Calabrese L, Taege AJ. HIV update 2005: origins, issues, prospects, and complications. *Cleve Clin J Med.* 2005; 72(1):73–78.
11. Hahn BH, Shaw GM, De Cock KM, et al. AIDS as a zoonosis: scientific and public health implications. *Science.* 2000; 287:607–614.
12. Castro BA, Cheng-Mayer C, Evans LA, et al. HIV heterogeneity and viral pathogenesis. *AIDS.* 1988; 2(Suppl 1):S17–S27.
13. Hirsch MS. Chemotherapy of human immunodeficiency virus infections: current practice and future prospects. *J Infect Dis.* 1990; 161:845–857.
14. Broder S, Mitsuya H, Yarchoan R, et al. Antiretroviral therapy in AIDS. *Ann Intern Med.* 1990; 113:604–618.
15. Altmeyer R. Virus attachment and entry offer numerous targets for antiviral therapy. *Curr Pharm Des.* 2004; 10(30):3701–3712.
16. Schols D. HIV co-receptors as targets of antiviral therapy. *Curr Top Med Chem.* 2004; 4(9):883–893.
17. Rubbert A, Ostowski M. Pathogenesis of HIV-1 infection. *HIV Medicine.* 2005; 59–81. Available at: http://www.hivmedicine.com. Accessed May 25, 2006.
18. Ho DD, Pomerantz RJ, Kaplan JC. Pathogenesis of infection with human immunodeficiency virus. *N Engl J Med.* 1987; 317:278–286.
19. The life cycle of HIV. Available at: http://www.tthhivclinic.com/lifecycle.htm. Accessed July 1, 2005.
20. Fauci AS. The human immunodeficiency virus: infectivity and mechanisms of pathogenesis. *Science.* 1988; 239:617–622.
21. Pantaleo G, Graziosi C, Fauci AS. The immunopathogenesis of human immunodeficiency virus infection. *N Engl J Med.* 1993; 328:327–335.
22. Fauci AS. Multifactorial nature of human immunodeficiency virus disease: implications for therapy. *Science.* 1993; 262:1011–1018.
23. Wei X, Ghosh SK, Taylor ME, et al. Viral dynamics in human immunodeficiency virus type 1 infection. *Nature.* 1995; 373:117–122.
24. Ho DD, Neumann AU, Perelson AS, et al. Rapid turnover of plasma virions and CD4 lymphocytes in HIV-1 infection. *Nature.* 1995; 373:123–126.
25. Perelson AS, Essunger P, Cao Y, et al. Decay characteristics of HIV-1-infected compartments during combination therapy. *Nature.* 1997; 387:188–191.

26. Chun TW, Stuyver L, Mizell SB, et al. Presence of an inducible HIV-1 latent reservoir during highly active antiretroviral therapy. *Proc Natl Acad Sci U S A.* 1997; 94:13193–13197.

27. Simon V, Ho DD. HIV-1 dynamics in vivo: implications for therapy. *Nat Rev Microbiol.* 2003; 1(3):181–190.

28. Phair JP. Variations in the natural history of HIV infection [keynote address]. *AIDS Res Hum Retroviruses.* 1994; 10:883–885.

29. Paranjape RS. Immunopathogenesis of HIV infection. *Indian J Med Res.* 2005; 121:240–255.

30. Yu VL, Weber R, Raoult D, eds. *Antimicrobial Therapy and Vaccines. Volume I: Microbes.* New York, NY: Apple Trees Productions, LLC; 2002.

31. Friedland GH, Klein RS. Transmission of the human immunodeficiency virus. *N Engl J Med.* 1987; 317:1125–1135.

32. Mastro TD, de Vincenzi I. Probabilities of sexual HIV-1 transmission. *AIDS.* 1996; 10:S75–82.

33. Holmberg SD, Horsburgh CR Jr, Ward JW, et al. Biologic factors in the sexual transmission of human immunodeficiency virus. *J Infect Dis.* 1989; 160:116–125.

34. Padian NS, Shiboski SC, Jewell NP. The effect of number of exposures on the risk of heterosexual HIV transmission. *J Infect Dis.* 1990; 161:883–887.

35. Tsai CC, Emau P, Follis KE, et al. Effectiveness of postinoculation ®-9-(2-phosphonylmethoxypropyl) adenine treatment for prevention of persistent simian immunodeficiency virus SIV infection depends critically on timing of initiation and duration of treatment. *J Virol.* 1998; 72:4265–4273.

36. Tsai CC, Follis KE, Sabo A, et al. Prevention of HIV infection in macaques by ®-9-(2-phosphonylmethoxypropyl)adenine. *Science.* 1995; 270:1197–1199.

37. Friedland GH, Klein RS. Transmission of the human immunodeficiency virus. *N Engl J Med.* 1987; 317:1125–1135.

38. Ward JW, Deppe DA, Samson S, et al. Risk of human immunodeficiency virus infection from blood donors who later developed the acquired immunodeficiency syndrome. *Ann Intern Med.* 1987; 106:61–62.

39. Ward JW, Holmberg SD, Allen JR, et al. Transmission of human immunodeficiency virus (HIV) by blood transfusions screened as negative for HIV antibody. *N Engl J Med.* 1988; 318:473–478.

40. Donegan E, Stuart M, Niland JC, et al. Infection with human immunodeficiency virus type 1 (HIV-1) among recipients of antibody-positive blood donations. *Ann Intern Med.* 1990; 113:733–739.

41. Donegan E, Lenes BA, Tomasulo PA, et al. Transmission of HIV-1 by component type and duration of shelf storage before transfusion. *Transfusion.* 1990; 30:839–840.

42. Centers for Disease Control and Prevention (CDC). U.S. Public Health Service Guidelines for Testing and Counseling Blood and Plasma Donors for Human Immunodeficiency Virus Type 1 Antigen. *MMWR Morb Mortal Wkly Rep.* March 1, 1996; (45) No. RR-2:1–9.

43. Tokars JI, Marcus R, Culver DH, et al. Surveillance of HIV infection and zidovudine use in health care workers after occupational exposure to HIV-infected blood. The CDC Cooperative Needlestick Surveillance Group. *Ann Intern Med.* 1993; 118:913–919.

44. Kaplan EH, Heimer R. A model-based estimate of HIV infectivity via needle sharing. *J Acquir Immune Defic Syndr.* 1992; 5:1116–1118.

45. Des Jarlais DC, Friedman SR, Stoneburner RL. HIV infection and intravenous drug use: critical issues in transmission dynamics, infection outcomes, and prevention. *Rev Infect Dis.* 1988; 10:151–158.

46. Cardo DM, Culver DH, Ciesielski CA, et al. A case-control study of HIV seroconversion in health care workers after percutaneous exposure. Centers for Disease Control and Prevention Needlestick Surveillance Group. *N Engl J Med.* 1997; 337:1485–1490.

47. Henderson DK, Fahey BS, Willy M, et al. Risk for occupational transmission of human immunodeficiency virus type 1 (HIV-1) associated with exposures. *Ann Intern Med.* 1990; 113:740–746.

48. Centers for Disease Control and Prevention (CDC). Updated U.S. Public Health Service Guidelines for the Management of Occupational Exposures to HBV, HCV, and HIV and Recommendations for Postexposure Prophylaxis. *MMWR Morb Mortal Wkly Rep.* 2001; 50:No. RR-11.

49. Henderson DK. Postexposure treatment of HIV—taking some risks for safety's sake. *N Engl J Med.* 1997; 337:1542–1543.

50. Connor EM, Sperling RS, Gelber R, et al. Reduction of maternal-infant transmission of human immunodeficiency virus type 1 with zidovudine treatment. Pediatric AIDS Clinical Trials Group Protocol 076 Study Group. *N Engl J Med.* 1994; 331:1173–1180.

51. U.S. Department of Health and Human Services. Public Health Service Task Force recommendations for use of antiretroviral drugs in pregnant women for maternal health and interventions to reduce perinatal HIV-1 transmission in the United States. Rockville, MD: HIV/AIDS Treatment Information Service. Available at: http://www.aidsinfo.org.nih.gov. Accessed July 3, 2005.

52. Cooper ER, Charuuat M, Mofenson C, et al. Combination antiretroviral strategies for the treatment of pregnant HIV-1-infected women and prevention of perinatal HIV-1 transmission. *J Acquir Immun Defic Syndr.* 2002; 29:484–494.

53. Bartlett JG, Gallant JE. 2005–2006 Medical Management of HIV Infection. Baltimore, MD: Johns Hopkins Medicine Health Publishing Business Group; 2005.

54. Busch MP, Satten GA. Time course of viraemia and antibody seroconversion following human immunodeficiency virus exposure. *Am J Med.* 1997; 102:117–124.

55. Tindall B, Cooper DA. Primary HIV infection: host responses and intervention strategies. *AIDS.* 1991; 5(1):1–14.

56. Niu MT, Stein DS, Schnittman SM. Primary human immunodeficiency virus type 1 infection: review of pathogenesis and early treatment interventions in humans. *J Infect Dis.* 1993; 168(6):1490–1501.

57. Kinlock-De Loes S, de Saussure P, Saurat JH, et al. Symptomatic primary infection due to human immunodeficiency virus type 1: review of 31 cases. *Clin Infect Dis.* 1993; 17(1):59–65.

58. Schacker T, Collier AC, Hughes J, et al. Clinical and epidemiologic features of primary HIV infections. *Ann Intern Med.* 1996; 125(4):257–264.

59. Hecht FM, Busch MP, Rawal B, et al. Use of laboratory tests and clinical symptoms for identification of primary HIV infection. *AIDS.* 2002; 16:1119–1129.

60. Kahn JO, Walker BD. Acute human immunodeficiency virus type 1 infection. *N Engl J Med.* 1998; 339:33–39.

61. Weinstock H, Dale M, Gwinn M, et al. HIV seroincidence among patients at clinics for sexually transmitted diseases in nine cities in the United States. *J Acquir Immune Defic Syndr.* 2002; 29:478–483.

62. Henrard DR, Phillips J, Windsor I, et al. Detection of human immunodeficiency virus type 1 p24 antigen and plasma RNA: relevance to indeterminate serologic tests. *Transfusion.* 1994; 34:376–380.

63. Panel on Clinical Practices for Treatment of HIV Infection convened by the Department of Health and Human Services (DHHS). Guidelines for the Use of Antiretroviral Agents in HIV-1-Infected Adults and Adolescents. May 4, 2006. Available at: http://www.aidsinfo.org.nih.gov. Accessed June 15, 2006.

64. Purdy BD, Plaisance KI. Infection with the human immunodeficiency virus: epidemiology, pathogenesis, transmission, diagnosis, and manifestations. *Am J Hosp Pharm.* 1989; 46:1185–1209.

65. Steckelberg JM, Cockerill FR. Subspecialty clinics: infectious diseases: serologic testing for human immunodeficiency virus antibodies. *Mayo Clin Proc.* 1988; 63:373–380.

66. Centers for Disease Control and Prevention (CDC). Interpretation and use of the Western blot assay for serodiagnosis of human immunodeficiency virus type 1 infections. *MMWR Morb Mortal Wkly Rep.* 1989; 38:S1–S7.

67. Horsburgh CR, Ou CY, Jason J, et al. Duration of human immunodeficiency virus infection before detection of antibody. *Lancet.* 1989; 2:637–640.

68. Rogers MF, Ou CY, Kilbourne B, et al. Advances and problems in the diagnosis of HIV infection in infants. In: Pizzo PA, Wilfert CM, eds. *Pediatric AIDS: The Challenge of HIV Infection in Infants, Children and Adolescents.* Baltimore, MD: Williams and Wilkins; 1991:159–174.

69. Centers for Disease Control and Prevention (CDC). Serologic testing for antibody to human immunodeficiency virus. *MMWR Morb Mortal Wkly Rep.* 1987; 36:833–845.

70. Sloand E, Pitt E, Chiarello RJ, et al. HIV testing state of the art. *JAMA.* 1991; 266:2861–2866.

71. Mylonakis E, Paliou M, Lally M, et al. Laboratory testing for infection with the human immunodeficiency virus: established and novel approaches. *Am J Med.* 2000; 109:568–576.

72. Marlink RG, Allan JS, McLane MP, et al. Low sensitivity of ELISA testing in early HIV infection. *N Engl J Med.* 1986; 315:1549.

73. Brust S, Duttman H, Feldner J, et al. Shortening of the diagnostic window with a new combined HIV p24 antigen and anti-HIV-1/2/O screening test. *J Virol Methods.* 2000; 90:153–165.

74. Saville RD, Constantine NT, Cleghorn FR, et al. Fourth-generation enzyme-linked immunosorbent assay for the simultaneous detection of human immunodeficiency virus antigen and antibody. *J Clin Microbiol.* 2001; 39:2518–2524.

75. Parks WP, Scott GB. An overview of pediatric AIDS: approaches to diagnosis and outcome assessment. In: Broder S, ed. *AIDS—Modern Concepts and Therapeutic Challenges.* New York: Marcel Dekker; 1987:245–262.

76. Centers for Disease Control and Prevention (CDC). Public Health Service guidelines for counseling and antibody testing to prevent HIV infection and AIDS. *MMWR Morb Mortal Wkly Rep.* 1987; 36:509–515.

77. van der Groen G, Vercauteren G, Piot P. Immunofluorescence tests for HIV antibody and their value as confirmatory tests. *J Virol Methods.* 1987; 17:35–43.

78. Steckelberg JM, Cockerill FR. Subspecialty clinics: infectious diseases: serologic testing for human immunodeficiency virus antibodies. *Mayo Clin Proc.* 1988; 63:373–380.

79. Centers for Disease Control and Prevention (CDC). Interpretation and use of the Western blot assay for serodiagnosis of human immunodeficiency virus type 1 infections. *MMWR Morb Mortal Wkly Rep.* 1989; 38:S1–S7.

80. Kessler HA, Baauw B, Spear J, et al. Diagnosis of human immunodeficiency virus infection in seronegative homosexuals presenting with an acute viral syndrome. *JAMA.* 1987; 258:1196–1199.

81. Wittek AE, Phelan MA, Wells MA, et al. Detection of human immunodeficiency virus core protein in plasma by enzyme immunoassay. Association of antigenemia with symptomatic disease and T-helper cell depletion. *Ann Intern Med.* 1987; 107:286–292.

82. Allain JP, Laurian Y, Paul DA, et al. Long-term evaluation of HIV antigen and antibodies to p24 and gp41 in patients with hemophilia. Potential clinical importance. *N Engl J Med.* 1987; 317:1114–1121.

83. Borkowksy W, Krasinski K, Paul D, et al. Human-immunodeficiency-virus infections in infants negative for anti-HIV by enzyme-linked immunoassay. *Lancet.* 1987; 1:1168–1171.

84. Chaisson RE, Allain J, Volberding PA. Significant changes in HIV antigen level in the serum of

patients treated with azidothymidine. *N Engl J Med.* 1986; 315:1610–1611.

85. Fahey JL, Taylor JMG, Detels R, et al. The prognostic value for cellular and serologic markers in infection with human immunodeficiency virus type 1. *N Engl J Med.* 1990; 322:166–172.

86. Ascher DP, Roberts C, Fowler A. Acidification modified p24 antigen capture assay in HIV seropositives. *J Acquir Immune Defic Syndr.* 1992; 5:1080–1083.

87. Nishanian P, Huskins KR, Stehn S, et al. A simple method for improved assay demonstrates that HIV p24 antigen is present as immune complexes in most sera from HIV-infected individuals. *J Infect Dis.* 1990; 162:21–28.

88. Rogers MF, Ou CY, Rayfield M, et al. Use of the polymerase chain reaction for early detection of proviral sequences of human immunodeficiency virus in infants born to seropositive mothers. *N Engl J Med.* 1989; 320:1649–1654.

89. Schochetman G. Diagnosis of HIV infection. *Clin Chim Acta.* 1992; 221:1–26.

90. Simmonds P, Balfe P, Peutherer JF, et al. Human immunodeficiency virus-infected individuals contain provirus in small numbers of peripheral mononuclear cells and at low copy numbers. *J Virol.* 1990; 64:864–872.

91. Frank AP, Wandell MG, Headings MD, et al. Anonymous HIV testing using home collection and telemedicine counseling: a multicenter evaluation. *Arch Intern Med.* 1997; 157:309–314.

92. Branson BM. Home sample collection tests for HIV infection. *JAMA.* 1998; 280:1699–1701.

93. Centers for Disease Control and Prevention (CDC). Rapid HIV testing. Available at: www.cdc.gov/hiv/rapid_testing. Accessed May 12, 2006.

94. ECRI Institute. Rapid HIV test kits. *Health Devices.* 2006; 35:157–177.

95. DeSimone JA, Pomerantz RJ. New methods for the detection of HIV. *Clin Lab Med.* 2002; 22:573–592.

96. Frerichs R, Eskes N, Htoon M. Validity of three assays for HIV-1 antibodies in saliva. *J Acquir Immune Defic Syndr.* 1994; 7:522–525.

97. Soto-Ramirez LE, Hernandez-Gomez L, Sifuentes-Osornio J, et al. Detection of specific antibodies in gingival crevicular transudate by enzyme-linked immunosorbent assay for diagnosis of human immunodeficiency virus type 1 infection. *J Clin Microbiol.* 1992; 30:2780–2783.

98. Gallo D, George JR, Fitchen JH, et al. Evaluation of a system using oral mucosal transudate for HIV-1 antibody screening and confirmatory testing. *JAMA.* 1997; 277:254–258.

99. Connell JA, Parry JV, Mortimer PP, et al. Preliminary report: accurate assays for anti-HIV in urine. *Lancet.* 1990; 335:1366–1369.

100. Cao YZ, Friedman KA, Mirabile M, et al. HIV-1 neutralizing antibodies in urine from seropositive individuals. *J Acquir Immune Defic Syndr.* 1990; 3:195–199.

101. Desai S, Bates H, Michalski FJ. Detection of antibody to HIV-1 in urine. *Lancet.* 1991; 337:183–184.

102. Urnovitz HB, Sturge JC, Gottfried TD, et al. Urine antibody tests: new insights into the dynamics of HIV-1 infection. *Clin Chem.* 1999; 45:1602–1613.

103. Mellors JW, Munoz A, Giorgi J, et al. Plasma viral load and CD4+ lymphocytes as prognostic markers of HIV-1 infection. *Ann Intern Med.* 1997; 126:946–954.

104. Mulder J, McKinney N, Christopherson C, et al. A rapid and simple PCR assay for quantification of HIV-1 RNA in plasma: application to acute retroviral infection. *J Clin Microbiol.* 1994; 32:292–300.

105. Van Gemen B, Kievits T, Schukkink R, et al. Quantification of HIV-1 RNA using NASBA during a primary HIV-1 infection. *J Virol Methods.* 1993; 43:177–188.

106. Pachl C, Todd JA, Kern DG, et al. Rapid and precise quantification of HIV-1 RNA in plasma using a branched DNA signal amplification assay. *J Acquir Immune Defic Syndr.* 1994; 8:446–544.

107. Lin H, Pedneault L, Hollinger B. Intra-assay performance characteristics of five assays for quantification of human immunodeficiency virus type 1 RNA in plasma. *J Clin Microbiol.* 1998; 36:835–839.

108. Revets H, Marissens D, DeWit S, et al. Comparative evaluation of NASBA HIV-1 RNA QT, Amplicor-HIV monitor, and Quantiplex HIV RNA assay, three methods for quantitation of human immunodeficiency virus type 1 RNA in plasma. *J Clin Microbiol.* 1996; 34:1058–1064.

109. Chew C, Zheng F, Byth K, et al. Comparison of three commercial assays for the quantification of plasma HIV-1 RNA from individuals with low viral loads. *AIDS.* 1999; 13:1977–2001.

110. Hirsch MS, Brun-Vezinet F, Clotet B, et al. Antiretroviral drug resistance testing in adults infected with human immunodeficiency virus type 1: 2003 recommendations of an International AIDS Society-USA panel. *Clin Infect Dis.* 2003; 37:113–128.

111. Benson CA, Kaplan JE, Masur H, et al. Treating opportunistic infections among HIV-infected adults and adolescents: recommendations from CDC, the National Institutes of Health, and the HIV Medicine Association/Infectious Disease Society of America. *Clin Infect Dis.* 2005; 40:S131–235.

112. Powderly W. Prophylaxis for opportunistic infections in an era of effective antiretroviral therapy. *Clin Infect Dis.* 2000; 31:597–601.

113. Jones JL, Hanson DL, Dworkin MS, et al. Surveillance for AIDS-defining opportunistic illnesses, 1992–1997. *MMWR CDC Surveil Summ.* 1999; 48(SS-2):1–22.

114. Hermsen ED, Wynn HE, McNabb J. Discontinuation of prophylaxis for HIV-associated opportunistic infections in the era of highly active antiretroviral therapy. *Am J Health-Syst Pharm.* 2004; 61:245–256.

115. Selik RM, Starcher ET, Curran JW. Opportunistic diseases reported in AIDS patients: frequencies, associations, and trends. *AIDS.* 1987; 1:175–182.

116. Guidelines for prophylaxis against *Pneumocystis carinii* pneumonia for patients infected with human immunodeficiency virus. *JAMA.* 1989; 262:335–339.

117. Phair T, Munoz A, Detels R, et al. The risk of *Pneumocystis carinii* pneumonia among men infected with human immunodeficiency virus type 1. *N Engl J Med.* 1990; 322:161–165.

118. Hughes WT. *Pneumocystis carinii* pneumonitis. *N Engl J Med.* 1987; 317:1021–1023.

119. Kovacs JA, Hiemenz JW, Macher AM, et al. *Pneumocystis carinii* pneumonia: a comparison between patients with the acquired immunodeficiency syndrome and patients with other immunodeficiencies. *Ann Intern Med.* 1984; 100:663–671.

120. Ognibene FP, Shelhamer J, Gill V, et al. The diagnosis of *Pneumocystis carinii* syndrome using subsegmental bronchoalveolar lavage. *Am Rev Resp Dis.* 1986; 133:226–229.

121. Bigby TD, Margolskee D, Curtis JL, et al. The usefulness of induced sputum in the diagnosis of *Pneumocystis carinii* pneumonia in patients with the acquired immunodeficiency syndrome. *Am Rev Resp Dis.* 1986; 133:515–518.

122. Kovacs JA, Hiemenz JW, Macher AM, et al. *Pneumocystis carinii* pneumonia: a comparison between patients with the acquired immunodeficiency syndrome and patients with other immunodeficiencies. *Ann Intern Med.* 1984; 100:663–671.

123. Allegra CJ, Chabner BA, Tuazon CU, et al. Trimetrexate for the treatment of *Pneumocystis carinii* pneumonia in patients with the acquired immunodeficiency syndrome. *N Engl J Med.* 1987; 317:978–985.

124. Ioannidis JP, Cappelleri JC, Skolnick PR, et al. A meta-analysis of the relative efficacy and toxicity of *Pneumocystis carinii* prophylactic regimens. *Arch Intern Med.* 1996; 156:177–188.

125. Bozzette SA, Finkelstein DM, Spector SA, et al. A randomized trial of three anti-pneumocystis agents in patients with advanced human immunodeficiency virus infection. *N Engl J Med.* 1995; 332:693–699.

126. Carr A, Tindall B, Brew BJ, et al. Low-dose trimethoprim-sulfamethoxazole prophylaxis for toxoplasmic encephalitis in patients with AIDS. *Ann Intern Med.* 1992; 117:106–111.

127. Powderly WG. Cryptococcal meningitis and AIDS. *Clin Infect Dis.* 1993; 17:837–842.

128. Kovacs JA, Kovacs AA, Polis M, et al. Cryptococcosis in the acquired immunodeficiency syndrome. *Ann Intern Med.* 1985; 103:533–538.

129. Zuger A, Louie E, Holzmann RS, et al. Cryptococcal disease in patients with the acquired immunodeficiency syndrome: diagnostic features and outcome of treatment. *Ann Intern Med.* 1986; 104:234–240.

130. Saag MS, Powderly WG, Cloud GA, et al. Comparison of amphotericin B with fluconazole in the treatment of acute AIDS-associated cryptococcal meningitis. *N Engl J Med.* 1992; 326:83–89.

131. van der Horst CM, Saag MS, Cloud GA, et al. Treatment of cryptococcal meningitis associated with the acquired immunodeficiency syndrome. *N Engl J Med.* 1997; 337:15–21.

132. Saag MS, Graybill JR, Lasen R, et al. Practice guidelines for the management of cryptococcal meningitis. *Clin Infect Dis.* 2000; 30:710–718.

133. Wong B, Gold JWM, Brown AE, et al. Central nervous system toxoplasmosis in homosexual men and parenteral drug abusers. *Ann Intern Med.* 1984; 100:36–42.

134. Leport C, Raffi F, Matheron S, et al. Treatment of central nervous system toxoplasmosis with pyrimethamine/sulfadiazine combination in 35 patients with the acquired immunodeficiency syndrome: efficacy of long-term continuous therapy. *Am J Med.* 1988; 84:94–100.

135. Katlama C, De Wit S, O'Doherty E, et al. Pyrimethamine-clindamycin vs. pyrimethamine-sulfadiazine as acute and long-term therapy for toxoplasmic encephalitis in patients with AIDS. *Clin Infect Dis.* 1996; 22:268–275.

136. Dannemann BR, McCutchan JA, Israelski DM, et al. Treatment of toxoplasmic encephalitis in patients with AIDS: a randomized trial comparing pyrimethamine plus clindamycin to pyrimethamine plus sulfadiazine. *Ann Intern Med.* 1992; 116:33–43.

137. Hawkins CC. Managing mycobacterial infections in AIDS patients. *Infect Med.* 1988; 5:157–159, 207–208.

138. Hawkins CC, Gold JWM, Whimbey E, et al. *Mycobacterium avium* complex infections in patients with the acquired immunodeficiency syndrome. *Ann Intern Med.* 1986; 105:184–188.

139. Young LS. *Mycobacterium avium* complex infection. *J Infect Dis.* 1988; 157:863–867.

140. Masur H. Recommendations on prophylaxis and therapy for disseminated *Mycobacterium avium* complex disease in patients infected with the human immunodeficiency virus infection. *N Engl J Med.* 1993; 329:898–904.

141. Chaisson RE, Slutkin G. Tuberculosis and human immunodeficiency virus infection. *J Infect Dis.* 1989; 159:96–100.

142. Glatt AE, Chirgwin K, Landesman SH. Current concepts: treatment of infections with human immunodeficiency virus. *N Engl J Med.* 1988; 318:1439–1448.

143. Klein RS, Harris CA, Small CB, et al. Oral candidiasis in high-risk patients as the initial manifestation of acquired immunodeficiency syndrome. *N Engl J Med.* 1984; 311:354–358.

144. Quinnan GV Jr, Masur H, Rook AH, et al. Herpes virus infections in the acquired immunodeficiency syndrome. *JAMA.* 1984; 252:72–77.

145. Jacobson MA, Mill J. Serious cytomegalovirus disease in the acquired immunodeficiency syndrome (AIDS): clinical findings, diagnosis, and treatment. *Ann Intern Med.* 1988; 108:585–594.

146. Drew WL. Cytomegalovirus infection in patients with AIDS. *J Infect Dis.* 1988; 158:449–455.

147. Smith CL. Local therapy for cytomegalovirus retinitis. *Ann Pharmacother.* 1998; 32:248–255.

148. Kempen JH, Jabs DA, Wilson LA, et al. Risk of vision loss with cytomegalovirus retinitis and the acquired immune deficiency syndrome. *Arch Opthamol.* 2003; 121:466–476.

149. Musch DC, Martin DF, Gordon JF, et al. Treatment of cytomegalovirus retinitis with a sustained release ganciclovir implant. *N Engl J Med.* 1997; 337:83–90.

150. Martin DF, Sierra-Madero J, Walmsley S, et al. A controlled trial of valganciclovir as induction therapy for cytomegalovirus retinitis. *N Engl J Med.* 2002; 346:1119–1126.

151. Martin DF, Kuppermann BD, Wolitz RA, et al. Oral ganciclovir for patients with cytomegalovirus treated with a ganciclovir implant. *N Engl J Med.* 1999; 340:1063–1070.

152. Palestine AG, Polis MA, de Smet MD, et al. A randomized controlled trial of foscarnet in the treatment of cytomegalovirus retinitis in patients with AIDS. *Ann Intern Med.* 1991; 115:665–673.

153. Studies of the Ocular Complications of AIDS Research Group. Mortality in patients with the acquired immune deficiency syndrome treated with either foscarnet or ganciclovir for cytomegalovirus retinitis. *N Engl J Med.* 1992; 326:213–220.

154. Studies of Ocular Complications of AIDS Research Group in Collaboration with the AIDS Clinical Trials Group. Parenteral cidofovir for cytomegalovirus in patients with AIDS: the HPMPC peripheral cytomegalovirus retinitis trial. *Ann Intern Med.* 1997; 126:264–274.

155. Macher AM, Reichert CM, Straus SE, et al. Death in the AIDS patient: role of cytomegalovirus. *N Engl J Med.* 1983; 309:1454.

156. Pau AK, Pitrak DL. Management of cytomegalovirus infection in patients with acquired immunodeficiency syndrome. *Clin Pharm.* 1990; 9:613–631.

157. Centers for Disease Control and Prevention (CDC). Kaposi's sarcoma and pneumocystis pneumonia among homosexual men—New York City and California. *MMWR Morb Mortal Wkly Rep.* 1981; 30:305–308.

158. Hymes KB, Cheung T, Greene JB, et al. Kaposi's sarcoma in homosexual men: a report of eight cases. *Lancet.* 1981; 2:598–600.

159. Denning P, Chu S, Fleming P. Current trends in the epidemiology of Kaposi's sarcoma. Paper presented at 35th Interscience Conference on Antimicrobial Agents and Chemotherapy (Abstract #I23); September 17–20, 1995; San Francisco, CA.

160. Moore PS, Chang Y. Detection of herpesvirus-like DNA sequences in Kaposi's sarcoma in patients with and those without HIV infection. *N Engl J Med.* 1995; 332:1181–1185.

161. Safai B, Lowenthal DA, Koziner B. Malignant neoplasms associated with the HTLV-III/LAV infection. *Antibiot Chemother Basel.* 1987; 38:80–98.

162. Groopman JE, Broder S. Cancer in AIDS and other immunodeficiency states. In: Devita VT, Hellman S, Rosenberg SA, eds. *Cancer: Principles and Practice of Oncology.* Vol. 2. Philadelphia, PA: JB Lippincott; 1989:1953–1970.

163. Jones JL, Hanson DL, Dworkin MS, et al. Incidence and trends in Kaposi's sarcoma in the era of effective antiretroviral therapy. *J Acquir Immune Defic Syndr.* 2000; 24:270–274.

164. Levine AM, Tulpule A. Clinical aspects and management of AIDS-related Kaposi's sarcoma. *Eur J Cancer.* 2001; 37:1288–1295.

165. Ziegler JL, Beckstead JA, Volberding PA, et al. Non-Hodgkin's lymphoma in 90 homosexual men. *N Engl J Med.* 1984; 311:565–570.

166. Levine AM, Meyer PR, Begandy MK, et al. Development of B-cell lymphoma in homosexual men. *Ann Intern Med.* 1986; 104:737.

167. Gill PS, Meyer PR, Pavlova Z, et al. B-cell ALL in adults: clinical, morphologic, and immunologic findings. *J Clin Oncol.* 1986; 4:747.

168. Kalter SP, Riggs SA, Cabanillas F, et al. Aggressive non-Hodgkin's lymphoma in immunocompromised homosexual males. *Blood.* 1985; 66:655–659.

169. Levine AM. Non-Hodgkin's lymphomas and other malignancies in the acquired immunodeficiency syndrome. *Semin Oncol.* 1987; 14(Suppl 3):34–38.

170. Bermudez MA, Grant KM, Rodvien R, et al. Non-Hodgkin's lymphoma in a population with or at risk for acquired immunodeficiency syndrome. *Am J Med.* 1989; 86:71–76.

171. Levine AM, Sullivan-Halley J, Pike MC, et al. Human immunodeficiency virus–related lymphoma: prognostic factors predictive of survival. *Cancer.* 1991; 68:2466–2472.

172. Kaplan LD, Abrams DI, Feigal E, et al. AIDS-associated non-Hodgkin's lymphoma in San Francisco. *JAMA.* 1989; 261:719–724.

SELF-ASSESSMENT QUESTIONS

1. Which of the following immune responses are affected by HIV infection?

   A. Humoral
   B. Cellular
   C. Both A and B
   D. None of the above

2. Which of the following is the initial event in the HIV replicative cycle?

   A. p24 attaches to reverse transcriptase
   B. The CD4+/CD8+ T-cell ratio is inverted

C. gp120 binds to the CD4 receptor
D. Viral proteins are assembled into a virion

3. The fastest-growing numbers of cases of HIV infection are in which of the following demographic groups?

A. Infants
B. Homosexuals
C. Heterosexuals
D. A and C

4. According to the 1993 revised classification for HIV infection, which of the following would be considered to have a diagnosis of AIDS?

A. An asymptomatic patient with a CD4+ T-cell count of 550 cells/mm³
B. An asymptomatic patient with a CD4+ T-cell count of 150 cells/mm³
C. A patient with oral candidiasis and a CD4+ T-cell count of 550 cells/mm³
D. A patient with persistent generalized lymphadenopathy and a CD4+ T-cell count of 600 cells/mm³

5. A newborn who shows two positive ELISAs and a positive Western blot over a 6-week period definitely has HIV infection.

A. True
B. False

6. PCR is used to detect:

A. Antibodies to HIV in the patient's blood
B. HIV proteins in the patient's blood
C. HIV viral DNA in the patient's blood
D. Replicating virus in culture

7. Malignancies that may be associated with HIV/AIDS include:

A. Kaposi's sarcoma
B. Non-small cell lung cancer
C. Non-Hodgkin's lymphoma
D. A and C
E. All of the above

8. All of the following are appropriate options for the treatment of *Pneumocystis jiroveci* pneumonia *except*:

A. Trimethoprim/sulfamethoxazole
B. Atovaquone
C. Dapsone
D. Pentamidine

9. Body fluids that may be used for HIV antibody testing include:

A. Blood
B. Urine
C. Saliva
D. A and C
E. All of the above

10. Chemoprophylaxis for opportunistic infections may be safely discontinued for:

A. *Pneumocystis jiroveci* pneumonia
B. Toxoplasmosis
C. Cryptococcal meningitis
D. A and B
E. All of the above

11. Appropriate therapy for the initial treatment of cryptococcal meningitis includes:

A. Amphotericin B
B. Flucytosine
C. Itraconazole
D. A and B only
E. All of the above

12. The majority of HIV-infected individuals harbor the chemokine coreceptor CXCR4.

A. True
B. False

13. Transmission of HIV may occur by which of the following routes?

A. Sexual
B. Parenteral
C. Perinatal
D. A and C only
E. All of the above

14. Quantitation of HIV viremia can be measured by which of the following?

A. Polymerase chain reaction (PCR)
B. Nucleic acid sequence-based amplification (NASBA)
C. Branched DNA signal amplification
D. All of the above

15. Toxoplasmosis is the most common cause of focal encephalitis in patients with AIDS.

A. True
B. False

CHAPTER 8

HIV Treatment Strategies

Beulah Perdue Sabundayo, Christopher W. James

CHAPTER OUTLINE

LEARNING OBJECTIVES

After completing this chapter, the reader should be able to:

1. Discuss the use of antiretroviral agents in the treatment of HIV infection.
2. Identify potential investigational targets for antiretroviral therapy.
3. Describe potential adverse drug reactions associated with antiretroviral therapy.
4. Discuss various approaches to immunologic therapy for HIV infection.
5. Identify various approaches to the development of AIDS vaccines.

ANTIRETROVIRAL THERAPY

Guidelines

In the United States, there are two major established guidelines for the treatment of HIV infection in adults and adolescents: the Department of Health and Human Services (DHHS) and the International AIDS Society–USA panel (IAS-USA).[1,2]

Goals of Therapy

Eradication of HIV infection or a cure is currently not possible. The goals of therapy are to achieve maximal and durable viral load suppression, restore and maintain immunologic function, reduce morbidity and mortality, and improve quality of life.[1]

When to Start Treatment

Both guidelines agree that patients with symptomatic HIV infection should receive antiretroviral treatment.[1,2] After this stage, however, the guidelines diverge in their recommendations for treatment. The 2006 DHHS guidelines for indications for antiretroviral therapy are outlined in **Table 8.1**.

When to Modify Therapy

Therapy should be modified for treatment failure, toxicity, or nonadherence.[1] *Treatment failure* is a suboptimal response to therapy associated with virologic failure, immunologic failure, or clinical progression.[1]

Virologic failure is either incomplete viral suppression (failure to obtain a viral load <400 or <50 copies/mL) or virologic rebound, with detectable viral loads after achieving viral suppression.[1] *Immunologic failure* is failure to increase CD4[+] T cell counts more than 25–50 cells/mm³ in the first year of therapy or a decrease to below the baseline CD4[+] T cell count.[1] *Clinical progression* is the occurrence or recurrence of an HIV-related event after at least 3 months on antiretroviral therapy.[1] Virologic, immunologic, and clinical parameters have distinct time courses and may occur independent of each other. Generally, virologic failure occurs first, followed by immunologic failure and then clinical progression.

Virologic failure may be the result of suboptimal pharmacokinetics, drug resistance, inadequate potency, drug toxicity or intolerance, or nonadherence.[1] Decreased drug levels, either due to nonadherence or suboptimal pharmacokinetics, can lead to drug resistance and subsequent failure of the regimen. Monitoring of pharmacokinetic parameters through therapeutic drug monitoring is a potential option.[1]

Resistance to one or more drugs in the regimen before initiation is an independent predictor of virologic outcome with that regimen. Use of drug resistance assays such as genotypes and phenotypes, and the knowledge to interpret the results, greatly increases the likelihood of successful outcomes.[1]

Drug toxicity has been shown to be a leading cause for nonadherence to therapy,[1,3,4] so management of adverse effects is crucial to the regimen's success. For patients experiencing toxicity in a successful regimen, it is appropriate to substitute a similar drug with a different adverse effect profile.

Intensification versus treatment interruption. *Intensification* is the addition of a drug to a regimen for a patient with a detectable viral load.[5] The goal is to provide viral suppression without changing the entire regimen, generally at lower viral loads (HIV RNA <10,000 copies/mL). Careful assessment and a detailed history of previous antiretroviral agents that the patient has taken are crucial to the success of intensification. Without close attention to previous regimens, the addition of a single drug could quickly lead to further resistance to the existing regimen as well as the added agent.[5]

Table 8.1. DHHS Guidelines: Indications for Initiation of Antiretroviral Therapy

Clinical Category	CD4[+] T Cell Count	Plasma HIV RNA	Recommendation
AIDS-defining illness or severe symptoms*	Any value	Any value	Treat
Asymptomatic	<200 cells/mm³	Any value	Treat
Asymptomatic	>200 cells/mm³ but ≤350 cells/mm³	Any value	Treatment should be offered following full discussion of risks and benefits with each patient
Asymptomatic	>350 cells/mm³	≥100,000 copies/mL	Most clinicians recommend deferring therapy, but some clinicians will treat
Asymptomatic	>350 cells/mm³	<100,000 copies/mL	Defer treatment

*AIDS-defining illness per CDC, 1993. Severe symptoms may also include unexplained fever or diarrhea for >2–4 weeks, oral candidiasis, or >10% unexplained weight loss.

Source: Panel on Clinical Practices for Treatment of HIV Infection convened by the Department of Health and Human Services (DHHS). Guidelines for the Use of Antiretroviral Agents in HIV-1-Infected Adults and Adolescents. October 10, 2006. Available at http://www.aidsinfo.nih.gov. Accessed February 10, 2007.

A once popular, but now mostly unfavorable, approach to management of the patient with persistently detectable viral load is treatment interruption. The theory was that interruption of therapy would replace resistant virus with wild-type virus and enhance a patient's response to retreatment with either the same regimen or a new one. Numerous studies have now shown this to be a risky approach in many patients, particularly those with CD4+ T-cell count nadirs of less than 200 cells/mm³ or high viral loads prior to treatment. Discontinuation of therapy has resulted in rapid declines in CD4+ T-cell counts, high viral loads with cases of acute seroconversion-like syndromes, and slow responses to reinitiation of therapy. This approach may be useful in patients who started therapy very early, with CD4+ T-cell count nadirs of more than 200 cells/mm³ or for patients experiencing severe drug toxicities.[1,5]

Antiretroviral Agents

The first drug for the treatment of HIV infection, zidovudine, was introduced in 1987.[6] Additional drugs in the class were approved over the following years, but it wasn't until the introduction of the protease inhibitor class in 1996 that truly potent combinations of medications—highly active antiretroviral therapy (HAART)—were used.

Classification. The stages in the viral replicative cycle that are potentially susceptible to antiviral intervention are shown in Figure 7.1 in Chapter 7. Potential targets may include entry of the virus into the cell, reverse transcriptase, integrase, protease, and viral maturation and release.[7,8]

Inhibitors of viral entry. The first drug from this class, enfuvirtide (T-20), was approved by the Food and Drug Administration (FDA) in 2003. Enfuvirtide, a fusion inhibitor, directly interferes with host and cellular membrane fusion, preventing entry of HIV-1 into the cell. The HIV-1 envelope contains surface glycoproteins (gp120) and transmembrane glycoproteins (gp41). The initial attachment between virus and cell is the coupling of the viral gp120 subunit to the CD4 cell, resulting in a conformational change that exposes the gp41 fusion peptide, which houses two N-terminal repeat domains (heptads) called HR1 and HR2. The changed gp41 springs outward toward the cell membrane, resulting in a hairpin structure that pulls the cell and viral membranes close, allowing fusion and viral entry.[9,10] Enfuvirtide binds to the region of gp41 normally responsible for the conformational change in the hairpin (HR1). This binding inhibits apposition and therefore fusion and viral entry.[1]

Enfuvirtide is not orally bioavailable; it is only given by subcutaneous injection, so it is typically reserved for treatment-experienced patients with few options for successful treatment. The most common adverse effect is injection site reactions (98% of patients). Rare cases of pneumonia have also been reported with its use; the cause is unknown at this time.[1]

Reverse transcriptase inhibitors. Because reverse transcriptase, which makes DNA from RNA, is an essential and relatively unique feature of HIV, inhibition of this enzyme was recognized early as an important target for antiretroviral therapy. In 1985, it was observed that the dideoxynucleosides had potent in-vitro activity against HIV.[7,8,11] Two classes of reverse transcriptase inhibitors have since been developed: nucleoside/nucleotide reverse transcriptase inhibitors and non-nucleoside reverse transcriptase inhibitors.

Nucleoside and nucleotide reverse transcriptase inhibitors. Nucleoside reverse transcriptase inhibitors (NRTIs) must be converted to the active triphosphate derivative by the biochemical machinery of the cell. This anabolic phosphorylation involves a three-step process. Substantial differences in the rates at which human cells phosphorylate these compounds are reflected in their antiretroviral activity.[7,8,11] NRTIs are modified compared to normal nucleosides in that they lack the essential 3'-hydroxyl group. Once reverse transcriptase adds these nucleotides to a growing chain of DNA, no additional nucleotides can be added. This results in chain termination and HIV replication is halted.[11] The nucleotide reverse transcriptase inhibitor tenofovir, unlike NRTIs, only requires two phosphorylation steps to produce its di-phosphorylated active moiety. It, too, incorporates into the growing chain of DNA and halts DNA synthesis.[6]

The NRTIs currently available for use in the United States are summarized in **Table 8.2**. All nucleosides and nucleotides except abacavir require dosage adjustments for renal insufficiency. Estimated glomerular filtration rates (GFR) should be calculated before starting patients on these drugs and periodically throughout treatment.[1]

Non-nucleoside reverse transcriptase inhibitors. Non-nucleoside reverse transcriptase inhibitors (NNRTIs) are summarized in Table 8.2.[1] Nevirapine was the first drug in the class to obtain FDA approval (1996). These non-nucleoside analogs are highly specific, direct noncompetitive inhibitors of HIV-1 reverse transcriptase and do not need cellular metabolism to be active.[12,13] They are not incorporated into the elongating strand of DNA and therefore do not cause chain termination. Because these agents only bind specifically to HIV-1,

Table 8.2. FDA-Approved Antiretroviral Drugs

Generic Name (Abbreviation)	Trade Name	FDA Pregnancy Category
Nucleoside Reverse Transcriptase Inhibitors (NRTIs)		
Abacavir (ABC)	Ziagen Trizivir with ZDV and 3TC Epzicom with 3TC	C
Didanosine (ddI)	Videx Videx Enteric Coated (EC) Generic didanosine EC	B
Emtricitabine (FTC)	Emtriva Truvada with TDF Atripla with EFV and TDF	B (D when used as Atripla due to EFV component)
Lamivudine (3TC)	Epivir Combivir with ZDV Trizivir with ZDV and ABC Epzicom with ABC	C
Stavudine (d4T)	Zerit	C
Zalcitabine (ddC)	Hivid	C
Zidovudine (ZDV, AZT)	Retrovir Generic zidovudine	C
Nucleotide Reverse Transcriptase Inhibitors		
Tenofovir (TDF)	Viread Truvada with FTC Atripla with EFV and FTC	B (D when used as Atripla due to EFV component)
Non-nucleoside Reverse Transcriptase Inhibitors (NNRTIs)		
Delavirdine (DLV)	Rescriptor	C
Efavirenz (EFV)	Sustiva Atripla with TDF and FTC	D
Nevirapine (NVP)	Viramune	C
Protease Inhibitors (PIs)		
Amprenavir (APV)	Agenerase	C
Atazanavir (ATZ)	Reyataz	B
Darunavir (DRV)	Prezista	B
Fosamprenavir (FPV)	Lexiva	C
Indinavir (IDV)	Crixivan	C
Lopinavir/Ritonavir (LPV/r)	Kaletra	C
Nelfinavir (NFV)	Viracept	B
Ritonavir (RTV)	Norvir	B
Saquinavir (SQV)	Invirase Fortovase	B
Tipranavir (TPV)	Aptivus	C
Fusion Inhibitors		
Enfuvirtide (T20)	Fuzeon	B

Sources: Panel on Clinical Practices for Treatment of HIV Infection convened by the Department of Health and Human Services (DHHS). Guidelines for the Use of Antiretroviral Agents in HIV-1-Infected Adults and Adolescents. October 10, 2006. Available at http://www.aidsinfo.org.nih.gov. Accessed February 10, 2007.

Yu VL, Edwards G, McKinnon PS, et al. *Antimicrobial Therapy and Vaccines.* Volume II: Antimicrobial Agents. Pittsburgh, PA: ESun Technologies, LLC; 2005.

U.S. Department of Health and Human Services. Public Health Service Task Force recommendations for use of antiretroviral drugs in pregnant women for maternal health and interventions to reduce perinatal HIV-1 transmission in the United States. Rockville, MD: HIV/AIDS Treatment Information Service. Available at http://www.aidsinfo.nih.gov. Accessed July 3, 2005.

they are not considered active against strains of HIV-2.[6,12,13]

The NNRTIs are inducers of cytochrome P450 enzyme system and result in many drug–drug interactions. Nevirapine is also responsible for its own metabolism. No renal adjustment is needed for these drugs since they are eliminated primarily via hepatic elimination.[1,6]

Protease inhibitors. HIV encodes for enzymes, in addition to reverse transcriptase, that are important in viral replication. The protease enzyme is essential for viral infectivity and the processing of core proteins. Protease cleaves the polyprotein precursors of viral proteins Gag and Pol, creating mature virion components. Protease inhibitors compete for the active cleavage site on the protease enzyme, inhibiting formation of mature core proteins and resulting in the release of a noninfectious virion from the host cell.[6–8]

Currently, there are 10 protease inhibitors (PIs) that are FDA-approved (see Table 8.2). Saquinavir was the first protease inhibitor to receive FDA approval in 1995.[1] Ritonavir and indinavir received approval in 1996, and the HAART revolution began. These drugs have complex pharmacologic profiles, especially when used together. Protease inhibitors are metabolized through the cytochrome P-450 system, and multiple drug interactions have been reported.[1,6] Because of ritonavir's potent inhibition of common pathways within this system and its lack of tolerability when used at standard doses, it is now primarily used as a "boosting" agent for the other protease inhibitors.[1]

No renal adjustment is needed for any of the protease inhibitors since they are all eliminated via hepatic metabolism. These agents should be used with caution in patients with moderate to severe hepatic impairment who may require dosage adjustments.[1,6]

Investigational targets. 2006 data on the emergence of new agents derived from stages in the life cycle of HIV (see Figure 7.1) is encouraging. These novel drug classes include various subcategories of HIV entry inhibitors such as the chemotactic cytokines or chemokines of CCR5 and CXCR4, integrase inhibitors, and maturation inhibitors. Newer agents with different resistance profiles for the current classes of medications are in development.

The class of entry inhibitors can be broken down into three subclasses based on discrete targets for viral entry: CD4 binding, chemokine receptor binding, and fusion.[9] The first and only FDA-approved drug from this class, enfuvirtide (a fusion inhibitor), was discussed in Chapter 7. Earlier attempts to prevent the initial binding of

HIV to CD4 with the soluble form of CD4, rsCD4, proved to have no antiviral effect. A new form, tetravalent CD4 that is linked to immunoglobulin (Ig) G, appears to inhibit HIV infection in vitro, and is in early stages of study.[9]

Most HIV isolates use CCR5 as a coreceptor that is critical for HIV entry. This discovery led to the investigation of new compounds with the first agents in clinic trials. These compounds act as antagonists at the CCR5 site by inhibiting chemotaxis in monocytes and macrophages caused by the beta-chemokine MIP-1 beta and by blocking chemokine-induced calcium flux. It is specific antagonism of CCR5 and does not inhibit CXCR4 infection. There is a theoretical concern that use of CCR5 inhibitors will cause the virus population to shift to CXCR4, a syncytium-inducing virus, which may cause a more rapid decline in CD4 counts.[14]

CXCR4 inhibitors have been investigated for many years without the success of the CCR5 inhibitors. The early compounds were withdrawn from investigation because they lacked efficacy and had serious side effects, including cardiac arrhythmias. Other compounds are currently being investigated.[14]

Another new class of drugs gaining momentum is the maturation inhibitors. These compounds block the catalytic conversion of a capsid precursor protein to the mature capsid form. Specifically, they produce a defect in Gag processing whereby the cleavage of p25 capsid protein is disrupted, blocking the release of capsid protein p24. The result is formation of defective condensation of the core structures and production of noninfectious viral particles that are incapable of infecting other cells.[14]

Adverse drug reactions. Lipodystrophy syndrome describes morphologic changes (lipoatrophy and lipohypertrophy) as well as metabolic complications (dyslipidemias and insulin resistance) associated with HIV infection and HAART. These disorders may occur together or independently.[1,15]

Lipoatrophy and lipohypertrophy. Lipoatrophy is fat loss in the face, extremities, and buttocks; it should not be confused with HIV wasting that involves overall fat and muscle loss. Lipohypertrophy is defined fat accumulation in the dorsocervical area ("buffalo hump"), breasts, or abdomen.[1,15]

Both conditions occur exclusively in the setting of antiretroviral treatment and with long-standing HIV infection. Specific risk factors for lipoatrophy may be use and duration of thymidine analog agents (particularly stavudine), overall duration of HAART, older age, lower CD4[+] T-cell counts, and white race.[1,5,15] Risk factors associated with the development of lipohypertrophy are similar and include duration of HAART, lower CD4[+] T-cell counts, older age, and use of protease inhibitor agents.[1,5,15] The mechanism by which these events occur is not fully elucidated, but is believed to be an interaction among the host, HIV disease, and the drugs used for HIV treatment.

No accepted uniform definition for these conditions exists and diagnosis is often subjective. The HIV Lipodystrophy Case Definition Study Group recently developed a complex case definition involving 10 variables and the use of dual-energy x-ray absorptiometry (DEXA) scans and computed tomography (CT) scans.[16] The model exhibits 80% accuracy and was developed as a research tool to allow more uniformity in the definition of HIV lipodystrophy syndrome or disease. Clinicians are also encouraged to use it as a guide when attempting to diagnose the disease.

Treatment generally involves discontinuing the offending agent since this is often not reversible. Thiazolidinediones are a treatment of interest, although convincing data are still needed. Surgical treatment options such as facial or buttocks implants and removal of buffalo humps have been performed. Facial fillers can be permanent or temporary and can make a significant difference. Although buffalo humps have been surgically removed, they tend to recur within a couple of years.[1,5,15]

Lactic acidosis. Lactic acidosis is defined as an arterial pH less than 7.35 in association with a venous lactate level of more than 5 mmol/L.[5] Other abnormal laboratory parameters include increased anion gap, elevated transaminases, lipase, amylase, and creatine phosphokinase (CPK). Lactic acidosis can occur during NRTI treatment and is associated with weight loss, fatigue, abdominal pain, tender hepatomegaly, nausea, vomiting, and respiratory distress. Untreated lactic acidosis has a mortality rate over 50%.[1,5]

Risk factors associated with development of lactic acidosis while taking an NRTI include female sex, pregnancy, obesity, and long-term use of an NRTI, in particular, stavudine.[1,5]

Treatment of lactic acidosis is primarily supportive care with the discontinuation of all NRTI drugs. In severe, acute cases, bicarbonate infusions, riboflavin and thiamine, vitamin C, co-enzyme-Q, and L-carnitine along with dialysis have been used, though data supporting their effectiveness is minimal. Rechallenge with a different NRTI should be undertaken cautiously under close supervision.[1,5]

Dyslipidemias. Increases in serum triglycerides, total and LDL cholesterol levels, and decreases in HDL cholesterol have been reported with the use of stavudine, to a lesser extent efavirenz, and all of the PIs except atazanavir.[1,5] The National Cholesterol Education Program (NCEP) guidelines are used as a general guide for treatment of lipid disorders, but they do not specifically address problems with HIV infection.[17] Specific guidelines for treatment of HAART-associated dyslipidemias have been published by the Adult AIDS Clinical Trials Group (ACTG) and the Infectious Disease Society of America (IDSA) Cardiovascular Disease Focus Group.[18] Other cardiac risk factors include smoking, hypertension, diabetes, family history of heart disease, menopause, obesity, and physical inactivity. Other possible confounding factors may include excessive alcohol use, cocaine use, hypothyroidism, renal disease, liver disease, hypogonadism, and use of other drugs such as corticosteroids, beta-blockers, and thiazide diuretics.[1,5]

Treatment for dyslipidemias always starts with diet and exercise. Depending on the degree of dyslipidemia, lipid-lowering medication may be needed early rather than after a trial of diet and exercise.[1,5]

Insulin resistance. Use of PIs in treatment of HIV infection has been associated with insulin resistance, hyperglycemia, and, in some cases, development of diabetes mellitus similar to type 2. As many as 40% of patients taking PIs may have insulin resistance, and 1% to 6% of patients will develop diabetes.[1,5]

Initial treatment of impaired fasting glucose or impaired glucose tolerance ("pre-diabetes") involves diet and exercise to lose weight. If hyperglycemia persists despite these successful measures, discontinuation of the PI should be considered if possible and metformin or rosiglitazone should be instituted. For diabetes mellitus, metformin or rosiglitazone should be started along with diet and exercise.[1,5]

Hepatotoxicity. Hepatotoxicity ranges from asymptomatic elevations in serum transaminases to clinical hepatitis. Asymptomatic serum transaminases elevations occur in 6% to 30% of patients on HAART.[1,5] Risk factors include co-infection with hepatitis B or C, alcoholism, concomitant use of hepatotoxic drugs, and (for certain patients) starting nevirapine.[1,5] For symptomatic patients, discontinue all antiretroviral drugs and other potentially hepatotoxic agents. After symptoms subside and serum transaminases return to baseline, a new antiretroviral regimen may be started.[1,5] In the asymptomatic patient (not on nevirapine) experiencing an increase in serum transaminases of 5–10 times the upper limit of normal, some clinicians would elect to continue therapy with close monitoring while others would discontinue therapy and start over with another regimen once transaminases return to normal.[1,5]

Nevirapine poses a particular risk for hepatotoxicity. Women with $CD4^+$ T-cell counts higher than 250 cells/mm^3 at the start of therapy, including pregnant women, are 12 times more likely to develop severe, life-threatening, and sometimes fatal hepatoxicity. Risk in men with $CD4^+$ T-cell counts higher than 400 cells/mm^3 at the start of therapy is 6.3% versus 1.2% in those with fewer than 400 cells/mm^3. Baseline serum transaminases should be obtained and closely monitored, every 2 weeks for the first 6 weeks of therapy, then monthly for the first 3 months, and every 3 months thereafter.[1]

Pancreatitis. Use of the NRTIs in HIV treatment has been associated with pancreatitis. The most common offender is didanosine (ddI) with rates of 1% to 7% when used alone, and 4–5 times that rate when used in combination with hydroxyurea.[1,5] There is also an increased frequency when ddI is used in combination with ribavirin, stavudine, or tenofovir. Early studies of lamivudine in children had rates of 14% to 18%, but subsequent studies revealed much lower rates of less than 1%.[1] Other risk factors include a history of pancreatitis, alcoholism, and hypertriglyceridemia. Initial complaints include abdominal pain, nausea, and vomiting. Laboratory abnormalities usually include elevations in serum amylase and lipase. Treatment involves discontinuation of the suspected agent and symptom management (bowel rest, intravenous hydration, and pain medications). Parenteral nutrition is rarely indicated since most patients can gradually resume oral intake shortly after onset with appropriate management. Didanosine should not be used in patients with a history of pancreatitis.[1,5]

Peripheral neuropathy. Peripheral neuropathy was initially described in untreated patients in the pre-HAART era and was associated with advanced disease. With HAART, it is most commonly associated with didanosine, stavudine, and zalcitabine, although it continues to be described in the untreated patient with advanced disease. It is primarily a sensory axonal neuropathy.[1,5]

Symptoms generally begin as numbness or paresthesias of the toes and feet and can progress up the calf; in rare cases, it can involve the upper extremities. It may be irreversible even with discontinuation of the offending drug. Other risk factors include preexisting peripheral neuropathy; combined use of didanosine, stavudine, or zalcitabine, or combinations with other known peripheral neuropathy-inducing drugs (e.g., dapsone, isoniazid); combining with drugs known to increase ddI intracellular activity

(e.g., hydroxyurea, ribavirin); advanced HIV infection (low $CD4^+$ T-cell counts <100 cells/mm^3); heavy alcohol consumption; nutritional deficiencies (e.g., vitamin B12); and diabetes mellitus.[1,5] Treatment involves discontinuation of the offending agent to slow the progression and pharmacologic management with gabapentin, tricyclic antidepressants, lamotrigine, oxcarbazepine, topiramate, or tramadol. Narcotic analgesics are generally reserved for more advanced cases that do not respond to the above drugs. Topical capsaicin cream and lidocaine have been used without much success.[1,5]

Renal/nephrotoxicity. Indinavir crystals or stones can form in the urine and cause obstruction between the renal tubules and urethra. About 10% of patients develop symptomatic nephrolithiasis when on indinavir alone; it may be even more common in ritonavir-boosted indinavir regimens. Rarely does this lead to an increase in serum creatinine, and it is completely reversible with discontinuation of the drug along with hydration. Patients are cautioned to drink more than 1.5 liters of water/fluids per day as a preventive measure. About 50% of patients experience a recurrence if indinavir is restarted.[1,5]

The frequency of tenofovir-associated nephrotoxicity is estimated to be between 0% and 7%. It generally occurs months after start of therapy, and ranges from asymptomatic increases in serum creatinine, proteinuria, hypophosphatemia, glycosuria, hypokalemia, and non-anion gap metabolic acidosis, to nephrogenic diabetes insipidus to Fanconi syndrome.[1] Treatment involves discontinuation of tenofovir, supportive care, and electrolyte replacement.[1]

Recently published guidelines for management of chronic kidney disease in HIV-infected patients[19] recommend that all newly diagnosed HIV-infected patients have urinalysis to evaluate their kidney function and estimations of glomerular filtration rate (GFR). For those patients with apparently normal renal function, yearly evaluations should be used to assess changes over time. But for patients with estimated GFRs less than 60 mL/min or proteinuria of grade one or higher, additional evaluations and referral to a nephrologist are recommended. The guidelines recommend biannual screening for patients who are at higher risk (those on indinavir or tenofovir).[19] In clinical practice, routine serum chemistries are often obtained every 3–6 months, so trends in serum creatinine and estimated GFR should be monitored.

Hypersensitivity reactions. Hypersensitivity reaction (HSR) resulting in skin rash may occur in patients on an NNRTI, abacavir, amprenavir, darunavir, fosamprenavir, or tipranavir.[1] Onset is usually within the first few days to weeks of initiation of therapy. Most are mild to moderate, diffuse, maculopapular, with or without pruritis, but the rash may progress to a more severe form such as Stevens-Johnson syndrome or toxic epidermal necrolysis.[1] These reactions are difficult to classify because of a lack of information supporting a predominant immunologic mechanism.

About 8% of patients who start abacavir will develop an HSR that begins as nonspecific gastrointestinal complaints, myalgias, fatigue, fever, shortness of breath, and rash.[1] Treatment is discontinuation of abacavir. Once a person has had an episode of HSR or suspected HSR, rechallenge is not possible since restarting therapy has been associated with severe reactions and death.[1]

Of the NNRTIs, nevirapine is the most common drug associated with rash.[1] Most patients can remain on therapy with close monitoring because the rash usually dissipates within days to weeks without the use of antihistamines or corticosteroids. In fact, use of corticosteroids during nevirapine dose escalation may actually increase the incidence of rash.[1] Rechallenge is possible with mild to moderate rashes, and cross-hypersensitivity between the NNRTIs is not complete unless a life-threatening reaction had occurred (e.g., Stevens-Johnson syndrome).[1,5] Patients on nevirapine who develop rash should receive intense monitoring of liver function since rash is associated with hepatotoxicity.

Amprenavir, darunavir, fosamprenavir, and tipranavir are sulfonamide drugs and therefore have the potential to cause rash. The cross-reactivity between sulfa drugs and these agents is unknown.[1,5]

Therapeutic Drug Monitoring

Interpatient variability in the pharmacokinetic parameters of protease inhibitors and NNTIs makes them likely candidates for therapeutic drug monitoring (TDM).[1,5] The NNTIs need intracellular phosphorylation for activation and their activity is not closely related to serum concentrations, so the utility of TDM with this class of drugs is limited.[1] Other factors can also influence the pharmacokinetics of the PIs and the NNRTIs, including adherence to dosing, food restrictions, and most notably, drug interactions.[5]

The rationale for using TDM is that subtherapeutic serum levels of antiretroviral drugs can lead to development of resistance and failure of the regimen. And some data show that supratherapeutic levels may also be related to drug toxicities.[1,5]

TDM use has been postulated to have potential in certain populations such as pregnant women; unknown or unstudied drug interactions; changes in pathophysiologic status (malabsorption of drugs); evaluation of unsatisfactory virologic responses; evaluation of unsuspected toxicities; once-daily regimens; and in patients on deep salvage regimens (higher than normal doses to overcome resistance).[1,5]

Antiretroviral Therapy during Pregnancy

Treatment during pregnancy involves not only mother-to-child transmission, but also the health and well-being of the HIV-infected mother. Without antiretroviral treatment, about 30% of infants born to infected mothers will be infected with HIV.[20,21] Infection can happen at any stage of pregnancy and postpartum through breastfeeding, but it is believed that most transmission occurs late in pregnancy, at the time of labor and delivery. Risk factors for increased rates of transmission include higher viral load, choice of treatment regimens, mode of delivery, duration of ruptured membranes, chorioamnionitis, fetal maturity or gestational age, and drug use by the mother.[21] The lower the mother's viral load, the less chance of transmission to the fetus, although there is still risk.

Current Public Health Force Task Force guidelines recommend triple combination regimens with zidovudine as a part of the regimen.[21] The mother's treatment history must also be taken into consideration. A past history of resistance should help guide the appropriate choices for treatment during pregnancy and prophylaxis for the infant afterwards. Because treatment during pregnancy and intrapartum dramatically decreases the likelihood of infection of the fetus, there has been a need for treatment of women who present in labor but did not receive prenatal care or did not know they were infected with HIV. Recent studies have shown efficacy with single doses of nevirapine.[21] But the concern has been development of resistance to nevirapine, even from a single dose, which effectively diminishes future treatment options with this class. Because of the rapid emergence of resistance, this jeopardizes the utility of this regimen as part of routine care.[21] Some of the available antiretroviral drugs have teratogenic effects and should not be used during pregnancy, or used with caution when risks outweigh benefits (see Table 8.2).[21] Also, the pharmacokinetics of some drugs may be altered by physiologic changes associated with pregnancy.[21]

In the absence of effective antiretroviral treatment during pregnancy, cesarean section can reduce the risk of transmission from about 20% to less than 10%.[5,21] When zidovudine is used during pregnancy and intrapartum, cesarean section can further reduce the likelihood of transmission from 4% to 7% to 1% to 2%.[5,21] The American College of Obstetrics and Gynecology has chosen a viral load of 1,000 copies/mL as the cutoff above which cesarean sections should be planned.[21] Below this limit, elective cesarean sections may be performed during weeks 38–39 or at the onset of labor to possibly further decrease risk of transmission.[21] The benefits of cesarean sections after rupture of membranes or in active labor are unknown.

Public Health Service guidelines recommend alternative forms of nutrition for infants other than breastfeeding. Breastfeeding increases the risk of transmission an additional 15% above the risk of pregnancy and appears to be related to duration of exposure or length of time the infant is fed.[21]

IMMUNOLOGIC THERAPY

The immunopathogenesis of HIV infection is a consequence of both chronic stimulation from persistent antigenic exposure and the resultant immunosuppression that accumulates over time. Strategies targeting the immune system could theoretically include methods to replace or enhance immune response and tactics that suppress the state of chronic activation. Although these two strategies appear diametrically opposed, containment of the destruction rendered by HIV may require each of these approaches to be used at specific points in the infection.

Immune Enhancement

Several strategies to enhance the immune deficiency caused by HIV infection have been evaluated. HIV-infected individuals have been administered HIV vaccines in an attempt to boost their immune response to the virus. This strategy is referred to as "therapeutic immunization" to differentiate it from vaccines administered to non-HIV-infected individuals in an attempt to prevent infection. The immune enhancement potential of various cytokines is also under evaluation. Hematopoietic growth factors may be able to minimize leukopenia, which occurs either as a consequence of HIV infection or medications.

Therapeutic immunization. Attempts at potentiating the immune response to HIV by immunizing HIV-infected individuals with a therapeutic vaccine are currently under investigation. A phase I trial conducted in subjects with early HIV infection (CD4+ T-cell count >400 cells/mL) evaluated a recombinant gp160 expressed in a baculovirus system (MicroGeneSys) at three different doses (40, 160, and 640 mg/L) and two different dosage schedules (three inoculations over 4 months or six inoculations over 6 months). Response was defined as a reproducible and selective potentiation of both cellular and humoral responses against specific HIV envelope epitopes associated with the timing of the inoculations. Response was noted in 19 of the 30 vaccine recipients, associated with both the number of injections and the baseline CD4+ T-cell count. Over a 10-month follow-up period, CD4+ T-cell counts remained stable in the responders whereas the CD4+ T-cell counts in the nonresponders declined by 7.3%. No systemic adverse effects from the vaccine were observed.[22]

The results of a phase II/III efficacy trial conducted in 103 asymptomatic HIV-infected individuals have been reported. The immunogen used in this trial was a gp120-depleted, inactivated HIV-1 presented in incomplete Freund's adjuvant. The control group received the adjuvant alone. Both humoral and cellular immune responses were observed, and both were significantly more pronounced in the immunogen recipients. Antibodies to p24 were maximal at 32 weeks (8 weeks after the last injection). Although a gradual decline was observed during the 1-year follow-up period, titers in the group receiving immunogen were still above baseline at the end of the study. Significant differences were also observed in viral burden (viral DNA) and progression of disease (CD4+ T-cell decline) between the immunogen recipients and the controls.[23]

These studies suggest that therapeutic immunization of HIV-infected individuals is safe and does stimulate a specific anti-HIV response. But a long-term follow-up study of the subjects is clearly needed to define the role of this strategy in affecting disease progression.

Cytokines. Defects in the production of various cytokines have been reported in patients with HIV infection. Replacement strategies initially focused on the interferons because of the triad of antiviral, immunomodulatory, and antiproliferative effects of these agents. Interferon (IFN)-α has been combined with zidovudine in patients with AIDS-related Kaposi's sarcoma. At a maximum tolerated dose of 600 mg/day of zidovudine and 18 MU/day of IFN-α, tumor regression was observed in 17 of 37 patients.[24] This combination yields higher regression rates than higher doses of IFN-α alone.[25]

The antiviral effects of IFN-α are complex, and the response to therapy is likely to depend on whether the patient has progressed to AIDS. Clinical isolates of HIV have variable susceptibility to IFN-α. Progression to AIDS has been associated with high circulating endogenous levels of IFN-α. It appears that IFN-α-resistant HIV occurs naturally at a low level, and its frequency is probably independent of endogenous IFN-α. As disease progresses, the higher levels of endogenous IFN-α select for the IFN-α-resistant phenotype. So patients in the later stages of HIV infection are likely to have a high prevalence of IFN-α-resistant HIV variants.[26] This suggests that the benefits of exogenous IFN-α therapy may be greatest at early stages of infection. In one study of asymptomatic HIV-infected individuals, both antiviral effects and stabilization in CD4$^+$ T-cell counts were observed in IFN-α recipients. But even in asymptomatic individuals, exogenous IFN-α was associated with significant toxicity. All the recipients experienced flu-like symptoms, and over half developed granulocytopenia. More than one third of the recipients withdrew from treatment because of toxicity.[27] These data together suggest that early intervention, perhaps using IFN-α gene therapy directed at HIV target cells, might have potential,[28] but toxicity may limit its usefulness.

Impaired production of interleukin (IL)-2 has also been described in patients with AIDS. Human CD4$^+$ T cells may be separated into two subsets, TH1 and TH2. TH1 cells secrete the cytokines important for enhancing cell-mediated immunity (IL-2, tumor necrosis factor [TNF]-β, and IFN-γ), and TH2 cells secrete cytokines that increase antibody production. Impaired production of IL-2 appears to result from a progressive, selective deficiency of TH1 responses and a predominance of TH2 responses (mediated by IL-4, IL-5, IL-6, and IL-10). This defect in TH1 response might be corrected by exogenous administration of IL-2 or IL-12.

Although immunoenhancing effects of IL-2 were observed in vitro, early results in patients were disappointing, perhaps because of suboptimal dosing.[28] Subsequent strategies focused on intermittent IL-2 therapy (5-day course, every 8 weeks). Randomized trials of intermittent intravenous IL-2 with antiretroviral therapy demonstrated sustained increases in CD4$^+$ counts without affecting plasma HIV RNA levels.[29,30] A preliminary evaluation of IL-2 observed that administration could increase viral replication, emphasizing the need for concomitant antiretroviral therapy.[31] Subcutaneous

administration of IL-2 has also been effective in "immunologic nonresponders" to antiretroviral therapy.[32,33] The immunologic efficacy of IL-2 has been demonstrated clinically, with a trend toward fewer opportunistic infections.[34]

Recent studies have also suggested that IL-12 therapy might be useful in managing HIV infection. Antigenic stimulation of peripheral blood mononuclear cells from subjects with HIV infection yields poor cell-mediated responses in vitro. This can be corrected by stimulating the cultures in the presence of IL-12. This finding suggests that IL-12 administration may be effective in restoring HIV-specific cell-mediated immunity, at least in vitro.[35]

Colony-stimulating factors—glycoprotein hormones that regulate cellular development from hematopoietic progenitors—might be useful in stimulating the production of both erythrocytes and leukocytes. Patients with AIDS who are receiving zidovudine and have low endogenous erythropoietin levels may benefit from epoetin alfa therapy. A reduction in red blood cell transfusion requirements has been observed in patients receiving concomitant therapy with recombinant epoetin alfa.[36,37] A phase I/II trial of granulocyte-macrophage colony-stimulating factor (GM-CSF) was undertaken in 16 patients with AIDS and leukopenia. This study revealed dose-dependent increases in circulating leukocytes. Mature neutrophils, band forms, and eosinophils accounted for the majority of the increase. Circulating monocytes increased two- to fourfold over baseline. Dose-related changes in lymphocyte counts were not observed.[38] The use of GM-CSF may reduce the morbidity associated with either disease-related or therapy-related leukopenia in patients with AIDS, but the ability of GM-CSF to stimulate HIV replication in monocytes is a cause for concern. Moreover, whether colony-stimulating factors will be able to sustain hematopoiesis in a setting of continued suppression is uncertain. A small study of GM-CSF, used as a single agent followed by an alternating regimen with zidovudine, supports these concerns. In that study, GM-CSF increased both circulating monocyte number and function and increased HIV replication (as measured by increased p24 antigen) in six of nine patients. Furthermore, bone marrow evaluations performed at 14 weeks revealed increased cellularity and increased myeloid precursors in only three of seven patients.[39] Because of the potential for enhancement of viral replication, the ultimate role of GM-CSF will likely be in combination with antiviral therapy. Although neither granulocyte colony-stimulating factor (G-CSF) nor GM-CSF is approved by the FDA for leukopenia in patients with AIDS, G-CSF has become widely used for bone marrow support in this setting.

Immune Suppression

Recently, investigators have targeted chronic activation of the immune system in an effort to preserve immune function. As reviewed in the discussion of immunopathogenesis above, chronic activation of the immune system enhances viral replication and promotes the destruction of CD4+ T cells. Although this approach may be reasonable (and preliminary data suggest promise), it is imperative that this strategy target patients unlikely to be harmed by additional immunosuppression.

Cyclosporine may be useful in blocking the state of chronic activation of the immune system promoted by HIV. Cyclosporine blocks the transcriptional activation of T lymphocytes by inhibiting nuclear factors, resulting in reduced HIV expression.[40] It may disrupt the production of infectious viral particles by interfering with the binding of cellular cyclophilin A and B to the Gag protein of HIV-1.[41] Clinical experience with cyclosporine has been mixed, with one trial suggesting improvement and another suggesting further deterioration of an already compromised immune system.[42] But one retrospective analysis of transplant recipients infected with HIV at about the time of transplantation suggested that cyclosporine administration soon after infection delayed the progression to AIDS. Of the 13 individuals who did not receive cyclosporine as part of the transplantation regimen, the 5-year cumulative risk of AIDS was 90%, compared with 31% in the 40 individuals who received it.[43] These data suggest the optimal time to administer immunosuppressives, such as cyclosporine, would be before the development of HIV-related immunosuppression. In patients who have already developed HIV immune dysfunction, less immunosuppressive analogs of cyclosporine may be of greater benefit.[42,44]

VACCINE DEVELOPMENT

Vaccine development is crucial to the ultimate containment of HIV, but the development of an effective and safe vaccine is a formidable challenge. The virus' ability to escape host immune responses has limited our success. Recent advances in the molecular understanding of viral variability and immunologic response to specific epitopes has created optimism. Meaningful progress in developing

a suitable animal model has been achieved with experimental trials of simian immunodeficiency virus (SIV) infection. These models permit evaluation of the cross-protection afforded to isolates dissimilar to those contained in the vaccine. Mucosal models of infection are also under development.[45] Although these are important advances in the evolution of a vaccine for HIV, several developmental considerations remain. The ideal vaccine would elicit strong immune responses to many different strains of HIV and confer long-lasting protection upon exposure to HIV.

Developmental Considerations

There are no documented cases of complete recovery from HIV infection or clearance of the virus. Despite HIV-specific cellular responses, HIV superinfection can occur, so we have no human model to guide research efforts. Instead, research has used long-term survivors and people who remain uninfected despite repeated exposures to HIV as their models. Long-term survivors are either long-term nonprogressors who are able to maintain normal steady state CD4+ T-cell counts for many years, or HIV-infected persons who have lost a significant proportion of their CD4+ T cells but remain healthy.[46] Despite the progress made in animal models, HIV is uniquely pathogenic for humans, so an exact animal model in which to study the spectrum of the disease does not exist. Chimpanzees, a close relative of humans, are susceptible to HIV infection.[46,47] Once infected, chimpanzees produce antibody profiles similar to those of humans, shed virus, and demonstrate cytopathic changes in CD4+ T cells. Chimpanzees occasionally develop lymphadenopathy and temporary CD4+ T-cell count depression, but development of an AIDS-like illness may take up to 10 years. The chimpanzee therefore is problematic as an adequate model in which to assess the efficacy of a vaccine against primary HIV infection.[46,47] Asian macaques can be infected with SIV and have been inoculated with a chimeric virus (SHIV) that is based on SIV and causes a serious illness similar to HIV.[46,47] This model appears to be the most useful in evaluating a pathogenic model system. Given these limitations, progress made with the SIV model has generated a great deal of excitement. However, genetic and biological differences between HIV and SIV may limit the value of this model, particularly with respect to extent of virus variability.[45,48]

HIV immunogenicity is produced via humoral and/or cellular immunity. Humoral or antibody-mediated immunity refers primarily to the action of neutralizing antibodies to the outer envelope of HIV (gp160 and gp120) that inactivate HIV or prevent it from binding and infecting cells.[46] The ideal HIV vaccine would need to produce sterilizing immunity early in the disease process. Other vaccines that produce sterilizing immunity do so by producing a strong neutralizing antibody response.[46] Research from this perspective has focused on recombinant technology to produce, purify, and test these vaccine candidates.

Cellular or cell-mediated immunity refers to the ability of cytotoxic T lymphocytes (CTLs) to destroy HIV-infected cells.[46] CTLs, also referred to as CD8+ T cells or "killer T cells," have surface CD8+ receptors that allow them to attach and destroy HIV-producing cells.[46] A CTL-mediated response vaccine would likely not produce sterilizing immunity but could possibly be used to limit viral replication and ultimately progression of the disease. Helper T (TH) cells, another component of cell-mediated immunity, are the main target of HIV. TH cells secrete cytokines that direct humoral and cellular immunity. A subset of TH cells, memory T cells, are produced after an initial exposure to an organism and serve as a quick, potent immune response on reexposure.[46] Mucosal immunity is also needed since most exposures are via sexual contact at the genital tract or rectum. The antibody IgA appears to be responsible for vaginal mucosal responses. Currently, only animal models exist to study how various AIDS vaccine candidates induce mucosal immunity.[46]

There is large variation in the strain of HIV due to genetic mutation and recombination. HIV isolates are categorized into three groups (M, N, and O), and then the M (Major) group is further subdivided into nine subtypes or clades.[46] Each M subtype varies about 30% from the others, and the predominant subtype in the United States and Europe is B. A successful vaccine would need to protect an exposed individual to many different subtypes; research efforts have focused on conserved regions of the HIV genes that are common to all or most subtypes.[46]

HIV vaccines that contain live, attenuated virus are deemed too dangerous for human testing. Vaccines for other viral diseases are made from whole virus that is either inactivated or attenuated. Inactivated HIV or SIV has been tested in animal models and has not been found to induce an effective immune response. Attenuated HIV has been tested in monkeys and found to induce protection, but it will not be tested in humans because of safety concerns.[46]

Strategies for optimizing the presentation of immunogen are being evaluated. Immunologic adjuvants are used to increase the type, strength, and durability of the vaccine response. The immunogenicity of the vaccine may be enhanced by several orders of magnitude if a potent adjuvant system is used. The only adjuvant approved by the FDA for human use is alum. Although alum is effective in some vaccines, a more efficient stimulator of humoral and cellular responses may be needed for a vaccine effective against HIV. Freund's adjuvant, along with alternative systems, such as muramyl dipeptides, liposomes, and immune-stimulating complexes such as IL-2-IgG, are under development.[46,49]

To test the efficacy of vaccine candidates, phase III studies of seronegative individuals who engage in high-risk behaviors are needed. Study participants may therefore be drawn from historically marginalized or disenfranchised groups who may have distrust of the government and the public health system. Investigators in these studies must balance their ability to obtain HIV vaccine efficacy data with their ethical obligation to inform and educate the subjects about the avoidance of risky behaviors. The implication of these conflicting goals is that the reported efficacy of the vaccine may be clouded by the impact of counseling. In addition, participants in the study may develop vaccine-induced HIV antibodies, which may lead to discrimination in insurance, employment, or medical care.[46,50]

Vaccine Approaches

Currently, there are four major approaches to human HIV vaccines (**Table 8.3**).[46] These approaches are generally not used alone; their primary utility will likely be found in combinations. The "prime-boost strategy" uses two vaccines, one after the other, to build a better immune response

Table 8.3. Major Approaches to HIV Vaccine Development

Live vector-based vaccine
DNA vaccine
Peptide vaccine
Modified envelope glycoprotein vaccine
Prime-boost strategy (involves combining two of the above vaccine approaches)

Sources: Spearman P. Current progress in the development of HIV vaccines. *Curr Pharm Des.* 2006; 12:1147–1167. Centers for Disease Control and Prevention (CDC). HIV vaccine unit. Available at http://www.cdc.gov/hiv/vaccine/hivvu.htm. Accessed July 9, 2005.

by "priming" the immune system with one type of vaccine and then boosting it with another type. An example of this strategy is to prime the immune system with a DNA vaccine followed by a live vector-based vaccine used as the boost to generate a strong and long-lived cellular immune response.[46]

A live vector vaccine is a common method of delivering vaccine to the body's cells. It is made up of genetically engineered HIV genes inserted into a vector that carries it into the body's cells; there, it can produce HIV protein that causes production of antibodies and T cells and then, an immune response. The live vector-based vaccine approach is hoped to produce a strong, long-lived cellular immune response. These vector-based vaccine approaches include adenoviral, attenuated poxvirus, alphavirus, adeno-associated virus (AAV), vesicular stomatitis virus (VSV)-HIV vaccines, and poliovirus-HIV vaccines. These viral vector approaches are only competent for a single round of infection within the host and are usually combined with heterologous immunogen boosters.[46]

DNA vaccines have been shown to produce both humoral and cellular immune responses. A small number of HIV genes are inserted into plasmids (self-replicating circles of DNA), which then produce proteins in the body's cells.[46] The potency of DNA vaccines is troubling, so adjuvants are critical to the success of this approach. An appropriate adjuvant is needed to enhance the uptake of the vaccine into the nucleus and produce a potent effect.[46]

Peptide vaccines have been shown to produce weak HIV-specific cellular immune responses. Again, the appropriate adjuvant will be critical to its success. Given its relative weak activity alone, peptide vaccines will need to be used in a prime-boost combination.[46]

Modified envelope glycoprotein approaches are being studied as a means of inducing neutralizing antibodies. The proposed combination of a CTL response generated by a live vector system, along with the induction of neutralizing antibodies via an oligomeric protein system, is very attractive.[46]

Human Trials

Over the past decade, at least 34 different HIV candidate vaccines have gone into phase I clinical trials, another three entered phase II, and the first phase III trial was completed.[50] All trials are closely monitored by Data and Safety Monitoring Boards as well as guidance from community advisory boards. The phase II trials of VAX003 and VAX004 evaluated the efficacy of gp-120-based vaccine candidates in both the United States as well as developing countries, but these vaccine candidates failed to prevent HIV infection.[50] The Centers for Disease Control and Prevention (CDC), along with the National Institutes of Health (NIH), the Department of Defense, and the NIH-funded HIV Vaccine Trials Network, as well as the Partnership for AIDS Vaccine Evaluation (PAVE), are collaborating on HIV vaccine development.[50] While development of an effective HIV vaccine or combination has been disappointing, lessons learned from these early trials have contributed significantly to our understanding of HIV immunology and our current approaches to finding an effective vaccine.

SUMMARY

With ongoing research defining the utility of various antiviral and immunomodulating strategies for HIV/AIDS, our approach to the management of patients continues to evolve. Given the heavy influence of complex medication regimens on the outcome of HIV disease with a special emphasis on adherence, pharmacists continue to be integral to the multidisciplinary care of HIV-infected patients in various settings.

REFERENCES

1. Panel on Clinical Practices for Treatment of HIV Infection convened by the Department of Health and Human Services (DHHS). Guidelines for the Use of Antiretroviral Agents in HIV-1-Infected Adults and Adolescents. October 10, 2006. Available at http://www.aidsinfo.nih.gov. Accessed February 10, 2007.
2. Yeni PG, Hammer SM, Hirsch MS, et al. Treatment for adult HIV infection: 2004 recommendations of the International AIDS Society—USA panel. *JAMA.* 2004; 292:251–265.
3. D'Arminio Monforte A, Lepri AC, Rezza G, et al. Insights into the reasons for discontinuation of the first highly active antiretroviral therapy (HAART) regimen in a cohort of antiretroviral naive patients. I.CO.N.A. Study Group. Italian Cohort of Antiretroviral-Naïve Patients. *AIDS.* 2000; 14(5):499–507.
4. Mocroft A, Youle M, Moore A, et al. Reasons for modification and discontinuation of antiretrovirals: results from a single treatment centre. *AIDS.* 2001; 15(2):185–194.
5. Yu VL, Weber R, Raoult D, eds. *Antimicrobial Therapy and Vaccines.* New York, NY: Apple Trees Productions, LLC; 2002:1249–1313.

6. Yu VL, Edwards G, McKinnon PS, et al. *Antimicrobial Therapy and Vaccines*. Pittsburgh, PA: ESun Technologies, LLC; 2005:817–833, 845–907.

7. Hirsch MS. Chemotherapy of human immunodeficiency virus infections: current practice and future prospects. *J Infect Dis*. 1990; 161:845–857.

8. Broder S, Mitsuya H, Yarchoan R, et al. Antiretroviral therapy in AIDS. *Ann Intern Med*. 1990; 113:604–618.

9. Altmeyer R. Virus attachment and entry offer numerous targets for antiviral therapy. *Curr Pharm Des*. 2004; 10(30):3701–3712.

10. Schols D. HIV co-receptors as targets of antiviral therapy. *Curr Top Med Chem*. 2004; 4(9):883–893.

11. Yarchoan R, Mitsuya H, Myers C, et al. Clinical pharmacology of 3'-azido-2',3'-dideoxythymidine (zidovudine) and related dideoxynucleosides. *N Engl J Med*. 1989; 321:726–738.

12. Mitsuya H, Yarchoan R. Development of antiretroviral therapy for AIDS and related disorders. In: Broder S, Merigan TC, Bolognesi D, eds. *Textbook of AIDS Medicine*. Baltimore, MD: Williams and Wilkins; 1994:721–742.

13. Fischl MA. Treatment of HIV infection. In: Sande MA, Volberding PA, eds. *The Medical Management of AIDS*. Philadelphia, PA: WB Saunders; 1995:141–160.

14. McNicholl IR, McNicholl JJ. On the horizon: promising investigational antiretroviral agents. *Curr Pharm Des*. 2006; 12:1091–1103.

15. Lichtenstein KA. Redefining lipodystrophy syndrome. Risks and impact on clinical decision making. *J Acquir Immun Defic*. 2005; 39:395–400.

16. Carr A. An objective case definition of lipodystrophy in HIV-infected adults: a case-control study. *Lancet*. 2003; 361:726–775.

17. NCEP. Executive Summary of the Third Report of the National Cholesterol Education Program (NCEP) Expert Panel on Detection, Evaluation, and Treatment of High Blood Cholesterol in Adults (Adult Treatment Panel III). *JAMA*. 2001; 285:2486–2497.

18. Dube MP, Stein JH, Aberg JA, et al for the Adult AIDS Clinical Trial Group Cardiovascular Subcommittee. Guidelines for the evaluation and management of dyslipidemia in human immunodeficiency virus (HIV)-infected adults receiving antiretroviral therapy: recommendations of the HIV Medicine Association of the Infectious Diseases Society of America and the Adult AIDS Clinical Trials Group. *Clin Infect Dis*. 2003; 37(4):613–627.

19. Gupta SK, Eustace JA, Winston JA, et al. Guidelines for the management of chronic kidney disease in HIV-infected patients: recommendations of the HIV medicine association for the Infectious Disease Society of America. *Clin Infect Dis*. 2005; 40:1559–1585.

20. Connor EM, Sperling RS, Gelber R, et al. Reduction of maternal-infant transmission of human immunodeficiency virus type 1 with zidovudine treatment. Pediatric AIDS Clinical Trials Group Protocol 076 Study Group. *N Engl J Med*. 1994; 331:1173–1180.

21. U.S. Department of Health and Human Services. Public Health Service Task Force recommendations for use of antiretroviral drugs in pregnant women for maternal health and interventions to reduce perinatal HIV-1 transmission in the United States. Rockville, MD: HIV/AIDS Treatment Information Service. Available at http://www.aidsinfo.nih.gov. Accessed July 3, 2005.

22. Redfield RR, Birx DL, Kettler N, et al. A phase I evaluation of the safety and immunogenicity of vaccination with recombinant gp160 in patients with early human immunodeficiency virus infection. *N Engl J Med*. 1991; 324:1677–1684.

23. Trauger RJ, Ferre F, Daigle AE, et al. Effect of immunization with inactivated gp120-depleted human immunodeficiency virus type 1 (HIV-1) immunogen on HIV-1 immunity, viral DNA, and percentage of CD4 cells. *J Infect Dis*. 1994; 169:1256–1264.

24. Krown SE, Gold JWM, Niedzwiecki D, et al. Interferon-alfa with zidovudine: safety, tolerance and clinical and virologic effects in patients with Kaposi sarcoma associated with the acquired immunodeficiency syndrome. *Ann Intern Med*. 1990; 112:812–821.

25. Krown SE. Approaches to interferon combination therapy in the treatment of AIDS. *Semin Oncol*. 1990; 17(suppl 1):11–15.

26. Kunzi MS, Farzadegan H, Margolick JB, et al. Identification of human immunodeficiency virus primary isolates resistant to interferon-alpha and correlation of prevalence to disease progression. *J Infect Dis*. 1995; 171:822–828.

27. Lane HC, Davey V, Kovacs JA, et al. Interferon-alfa in patients with asymptomatic human immunodeficiency virus infection. *Ann Intern Med*. 1990; 112:805–811.

28. Lotze MT, Franan LW, Sharrow DO, et al. In vivo administration of purified human interleukin 2. I. Half-life and immunologic effects of the Jurkat cell line-derived interleukin-2. *J Immunol*. 1985; 134:157–166.

29. Kovacs JA, Vogel S, Albert JM, et al. Controlled trial of interleukin-2 infusions in patients with the human immunodeficiency virus. *N Engl J Med*. 1996; 335:1350–1356.

30. Carr A, Emery S, Lloyd A, et al. Outpatient continuous intravenous interleukin-2 or subcutaneous, polyethylene glycol-modified interleukin-2 in human immunodeficiency virus-infected patients: a randomized, controlled, multicenter study. *J Infect Dis*. 1998; 178:992–999.

31. Kovacs JA, Baseler M, Dewar RJ, et al. Increases in CD4 T lymphocytes with intermittent courses of interleukin-2 in patients with human immunodeficiency virus infection: a preliminary study. *N Engl J Med*. 1995; 332:567–575.

32. Arno A, Ruiz L, Juan M, et al. Efficacy of low-dose subcutaneous interleukin-2 to treat advanced human immunodeficiency virus type 1 in persons with ≤250/μL CD4 T cells and undetectable plasma virus load. *J Infect Dis.* 1999; 180:56–60.

33. David D, Nait-Ighil L, Dupont B, et al. Rapid effect of interleukin-2 in human immunodeficiency virus infected patients whose CD4 cell counts increase only slightly in response to combined antiretroviral treatment. *J Infect Dis.* 2001; 183:730–735.

34. Emery S, Capra WB, Cooper DA, et al. Pooled analysis of 3 randomized, controlled trials of interleukin-2 therapy in adult human immunodeficiency virus type 1 disease. *J Infect Dis.* 2000; 182:428–434.

35. Clerici M, Lucey DR, Berzofsky JA, et al. Restoration of HIV-specific cell-mediated immune responses by interleukin-12 in vitro. *Science.* 1993; 262:1721–1724.

36. Fischl M, Galpin JE, Levine JD, et al. Recombinant erythropoietin for patients with AIDS treated with zidovudine. *N Engl J Med.* 1990; 322:1488–1493.

37. Henry DH, Beall GN, Benson CA, et al. Recombinant human erythropoietin in the treatment of anemia associated with human immunodeficiency virus infection and zidovudine therapy: overview of four clinical trials. *Ann Intern Med.* 1992; 117:739–748.

38. Groopman JE, Mitsuyasu RT, DeLeo MJ, et al. Effect of recombinant human granulocyte-macrophage colony-stimulating factor in the acquired immunodeficiency syndrome. *N Engl J Med.* 1987; 317:593–598.

39. Pluda JM, Yarchoan R, Smith PD, et al. Subcutaneous recombinant granulocyte-macrophage colony-stimulating factor used as a single agent and in an alternating regimen with azidothymidine in leukopenic patients with severe human immunodeficiency virus infection. *Blood.* 1990; 76:463–472.

40. Fliri H, Baumann G, Enz A, et al. Cyclosporins: structure-activity relationships. *Ann NY Acad Sci.* 1993; 696:47–53.

41. Luban J, Bossolt KL, Franke EK, et al. Human immunodeficiency virus type 1 gag protein binds to cyclophilins A and B. *Cell.* 1993; 73:1067–1078.

42. Fauci AS. Multifactorial nature of human immunodeficiency virus disease: implications for therapy. *Science.* 1993; 262:1011–1018.

43. Schwarz A, Offermann G, Keller F, et al. The effect of cyclosporine on the progression of human immunodeficiency virus type 1 infection transmitted by transplantation—data on four cases and review of the literature. *Transplantation.* 1993; 55:95–103.

44. Lederman MM. Host-directed and immune-based therapies for human immunodeficiency virus infection. *Ann Intern Med.* 1995; 122:218–222.

45. Bolognesi DP. AIDS vaccines: progress and unmet challenges. *Ann Intern Med.* 1991; 114:161–162.

46. Spearman P. Current progress in the development of HIV vaccines. *Curr Pharm Des.* 2006; 12:1147–1167.

47. Goudsmit J, Smit L, Krone WJA, et al. IgG response to human immunodeficiency virus in experimentally infected chimpanzees mimics the IgG response in humans. *J Infect Dis.* 1987; 155:327–331.

48. Fauci AS, Gallo RC, Koenig S, et al. Development and evaluation of a vaccine for human immunodeficiency virus (HIV) infection. *Ann Intern Med.* 1989; 110:373–385.

49. Koff WC, Hoth DF. Development and testing of AIDS vaccines. *Science.* 1988; 241:426–432.

50. Centers for Disease Control and Prevention (CDC). HIV vaccine unit. Available at http://www.cdc.gov/hiv/vaccine/hivvu.htm. Accessed July 9, 2005.

SELF-ASSESSMENT QUESTIONS

1. Which of the following is *not* a goal of current HIV therapy?

   A. Achieve maximal and durable viral load suppression
   B. Restore and maintain immunologic function
   C. Eradicate HIV infection
   D. Improve quality of life

2. HIV therapy should be modified for the following reasons:

   A. Treatment failure
   B. Treatment toxicity
   C. Nonadherence to treatment regimen
   D. All of the above

3. Nevirapine poses a particular risk for hepatotoxicity and should only be initiated in the following patients with caution:

   A. Women with CD4$^+$ T cell count >250 cells/mm^3
   B. Men with CD4$^+$ T cell count >400 cells/mm^3
   C. Both A and B
   D. None of the above

4. A leading cause for nonadherence to antiretroviral therapy is:

   A. African-American race
   B. Past history of illicit drug use
   C. HIV treatment toxicity
   D. Age >50 years

5. The treatment of choice for HIV-infected pregnant women is a single dose of zidovudine at the time of delivery.

   A. True
   B. False

6. Currently FDA-approved antiretroviral drugs work by which of the following mechanism(s)?

   A. Inhibition of viral fusion with the host cell
   B. Inhibition of maturation
   C. Inhibition of integrase
   D. Inhibition of the chemokines CCR5 and CXCR4

7. Lipodystrophy syndrome associated with HIV infection and HAART describes which of the following?

   A. Renal failure (increases in serum creatinine and BUN)
   B. Morphologic changes (fat atrophy and hypertrophy)
   C. Development of muscular dystrophy
   D. The individual is not infectious to others

8. Which of the following agents inhibits reverse transcriptase?

   A. Stavudine
   B. Enfuvirtide
   C. Saquinavir
   D. Tipranavir

9. The "prime-boost strategy" of preventive HIV vaccines uses the following approach(es):

   A. Two different vaccines, given one after another, to build a better immune response
   B. Repeated doses of the same vaccine over long periods of time
   C. Both A and B
   D. Neither A nor B

10. Recently published guidelines for the management of chronic kidney disease in HIV-infected patients recommend that all newly diagnosed patients have what?

    A. Monthly urinalyses for patients on tenofovir
    B. Urinalysis and estimation of glomerular filtration rate (GFR) performed at baseline
    C. Referral to nephrologist for kidney biopsy
    D. Use of an ACE inhibitor

11. About 8% of patients who start abacavir will develop a hypersensitivity reaction that *does not* involve the following:

    A. Renal failure
    B. Myalgias
    C. Rash
    D. Fever

12. Potential immune-based therapies for HIV include all of the following *except*:

    A. Therapeutic vaccination
    B. Corticosteroids
    C. TIBO compounds
    D. IFN-α

13. Strategies that either suppress or enhance the immune response to HIV infection are under evaluation.

    A. True
    B. False

14. The rationale for using therapeutic drug monitoring (TDM) is that subtherapeutic serum levels of protease inhibitors can lead to the development of drug toxicity.

    A. True
    B. False

15. Immunologic adjuvants are used for which of the following reasons?

    A. Decrease response to live, attenuated virus
    B. Inhibit the genetic mutation and recombination of the HIV strain
    C. Increase the type, strength, and durability of the vaccine response
    D. Decrease bias introduced by society

CHAPTER 9

Solid Organ Transplantation

Nicole Sifontis, Debra Tucker Sierka

CHAPTER OUTLINE

INTRODUCTION

For many years, scientists were unsuccessful in their attempts to replace diseased and injured organs with donated healthy organs. Historically, only an organ donated from an identical twin was acceptable to the host's immune system. Organs donated from family members, unrelated donors, or deceased donors were insufficiently compatible to avoid rejection. With the introduction of newer immunosuppressive agents, advancements in surgical procedures, improved management in intensive care units, better op-

tions for treating posttransplant complications, and an increased understanding of the immune system, organ transplantation has been elevated from an experimental procedure to an accepted treatment for end-stage organ failure. Despite excellent 1-year graft survival rates, problems still remain in preventing chronic rejection and ultimately extending long-term graft survival. Furthermore, toxicities of immunosuppressive agents add their own array of complications to a patient's therapy. Suppressing the immune system reduces the incidence of graft rejection but leaves the patient vulnerable to opportunistic infections and malignant disorders. And immunosuppressive agents have detrimental side effects that increase the patient's risk for other complications. The long-term survival of solid organ allografts is usually complicated by development of chronic rejection processes that in most cases can be treated only by retransplantation.

The pharmacist's role in providing pharmaceutical care for the transplant patient is very important. There are many opportunities for involvement: optimizing immunosuppressive and other concomitant drug therapy, developing protocols for preventive and palliative therapy for adverse reactions, monitoring and adjusting drug concentrations, managing drug interactions, providing advice about appropriate investigational agents, and counseling patients to ensure compliance and adherence. In addition to understanding potential pharmacokinetic changes that may occur in transplant recipients, the pharmacist must have a thorough understanding of the physiologic consequences of organ transplantation.

This chapter begins with a brief overview of the development and current state of solid organ transplantation and the basic immunology of allograft rejection. Immunosuppressive agents are categorized according to their primary mechanism of action. A discussion of the clinical use, dosing, monitoring, and adverse effects of these agents is included.

In Part II, specific complications encountered after solid organ transplantation are discussed, along with management strategies for preventing or treating these common problems.

LEARNING OBJECTIVES

After completing this chapter, the reader should be able to:

1. Describe the basic immune response involved in an acute rejection episode and identify the sites of action of the various immunosuppressive agents.
2. Discuss the immunosuppressive therapies for solid organ transplantation procedures and explain how to monitor for efficacy and toxicity.
3. Compare rescue therapies available for the treatment of acute organ rejection.
4. Describe management strategies for dealing with immunosuppressant drug interactions.
5. Recognize postoperative transplant complications and describe treatment plans for immunotherapy-related adverse effects.

PART I—TRANSPLANT IMMUNOLOGY AND IMMUNOTHERAPY

Although the idea of solid organ transplantation dates back to ancient times, the first attempt at kidney transplantation occurred in 1933. But it was not until 1954, in Boston, that the first long-term surviving kidney transplant was performed between identical twins without immunosuppression. The first successful attempts at intentionally suppressing the immune system in humans occurred between 1958 and 1962, when Murray in Boston[1] and Hamburger in Paris used varying dosages of total body irradiation to circumvent rejection of transplanted kidneys in nonidentical twins.[2] This was the beginning of immunosuppression, and the advances in transplantation have paralleled those in immunosuppressive therapy.

Subsequent major milestones in organ transplantation occurred in the 1960s with the development of tissue-typing techniques and new immunosuppressive agents. Early work with the antimetabolite 6-mercaptopurine (6-MP) by Schwartz and Dameshek[3] led to the development of an imidazole derivative of this drug, azathioprine (AZA), by Hitchings and Elion.[4] The combination of this agent with corticosteroids demonstrated increased efficacy in preventing rejection.[5] During the next decade, a variety of techniques and agents were used in attempts to suppress the immune response: thoracic duct drainage, splenectomy, thymectomy, lymphoid or graft irradiation, cyclophosphamide (CTX), and the polyclonal antilymphocyte and antithymocyte globulins.[2] The next major milestone occurred in the mid-1970s with the discovery of cyclosporine (CsA). By the mid-1980s, combinations of two, three, and four drugs in combination with CsA were being used to augment immunosuppression while minimizing the toxicity of the individual agents. The success of heart, liver, pancreas, pancreas–kidney, heart–lung, and lung transplantation during the 1990s has been credited to the introduction of CsA.

The immunosuppressive armamentarium has doubled in the past 10 years, and clinicians now have several options available in combination immunosuppressive protocols. Many of these agents complement each other because of their degree of specificity to different targets in the immune response, as well as their varied side effect profiles. Improvements in immunosuppressive therapy have resulted in impressive increases in allograft and patient survival in the past; these statistics have been stable for several years (**Tables 9.1 and 9.2**).[6] Moreover, more

Table 9.1. One-Year Adjusted Graft Survival by Organ and Year of Transplant

Graft Survival, %	Year of Transplant		
	1995	2000	2004
Kidney: deceased donor	85	88	90
Kidney: living donor	92	94	95
Pancreas transplant alone	65	75	78
Pancreas after kidney	72	74	79
Kidney–pancreas	89	93	92
Liver: deceased donor	78	81	83
Liver: living donor	71	77	84
Intestine	59	69	77
Heart	84	85	88
Lung	75	76	84
Heart–lung	79	64	75

(Source: Organ Procurement and Transplant Network (OPTN)/Scientific Registry of Transplant Recipients (SRTR) data as of May 1, 2006.)

Table 9.2. One-Year Adjusted Patient Survival by Organ and Year of Transplant

Patient Survival, %	Year of Transplant		
	1995	2000	2004
Kidney: deceased donor	94	94	96
Kidney: living donor	97	98	98
Pancreas transplant alone	92	Unknown	96
Pancreas after kidney	96	96	96
Kidney–pancreas	94	95	95
Liver: deceased donor	84	86	87
Liver: living donor	88	87	92
Intestine	68	75	80
Heart	85	86	88
Lung	76	77	86
Heart–lung	80	64	76

(Source: Organ Procurement and Transplant Network (OPTN)/Scientific Registry of Transplant Recipients (SRTR) data as of May 1, 2006.)

transplants are being performed each year due in large part to improved patient outcomes with newer immunosuppressive therapies and advancements in transplant techniques (**Table 9.3**).[6] In 2005, more than 25,000 organs were transplanted in the United States, an increase of 3.7% over 2004.[6] The number of patients on the organ transplant waiting list has more than doubled from 35,751 at the end of 1994 to more than 94,000 at the end of 2005. **Table 9.4** demonstrates the increased number of candidates by organ, comparing 2004 and 2005. Notably, there was a significant decrease in the number of lung and heart–lung transplants on the waiting list because of the improvements and increased use of mechanical devices to prolong survival in these patients. Long wait times for transplant recipients and continued growth of the waiting list exacerbate the shortage of organs.

The number of people awaiting a kidney transplant in the United States based on the United Network for Organ Sharing (UNOS) data exceeded

Table 9.3. Growth in Number of Transplanted Organs, 2002–2003

	Year of Transplant		Percent Change
	2004	2005	
Total	26,541	27,527	3.7
Deceased donor	19,551	20,635	5.5
Living donor	6,990	6,892	−1.4
Kidney	15,674	16,072	2.5
Deceased donor	9,027	9,509	5.3
Living donor	6,647	6,563	−1.2
Pancreas transplant alone	130	129	No change
Pancreas after kidney	419	343	−18.0
Kidney–pancreas	880	896	1.8
Liver	5,779	6,000	3.8
Deceased donor	5,457	5,679	4.0
Living donor	322	321	−11.4
Intestine	52	68	30.0
Heart	1,961	2,063	5.2
Lung	1,168	1,405	20.0
Heart–lung	37	32	−13.5

(Source: Organ Procurement and Transplant Network (OPTN)/Scientific Registry of Transplant Recipients (SRTR) data as of May 1, 2006.)

Table 9.4. Growth in Number of Patients on the Waiting List, 2004–2005

	End of Year		Percent Change
	2004	2005	
Total	90,090	94,086	4.4
Kidney	61,283	65,859	7.4
Pancreas transplant alone	507	529	4.3
Pancreas after kidney	983	987	No change
Kidney–pancreas	2,446	2,544	4.0
Liver	17,411	17,673	1.5
Intestine	196	203	3.6
Heart	3,223	2,980	−7.5
Lung	3,870	3,170	−18.0
Heart–lung	171	141	−17.5

(Source: Organ Procurement and Transplant Network (OPTN)/SRTR data as of May 1, 2006.)

60,000 for the first time in 2004, making it by far the most common transplant and most commonly needed organ. As the kidney waiting list continues to grow, input on expanded criteria donors (ECD) and ways to facilitate living unrelated donation continue to be explored. According to data from the Organ Procurement and Transplant Network (OPTN), transplant operations using an organ donated by a living person hit a new high (27%) in 2004, a 2.3% increase over 2003. Because of the huge disparity between the supply and demand for organ transplants, several strategies have been considered. One approach is to use ECD organs for kidney transplants. OPTN defines ECD as a kidney donor older than 60 or between 50 and 59 with one or more of the following medical criteria: died from a stroke, had a history of hypertension, or had a serum creatinine >1.5 mg/dL at the time of death. ECD kidneys have increased from about 11% of transplants in 1994 to 16% in 2003. Another approach to meeting the organ shortage crisis includes transplanting across ABO barriers. Historically, incompatible ABO transplants had a low graft survival rate because of a high incidence of hyperacute rejection so specific protocols were developed. These protocols use preemptive steps such as plasmapheresis, intravenous immune globulin therapy (with or without monoclonal antibodies like rituximab), and splenectomy in the recipient. A third approach includes using two sets of donors and recipients who are incompatible, in

a paired donor exchange program (kidney transplant only). A fourth approach involves expanding the use of altruistic donors, or living donation to an unknown recipient (nondirected kidney donation); some have even suggested direct payment for suitable kidney donors.[7] Today in the United States it is illegal to pay for organs for transplantation.

Although acute rejection and early graft loss have become relatively uncommon, late graft loss and premature death (primarily resulting from cardiovascular diseases), as well as the organ shortage crisis, remain major challenges.

TRANSPLANT IMMUNOLOGY

Allograft rejection is the major barrier to long-term patient and graft survival after solid organ transplantation. The process of rejection is a normal immune response in which the allograft is recognized as foreign, resulting in the activation of cytotoxic responses. Significant advances have been made in understanding the immunologic mechanisms of rejection and how to interrupt these processes with various pharmacologic and immunologic interventions. Experience gained using these agents for the prevention and reversal of rejection has helped to expand our understanding of the specific molecular processes involved in this complex immune response. Yet the development of graft acceptance without immunosuppressive therapy (i.e., tolerance) remains an elusive goal in clinical transplantation.

Basic Components of the Immune System

Acute rejection episodes are primarily regulated by cell-mediated immunity. To develop appropriate antirejection or tolerance-inducing strategies, an understanding of the specific roles and complex relationships among these components during an acute rejection episode is required.

Major Histocompatibility Complex

The major histocompatibility complex (MHC), or human leukocyte antigen (HLA) complex, is a specific cluster of genes that controls the expression of class I and II HLA proteins, the primary antigens of the immune response pathways.[8] T-cell recognition of foreign antigens is determined by class I and class II HLA molecules. Class I HLAs are cell-surface proteins—HLA-A, -B, and -C—that serve as primary targets for cytotoxic lymphocytes, as well as direct activators of cytotoxic cell responses.

These proteins are expressed in varying degrees on the surface of most somatic cells. Conversely, expression of class II HLA proteins, known as HLA-DP, -DQ, and -DR, is more restricted, and these antigens are found primarily on macrophages (antigen-presenting cells [APC]), monocytes, B lymphocytes, and dendritic cells. Class I and II HLAs serve as primary activators of the helper T-cell response in initiating the immune response to foreign tissue. Both classes of HLA molecules are responsible for the binding, processing, and presentation of key antigens associated with acute rejection response. Other clusters of genes have been associated with the pathogenesis of rejection, but they encode for only minor antigens.[8,9]

T-Cell, CD4, and CD8 receptors. The specific immune response to allograft tissue depends on donor antigens (alloantigens) presented by class I and II HLA molecules to the T-cell receptor (TCR). The TCR is directly associated with the CD3 complex and is clonally restricted in its expression and antigen recognition properties. The TCR is responsible for direct (class I) and indirect (class II) alloantigen recognition.[9] The CD4 marker is expressed exclusively on helper T cells and preferentially interacts with class II HLA molecules. Conversely, the CD8 marker is expressed on the surface of cytotoxic T cells, which react with class I HLA molecules.[9]

Cytokine mediators. Cytokines, including interleukins (IL), interferons (IFN), colony-stimulating factors, and growth hormones, are the chemical mediators of most immune responses.[10] These cytokines mediate their activity through both self-regulating and direct stimulatory or inhibitory pathways. Increased concentrations of IL-1, IL-2, IL-6, tumor necrosis factor alpha (TNF-α), and IFN-γ are observed within the allografts of patients having a rejection episode. The activating properties of cytokines are exemplified by the up-regulation of class I and class II HLA expression on endothelial cells exposed to TNF-α and IFN-γ. Other examples include the roles of IL-1, IL-2, and IL-6 in T-cell postantigenic differentiation, activation, and proliferation. In contrast, other cytokines (IL-4, IL-5, IL-10) suppress T-cell activation and may be clinically relevant in the induction of tolerance.

Mechanisms Involved in Graft Rejection

Rejection of a transplanted organ occurs when the recipient's immune system recognizes the allograft as foreign. The MHC molecules described above are proteins that allow the immune system to differentiate self from nonself, and are important in HLA antigen matching of the donor and recipient in transplantation. The ideal donor–recipient match in genetically nonidentical people would be a zero-antigen mismatch (0-antigen mismatch). The HLA antigens considered most important for the likelihood of a successful outcome are the HLA-A, -B, and -DR antigens.[11] The phenomenon of graft rejection is complex, but it offers a multitude of potential targets for pharmacological interference. The mechanisms involved in allograft rejection include alloantigen recognition, T-cell activation with costimulatory pathway involvement, clonal expansion, and graft inflammation.

Alloantigen recognition. It is thought that alloantigen recognition may be achieved by direct and indirect processes. Recipient CD4$^+$ T cells and CD8$^+$ T cells have TCRs consisting of variable antigen binding sites for a particular antigen, in this case the transplanted organ. Foreign antigen recognition is only achieved in the presence of MHC. Molecules of MHC I and II have an antigen binding cleft. After processing of foreign protein by APCs, pieces of that protein are mobilized to the MHC cleft for presentation. Helper T cells specialized to direct the immune system can only recognize foreign antigen in the presence of MHC II, while cytotoxic T cells specialized to destroy infected or cancerous cells can only recognize antigen in the presence of MHC I. Direct recognition of donor MHC may be responsible for acute rejection episodes. Indirect activation may be responsible for acute and chronic episodes.[11]

T-cell activation. T-cell activation requires at least two signals: an antigen-dependent T-cell receptor–mediated signal 1, and an antigen-independent costimulatory signal 2. T-cell activation occurs due to interactions among TCRs and the MHC, cellular adhesion molecules, and costimulatory molecules. After TCR and MHC recognition and binding, conformational changes and coupling of the TCR CD3 complex and CD4 or CD8 molecules occur. This change allows for phosphorylation of tyrosine residues attached to the intracellular domains of several cell surface receptors. Calcineurin is activated after interaction with calcium and calmodulin. Activated calcineurin is a phosphatase that serves to dephosphorylate nuclear factor of activated T cells (NFAT), allowing NFAT to transverse the nuclear membrane and bind to promoter regions specific for regulatory proteins such as IL-2. Calcineurin is implicated in the pharmacologic mechanism of CsA and tacrolimus.[11]

Costimulatory pathways. In the absence of a second signal induced by co-stimulatory molecules, activation of T cells does not occur. The B7/CD28:CTLA4 interaction has been explored. The B7 receptor is located on APCs, whereas the CD28 and CTLA4 receptors are located on T cells. Binding of the B7 receptor to CD28 induces T-cell activation in the presence of TCR and MHC interaction, allowing for synthesis of cell-regulating proteins. If the B7 receptor binds to CTLA4, the opposite occurs and T-lymphocyte activation is antagonized.[11]

Adhesion molecules are also important for APC and T-cell interactions because they promote cell-to-cell recognition and stabilization. Adhesion molecules are expressed on vascular endothelial cells during inflammation, allowing effector cells to migrate to the proper anatomic location. After initial T-cell activation, the process of clonal expansion and immunologic progression is mediated by cytokines. The ultimate result is the infiltration of T cells into the allograft, which can result in an acute rejection episode.

Clinical Manifestation of Graft Rejection

Inflammation of the allograft results from the processes described above through specific and nonspecific mechanisms. These immunologic and inflammatory events may lead to acute rejection. Despite the use of multidrug immunosuppressive regimens, the incidence of acute rejection in the United States is about 5% to 20%. There are four major types of rejection episodes based on time of onset, clinical criteria, histologic findings, and response to antirejection.

Hyperacute rejection occurs within minutes to a few hours of transplantation, before the patient has left the operating room, and is related to previous antigen exposure or ABO incompatibility.

This phenomenon rarely occurs today because of extensive pretransplantation screening. When it does occur, rapid necrosis and failure of the transplanted organ follow. To alleviate the organ shortage, ABO-incompatible transplants are being performed with the assistance of preemptive protocols incorporating plasmapheresis and intravenous immune globulin. Advances in tissue typing and immunosuppression have made hyperacute rejection an uncommon phenomenon (**Table 9.5**).

Accelerated acute rejection usually occurs within 6 days of transplantation.[12] Initial function can progress to acute allograft dysfunction because of previous sensitization to minor donor antigens through blood transfusions, multiple pregnancies, or a previous transplant. Most patients who experience accelerated acute rejection do not respond to antirejection therapy, but antilymphocyte antibody preparations like OKT3 or thymoglobulin therapy are occasionally effective.

Acute cellular rejection is the most common manifestation of immunologic incompatibility in transplant recipients and usually presents within 1 week to 6 months after the transplant, although it can occur at anytime during the life of the allograft.[12] Clinical manifestations may vary from an asymptomatic, mild reduction in allograft function to frank allograft failure. Other clinical events associated with acute cellular rejection include fever, malaise, anorexia, and myalgia. Acute rejection episodes are ultimately confirmed by biopsy, which shows lymphocyte infiltrates. This type of rejection episode typically responds to antirejection therapy.

Chronic rejection implies gradual, yet irreversible, functional and structural deterioration of an organ allograft occurring over months or years after transplantation. This complex process affects all organ types; both immunologically directed antigen-dependent risk factors and non-

Table 9.5. Types of Rejection Episodes

Type	Time of Onset	Cause	Response to Anti-rejection Therapy
Hyperacute	Minutes to hours	Preformed cytotoxic antibodies directed against donor antigens	No
Accelerated	2–5 days	Previous sensitization to donor antigens	Occasionally
Acute	7–180 days, but may occur at anytime	Development of allogenic reaction to donor antigens	Yes
Chronic	Months–years	Allogen dependent and independent factors	No

Table 9.6. Factors Implicated in Chronic Rejection

Allogen-Dependent Risk Factors	Allogen-Independent Risk Factors
Acute rejection	Ischemic injury and delayed graft function
HLA mismatch	Older donor age
Prior sensitization	Donor and recipient size mismatching
Suboptimal immunosup-pression	Hyperlipidemia
Medication noncompliance	Hypertension
	Cigarette smoking
	Hyperhomosysteinemia
	Infection (particularly CMV/BK virus)

immunologically dependent antigen-independent risk factors have been implicated (**Table 9.6**).[13,14] Because there is no effective treatment for chronic rejection other than retransplantation, therapy attempts to delay the progression. Histologically, biopsy specimens reveal intimal thickening and fibrosis of the vasculature. In the kidney, these effects can be seen as glomerulosclerosis, tubular atropy, and fibrosis. In the heart, changes are noted as arteriosclerosis of the coronary vessels. In the lung, chronic rejection can be noted as bronchiolitis obliterans, and in the liver as vanishing bile duct syndrome (**Table 9.7**).[14] Because of chronic rejection, long-term allograft survival has not changed substantially over the years.[13]

Tolerance

Although improvements in immunosuppressive therapy have drastically increased the success of solid organ transplantation, chronic rejection is still a major problem leading to constant attrition of all organ types.[15] Induction of donor-specific tolerance with preservation of otherwise normal immune responses is therefore a major goal of transplantation research. Tolerance broadly refers to the absence of immune responses to specific antigens. In transplantation, tolerance can be defined as the absence of a destructive immune response to a graft in a host with otherwise intact immunity. The imbalance between solid organ transplant supply and demand also drives the interest in tolerance strategies. The holy grail of transplantation, as predicted by Peter Medawar in the 1950s, remains the development of donor-specific tolerance.[7]

TRANSPLANT IMMUNOTHERAPY

Before the 1980s, immunosuppression for solid organ transplantation was accomplished with only four drugs: cyclosporine, azathioprine, corticosteroids, and polyclonal antilymphocyte antibodies. Since then, the number of agents available for use has more than tripled, allowing for varied

Table 9.7. Characteristics of Chronic Rejection

Organ	Clinical Characteristics	Histological Characteristics	Incidence at 5 Years
Kidney	Decline in renal function Protenuria Hypertension	Interstitial fibrosis Tubular atrophy Occlusive vasculopathy Glomerulosclerosis	40% to 50%
Liver	Cholestasis	Absence of interlobular septal bile ducts in 50% or more portal tracts Obliterative arteritis	<5% to 10%
Heart	Left ventricular arterio-sclerosis	Endarteritis obliterans in epicardial and smaller branch vessels Endothelialitis	50%
Lungs	Cough Dyspnea on exertion Decreased FEV1	Submucosal fibrosis Partial or total obliteration of the bronchiolar lumen	75% to 85%

(Source: Adapted from Goodman J, Mohanakumar T. Chronic rejection: failure of immune regulation. *Front Biosci*. 2003; 8:s838–844.)

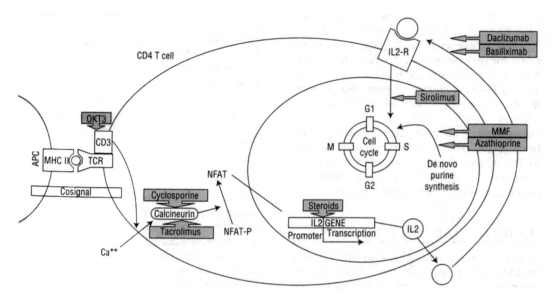

Figure 9.1. Mechanism of action. Stages of CD4 T-cell activation and cytokine production with identification of the sites of action from different immunosuppressive agents. Antigen-major histocompatibility complex (MHC) II molecule complexes are responsible for initiating the activation of CD4 T cells. These MHC-peptide complexes are recognized by the T-cell recognition complex (TCR); a costimulatory signal initiates signal transduction with activation of second messengers, one of which is calcineurin. Calcineruin removes phosphates from the nuclear factors (NFAT-P) allowing them to enter the nucleus. These nuclear factors specifically bind to an interleukin-2 (IL-2) promoter gene facilitating IL-2 gene transcription. Interaction of IL-2 with IL-2 receptor (IL-2R) on the cell membrane surface induces cell proliferation and production or cytokines specific to the T cell. APC = antigen-producing cells; MMF = mycophenolate mofetil. (Reprinted, with permission, from Mueller XM. Drug immunosuppression therapy for adult heart transplantation. Part 1: immune response to allograft and mechanism of action of immunosuppressants. *Ann Thorac Surg.* 2004; 77:354–362.)

combinations to optimize drug efficacy while minimizing potential toxicities. Many of these new immunosuppressants target novel mechanisms of action with greater specificity, while others offer moderate advantages to previously existing agents (**Figure 9.1**).[16] Use of these agents remains an exciting and evolving science.

The pharmacology, pharmacokinetics, and toxicology of immunosuppressant drugs used in solid organ transplant as well as practical guidelines for their therapeutic use are addressed below; specific organ transplant complications and their management strategies are discussed later in this chapter.

Corticosteroids

Pharmacology and clinical uses. The utility of corticosteroids in solid organ transplantation results from three of their pharmacologic effects: (1) a direct effect on circulating lymphocytes, (2) modulation of specific cellular immune functions, and (3) a nonspecific anti-inflammatory effect.

Corticosteroids cause a rapid and profound drop in circulating T lymphocytes by sequestering lymphocytes in the bone marrow; direct destruc-

tion of the lymphocytes does not occur. Besides decreasing the number of circulating monocytes and lymphocytes (particularly CD4+ T lymphocytes) and increasing the number of circulating neutrophils, corticosteroids have major effects on the function of these cells. Corticosteroids bind to an intracytosolic steroid receptor and are transported to the nucleus, where they alter DNA and RNA synthesis. They also potently inhibit phosphodiesterase, leading to accumulation of intracellular cyclic adenosine monophosphate and inhibition of lymphocyte activation. Inhibition of IL-1 secretion from macrophages and IL-2 secretion from T lymphocytes inhibits the generation of cytotoxic T lymphocytes. The nonspecific, potent anti-inflammatory effect is a result of the inhibition of arachidonic acid release and suppression of macrophage phagocytosis.

Dosing and monitoring. Corticosteroids are used to prevent and treat graft rejection. Dosing protocols for corticosteroids in combination with other immunosuppressants have changed dramatically as many transplant centers are attempting to minimize, circumvent, or eliminate steroid use to avoid long-term side effects. In 2003, 15% of kidney transplant recipients were discharged on steroid-free regimens compared to 3% in 1999. Similar trends have also been noted in pancreas, intestinal, and liver transplantation, but corticosteroids remain an integral part of immunosuppression for lung and heart transplantation.[17] High-dose methylprednisolone induction (250–1000 mg) is still used in most organ transplants preoperatively or intraoperatively immediately before revascularization of the newly placed allograft. Dosing thereafter varies widely; steroids may be rapidly tapered to 5 mg of oral prednisone per day by 1 week, discontinued after postoperative day 1 or 2, or continued as a component of long-term maintenance immunosuppression at a dose of 0.1–0.3 mg/kg/day of oral prednisone. Dosing requirements are consistently higher in pediatric recipients and may vary by race.[18] High-dose corticosteroids remain the first-line treatment of choice for acute rejection episode for all types of solid organ transplantation.[17] Pulse doses of 250–1000 mg of methylprednisolone once daily for 2–4 days successfully aborts 60% to 80% of acute rejection episodes. Large doses of oral prednisone (100–200 mg) have also been used for "pulse" treatment of rejection.[18,19]

Adverse effects and toxicities. The wide array of acute and chronic side effects of corticosteroids stems from the presence of steroid receptors on nearly every cell in the body. Because of the significant toxicities with long-term corticosteroid use, other immunosuppressive agents are being used so that lower doses of steroids can be given.[17,20–22] **Table 9.8** lists some of the most common side effects of corticosteroid use.

Inhibitors of Early T-Cell Activation

Cyclosporine. CsA is an 11–amino acid cyclic peptide with reversible immunosuppressive activity. This agent is a naturally occurring metabolic product of the soil fungus *Tolypocladium inflatum gams*, first isolated in the early 1970s and introduced into human use in transplantation in 1978. Since 1982, it has formed the basis for a new era in organ transplantation, resulting in a dramatic improvement in renal allograft survival and allowing the widespread growth of extrarenal transplantation. The discovery and development of CsA as an immunosuppressive agent brought with it new insights into the mechanisms of alloimmunity and opened a floodgate of investigation into further drug innovations.

Pharmacology and clinical uses. The mechanism of action of CsA is unique; CsA binds to cyclophilin, a cytosolic binding protein that is key to signal transmission for de novo IL-2 production. The CsA-

Table 9.8. Selected Side Effects of Corticosteroid Therapy

Central nervous system
Euphoria
Depression
Adrenal axis suppression
Hypertension
Sodium and water retention
Myopathy
Avascular necrosis
Infection
Impaired wound healing
Increased appetite and weight gain
Osteoporosis
Cataracts
Hyperglycemia
Hyperlipidemia
Impaired growth and sexual maturation

cyclophilin complex binds competitively to and inhibits calcineurin, a phosphatase whose activity depends on binding to calcium and calmodulin. Inhibition of calcineurin is believed to mediate the immunosuppressive activity of both CsA and tacrolimus. Calcineurin activity activates the promoter region for the gene encoding IL-2, which leads to transcription; inhibition of calcineurin activity by CsA inhibits transcription. CsA interferes with transcription of the genes encoding for the enzyme peptidyl-prolyl cis-trans isomerase, blocking signal transduction for lymphokine synthesis from the cytoplasm to the nucleus. The production of IL-2 from CD4+ T cells is inhibited with no apparent direct effect on CD8+ T cells, B cells, macrophages, or granulocytes. Clonal expansion of allosensitized T cells is also reduced by inhibiting expression of IL-2 surface receptors. Because CsA selectively inhibits the synthesis of other lymphokines (including IFN-γ, the lymphokine that provides an amplification signal activating macrophages and monocytes), preformed cytotoxic (CD8+) T lymphocytes are not affected by CsA. Hyperacute rejection and other humorally mediated processes are also not affected.[23,24]

CsA exhibits wide inter- and intrapatient variation in its pharmacokinetic profile. Oral absorption, which occurs primarily in the duodenum, is slow and incomplete (mean bioavailability 30%), in part because of presystemic metabolism by cytochrome P-450 (CYP450) in the gut wall. Absorption is influenced by biliary diversion (see the discussion on bile duct anastomosis after liver transplantation below), cholestasis, delayed gastric emptying, dietary fat content, increased gastrointestinal motility, and reduced pancreatic exocrine secretions. After administration, CsA is widely distributed, with more than 90% of total drug bound to serum lipoproteins and erythrocytes (volume of distribution reported 3.5–13.0 L/kg). Biotransformation of the parent compound occurs through the hepatic and gut microsomal mixed-function oxidase enzyme system (CYP450-3A4) and results in the formation of at least 21 metabolites. The mean terminal half-life is 10–27 hours; it varies widely according to patient age and liver function and the effects of interacting drugs that induce or inhibit the CYP450 system. The pharmacokinetics of CsA are not influenced by hemodialysis, peritoneal dialysis, or continuous venovenous hemofiltration.

In the traditional regimen, CsA is used with corticosteroids and an adjunctive agent (mycophenolate mofetil or azathioprine). Because of the nephrotoxicity associated with CsA, newer regimens have evolved using CsA in combination with sirolimus or mycophenolate, with or without steroids. It is also used in steroid-sparing regimens with sirolimus.

Dosing and monitoring. CsA pharmacokinetics are complex and vary among transplant populations.[24,25] Red blood cells (RBCs) bind CsA; because of its low-to-intermediate extraction ratio, clearance increases with decreased binding. CsA pharmacokinetics may therefore be altered in patients with low hematocrit. Age also seems to be an important factor in the disposition of CsA; pediatric patients have higher clearance values than older patients. One study has suggested that this age-related difference in clearance may result from lower serum lipoprotein concentrations and CsA binding in younger patients.[26] In addition, many drugs are capable of altering the clearance of CsA (Table 9.10).[27-29]

Cyclosporine absorption and disposition from the commercially available oral formulations are markedly variable; this complicates dosing and monitoring strategies with respect to maintenance of desired target blood concentrations and avoidance of toxicity. A microemulsion concentrate of CsA (Neoral; Novartis) was developed and has demonstrated an increased rate and extent of drug absorption with lower intra- and interindividual pharmacokinetic variability when compared with the original formulation (Sandimmune).

Neoral is well tolerated and exhibits greater relative bioavailability (faster time to peak [T_{max}] and maximum concentration [C_{max}]), greater area under the plasma drug concentration-versus-time curve (AUC), and less intra- and interindividual variability than Sandimmune.[30-32] Two generic formulations of CsA microemulsion are also available: Gengraf (Abbott) and cyclosporine (modified) (Eon Labs).

Trough measurements traditionally have been used to determine drug exposure and to guide appropriate dosing of cyclosporine. More recently C2 levels, or ones drawn 2 hours postdose, have been shown to be better predictors of AUC.[33,34] The clinical utility of C2 monitoring has been validated by studies demonstrating a lower incidence of early acute allograft rejection and a decrease in hypertension, dyslipidemia, and chronic renal allograft dysfunction.[35-37] But it has also been demonstrated that C2 monitoring may not detect toxicity in poor or slow absorbers.[38] Suggested C2 levels for renal transplant recipients immediately posttransplant are 1300–1700 ng/mL; maintenance C2 target levels are 800–1000 ng/mL.[35,36]

Adverse effects and toxicity. CsA has a number of important toxicities (**Table 9.9**); the most common and clinically relevant is renal dysfunction. CsA nephrotoxicity can manifest as acute renal failure or as chronic nephrotoxicity. The acute renal dysfunction associated with CsA is characterized by decreased glomerular filtration within days of starting the drug.

In addition to nephrotoxicity, CsA can cause liver dysfunction, neurotoxicity, hirsutism, gingival hyperplasia, and infusion-related reactions characterized by burning of the soles and palms.[39] Hypertension occurs as a result of CsA administration in 50% to 90% of transplant patients. The requirement for effective treatment of hypertension cannot be overemphasized because uncontrolled blood pressure will result in premature loss of allograft function. This complication will be discussed later.

Tacrolimus. Tacrolimus (FK506, Prograf; Astellas) is a naturally occurring macrolide product of the soil fungus *Streptomyces tsukubaensis* and has immunosuppressive ability similar to that of CsA.

Pharmacology and clinical uses. Clinical use of tacrolimus began in February 1989 at the University of Pittsburgh. Multicenter, randomized, prospective clinical trials comparing a tacrolimus-based regimen with CsA-based regimens in liver transplantation began in the fall of 1990, resulting in Food and Drug Administration (FDA) approval

Table 9.9. Incidence of Adverse Events with Tacrolimus and Cyclosporine[a]

Adverse Event[b]	Tacrolimus (n = 263)	Cyclosporine (n = 266)	P Value
Alopecia	20	6	<.001
Anemia	47	38	.047
Anorexia	34	24	.01
Diarrhea	72	47	<.001
Fever	48	56	.089
Headache	64	60	.408
Hirsutism	7	31	<.001
Hyperglycemia	47	38	.07
Hyperkalemia	45	26	<.001
Hypertension	47	56	.06
Nausea	46	37	.046
Paresthesia	40	30	.039
Pruritus	36	20	<.001
Rash	24	19	.101
Tremor	56	46	.032
Vomiting	27	15	.001

[a]Values are the percentages of patients reporting the first occurrence of any treatment-related event on the basis of history, physical examination, or laboratory examination or diagnostic tests during the 1-year follow-up.

[b]Hypertension was defined as elevated blood pressure (regardless of the specific value) that was being treated with at least one medication. Anemia, hyperglycemia, and hyperkalemia were defined at each study site on the basis of accepted laboratory values at that institution.

(Source: Reprinted from U.S. Multicenter FK506 Liver Study Group. N Engl J Med. 1994; 331(17):1110–1115.)

in April 1994.[40,41] Tacrolimus has also been shown to be an effective agent for prevention of allograft rejection in noncomparative trials in primary renal,[42,43] lung,[44] and cardiac[45] transplantation and as rescue therapy for patients experiencing persistent allograft rejection during primary immunosuppression with CsA.[46,47] Reviews of its extensive clinical use are presented elsewhere.[48,49]

Tacrolimus shares a mechanism of action similar to that of CsA but binds to a specific cytoplasmic immunophilin (FK binding protein 12) different from the calcineurin binding site of CsA. Both agents inhibit calcium-dependent signal transduction pathways in T cells, blocking the secretion of IL-2 and other lymphokines.[50–52] Their pharmacokinetic profiles are also similar. Reported clinical pharmacokinetic parameters for tacrolimus include a half-life of 8.7 hours (range, 5.5–16.6 hours), mean volume of distribution of 19.4 L/kg, and mean clearance of 143 L/h (range, 88–269 L/h). After oral administration, tacrolimus is poorly, erratically, and incompletely absorbed. The mean bioavailability is 27%; wide interpatient variability is observed, particularly among pediatric patients.[53] Unlike CsA, it does not require bile to ensure adequate absorption.[54] An oral dose of 0.15 mg/kg achieves peak plasma concentrations of 0.4–3.7 ng/mL in 1–4 hours. Tacrolimus is metabolized by the CYP450 enzyme system, as is CsA,[54] which accounts for the similar drug interaction profile.[54–56] Metabolism is significantly impaired in the presence of poor hepatic function, requiring close attention to blood concentration monitoring and careful dosage adjustment. A modified-release tacrolimus allowing for once-daily dosing is under development. This extended-release formulation demonstrated similar AUCs and trough levels as conventional tacrolimus dosed twice daily in both healthy volunteers and kidney or liver recipients.[57]

Clincial use of tacrolimus has mirrored that of CsA. Originally it was used as the primary component of a triple-drug regimen with corticosteroids and azathioprine or mycophenolate. More recent protocols have used tacrolimus with sirolimus to avoid or minimize the use of corticosteroids or to minimize long-term exposure and the development of tacrolimus-associated nephrotoxicity.

Dosing and monitoring. Therapy with tacrolimus is initiated with a dose of 0.05–0.1 mg/kg administered orally twice daily.[58] Tacrolimus is adequately absorbed in the immediate posttransplant period; routine parenteral administration is neither required nor desirable, because of the potentially greater neurotoxicity and nephrotoxicity associated with the intravenous dosage form. But for those patients who cannot receive oral medication, tacrolimus may be administered at initial doses of 0.05–0.075 mg/kg/day as a continuous intravenous infusion over 24 hours. Therapy is adjusted based on whole blood or plasma trough concentrations as measured by enzyme-linked immunosorbent assay (ELISA) or by microparticle enzyme immunoassay (IMX).[59,60] Typical whole blood trough concentrations range from 5–15 ng/mL depending on time posttransplant, type of organ transplanted, and concomitant medications. As with CsA, the optimal target blood concentrations for tacrolimus have not been determined and the clearance of tacrolimus is altered by many other drugs (**Table 9.10**).

Table 9.10. Drugs That Interact With CsA, Tacrolimus, and Sirolimus[*]

Increased Concentrations	Decreased Concentrations
Diltiazem, nicardipine, verapamil	Phenytoin
Ketoconazole, itraconazole, fluconazole, voriconazole	Phenobarbital
Erythromycin, clarithromycin, troleandomycin	Carbamazepine
Metaclopromide	Rifampin, rifabutin, isoniazid
Cisapride	Nafcillin
Cimetidine	Sulfadimidine
Omeprazole, lansoprazole, esomeprazole, rabeprazole	Caspofungin
Magnesium-aluminum hydroxide	Octreotide
Protease inhibitors	Probucol
Nefazadone	Primidone
Oral contraceptives	St. John's wort
Danazole	
Bromocriptine	
Grapefruit juice	

[*]This table includes some of the most common drugs known to interact with or with the potential to interact with CsA, tacrolimus, and sirolimus.

Adverse effects and toxicity. Table 9.9 compares the adverse effects of tacrolimus with those of CsA. Tacrolimus may have a lesser incidence of certain side effects (e.g., hypertension, hypercholesterolemia, hirsutism, and gingival hyperplasia) than CsA.[61] The propensity of tacrolimus to cause nephrotoxicity and diabetes and predispose patients to opportunistic infections is similar to that of CsA.[62-64] A variety of neurotoxic effects have been reported, including akinetic mutism, expressive aphasia, seizures, confusion, psychosis, encephalopathy, coma, tremors, headache, and sleep disturbances.[48] Gastrointestinal toxicity may manifest as nausea or diarrhea. Many patients will respond to dosage reductions, but in other cases neurotoxicity may necessitate withdrawal of this agent and conversion to CsA.[65-67]

Inhibitors of Late T-Cell Function

Sirolimus. Sirolimus (rapamycin, Rapamune; Wyeth) was discovered in the mid-1970s during a screening program intended to identify novel antifungal agents, although further development was not pursued at that time. When the structure of tacrolimus was explained, sirolimus was found to be structurally similar, and investigations began into its use as an antirejection agent.

Pharmacology and clinical uses. The immunosuppressive activity of sirolimus is mediated through a mechanism distinct from that of tacrolimus or CsA. Sirolimus markedly suppresses IL-2- and IL-4-driven T-cell proliferation by forming a complex with FKBP 12, which inhibits the protein kinase mammalian target of rapamycin (TOR), acting at a later phase of the cell cycle (G1) than tacrolimus or CsA. Sirolimus inhibits the response to activating cytokines IL-2 and IL-6, rather than the direct synthesis and secretion of these mediators. This agent also inhibits IL-6-supported proliferation and IFN-α and IFN-β activity.[68,69] Sirolimus has been shown to compete with tacrolimus for binding to FKBP12 in vitro, though this effect is not clinically relevant in vivo since about 95% of FKBP12 remains unbound when both drugs are used at immunosuppressant doses. The potency of sirolimus increases markedly in combination with CsA, permitting at least threefold reduction of the dose of each agent.[70]

Sirolimus is rapidly absorbed after oral administration with a time to peak of about 1–2 hours. The systemic availability of sirolimus is reportedly

10% to 27% and increases with the administration of high-fat foods. It is recommended that sirolimus be administered consistently with or without food. The volume of distribution is 12 ± 8 L/kg, and it is 97% plasma protein bound. Sirolimus is a substrate for both CYP450-3A4 and P-glycoprotein, and its pharmacokinetic profile is affected by the concomitant administration of drugs that affect these proteins. It is extensively metabolized by O-demethylation and hydroxylation, resulting in seven major metabolites. Sirolimus has a long half-life of 62 ± 16 hours, and the AUC correlates well with whole blood trough concentrations.

Clinical trials support the use of sirolimus in a variety of combinations. Initial trials documented its use as an adjunctive agent to the calcineurin inhibitors cyclosporine and tacrolimus; early evidence now supports a new role as primary immunosuppressant to minimize or avoid the use of calcineurin inhibitors and corticosteroids.[21,71]

The antiproliferative effects of sirolimus have led to use outside transplantation. Sirolimus-eluting stents used in the treatment of coronary artery disease have been proven to decrease the extent of restenosis compared to conventional stents up to 8 months after implantation.[72] The effects of sirolimus and its analog temsirolimus, also known as CCI-997, on various malignancies are being evaluated.[73-75]

Dosing and monitoring. The optimal time to begin sirolimus therapy is somewhat controversial. Initial recommendations dictated initiation of therapy immediately after transplantation, with a loading dose of 6–15 mg followed by maintenance doses of 2–5 mg per day. Subsequent experience with sirolimus has correlated its use with an increase in delayed wound healing and development of lymphocele in kidney and liver recipients.[76] This may suggest the need to delay initiation of the drug by 5–7 days. The concomitant administration of CsA with sirolimus results in elevations in all pharmacokinetic parameters of sirolimus; it is recommended that CsA be administered 4 hours before sirolimus. Therapeutic drug monitoring of sirolimus is not essential to use, but may help ensure efficacy, prevention of side effects, and the identification of drug interactions. The pivotal phase III clinical trials that used full-dose cyclosporine, corticosteroids, and fixed doses of sirolimus resulted in whole blood levels of 8.59 ± 4.0 ng/mL and 17.3 ± 7.4 ng/mL for the 2 mg and 5 mg doses, respectively.[77] For regimens using sirolimus as the primary immunosuppressant and minimizing the use of calcinuerin inhibitors or corticosteroids, a target range of 10–20 ng/mL has proven effective for prevention of acute kidney rejection.[21] Table

9.10 also includes agents that alter the drug levels of sirolimus.

Adverse effects and toxicity. The most frequently reported side effects of sirolimus are thrombocytopenia, leukopenia, hypercholesterolemia, hypertriglyceridemia, and diarrhea. When used in conjunction with full-dose tacrolimus or cyclosporine, sirolimus results in an increased incidence of drug-related nephrotoxicity and may result in tubular collapse, vacuolization, and nephrocalcinosis.[78] This effect appears to be ameliorated by reducing exposure to the calcineurin inhibitor.[21] Sirolimus has also been reported to cause pneumonitis, bronchiolitis obliterans-organizing pneumonia (BOOP), and decreases in total testosterone levels in males.[79-81] As mentioned earlier, sirolimus use has been correlated with an increased incidence of delayed wound healing and lymphocele development.[76] These complications may be minimized by avoiding corticosteroids before and after transplantation.[82]

Everolimus. Everolimus (Certican; Novartis) is a derivative of sirolimus, which has a stable 2-hydroxy-ethyl chain substitution at position 40. It has a similar mechanism of action, drug interaction, and side-effect profile as its parent compound. Everolimus has a slightly higher bioavailability than sirolimus (16% versus 10%) and a shorter half-life (18.1–35.0 hours) requiring twice-daily dosing.[83,84] Therapeutic drug monitoring is needed for appropriate use of everolimus, and blood concentrations are predictive of the immunosuppressant activity and severity of adverse effects. Steady-state trough concentrations of everolimus correlate well with AUC and should be used to guide dosing.[84]

Everolimus has proven as effective as mycophenolate mofetil in preventing graft rejection in de novo renal transplant recipients when used with full-dose cyclosporine.[85] Although everolimus exerts a synergistic immunosuppressant effect with cyclosporine, it also appears to increase the drug's nephrotoxicity. Using a reduced cyclosporine exposure protocol in conjunction with everolimus demonstrated decreased nephrotoxicity while maintaining efficacy.[85] Due to the similar mechanism of action, the clinical use of everolimus is expected to mirror that of sirolimus.

Like sirolimus, everolimus has antiproliferative effects that have been documented to decrease the vascular remodeling and hyperplasia of vascular smooth muscle. These positive effects have led to the development and use of everolimus in the treatment of coronary artery disease outside the context of transplantation. Stents that elute sirolimus or everolimus have led to significant decreases in the slow vascular remodeling and restenosis that may occur with standard devices.[86,87] Recently everolimus has shown to help prevent allograft rejection and vasculopathy when used with maintenance cyclosporine and corticosteroids, documented by intravascular ultrasonography in cardiac transplant recipients. Both allograft rejection and vasculopathy decreased significantly in patients receiving everolimus versus those receiving azathioprine.[88] Everolimus is currently not available for use in the United States.

Leflunomide. Leflunomide (Arava; Sanofi-Aventis) was approved by the FDA for use in rheumatoid arthritis in 1998 and has shown promise as an alternative to the conventional transplant armamentarium.

Pharmacology and clinical uses. After oral absorption, leflunomide undergoes metabolism in the liver to the active compound A77-1726, which constitutes more than 90% of the parent and its derivatives. There are two proposed mechanisms of action of this active metabolite. The first is reversible blockade of dihydro-orotate dehydrogenase, an enzyme needed for de novo pyrimidine synthesis in lymphocytes and other cells. It also inhibits tyrosine kinases. In addition to immunosuppressant properties, A77-1726 has demonstrated substantial in-vitro antiviral activity.[89] The metabolite has a volume of distribution of 0.13 L/kg and is extensively plasma protein bound (>99.3%). The specific site of leflunomide metabolism is unknown. The active metabolite is further metabolized and ultimately eliminated in the kidney and by direct biliary excretion. The half-life of leflunomide is reportedly 15–18 days. Leflunomide and its metabolites are not dialyzable, and there have been no reported drug interactions with other immunosuppressive agents.

Use in clinical transplantation to date has been limited to patients with inadequate response or toxicity to current immunosuppressant therapy and to transplant patients with polyomavirus type BK nephropathy or cytomegalovirus infections.[90-92] FK778, an analog of leflunomide, has demonstrated promise in animal models and phase II clinical trials are under way for kidney transplantation.[93,94]

Dosing and monitoring. The safe and effective dose for the use of leflunomide in solid organ transplant has yet to be determined. Based on the active level of drug needed to inhibit assays of in vitro immune activity and experience from dosing for rheumatoid arthritis and cancer patients, target serum levels of 100 µg/mL were initially suggested. Loading doses of 200 mg/day and maintenance

doses of 40–60 mg/day have been used to achieve this target range. Experience with this dosing regimen in kidney or liver recipients, while effective in preventing acute rejection, revealed dose-limiting side effects in 25% to 35% of patients; reduction of target serum levels to ≤60 µg/mL decreased these toxicities to less than 15%.[95]

The long half-life of the active metabolite of leflunomide makes dose adjustments difficult in patients with adverse effects. The leflunomide analog FK778 may offer advantages in dosing; early evidence indicates a shorter half-life in animal models.[94] No dosing recommendations are available for leflunomide in patients with renal or hepatic insufficiency; close monitoring for efficacy and toxicity is prudent in patients with acute or severe impairment.

Adverse effects and toxicity. As previously explained, the adverse effects and toxicity of leflunomide have been correlated with high serum levels of the active metabolite A77-1726. The most common adverse effects of leflunomide are diarrhea, abdominal pain, leucopenia, anemia, and elevated liver enzymes. Anemia is the most commonly reported dose-limiting side effect in transplant recipients.[90] In other patient populations, severe and potentially fatal cases of interstitial lung disease, hepatotoxicity, and Stevens-Johnson syndrome have been reported. In case of serious drug toxicity with leflunomide, the drug should be discontinued. Emergent need for drug elimination requires administration of cholestyramine and activated charcoal.

Inhibitors of Cell Proliferation

Azathioprine. Azathioprine (AZA) is a purine analog that has been used in immunosuppressive regimens since 1961.[2] Its popularity has waned through the decades as new immunosuppressive agents have been introduced, but it has played a major role in the evolution of clinical transplantation.

Pharmacology and clinical uses. AZA is an imidazolyl derivative of 6-MP and is readily converted to this active metabolite.[95] It incorporates into cellular DNA and inhibits purine synthesis; purines are needed for both DNA and RNA synthesis. AZA is most toxic to rapidly proliferating cells that are making new DNA. It inhibits humoral and cellular immunity during the initial stages of lymphoid differentiation, so it is useful in prevention, but not treatment, of acute rejection. AZA may also reduce neutrophil production and macrophage function, reducing the nonspecific inflammatory aspect of the immune reaction.[96]

Dosing and monitoring. Even though AZA has been used for decades, its pharmacokinetics have not been fully understood. The development of more sensitive and specific assays has given a better understanding of the pharmacokinetics of AZA and its metabolites.[97–101] Orally administered AZA is absorbed rapidly but incompletely. It is quickly converted by glutathione to 6-MP in the liver and RBCs.[97–99,102,103] Both AZA and 6-MP have short half-lives: 12.5 ± 3.0 and 50.4 ± 36.6 minutes, respectively. Bioavailability of 6-MP after administration of AZA has been estimated to be 41% to 44%.[104] Based on these findings, it has been suggested that the AZA dose be reduced by 50% when converting from oral to intravenous administration.[95] Because the immunologic activity is actually conveyed by its metabolites, it is unclear whether dosage adjustments of the prodrug (i.e., AZA) are needed. 6-MP is either transformed intracellularly to thioinosinic acid and 6-thioguanine nucleotides (TGNs) or further broken down to 6-thiouric acid, an inactive end product primarily eliminated by the kidneys.[102] Thioinosinic acid is an inhibitor of purine synthesis. The TGNs incorporate into DNA and probably are toxic to dividing cells. The half-life of RBC TGN appears to be quite long (about 13 days), allowing for once-daily dosing of AZA[102] but also contributing to delayed reversal of toxicity. The concentration of TGN in the tissues may be the more clinically relevant level to be measured, but at this time therapeutic drug monitoring is only investigational. Clearance of AZA is not affected by renal impairment, but its metabolite 6-thioguanine may accumulate, with renal impairment contributing to enhanced toxicity.[99] Dosing guidelines for renal impairment are not available.

AZA has been used extensively in double- (also known as "conventional therapy"), triple-, and quadruple-drug regimens for organ transplantation. An initial, one-time dose of 3–5 mg/kg per day of AZA is administered preoperatively. Immediately after transplantation, the dose is usually tapered to a maintenance dose of 1–3 mg/kg per day or titrated to patient tolerance as determined by a desired white blood cell (WBC) count of 3500–6000 cells/mm³.[95] WBC counts below 3000 usually necessitate temporary discontinuation of the drug or subsequent dosage reduction (e.g., 25 mg/day). Infectious complications (e.g., cytomegalovirus [CMV]) and other medications commonly used in transplant patients (e.g., trimethoprim–sulfamethoxazole, ganciclovir) may further confound the differential diagnosis of leukopenia observed in patients treated with AZA.

A reduction of 75% to 80% of the AZA dose is needed in patients receiving the xanthine-oxidase inhibitor allopurinol, which blocks the metabolism of AZA's metabolites.[105–107] This interaction can cause life-threatening pancytopenia, which may not become clinically apparent until after a month of concomitant therapy. Administration of granulocyte colony-stimulating factor may be needed to decrease the risk of infection and other complications of profound marrow suppression. AZA has been associated with increased need for the nondepolarizing muscle relaxant pancuronium, but it potentiates the activity of succinylcholine, a depolarizing muscle relaxant.[108,109] Increased warfarin requirements have been reported for patients receiving 6-MP and may be expected with AZA.[110]

Adverse effects and toxicity. The primary toxicity of AZA is its dose-related bone marrow suppression, appearing 7–14 days after initiation of therapy.[111] The myelosuppression is characterized by leukopenia,[112,113] thrombocytopenia, macrocytic anemia, pure red cell aplasia, and reticulocytopenia.[114] Other adverse effects include increased predisposition to infections (viral, bacterial, and fungal),[115] hepatic dysfunction and jaundice,[116,117] alopecia, stomatitis,[118] acute pancreatitis,[119] and increased risk of malignancy.[120]

Mycophenolate mofetil and mycophenolic sodium.
Pharmacology and clinical uses. Mycophenolate mofetil (CellCept, Roche Pharmaceuticals) is a semisynthetic agent derived from the fermentation of several Penicillum species. The compound is the morpholino-ethyl ester of mycophenolic acid, the active form of the drug, and is rapidly hydrolyzed to this compound in vivo.[121] Mycophenolic acid selectively blocks human B- and T- lymphocyte proliferative responses by inhibiting de novo pathways of purine biosynthesis. This results in decreased intracellular pools of guanosine ribonucleotides and dGTP, which are needed for the regulation of DNA polymerase activity and subsequent lymphocyte proliferation. De novo purine synthesis is specific to lymphocytes, so the antiproliferative effects on other cell types are significantly lower with mycophenolic acid than with other agents. Secondary immunologic effects include decreased B-lymphocyte antibody production and reduced expression of selective adhesion molecules responsible for key cellular interactions. Unlike CsA and tacrolimus, mycophenolic acid does not affect production of IL-1 and IL-2, the key cytokines associated with early T-cell signal transduction.

Mycophenolic acid undergoes hepatic conjugation to the inactive metabolite mycophenolic acid glucuronide (MPAG).[121,122] However, this compound undergoes enterohepatic recirculation and can be hydrolyzed back to mycophenolic acid by intestinal and cellular β-glucuronidase enzymes. Pharmacokinetic studies after oral administration demonstrated 94% bioavailability, T_{max} of 1.0 hour, a dose-dependent C_{max} of 2.0–18.7 mg/mL, and a plasma half-life of 15.8 hours.[122] The agent undergoes extensive metabolism and enterohepatic recirculation: more than 90% of mycophenolic acid is excreted in the urine. The apparent lack of effect on human CYP450 activity is supported by the absence of a pharmacokinetic drug interaction with CsA.[121,122]

Initially evaluated in the late 1970s as an immunosuppressant for several autoimmune indications, clinical investigations with mycophenolate mofetil in solid organ transplant recipients did not begin until 1991.[122] Subsequently, mycophenolate mofetil, combined with CsA and prednisone, has undergone extensive phase I–III trials for the prevention of rejection after kidney,[122–124] liver,[125] and heart[126] transplantation and was approved by the FDA in the summer of 1995 for renal allograft recipients. The efficacy and tolerability of mycophenolate mofetil has withstood the test of time; in the past decade, it has become the most commonly administered immunosuppressant agent in solid organ transplant.[17] It is primarily used in conjunction with a calcineurin inhibitor and corticosteroids.

An enteric-coated formulation of mycophenolate sodium (Myfortic; Novartis Pharma) was developed in an effort to improve the upper gastrointestinal tolerability of mycophenolic acid. This formulation was approved by the FDA in 2004 and has proven to be safe and therapeutically equivalent to mycophenolate mofetil, offering an alternative to patients with tolerance issues to mycophenolate mofetil.[127–129]

Dosing and monitoring. The immunosuppressive activity of mycophenolate mofetil, as well as adverse effects, appear to be dose-dependent, with doses ranging from 100–3500 mg/day evaluated in various clinical settings.[123] Doses of 2000 mg/day appear necessary to prevent kidney transplant rejection and provide optimal immunosuppression with minimal adverse effects.[123,130,131] The agent can be administered orally twice a day and is generally adjusted based on adverse effects or intolerance. Intravenous administration of mycophenolate mofetil follows the same guidelines as that of oral dosing. The mycophenolic acid content and exposure of 720 mg of enteric-coated mychophenolate sodium is equivalent to 1000 mg of mycophenolate mofetil.[129] Preliminary results from conversion trials suggest that substituting the enteric-coated product for conventional mycophenolate mofetil

appears to be well tolerated in maintenance renal transplant patients.[129] Recent studies have demonstrated a role for therapeutic drug monitoring of mycophenolic acid. Data describing a wide interpatient variability of MPA steady-state concentrations and correlations of MPA AUCs with the risk for acute rejection support this role.[132,133] Multicenter trials are needed to identify target levels for MPA and the appropriate method of therapeutic drug monitoring to predict drug efficacy.

There are several drug–drug interactions documented with mycophenolate mofetil.[132] Acyclovir and probenecid appear to compete for renal tubular secretion with MPAG, increasing the AUC of theses agents and MPAG. Cholestyramine and aluminum- or magnesium-based antacids significantly reduce the bioavailability of mycophenolate mofetil; these agents should not be administered concomitantly. Though no formal dosing guidelines exist for renal insufficiency, patients with significant acute or chronic failure should be monitored closely for toxicity. Preliminary studies have demonstrated that cirrhosis has no effect on the metabolism of mycophenolate mofetil.

Adverse effects and toxicity. Mycophenolate mofetil is generally well tolerated, with fewer dose-limiting effects than other antiproliferative agents.[123–126,130–131,135] Gastrointestinal effects, such as gastritis, nausea, anorexia, and abdominal cramping, are most frequently reported at standard doses (2–3 g/day).[123,130,131,134] Rare cases of gastrointestinal ulceration and bleeding have been reported with larger doses (above 3.5 g/day). These side effects have also been reported with enteric-coated mycophenolate sodium.[129,130] Hematologic toxicities, including neutropenia, thrombocytopenia, and anemia, occur at similar or less frequent rates than with standard AZA therapy. Incidence of viral infections is at least equivalent to AZA, with several studies demonstrating an increase in CMV disease in patients treated with mycophenolate mofetil. The incidence of Epstein-Barr virus (EBV)–related lymphoma and malignancy appears similar to that of AZA when combined with CsA and prednisone.[123–126,130,131,134–136]

Polyclonal Antilymphocyte Antibodies

The immunosuppressive qualities of antilymphocyte serum were first described by Woodruff in 1963.[137] Antilymphocyte antibodies were the first form of selective immunosuppression to be used as anti-T-cell therapy. Polyclonal antilymphocyte antibodies have since been used—both alone and in combination with other immunosuppressive agents—to prevent and treat rejection episodes in organ transplantation.[138–146] They are commonly used as induction agents in the early post-transplant period to reduce or modify early immune system activity against the transplanted organ.[17]

Pharmacology and clinical uses. Antilymphocyte globulin (ALG) and antithymocyte globulin (ATG) are produced by first injecting a series of human spleen cells (ALG) or thymocytes (ATG) into various animals (horse, goat, rabbit). Antibodies are then isolated from the animal sera.[147,148] Their potency lies primarily in the immunoglobulin G (IgG) antibody fraction. Their action is directed not only against T cells but also against B cells, causing marked lymphocytopenia. Additional binding to nonlymphoid cells (platelets, RBCs, and WBCs) can also occur, resulting in various blood dyscrasias. ALG acts by binding to surface antigens on host T or B lymphocytes, causing (1) opsonization and removal by the reticuloendothelial system or (2) direct, complement-assisted lysing of lymphocytes.

Dosing and monitoring. The pharmacokinetics of ATGs have not been fully explained. The plasma half-life of equine IgG averages 6 days (range, 1.5–12.0 days). The plasma concentrations and half-life of IgG vary, depending on the patient's ability to catabolize foreign IgG. Concentrations of ATG have been detected up to 30 days after administration. About 1% of a dose of ATG is excreted in urine as unchanged equine IgG. The distribution and selective binding to different binding sites vary from product to product.[149] The half-life of rabbit ATG is 2–3 days after the first dose. Measurable concentrations of rabbit ATG are detectable up to 90 days after completion of therapy.[150]

Rabbit anti-thymocyte globulin (Thymoglobulin; Genzyme) is the most commonly used induction agent for all solid organ transplants in the United States. The use of equine anti-thymocyte globulin (Atgam; Pharmacia) for induction in kidney transplant recipients decreased to 1.1% in 2003. Rabbit ATG is also the antilymphocyte therapy of choice for treating rejection episodes.[17] The recommended dose of rabbit ATG for induction therapy is 1 mg/kg/day administered perioperatively through a central line over 4–6 hours for 3–6 doses.[151] The recommended dose for rejection episodes is 1–1.5 mg/kg/day for 7–14 days.[150] The recommended dose for equine preparations is usually 10–20 mg/kg per day for up to 14 days but varies according to institutional protocol and type of transplant. The required dose should be diluted in saline at a maximum concentration of 4 mg/mL and administered through a central line over 4–8 hours.[152] For all these agents, efficacy

can be monitored by measuring the T-cell count. Controversy exists as to the most appropriate lymphocyte population to monitor the efficacy of polyclonal antibodies. Each preparation has a different binding specificity for CD2, CD3, CD4, CD8, and other specific epitopes.[153] Several studies have used variable dosing of polyclonal antibodies based on reduction in $CD2^+$ or $CD3^+$ T-cell counts during sequential induction.[153] Other centers have used reduction in total lymphocyte counts as a marker of response.[154] In general, a 90% reduction in $CD2^+$ or $CD3^+$ T cells from baseline correlates with an adequate response.[155]

Adverse effects and toxicity. ATGs are composed of antibodies directed against multiple-surface antigens. This nonspecificity predisposes the patient to significant side effects from the products' cross-reactivity with nonlymphocytic blood cells and other human tissues.[156,157] Side effects of these agents include fever, chills, erythema, pruritus, leukopenia, thrombocytopenia, arthralgias, myalgias, and (rarely) allergic reactions, such as anaphylaxis and serum sickness. Premedication with acetaminophen, antihistamines, and steroids decreases the incidence of adverse reactions. Doses are reduced by 50% if the platelet count falls between 50,000 and 70,000 per microliter or if the total white blood cell count is between 2000 and 3000 per microliter. Like other immunosuppressants, these agents have also been associated with increased incidence of infections (particularly cytomegalovirus) and neoplasms.[150,158]

Monoclonal Antibodies

Muromonab-CD3 (Orthoclone-OKT3; Ortho Biotech), approved by the FDA in 1986, was the first monoclonal antibody (mAb) approved for therapeutic use in humans. This agent was biologically engineered using murine- (mouse-) derived protein and, although highly effective for prevention and treatment of acute rejection, has been associated with development of host responses to the foreign protein as well as significant side effects. Almost 10 years after the approval of OKT-3, two more mAbs, daclizumab (Zenapax; Roche Pharmaceuticals) and basiliximab (Simulect; Novartis), were approved for the prevention of acute rejection in solid organ transplantation. These agents represent the future of immunosupression with more specific mechanisms of action and decreased immunogenicity than OKT3.

OKT3. *Immunologic effects.* Muromonab OKT3 is a murine mAb of the IgG2a isotype that binds to the CD3 receptor found on mature circulating T cells and medullary thymocytes.[159,160] The CD3 receptor complex is next to the T-cell antigen-recognition site. By binding to the CD3 receptor, OKT3 blocks the cells' ability to become stimulated by foreign antigens, inhibiting both the generation and function of cytotoxic T cells responsible for graft rejection. After the initial dose of OKT3, T cells virtually disappear from the circulation within minutes to hours. During treatment with OKT3, T cells bearing the usual array of surface markers (CD2, CD4, CD8) reappear but are devoid of the OKT3 target, the CD3 receptor.[161–163] Within 48 hours of discontinuing therapy, however, the normal array of surface markers, including CD3, reappears on T cells. Proposed mechanisms for OKT3's action include opsonization of circulating T cells and subsequent removal by the reticuloendothelial system[164]; modulation (internalization) of the T-lymphocyte antigen receptor (CD3 complex), which would render the T cell nonfunctional[165]; and coating of the TCR, which would inhibit T-lymphocyte antigen recognition for the duration of the therapy.[166,167] The therapeutic effectiveness of OKT3 in reversing acute allograft rejection is related to its ability to block the action of cytotoxic T lymphocytes against the allograft. Potential causes for failure of OKT3 or subsequent need for higher OKT3 doses include immune clearance of the agent as a result of human antimurine antibody (HAMA) production, increased consumption from high antigen production rates, an abnormally high clearance rate of mouse immunoglobulin, and lack of T-cell functional dependence on the CD3 antigen.[163]

Dosing and monitoring. The clinical efficacy of OKT3 is well established for the treatment of rejection, steroid-resistant rejection, and rejection prophylaxis (induction) in most solid organ transplant populations though the use of this agent has declined in favor of newer, less toxic immunosuppressants.[17,168] The usual dosage regimen for OKT3 is 5 mg intravenously daily for 10–14 days for rejection and 7–10 days for induction. Before administration, OKT3 must be filtered through a 0.20- to 0.22-μm low-protein-binding filter to remove particulate matter. After filtering, OKT3 should be administered as an intravenous bolus via either peripheral or central access. Lower doses have proven equally effective in some patients for rejection prophylaxis.[169] The manufacturer recommends a dose of 2.5 mg be administered daily in children who weigh less than 30 kg, but it has been observed that children may actually require larger doses (5–7.5 mg daily) to achieve similar immunosuppressive efficacy.[170–172] The efficacy of OKT3 therapy can be monitored by measuring peripheral lymphocyte subsets (CD3$^+$ T cells), serum OKT3

concentrations, and the production of HAMAs.[173] Based on the alterations of CD3 expression during OKT3 therapy, lymphocyte subset populations have been the mainstay of monitoring immunologic response to OKT3. The absolute number and percentage of peripheral CD3$^+$ T cells/mm^3 have been correlated with effective immunosuppression. Absolute CD3$^+$ T cell counts below 10–50 cells/mm^3 or percentages of total lymphocyte below 3% to 5% indicate adequate immunosuppression.[174–177] A consistent increase in CD3$^+$ T cells during treatment reflects therapeutic failure. Although monitoring peripheral circulating CD3$^+$ T cells does not detect lymphocytes infiltrating the allograft or lymphoid tissue, most courses of OKT3 are successfully monitored using this method in conjunction with other biochemical or clinical parameters.

Adverse effects and toxicity. Most patients experience a mild to severe flu-like syndrome with the first several doses of OKT3. Symptoms include fever, chills, headache, nausea, vomiting, diarrhea, and myalgias. This reaction is related to the activation of T cells and monocytes by OKT3, which results in the release of cytokines such as IL-2, IL-6, IFN-γ, and TNF.[178–180] With subsequent doses, the severity of the reaction is lessened or the syndrome disappears because of the substantial reduction in the number of circulating CD3$^+$ T cells, the amount of cytokines released, and the depletion of cytokine receptors. Less frequent side effects include pulmonary edema in fluid-overloaded patients (more than 3% over dry weight),[178–181] marked hypotension,[182] aseptic meningitis,[183–185] and seizures.[186] An acute decline in glomerular filtration rate, causing a reversible rise in serum creatinine during the first 1–3 days of OKT3 therapy, may be the result of cytokine-induced renal toxicity.[187] Initial attempts to prevent these cytokine-mediated toxicities with acetaminophen, antihistamines, and low doses of corticosteroids proved relatively ineffective.[188,189] High doses of corticosteroids given 1 hour before the administration of OKT3 significantly reduce cytokine release and subsequent side effects in both murine and human models.[190] Current guidelines recommend administering 500–1000 mg of methylprednisolone intravenously in combination with acetaminophen and diphenhydramine 1 hour before the first two doses of OKT3 for optimal management of cytokine release syndrome. A recent study demonstrated that dividing the steroids into two doses and administering them at 6 hours and 1 hour prior to OKT3 may further reduce clinical symptoms.[191] Other adjunctive agents, such as pentoxifylline, indomethacin, and anti-TNF mAbs, have demonstrated variable clinical effects.[192–194]

As with other antilymphocyte agents, a higher incidence of viral infections and malignancy has been observed after OKT3 therapy.[195] This finding is most likely related to the degree and duration of the overall concentration of immunosuppression that predisposes patients to viral reactivation and compromises the T-cell–mediated immunity needed for combating viral pathogens. Although antiviral prophylaxis with ganciclovir or acyclovir may reduce the incidence and severity of these secondary viral complications, induction therapy with OKT3 has fallen out of favor in non–high-risk patients because of these increased risks of overimmunosuppression.

Other monoclonal antibodies. The use of monoclonal antibodies approved for nontransplant indications in the realm of transplantation is emerging in single-center clinical trials and case reports. Although these agents show promise in a wide range of transplant-related indications, caution must be used before incorporating them into routine clinical practice because of their potentially serious side effect profiles.

Alemtuzumab (Campath-1H; Berlex Medical) is a humanized anti-CD52 mAb currently approved for the treatment of chronic B-cell lymphocytic leukemia. The CD-52 antigen is a glycoprotein expressed on circulating T and B lymphocytes and NK cells. Alemtuzumab profoundly depletes circulating lymphocytes long term and causes a transient depletion of B cells and monocytes.[196] Preliminary studies in simultaneous pancreas and kidney transplantation and kidney transplantation alone suggest that alemtuzumab may be useful as an induction agent followed by calcineurin-inhibitor or corticosteroid-free maintenance regimens.[197,198] Larger, randomized controlled trials are needed to accurately define the role of alemtuzumab in solid organ transplantation.

Rituximab (Rituxan; Genentech, Inc) is a chimeric human/murine mAb with a high affinity for CD-20, a protein expressed on B lymphocytes. Rituximab is approved for the treatment of refractory or relapsed B-cell non-Hodgkin's lymphoma. Many potential complications following organ transplantation, including posttransplant lymphoproliferative disorder and refractory acute rejection, may be partially mediated by an uncontrolled proliferation of B lymphocytes. Promising evidence to support the use of rituximab in treating these complications has been reported in single and small series case reports.[199,200] Rituximab also has been included in preconditioning protocols to allow ABO-incompatible transplantation.[201]

Interleukin-2 Receptor Antagonists

Pharmacology and clinical uses. The interleukin-2 receptor antagonists (IL-2Ra), daclizumab and basiliximab, are mAbs to the alpha subunit of the IL-2 receptor which is present on activated T lymphocytes; they do not bind to resting T lymphocytes. By competitively binding to the α subunit, also known as CD25 or Tac, they prevent the formation of the complete binding site required for IL-2 to transmit messages which otherwise result in the proliferation of cytolytic T cells. Their proposed mechanisms of action include promotion of antibody dependent cytotoxicity, T-cell elimination by long-term IL-2 deprivation, down-regulation of IL-2 receptor expression, increased shedding of the bound IL-2Rα chain, and alterations to lymphocyte recirculation.[202]

Daclizumab is a humanized mAb with 90% of the protein mass consisting of human gene regions; the remaining 10% are murine and are present only in the hypervariable regions of the antibody responsible for antigen recognition.[203] Basiliximab, on the other hand, is a chimeric mAb in which the variable regions of the murine portion responsible for binding to the IL-2Rα are combined with the constant human portions.[204] Both drugs have a high affinity and specificity for IL-2Rα and have low immunogenicity compared with murine or rat antibodies.

The interleukin-2 receptor antagonists are primarily used as induction agents in combination with triple-drug maintenance regimens.[202] They have been proven to significantly reduce acute rejection within the first year in renal transplant patients, though no significant difference has been demonstrated in long-term graft survival. There is no clinical evidence to support differences in efficacy between basiliximab and daclizumab, though no head-to-head trials have been conducted.[205]

Dosing and monitoring. Saturation of IL-2Rα and subsequent suppression of IL-2 activity requires serum levels of 5–10 μg/mL of daclizumab or 0.2 mcg/mL of basiliximab.[202] The recommended dosing regimen for basiliximab in adults is 20 mg infused over 20–30 minutes. The first dose is given on induction of anesthesia and repeated once on postoperative day 4. The pediatric dose for patients weighing 40 kg or less is 10 mg on days 0 and 4. These dosing regimens have been reported to achieve adequate serum levels of basiliximab in 97% of renal transplant recipients.[204] The FDA-approved dosing regimen for daclizumab in renal transplant recipients is 1 mg/kg infused over 15 minutes on induction of anesthesia and repeated once every 2 weeks for a total of five doses. This dosing regimen sustains serum concentrations needed to saturate IL-2 receptors for 12 weeks after transplantation. Since approval, the desire for a more practical and economic dosing regimen for daclizumab has led to the practice of using one or two doses of 2 mg/kg.[206,207]

Adverse effects and toxicity. The specificity and low immunogenicity of the IL-2Ra translate into agents with low toxicity. Placebo-controlled trials in renal transplant recipients for both basiliximab and daclizumab have revealed no significant differences in the incidence of all reported adverse events. The risk for opportunistic infections or development of lymphoproliferative disorders or malignancies is also unchanged. No instances of hypersensitivity or anaphylaxis were reported with either agent in pre-marketing studies. Since approval, rare cases (<1 per 1000 patients) of acute hypersensitivity reactions, including anaphylaxis, have been reported following initial exposure to basiliximab or after repeated courses of therapy separated by several months. Hypersensitivity reactions have included hypotension, tachycardia, wheezing, cardiac failure, dyspnea, bronchospasm, pulmonary edema, respiratory failure, urticaria, rash, pruritis, sneezing, and capillary leak syndrome. It is recommended that patients receiving subsequent courses of basiliximab do so only with extreme caution.[203,204]

Novel Immunosuppressant Mechanisms

Development of new immunosuppressives that target novel mechanisms of action is growing rapidly because of the increasingly detailed understanding of immune events that occur after solid organ transplantation. The critical steps that have been identified allow the creation of new agents that selectively target the signal pathways of these events. These new agents are potentially more selective to prevent and treat acute rejection and, therefore, offer the hope of decreased toxicity while improving efficacy.[208,209]

Sphingosine 1-phosphatase receptor agonists. FTY720 (Novartis) is first in a new class of novel immunomodulators known as sphingosine 1-phosphate receptor (S1P-R) agonists. Stimulation of S1P-Rs by FTY720 prevents the infiltration of lymphocytes into transplanted organs and inflammatory sites by reducing their recirculation from lymphatic tissue to blood and peripheral tissues.[210–212] The effect of FTY720 appears to be completely reversible; it does not impair T-cell activation, expansion, or memory to

viral infections, leaving the host's ability to combat these infections intact.[210] Early clinical trials in kidney transplant recipients demonstrate synergistic effects of FTY720 when used in combination with cyclosporine and everolimus[213,214] without any increase in renal, hepatic, or bone marrow toxicities. A transient decrease in heart rate by an average of 10% from baseline has been reported; heart rates return to baseline within 7–14 days with continued FTY720 dosing.[212] A recent phase III study demonstrated that 2.5 mg of FTY720 plus full-dose cyclosporine provided comparable rejection prophylaxis in de novo renal transplant recipients compared to mycophenolate mofetil. In this trial, FTY720 was associated with lower renal function and macular edema.[215] While the novel mechanism of action of FTY720 may offer potential advantages to current immunosuppressant protocols, the side-effect profile and long-term effects of the drug have yet to be determined. FTY720 is currently an investigational agent not approved in the United States for use in solid organ transplant recipients.

Nondepleting proteins. LEA29Y (Belatacept; Bristol Meyers-Squibb) is a fusion protein combining CTLA-4 with the Fc portion of IgG. It inhibits T-cell activation via selective inhibition of the CD28, CD80, and CD86 costimulatory pathways. Preliminary results of phase II trials in kidney transplant recipients show promise in the efforts to develop calcineurin inhibitor-free immunosuppression protocols.[216–218]

Janus kinase 3 inhibitors. Janus kinase 3 (Jak3) mediates signal transduction via the gamma common chain of lymphokine surface receptors; it is involved in the signaling of IL-2, -4, -7, -9, -15, and -21. It is postulated that inhibition of Jak3 would not cause side effects in other organ systems as the enzyme appears to be restricted to the lymphoid system. The development of Jak3 inhibitors is under way, and early animal studies indicate some success in nonhuman primate models of renal transplantation.[219]

Drug Interactions

The pharmacist plays an important role on the transplant team by providing pharmaceutical care to solid organ transplant recipients. One important component of this service is to monitor and manage drug interactions. Pharmacists are also in a unique position to assist in patient care by coordinating the drug therapy of the transplant patient who is cared for by multiple specialists outside the transplant clinic. The inherent possibility of a drug interaction is magnified not only by the multitude of drugs prescribed for these patients but also by multiple prescribers. It is important to remember that in addition to drug–drug interactions, medications can interact with food or alcohol and that a drug's pharmacokinetics can be altered by the coexisting disease states seen in transplant patients.[220]

It is impossible to be familiar with all potential interactions, so it is important for the practitioner to have a thorough understanding of the fundamental mechanisms of these interactions. Anticipation of potential problems allows for early detection and/or avoidance of troublesome regimens whenever possible. In addition, pharmacists should use their knowledge and understanding of substantiated drug interactions to predict the interactive potential of new compounds.

All immunosuppressive drugs are known to interact with at least a few compounds.[29,221] The consequences of drug interactions in the transplant patient can vary from minor inconveniences, such as more frequent drug concentration monitoring or dosage adjustments, to more life-threatening complications, such as graft rejection, nephrotoxicity, or infection.[222–224] The best documented interactions in the transplant patient are typically pharmacokinetic in origin (based on alterations in the absorption, distribution, metabolism, or excretion of the immunosuppressant, resulting in an alteration in the drug concentration); however, pharmacodynamic interactions (those resulting in altered physiologic or toxicologic effects of the drug) also occur.

Pharmacokinetic interactions. The majority of pharmacokinetic interactions seen in transplant patients are mediated through cytochrome P450 3A4/5, UDP-glucuronyltransferases (UGTs), xanthine oxidase, or the P-glycoprotein (P-gp) system. CsA, tacrolimus, sirolimus, and everolimus are all metabolized or affected by CYP450 3A4/5 and P-gp. They are inducers, substrates, or inhibitors of these two important enzymatic systems as are the majority of drugs they interact with.[77,83,225–229] Mycophenolic acid is primarily metabolized by UGTs.

The liver is the predominant site of metabolism for CsA, tacrolimus, and sirolimus, although human intestinal mucosa also contain high concentrations of the enzymes responsible for metabolism of these drugs.[77,230–232] Presystemic metabolism of these compounds in the small intestine is most likely responsible for their poor bioavailability (CsA 30%, tacrolimus 26%, sirolimus 15–27%).[23,77,231–233] Thus, CYP450 inducers (e.g., phenytoin[234] and rifampin[235–237]) and inhibitors (e.g., erythromycin[238–240]) first alter the

absorption of the compound from the gut and then alter its metabolism by affecting similar enzymes in the liver. Interactions with these compounds are less problematic when either of these agents is administered intravenously, again providing evidence that the interactions occur at sites other than just the liver.[240,241]

Grapefruit juice has been shown to facilitate the absorption of CsA and that of other drugs, presumably by inhibiting its gut metabolism.[242–244] Grapefruit juice does not affect systemic clearance when CsA is administered intravenously.[245] The exact mechanism is not known, but flavanoids (particularly naringin) in grapefruit juice may inhibit CYP450-3A4.[242] Another consideration is that interactions involving absorption (i.e., altered CYP450 activity in the small intestine) are more problematic when two interacting agents are administered simultaneously rather than at different dosing intervals.[246,247] This may also account for some of the intra- and interpatient variability seen when patients alter the timing of medication administration to accommodate lifestyle changes.

Other interactions, such as those between AZA and concomitant allopurinol, also occur predominantly in the small intestine; allopurinol blocks xanthine oxidase function in the gut, causing a three- to fourfold increase in AZA absorption. This interaction is also far less significant when AZA is administered intravenously.[248,249]

Pharmacodynamic interactions. Nephrotoxicity is the primary side effect observed in all patients maintained on CsA[250,251] and tacrolimus.[63] Theoretically, any drug capable of causing nephrotoxicity may exacerbate CsA's and tacrolimus's nephrotoxicity. Whether the effects of administering two or more nephrotoxic agents is additive or synergistic remains to be determined.

Several drugs, including aminoglycosides, amphotericin B, acyclovir, ganciclovir, diclofenac, ibuprofen, indomethacin, sulindac, melphalan, and others, have been reported to increase CsA's nephrotoxicity.[252]

Acute CsA nephrotoxicity is concentration-dependent and is usually reversible following dosage reduction. Chronic nephrotoxicity is irreversible and may be a consequence of persistent renal vasoconstriction and mesangial cell proliferation with resultant glomerulosclerosis. The vasoconstriction appears to be mediated by an increased production of thromboxane A_2 and endothelin. A number of agents, including captopril, enisoprostil, misoprostil,[253] and pentoxifylline,[254] have been studied for their potentially beneficial renal-protective effects. The calcium-channel antagonists (e.g., verapamil, diltiazem, felodipine, nifedipine, nicardipine, and isradipine) appear to be most promising.[255,256] These agents may block the endothelin-induced constriction of smooth muscle cells that is dependent on the influx of calcium.[257] This mechanism may also explain, at least in part, the efficacy of calcium antagonists for the treatment of CsA-induced hypertension.

In addition to a decrease in glomerular filtration rate and an increase in serum creatinine and blood urea nitrogen, other CsA-induced laboratory abnormalities include hypomagnesemia, hyperkalemia, and hyperuricemia. Patients treated with CsA commonly require aggressive magnesium supplementation to maintain serum magnesium concentrations at the lower end of the normal range. In addition, a number of other medications used concomitantly in CsA-treated patients may exacerbate these fluid and electrolyte derangements (e.g., diuretics may cause hyperuricemia and gout, hypomagnesemia, or enhanced nephrotoxicity with volume depletion). Potassium-sparing diuretics (e.g., spironolactone, amiloride, and triamterene), β-blockers, and angiotensin-converting enzyme inhibitors may exacerbate hyperkalemia.

Other complications of CsA that are difficult to manage include hypertension and hyperlipidemia. Both these conditions can be complicated by the administration of other drugs capable of exacerbating hypertension (e.g., corticosteroids) and hyperlipidemia (e.g., diuretics, β-blockers) in CsA-treated patients. These disorders require aggressive strategies, including dietary modifications, multidrug regimens, and, if necessary, reduction of CsA concentration or discontinuation of therapy. CsA has also been associated with a number of benign but troublesome dose-related side effects, such as hirsutism, neurotoxicity, and gingival hyperplasia.

Other pharmacodynamic interactions with immunosuppressive agents include enhanced bone marrow toxicity observed with the antiproliferative agents and drugs known to suppress the bone marrow (e.g., trimethoprim–sulfamethoxazole and ganciclovir) that are also commonly used in transplant recipients. Minoxidil and other drugs may exacerbate the hypertrichosis and hirsutism seen with CsA and steroids.

Management of drug interactions. Managing confirmed immunosuppressant drug interactions requires proactive measures, such as altering the dose of the affected drug on either initiation or discontinuation of the interacting agent; measuring drug concentrations; and monitoring renal function tests, creatinine phosphokinase concentrations, and any other tests indicative of pharmacologic or toxic response.

Because of the number of drug interactions reported with CsA, tacrolimus, and sirolimus, it is useful to categorize the interactions based on severity to assist the pharmacist in making therapeutic decisions. Table 9.10 lists drugs known to increase or decrease the concentrations of these immunosuppressants.

Serious interactions. Serious interactions are those that cause the serum concentrations of the object drug to increase at least three- to fourfold, which usually correspond to a significantly increased risk of toxicity. The most serious interactions require immediate intervention on initiation of the concomitant interactant. One such interactant is ketoconazole, which inhibits the metabolism of CsA, tacrolimus, and sirolimus. Of the azole antifungals, ketoconazole is the most potent inhibitor of the CYP450 system, and, as expected, CsA dosage reductions of up to 80% are necessary during concomitant therapy.[258,259] Unless the CsA dose is reduced at the outset of concomitant therapy, CsA concentrations rise dramatically within 24–48 hours, placing the patient at unnecessary risk for nephrotoxicity. Similar reductions in tacrolimus and sirolimus doses would be needed to avoid toxicity.

Tacrolimus concentrations have been reported to rise with fluconazole[260,261] and clotrimazole,[262] so suspicion should be high for all of the azole antifungals, just as it is with CsA.[258] Because tacrolimus has such a narrow therapeutic index, it may be even more susceptible to potentially negative interactions. With tacrolimus (as well as with CsA), a doubling of the drug concentration may cause serious consequences in a patient maintained on concentrations at the higher end of the therapeutic range. Other CYP450 enzyme inhibitors with documented serious interactions with immunosuppressants include the protease inhibitors, specifically ritonavir.[263]

Enzyme inducers, such as phenytoin, phenobarbital, rifampin, and highly active antiretroviral therapy (HAART), can also cause serious interactions with CsA, tacrolimus, and sirolimus.[261,263–265] Before these drug interactions were well recognized, a number of patients experienced acute rejection episodes and lost their grafts when their CsA concentrations were found to be undetectable. In contrast to the concomitant administration of enzyme inhibitors, during which the dosage of these immunosuppressants must be reduced dramatically to counterbalance decreased metabolism, with concurrent enzyme-inducer therapy the dosage must be increased at least two- to threefold to maintain therapeutic drug concentrations.

The other important point to remember about these interactions is that when the enzyme inducer is discontinued, the effect may persist up to 2–3 weeks, necessitating more frequent drug concentration monitoring not only when initiating therapy but also after discontinuing the interacting drug. The timeframe for reversal of enzyme inhibition depends on whether it is because of actual inhibition of enzyme function or competition for the same metabolic site; the latter will reverse upon elimination of the competing drug from the site of metabolism.

Another serious interaction occurs between AZA and allopurinol.[96] The dosage of AZA needs to be reduced by 75% when allopurinol is added to the regimen. The serious consequences of this interaction (e.g., profound pancytopenia) are not usually clinically evident for 4–6 weeks because of the prolonged half-life of the TGNs and delayed impact on marrow production. Toxicity can be detected by frequent complete blood count monitoring, though it is better to prevent the consequences of profound marrow suppression than to deal with them after they occur.

Because of the potentially serious consequences of these interactions, the need to alter the dosage of the object drug (e.g., CsA, tacrolimus, sirolimus, or AZA) must be taken into consideration when initiating concomitant therapy.

Moderately serious interactions. Moderately problematic interactions include those that can cause a twofold rise in drug concentrations of the object drug. Some of the drugs that have this effect with CsA, tacrolimus, and sirolimus—presumably by competing for the same CYP450 substrate—include erythromycin[238-240] and some of the calcium-channel blockers. Diltiazem, verapamil, and nicardipine inhibit CsA's metabolism; diltiazem is the most potent.[266-272] Dosage reductions of about 50% can be expected with diltiazem, and smaller reductions are needed with the other drugs. With moderately problematic drug interactions, the time to alter the dosage of the drug may depend on the initial drug concentrations. For instance, when adding diltiazem therapy to a patient who has a low therapeutic CsA concentration, it may be better to alter the CsA dosage once the concentrations begin to rise rather than at the outset of therapy. This increases the inconvenience for the patient as more frequent monitoring is required, but the risk for rejection would be minimized.

Minor interactions. These interactions occur when an increase in CsA concentration of less than 50% is observed during concomitant therapy. In this situation, awareness of the interaction is important and must be considered in light of the clinical status of the patient. Unless the patient has very labile renal function or high therapeutic levels, dosage adjustments of immunosuppressants can usually be made once the interaction becomes evident, rather than at the outset of therapy.

Other considerations. When selecting agents to treat the various medical problems of transplant patients, it is important to consider whether the treatment is for an acute (requiring less than 2–3 weeks of therapy) or a chronic medical condition. In acute cases, it is preferable to avoid drug interactions because of the inconvenience associated with dosage adjustments and more frequent monitoring. The use of alternative (noninteracting) agents is usually preferable in the short-term (e.g., 7–14 days) when equally effective agents are available. Obviously, if therapeutically equivalent products are not available, then it is most appropriate to use the drug of choice for the condition and deal with the resulting drug interaction. For example, short-term erythromycin therapy (e.g., a 10- to 14-day course) is usually discouraged because it is inconvenient to adjust the dose of immunosuppression for a short period of time and then readjust it. But in the case of endocarditis prophylaxis in a penicillin-allergic patient, it may be appropriate to administer the standard two doses of erythromycin if the patient's CsA, tacrolimus, or sirolimus concentration is moderately low. The increased absorption and inhibited metabolism of these immunosuppressants following one or two doses of erythromycin should not have a major effect on the patient's kidney function unless renal dysfunction is already present. In the case of enzyme inducers, if chronic anticonvulsant drug therapy is needed in a transplant patient, then it is best to use the agent of choice for the seizure type and deal with the drug interaction to ensure optimal immunosuppressive and anticonvulsant efficacy.

The impact on the patient's quality of life should also be considered in drug interactions. Additional monitoring, more frequent clinic visits, and dosage adjustments may cause an unnecessary burden in a long-term patient who returns to the clinic infrequently. Because calcium-channel blockers are often used in transplant patients and a number of calcium-channel blockers are available, it seems prudent to consider what impact the drug interaction will have on the patient's quality of life. The initiation of interacting agents (e.g., diltiazem or nicardipine) is most easily accomplished soon after transplantation, when patients generally need more frequent monitoring. But several years after a transplant, when a patient has returned to work or school, the increased frequency of monitoring and corresponding dosage adjustments may be inconvenient. For these patients it may be preferable to initiate a noninteracting calcium-channel blocker, such as nifedipine, amlodipine, or felodipine.[221]

Finally, patient compliance must be considered, especially when dealing with serious interactions. Utmost compliance is necessary when a drug interaction results in a significant dosage reduction of the immunosuppressive agent. The most dramatic impact would be seen in a patient on concomitant CsA, tacrolimus, or sirolimus and ketoconazole in whom the immunosuppressant dosage has been reduced to 20% of the previous steady-state dose. Many of these patients are maintained on very low doses, so if the patient either stops taking ketoconazole or takes it sporadically, the level of immunosuppression may drop precipitously, predisposing the patient to rejection. Similar problems can occur even if the immunosuppressant dosage has only been reduced by 50% (e.g., by interaction with diltiazem), especially if the patient is running borderline low concentrations. Compliance is a critical factor for transplant patients, so consideration must be given when adding drugs that interact and mandate dosage alterations of the immunosuppressant. Compliance is equally important in a patient on an enzyme inducer (e.g., phenytoin) in whom the CsA, tacrolimus, or sirolimus dose has been tripled to achieve therapeutic concentrations. At these high doses, the cost of therapy may become prohibitive and patients may not be able to afford prolonged concomitant therapy.

When making recommendations about drug interactions, pharmacists must be familiar with the available drug interaction literature and have a thorough understanding of pharmacokinetic and pharmacodynamic principles of drug interactions. Pharmacists also need to rely on their expertise and practical experience when trying to predict whether an interaction may occur with a new drug. Anticipating drug interactions promotes the development of a monitoring strategy for the patient when it is not known whether new compounds interact with immunosuppressive drugs. Being aware of some of the problematic therapeutic classes (e.g., azole antifungals, calcium-channel blockers, and nephrotoxic drugs) is useful when considering the likelihood of an interaction. Even though it is difficult to predict the extent of an interaction in an individual patient, being aware of whether the drug is metabolized via the same CYP450 enzymes as the immunosuppressive agent at least raises the level of suspicion and allows the pharmacist to develop a monitoring strategy for the transplant patient.

PART II—COMPLICATIONS AFTER SOLID ORGAN TRANSPLANTATION

Graft and patient survival following solid organ transplantation have increased dramatically because of a variety of factors: identification of better patient selection parameters; improvements in tissue-typing techniques; development of more specific immunosuppressive regimens; improvements in organ preservation; refinement of surgical technique; improvements in the recognition, distinction, and treatment of allograft rejection; and introduction of effective agents for the prophylaxis and treatment of all types of opportunistic infections.[273–279] Major complications arise from an imbalance in the recipient's overall level of immunosuppression. Preventing rejection with immunosuppressants may increase the risk of infection and malignancy. The ultimate goal of immunosuppressive therapy is to develop tolerance to the graft while leaving intact the host's defenses against microbial pathogens and tumors.

INFECTIOUS COMPLICATIONS

The clinical approach to infectious complications after solid organ transplant involves a careful analysis of clinical presentation, diagnostic tests and procedures, specific risk factors, and preventive strategies used.[280] Risk factor analysis is key in determining the likely pathogen as well as appropriate clinical interventions and anti-infective treatments. The use of various anti-infective agents in transplant recipients is generally classified into three treatment strategies: prophylaxis, preemptive therapy, and treatment. *Prophylaxis* refers to the administration of preventive agents to all individuals and implies a low-toxicity regimen for a high-risk group. *Preemptive therapy* is the selective administration of preventive agents based on specific indicators of high risk for infection. *Treatment* indicates therapeutic intervention with curative agents for an established infection. Pharmacologic, pharmacoeconomic, and anti-infective resistance considerations have pressured the transplant clinician to evolve from generalized prophylaxis to selective preemptive therapy.

Bacterial Infections

Strategies for prevention and treatment should focus on the most common pathogens at the suspected or potential site of infection in conjunction with the specific risk factors of the type of organ transplant or the intended procedure. Although immunosuppression compromises the host's ability to fight active infections, specific agents have not been linked to an increased risk of bacterial infections.

The prevention of posttransplant infection should focus on discriminate pre- and posttransplant antibiotic therapy. Unnecessary use of long courses of therapy and broad-spectrum antibiotics can result in significant resistance and predispose patients to other pathogenic organisms. Increasing reports of enterococcal and gram-negative rod bacterial resistance in transplant recipients are most likely because of indiscriminate and prolonged antibiotic therapy in this population. Other preventive strategies have focused on specific populations of transplant patients. Prophylaxis against viral pathogens and other opportunistic infections appears to contribute to a lower incidence of concurrent bacterial infections.

Viral Infections

Posttransplant viral infections are generally divided into the herpes group viruses, rare pathogens, and the hepatotrophic viruses. Only the herpes viruses and the rare pathogens will be discussed here; the most common pathogens in each classification are listed in **Table 9.11**. These viral pathogens have a significant clinical impact on patient and graft survival, causing clinical infection and disease, increased susceptibility to other bacterial or fungal pathogens because of secondary immunosuppression, indirect and direct allograft injury, and increased risk of malignancy.[281,282] There is growing evidence of the relationship between CMV infection and the subsequent development of acute and chronic rejection.[283] So preventive strategies against common viral pathogens are key focuses of clinical practice and research in solid organ transplant recipients.

Herpes group viruses. *Cytomegalovirus.* CMV remains the most prevalent viral pathogen in transplant recipients, causing symptomatic infection in up to 60% of this population.[284] CMV presents either latently, without viral replication, or as active infection, with subsequent viral shedding and immune activation.[289] CMV infection is often classified on the basis of donor and recipient CMV IgG antibody status at the time of transplant, the highest risk being the CMV-positive donor/CMV-negative recipient patient. Symptomatic CMV infection generally presents as a flu-like syndrome, often in combination with leukopenia. CMV disease is the progression to invasive infection with biochemical, histopathologic, or radiographic evidence of organ involvement.

Table 9.11. Prophylaxis and Treatment of Posttransplant Infections

Infection	Prophylaxis	Treatment
Cytomegalovirus	Valganciclovir	IV Ganciclovir
	Ganciclovir	Valganciclovir
	Cytogam	Cytogam
		Foscarnet
		Cidofovir
Herpes virus	Acyclovir	Acyclovir
		Valacyclovir
Varicella virus	Vaccination?	Acyclovir
Epstein Barr virus	Unknown	Reduced immunosuppression
		Rituximab
Polyoma virus	Reduction in immunosuppression	Cidofovir
P jiroveci	SMZ/TMP	SMZ/TMP
	Dapsone	
	Atovaquone	
	Pentamidine	
Fungal	Nystatin	Triazoles
	Triazoles	Polyenes (Amphotericin B; lipid formulations)
		Echinocandins (caspofungin, micafungin)

SMZ/TMP = sulfamethoxazole/trimethoprim.

The greatest risk for symptomatic CMV infection is during the first 2–3 months following transplantation.[284] In addition to donor and recipient serology, other risk factors for CMV infection include net immunosuppression, type of organ transplanted, blood product exposure, recipient age, HLA phenotyping, cadaveric transplants, and retransplants.[284–286] The specific role of immunosuppression depends on the ability of the agent to either stimulate reactivation or amplify viral replication.[285] Antilymphocyte antibody preparations (OKT3, ATG, and thymoglobulin) are associated with a high risk of CMV reactivation from latency, whereas steroids, AZA, mycophenolic acid, CsA, tacrolimus, and sirolimus are associated with a low-to-moderate risk of viral reactivation.[285] Conversely, cyclosporine, tacrolimus, and sirolimus potently amplify viral replication after reactivation has occurred. So the sequence and duration of specific immunotherapeutic agents are keys to the subsequent development of CMV disease.

General strategies for the prevention of CMV infection have focused on avoidance of viral exposure, use of preemptive indicators to predict high-risk patients, and immunologic and pharmacologic inhibition of viral reactivation and replication. Strategies for avoiding viral exposure include donor/recipient serologic matching as well as serologic screening or leukocyte filtration of blood products.[285] Primary attention has been directed at the use of various antiviral agents such as acyclovir and ganciclovir and valganciclovir in the prevention and treatment of CMV infection.

High-dose oral acyclovir (3200 mg/day) initially demonstrated protection against CMV in renal transplant recipients.[287] But subsequent studies failed to demonstrate efficacy in high-risk recipients, so this regimen has been abandoned in the prevention of CMV infection. Prevention strategies include ganciclovir 5 mg/kg iv q12 and oral ganciclovir at 1000 mg po tid x 100 days.[288] Valganciclovir is a valine ester prodrug of ganciclovir with improved bioavailability compared with oral ganciclovir. This allows for convenient once-daily dosing for CMV prophylaxis at a dose of 900 mg.[288]

The new era of CMV diagnosis is based on the pp65 antigenemia assay, a semiquantitative fluorescent assay based on detection of infected cells in peripheral blood. This assay has higher sensitivity and specificity than culture-based methods and is comparable in sensitivity to some CMV PCR assays. Both the pp65 antigenemia assay and the CMV nucleic acid testing can be used to follow the time course of resolution of a CMV episode.[288] Preemptive therapy is a suitable option for patients at low or intermediate risk for CMV disease. The best lab test for monitoring is either a nucleic acid detection test (DNA or RNA) or a CMV antigenemia assay. The optimal monitoring strategy is unknown, but weekly testing for 12 weeks posttransplant is suggested.[288] The optimal drug for preemptive therapy is unknown but could include IV ganciclovir 5 mg/kg bid or oral valganciclovir 900 mg bid.[288] Oral ganciclovir can be used but should be avoided in patients with high-level viremia because of the risk of drug resistance.[288] Drug therapy should be continued for a minimum of 1 week and preferably until the CMV detection test is negative.

Therapeutic options for treating CMV disease include IV ganciclovir, oral ganciclovir, or oral valganciclovir. Currently IV ganciclovir is the preferred agent for treating CMV disease in solid organ transplant recipients. Established CMV disease is generally treated with therapeutic doses of intravenous ganciclovir (5 mg/kg twice daily) for 14–28 days, depending on the severity of illness. In cases of life-threatening disease, adjunctive therapy with immune globulin preparations is recommended. Oral valganciclovir at a dose of 900 mg bid has been shown to be equivalent to IV ganciclovir 5 mg/kg q12. Ganciclovir-resistant CMV appears to be an increasing problem in solid organ transplant recipients; resistance is most commonly due to mutations in the CMV UL97 gene, which codes for a viral protein kinase responsible for initial phosphorylation of ganciclovir.[288] Risk factors for development of resistance include CMV+/– serostatus, more potent immunosuppression, and prolonged use of oral ganciclovir. Cidofovir and foscarnet can be used to treat ganciclovir resistant CMV disease in solid-organ transplant recipients. Both agents are limited by their toxicity profiles, which include nephrotoxicity.

Epstein-Barr virus. Epstein-Barr virus (EBV), a member of the herpes family of viruses, infects B lymphocytes and squamous epithelial cells and has been linked to the development of posttransplant lymphoproliferative disease (PTLD).[289] After acute EBV infection, immunocompetent patients develop an asymptomatic persistent infection in which cytotoxic T cells suppress the acute infection into a latent state. But in transplant recipients, immunosuppression results in loss of this immune control, which can lead to uncontrolled B-cell proliferation and eventual lymphoma formation.[290] The clinical presentation of PTLD can vary widely from a mild viral illness to a fulminant, rapidly fatal disease. The mild form may present with fever, malaise, and lymphadenopathy. Tumors in the gastrointestinal tract often present as acute abdominal pain with subsequent perforation, obstruction, or bleeding.[291,292] PTLD also commonly presents as tumors in the central nervous system or the allograft.

The two primary factors contributing to EBV-related PTLD are pretransplant immune status to the virus and the net level of immunosuppression.[293] Transplant patients naive to the virus are at a greater risk for primary infection and progression to PTLD secondary to personal contact, exposure to blood products, or infection by the transplanted organ. In patients previously infected with EBV, reactivation of the latent virus appears to be directly related to the immunosuppressive regimen administered. The incidence of lymphoma appears closely correlated with the overall intensity of immunosuppression. This is reflected by higher lymphoma rates in cardiac and liver transplant recipients, who receive more intense immunosuppression than do renal transplant patients.[294] As with CMV, antilymphocyte agents appear to be associated with significant reactivation of EBV and resultant PTLD. Initial reports suggested OKT3 was associated with a greater risk than polyclonal preparations, but subsequent analyses have established equivalent risk with monoclonal and polyclonal antibody therapy.[295–298] More important, the duration of therapy and the proximity of multiple courses of antilymphocyte preparations appear to be the primary risk factors, not the total dose.

The term PTLD refers to a highly diverse spectrum of disease states that varies greatly in clinical presentation. The disease may be nodal or extranodal, localized often in the graft, or widely disseminated.[299] Patients may be symptomatic or asymptomatic, and pathology remains the definitive diagnosis. In the absence of reliably effective therapy for all stages of PTLD, the optimal strategy for management currently focuses on prevention. Both acyclovir and ganciclovir may be useful as prophylactic antiviral agents for the prevention of PTLD, although this is more theoretical than proven.[299] It has been observed that PTLD spontaneously regresses in 23% to 50% of cases following decrease in immunosuppression, making reduction of immunosuppression the primary approach to management.[299–301] The duration of immunosuppression decrease or discontinuance is unclear, so monitoring for rejection is paramount. Surgical resection for tumor debulking as management for local complications associated with PTLD has been used as adjunctive therapy with immunosuppression reduction. If reduction in immunosuppression fails, the B-cell monoclonal antibody targeted against the CD20 receptor is an attractive second-line therapeutic option because of low toxicity. Rituximab (anti-CD 20 antibody) at a dose of 375 mg/m[2] weekly for 4 weeks based on clinical response has shown response rates of 61% to 76% in solid organ transplant recipients with PTLD.[301,302]

Other herpes group viruses. Infection with herpes simplex virus (HSV-1, -2) is generally confined to latent infections reactivated by immunosuppression or other stress factors.[303] Most infections are confined to mucocutaneous sites, but occasional rare invasive infections can occur. Prevention or treatment with standard doses of acyclovir (oral or intravenous) or oral valacyclovir is generally effective. A significant decrease in HSV infections is a secondary result of using CMV preventive strategies.[304]

Varicella-zoster virus (VZV) infections present as a primary infection (chickenpox) or as reactivation (shingles).[305] VZV will occasionally present as severe hepatitis, pneumonitis, or encephalitis. Recent advances in prevention of primary VZV infection include using the varicella-zoster vaccine. Further data are needed regarding its use in transplant recipients. Treatment of established infections with high-dose acyclovir offers variable results with chicken pox but appears to attenuate the duration and severity of other VZV infections.

Polyomavirus. Infection with BK virus (a polyoma virus) occurs worldwide with seroprevalence rates as high as 60% to 80% reported among adults in the United States and Europe.[306,307] In recent years, polyomavirus-associated nephropathy (PVAN) has become a major complication of renal transplantation; estimated prevalence is 1% to 10% of all renal transplant recipients.[306,307] The majority of cases appear to result from reactivation of latent virus. Among renal transplant recipients, tubulointerstitial nephritis is the most common manifestation of BK disease and typically manifests as elevation in serum creatinine, which can be misdiagnosed as rejection or drug toxicity.[306,307] Definitive diagnosis of BK virus infection requires a renal biopsy. To date there is no consensus on the optimal management of BK virus disease. Published data suggest that reduction of immunosuppression is the first-line approach.[310–314] Intravenous cidofovir 0.25–1.0 mg/kg every 2–3 weeks for a total of 1–4 doses has been shown to be a potent and highly selective inhibitor of BK virus and has greater activity than other nucleoside analog agents in vitro.[306–310] But cidofovir's nephrotoxicity profile may limit its use. Further research is needed to delineate the role of various screening tools and the role of other agents in the treatment of BK virus disease.

Fungal Infections

Fungal infections following solid organ transplantation are a major cause of morbidity and mortality. Management of fungal infections varies widely among different transplant centers. Large multicenter, randomized controlled trials evaluating risk factors, diagnosis, prophylaxis, and treatment strategies in organ transplant recipients are lacking, so no uniform consensus exists. *Candida* and *Aspergillus* species account for the majority of these infections, although the incidence is higher among recipients of organs other than kidneys because those patients receive more immunosuppressive therapy.[311] Attack rates range from 5% among kidney allograft recipients to 40% among liver graft recipients. Risk factors that predispose to fungal infection in the latter group include renal insufficiency, length of the transplant operation, and the need for re-exploration or retransplantation.[312] *Aspergillus* infection in these patients is characterized by pulmonary localization with subsequent dissemination; infection with *Candida albicans* is most often disseminated but rarely involves the lungs. *Aspergillus* infection of the lungs is associated with high mortality despite aggressive treatment with amphotericin B. Superficial infections may also occur in the oropharynx with *Candida* species, or on the skin or nail beds with dermatophytes. The latter may be particularly resistant to treatment and can be a cause of considerable discomfort and concern to patients.

Although amphotericin B remains the drug of choice for treatment of invasive aspergillosis, its toxicity limits its widespread use. Liposomal formulations of amphotericin B have shown promise in ameliorating the toxicity associated with amphotericin B deoxycholate and may be preferred for transplant recipients.[313] Newer agents such as the echinocandins (caspofungin and micafungin) have also shown promise in the treatment of invasive aspergillosis infection in solid organ transplant recipients.[314] Recent experience suggests that fluconazole may be a safe and effective alternative for the treatment of fungal infections caused by *Candida* species or *Cryptococcus neoformans*. Prevention of fungal infections remains one of the most important goals in transplantation. New approaches, such as the use of prophylactic or preemptive therapy for patients at greatest risk of developing infection, may help.[304,315]

Nystatin administered as swish-and-swallow suspension or clotrimazole troches three times daily for 6 months are used to prevent fungal colonization and infection. Clinicians must be aware of potential drug interaction with the new antifungal agents (such as caspofungin) and maintenance immunosuppressive therapy, particularly cyclosporine and tacrolimus. The azole antifungal agents also have documented drug interactions with cyclosporine and tacrolimus that must be taken into account when optimizing therapy in transplant recipients.

Opportunistic Infections

Opportunistic infections after organ transplantation may occur with *Pneumocystis jiroveci* (formerly *Pneumocystis carinii*) or *Toxoplasma gondii*. In most solid organ transplant recipients treated with standard immunosuppression, the risk of *P jiroveci* is 5% to 15%.[316] Pneumocystis pneumonia is usually subacute to acute in onset and develops over a few days to weeks. Patients may develop progressive dyspnea, tachypnea, cyanosis, and a nonproductive cough. Prophylaxis with trimethoprim–sulfamethoxazole one single-strength tablet daily or three times a week or one double-strength tablet daily or three times a week for 6 months seems appropriate, but duration of prophylactic regimen varies among transplant centers.[316] Dapsone 100 mg daily, pentamidine 300–600 mg inhaled once a month, and atovaquone 1500 mg daily are recommended alternatives for prophylaxis of *P jiroveci* in patients with a true sulfur allergy. Treatment for *P jiroveci* includes trimethoprim–sulfamethoxazole 15–20 mg/kg/day IV ± corticosteroids for patients with significant hypoxemia.

HYPERTENSION

Hypertension, a significant risk factor for morbidity and mortality in the general population, is a factor in at least 60% to 80% of transplant cases.[317] Cardiovascular disease is the primary cause of death in 30% to 40% of patients with functioning renal allografts.[317] Treatment of hypertension usually mandates the use of multiple drugs, some of which interact with immunosuppressive therapy, further increasing the risk of drug-related complications and noncompliance.

The pathogenesis of hypertension in solid organ recipients is multifactorial and includes immunosuppressive therapy (e.g., CsA, steroids, tacrolimus), renal disease (including CsA or tacrolimus-induced nephrotoxicity), recurrent essential hypertension, or other causes of secondary hypertension. Renal transplant recipients may become hypertensive with chronic rejection or recurrence of their diabetic nephropathy.[317]

The complications of posttransplant hypertension are presumed to be a heightened risk of cardiovascular disease and allograft failure, so hypertension should be aggressively treated in all patients. The Seventh Report of the Joint National Committee on Prevention, Detection, Evaluation and Treatment of High Blood Pressure (JNC VII) guideline for managing hypertension in the setting of chronic kidney disease recommends a target blood pressure of less than 130/80 mm Hg. Nonpharmacologic measures such as weight loss, moderation of sodium intake, moderation of alcohol intake, and increased exercise should be emphasized. The dosage of corticosteroids, cyclosporine, and tacrolimus should be minimized when possible.[317] Many patients need more than one antihypertensive agent to control blood pressure. Calcium-channel blockers and β-blockers are considered first-line therapy. Diuretics, angiotensin-converting enzyme inhibitors, and angiotensin-receptor blockers should be used with caution in the first 3 months posttransplantation in kidney recipients; they have been known to cause elevations in serum creatinine and potassium levels. But these agents may be appropriate as first-line therapy in other organ transplant recipients.[317]

Calcium-channel blockers, particularly those of the dihydropyridine class, are preferred antihypertensive agents because of their favorable effects on renal blood flow and serum lipid profile.[255] Angiotensin-converting enzyme inhibitors are also effective, but they can compromise renal blood flow and exacerbate the hyperkalemia associated with CsA in the early posttransplant period.

HYPERLIPIDEMIA

Hyperlipidemia occurs in the majority of solid organ recipients following transplantation.[318–323] The prevalence of hypercholesterolemia and hypertrigylceridemia after transplantation has been estimated at 60% and 35%, respectively. Many renal and cardiac transplant recipients have preexisting hyperlipidemia, which may have contributed to their end-stage organ disease, and transplantation of the corresponding organ does not correct their hyperlipidemia. Following transplantation, these patients receive medications such as corticosteroids, cyclosporine, and sirolimus as maintenance therapy that may further exacerbate their hyperlipidemia.[317] Because cardiovascular disease is so prevalent in these patients, it is reasonable to consider the renal transplant recipient's status a "coronary heart disease risk equivalent" when applying the guidelines. This implies targeting plasma low-density lipoprotein cholesterol levels <100 mg/dL through a combination of therapeutic lifestyle changes and drug therapy. Statins are the cholesterol-lowering agent of choice in transplant recipients. Because the metabolism of statins is partly inhibited by calciuneurin inhibitors such as cyclosporine, blood concentrations of statins may be increased in transplant recipients, increasing the risk for adverse effects such as rhabdomyolysis. Measures to minimize the risk of statin toxicity include starting with low statin doses; using pravastatin or fluvastatin (which appear to have the least interactions with cyclosporine); and avoiding other inhibitors of the CYP3A4 system. Rarely, nonstatin drugs are used to lower plasma lipids in transplant patients. Fibrates and ezetimibe should be prescribed with caution because of their drug interaction with cyclosporine.[324,325] Cholestyramine is not effective in lowering plasma lipids in transplant recipients and should be avoided.

NEW ONSET DIABETES AFTER TRANSPLANTATION

Diabetes mellitus is the leading cause of end-stage renal disease in the U.S. Glucose control worsens after transplantation because of long-term corticosteroid use, increased food intake, weight gain, and restoration of kidney function. Risk factors for posttransplant diabetes include greater recipient age, nonwhite ethnicity, steroid treatment for rejection, and high doses of CNI (particularly high-dose tacrolimus, which is diabetogenic).[317] The incidence of native diabetes mellitus in solid organ recipients varies with the type of organ transplanted. The significance of new-onset diabetes after transplantation (NODAT) is the development of diabetic micro- and macrovascular complications (e.g., coronary heart disease, stroke, retinopathy, nephropathy, or neuropathy) and the higher incidence of infections—all of which can increase morbidity and mortality. This is especially worrisome because it appears that many immunosuppressive agents pose a triple threat by causing hyperlipidemia, hypertension, and hyperglycemia, increasing the risk of death by coronary disease or stroke.[326]

Corticosteroids have been reported to decrease insulin receptor number and affinity, impair peripheral glucose uptake in the muscle, impair suppression of endogenous glucose production, impair activation of the glucose/fatty acid cycle,[327] and induce insulin resistance.[326] Because reducing steroid dosages has a beneficial effect on PTDM, some centers have advocated the use of steroid-weaning protocols in their diabetic patients; this must be weighed against the risks of both acute and chronic rejection.

Both CsA and tacrolimus are diabetogenic. An increased incidence of PTDM (11% to 14%) was seen following the introduction of CsA-based regimens, despite a reduction in steroid dosage. CsA may inhibit the clearance of steroids, potentiating their diabetogenic effects[328]; but studies have shown that CsA also affects glycemic control in patients not receiving steroids.[329] CsA has been shown to directly inhibit pancreatic islet cell function and insulin release.[330] Initially, because of tacrolimus's steroid-sparing effects, it was assumed that NODAT would be less problematic with this agent. In fact, the incidence appears to be similar or higher than with CsA-based regimens.[331] With the recent use of lower tacrolimus target trough concentrations, the incidence of NODAT in tacrolimus-based regimens is comparable to that of CSA-based regimens. These agents may impair insulin secretion, increase insulin resistance, or be directly toxic to beta cells in the pancreas. Finally, it is important to remember that, in addition to the primary immunosuppressive agents, many transplant patients may receive other drugs known to exacerbate glycemic control, including thiazide diuretics and β-blockers. Pharmacists can play an important role by identifying drug therapy that can impair glucose tolerance and providing recommendations for alternative agents in these patients. Treatment of diabetes in the transplant patient is similar to that for other diabetic patients; meticulous diabetic control should be the goal in these patients, and a thorough understanding of the added risks and complications is needed to ensure survival comparable to nondiabetic organ transplant recipients.[317]

BONE AND MUSCLE DISORDERS

Bone loss following transplantation is usually rapid in the early phase posttransplantation with stabilization after 1 year; fracture rates are variable and often extremely high.[332] Compared with expected rates in the normal population, fracture incidence was five times higher in male kidney recipients[332] and 18–34 times higher in female kidney recipients. Kidney transplant recipients lose bone early from sites rich in trabecular bone. Bone mineral density (BMD) decreased in the lumbar spine by 5% in the first year, and longitudinal studies showed lumbar spine bone loss of 1.7% annually.[333] Bone loss following cardiac, liver, and lung transplantation is strikingly high during the first 6 months posttransplant with fracture rates to match, ranging from 22% to 36%, 24% to 65%, and as high as 73%, respectively.[332] Reduction in BMD is now recognized as a very common complication of solid organ transplantation. The principal cause is long-term corticosteroid use resulting in direct inhibition of osteoblastogenesis, induction of apoptosis in bone cells, inhibition of sex hormone production, and increased urinary calcium excretion.[317] Corticosteroid complications include osteoporosis, osteopenia, avascular necrosis, and growth retardation.

Early intervention with bisphophonates, which remain bound to skeletal tissues for years, may benefit renal transplant patients for a long time after the bisphophonates therapy has ceased. Bisphosphonates also show promise in cardiac, lung, and liver transplantation. Use of bisphosphonates like intravenous pamidronate has shown excellent results in prevention strategies, with prolonged benefit up to 4 years. IV pamidronate was clearly more effective than nasal calcinonin plus calcitriol

in patients following cardiac transplantation. The use of vitamin D, supplemental calcium, and activated vitamin D such as calcitriol has been evaluated in a number of studies. No regimen has yet reported convincing reduction of fracture rates in these patients.[317] Steroid withdrawal protocols are being investigated as a strategy to decrease the risk of osteopenia and osteoporosis in transplant recipients.

Guidelines for prevention and management of osteoporosis in transplant recipients include measuring hip and spine BMD prior to transplantation. If BMD is low, patients should receive calcium and vitamin D (1000–1500 mg/day of calcium and 400–800 international units per day of vitamin D). Studies show that bone loss is most rapid immediately after transplantation and fractures may occur very early. Bisphosphonates have been shown to be the most promising approach for the prevention and treatment of posttransplant osteoporosis.[333]

SUMMARY

Recent advances in solid organ transplantation can be attributed to a number of factors, especially immunosuppressive therapy. The introduction of cyclosporine in the late 1970s allowed the successful transplantation of many previously untransplantable organs. In the past decade, newer agents such as tacrolimus and mycophenolate mofetil have offered significant reduction in acute rejection rates. Development of polyclonal antilymphocyte antibodies such as thymoglobulin has yielded great strides in delayed graft function and in strategies that delay the use of calcineurin inhibitors early posttransplantation. New monoclonal antibodies are being investigated for treating PTLD and polyomavirus. Pharmacists play a key role on the transplant team by serving as the drug experts and providing pharmaceutical care to transplant recipients. The number of successful heart, lung, liver, kidney, pancreas, and islet cell transplants has increased during the past decade. Improvements have been made in immunomodulating agents, surgical techniques, and organ donor programs.

Postoperative complications following solid organ transplantation can include acute or chronic rejection, infections, hypertension, hyperlipidemia, diabetes, and bone disease. Acute rejection is frequently treated with an intravenous steroid pulse with or without a prednisone taper. To date, there are no effective therapies for the treatment of chronic rejection even though preventing delayed graft function and minimizing acute rejection episodes may be advantageous.

REFERENCES

1. Murray JE, Merrill JP, Dammin GJ, et al. Studies on transplantation immunity after total body irradiation: clinical and experimental investigations. *Surgery.* 1960; 48:272–284.

2. Flye MW. History of transplantation. In: *Principles of Organ Transplantation.* Philadelphia, PA: WB Saunders; 1989:1–17.

3. Schwartz R, Dameschek W. Drug-induced immunological tolerance. *Nature.* 1959; 183:1682.

4. Hitchings GH, Elion BG, Falco EA, et al. Antagonists of nucleic acid derivatives. I. The lactobacillus case model. *J Bio Chem.* 1950; 183:1.

5. Starzl TE, Marchioro TL, Waddell WR. The reversal of rejection in human renal homografts with subsequent development of homograft tolerance. *Surg Gynecol Obstet.* 1963; 117:385–395.

6. Scientific Registry of Transplant Recipients. Available at: www.ustransplant.org. Accessed March 22, 2007.

7. Doyle AM, Lechler RJ, Turka LA. Organ transplantation: halfway through the first century. *J Am Soc Nephrol.* 2004; 15(12):2965–2971.

8. Bach FH, Sachs DH. Transplant immunology. *N Engl J Med.* 1987; 317:482–492.

9. Halloran PF, Broski AP, Batiuk TD, et al. The molecular immunology of acute rejection: an overview. *Transplant Immunol.* 1993; 1(1):3–27.

10. Krams SM, Ascher NL, Martinez OM. New immunologic insights into mechanisms of allograft rejection. *Gastroenterol Clin North Am.* 1993; 22(2):381–400.

11. Bush W, Bartucci MR, Cupples SA. Overview of transplantation immunology and the pharmacotherapy of adult solid organ transplant recipients: Focus on immunosuppression. *AACN Clin Issues ADV Pract Acute Crit Care.* 1999; 10(2):253–269.

12. Rao KV. Mechanism, pathophysiology, diagnosis, and management of renal transplant rejection. *Med Clin North Am.* 1990; 74(4):1039–1057.

13. Tilney NL. Chronic rejection. *Transplantation Proc.* 1999; 31(suppl 1/2A):41S–44S.

14. Goodman J, Mohanakumar T. Chronic rejection: failure of immune regulation. *Frontiers in Bioscience.* 2003; 8:s838–844.

15. Fehr T, Sykes M. Tolerance induction in clinical transplantation. *Transplant Immunology.* 2004; 12:117–130.

16. Mueller XM. Drug immunosuppression therapy for adult heart transplantation. Part I: immune response to allograft and mechanism of action of immunosuppressants. *Ann Thorac Surg.* 2004; 77 354–362.

17. Shapiro R, Young JB, Milford EL, et al. Immunosuppression: evolution in practice and trends, 1993–2003. *Am J Transplant.* 2005; 5(pt 2):874–886.

18. Tornatore KM, Reed KA, Venuto RC. Racial differences in the pharmacokinetics of methylprednisolone in black and white renal transplant patients. *Pharmacotherapy.* 1993; 13(5):481–486.

19. Kobashigawa JA, Stevenson LW, Moriguchi JD, et al. Is intravenous glucocorticoid therapy better than an oral regimen for asymptomatic cardiac rejection? A randomized trial. *J Am Coll Cardiol.* 1993; 21(5):1142–1144.

20. Fryer JP, Granger DK, Leventhal JR, et al. Steroid-related complications in the cyclosporine era. *Clin Transplant.* 1994; 8:224–229.

21. Chueh SJ, Kahan B. Clinical application of sirolimus in renal transplantation: an update. *Transplant Int.* 2005; 18:261–277.

22. Kumar MSA, Xiao SG, Fyfye B, et al. Steroid avoidance in renal transplantation using basiliximab induction, cyclosporine–based immunosuppression and protocol biopsies. *Clin Transplantation.* 2005; 19(1):61–69.

23. Schreiber SL, Crabtree GR. The mechanism of action of cyclosporin A and FK506. *Immunol Today.* 1992; 13:136–142.

24. Kahan BD. Cyclosporine. *N Engl J Med.* 1989; 321(25):1725–1738.

25. Canafax DM. Minimizing cyclosporine concentration variability to optimize transplant outcome. *Clin Transplant.* 1995; 9(1):1–13.

26. Yee GC, McGuire TR, Gmur DJ, et al. Blood cyclosporine pharmacokinetics in patients undergoing marrow transplantation. *Transplantation.* 1988; 46:399–402.

27. Lake KD. Update and management of CsA drug interactions. *Pharmacotherapy.* 1991; 11(5):110S–118S.

28. Lake KD. Drug interactions in transplant patients. In: Emery RW, and Miller LW, eds. *Handbook of Cardiac Transplantation.* Philadelphia, PA: Hanley & Belfus; 1995:147–164.

29. Yee GC, McGuire TR. Pharmacokinetic interactions with cyclosporine. Parts I and II. *Clin Pharmacokinet.* 1990; 19:319–332.

30. Kahan BD, Dunn J, Fitts C, et al. Reduced inter- and intrasubject variability in cyclosporine pharmacokinetics in renal transplant recipients treated with a microemulsion formulation in conjunction with fasting, low-fat meals, or high-fat meals. *Transplantation.* 1995; 59(4):505–511.

31. Kovarik JM, Mueller EA, van Bree JB, et al. Cyclosporine pharmacokinetics and variability from a microemulsion formulation—a multicenter investigation in kidney transplant patients. *Transplantation.* 1994; 58(6):658–663.

32. Mueller EA, Kovarik JM, van Bree JB, et al. Pharmacokinetics and tolerability of a microemulsion formulation of cyclosporine in renal allograft recipients—a concentration-controlled comparison with the commercial formulation. *Transplantation.* 1994; 57(8):1178–1182.

33. Mahalati K, Belitsky P, Sketris I, et al. Neoral monitoring by simplified sparse sampling area under the concentration-time curve: its relationship to acute rejection and cyclosporine nephrotoxicity early after kidney transplantation. *Transplantation.* 1999; 68(1):55–62.

34. Holt DW, Johnston A. The impact of cyclosporin formulation on clinical outcomes. *Transplantation Proc.* 2000; 32(7):1552–1555.

35. Citterio F, Scata MC, Romagnoli J, et al. Results of a three-year prospective study of C2 monitoring in long-term renal transplant recipients receiving cyclosporine microemulsion. *Transplantation.* 2005; 79(7):802–806.

36. Birsan T, Loining C, Bodingbauer M, et al. Comparison between C0 and C2 monitoring in de novo renal transplant recipients: retrospective analysis of a single-center experience. *Transplantation.* 2004; 78(12):1787–1791.

37. Stefoni S, Mictved K, Cole E, et al. Efficacy and safety outcomes among denovo renal transplant recipients managed by C2 monitoring of cyclosporine a microemulsion: results of a 12-month, randomized, multicenter study. *Transplantation.* 2005; 79(5):577–583.

38. Einecke G, Schutz M, Mai I, et al. Limitations of C2 monitoring in renal transplant recipients. *Nephrol Dial Transplant.* 2005; 20(7):1463–1470.

39. Scott JP, Higenbottam TW. Adverse reactions and interactions of cyclosporin. *Med Toxicol.* 1988; 3:107–127.

40. U.S. Multicenter FK506 Liver Study Group. A comparison of tacrolimus (FK 506) and cyclosporine for immunosuppression in liver transplantation. *N Engl J Med.* 1994; 331(17):1110–1115.

41. European FK506 Multicentre Liver Study Group. Randomized trial comparing tacrolimus (FK506) and cyclosporin in prevention of liver allograft rejection. *Lancet.* 1994; 344:423–428.

42. Shapiro R, Jordan ML, Scantlebury VP, et al. A prospective, randomized trial of FK-506 in renal transplantation—a comparison between double- and triple-drug therapy. *Clin Transplant.* 1994; 8:508–515.

43. Shapiro R, Jordan ML, Scantlebury VP, et al. A prospective randomized trial of FK506-based immunosuppression after renal transplantation. *Transplantation.* 1995; 59(4):485–490.

44. Griffith BP, Bando K, Hardesty RL, et al. A prospective randomized trial of FK506 versus cyclosporine after human pulmonary transplantation. *Transplantation.* 1994; 57(6):848–851.

45. Armitage JM, Kormos RL, Morita S, et al. Clinical trial of FK 506 immunosuppression in adult cardiac transplantation. *Ann Thorac Surg.* 1992; 54:205–211.

46. Egawa H, Esquivel CO, So SK, et al. FK506 conversion therapy in pediatric liver transplantation. *Transplantation.* 1994; 57(8):1169–1173.

47. Jordan ML, Shapiro R, Vivas CA, et al. FK506 "rescue" for resistant rejection of renal allografts under primary cyclosporine immunosuppression. *Transplantation.* 1994; 57(6):860–865.

48. Peters DH, Fitton A, Plosker GL, et al. Tacrolimus: a review of its pharmacology, and therapeutic potential in hepatic and renal transplantation. *Drugs.* 1993; 46(4):746–794.

49. Klintmalm G. A review of FK506: a new immunosuppressant agent for the prevention and rescue of graft rejection. *Transplant Rev.* 1994; 8(2):53–62.

50. Kino T, Hatanaka H, Miyata S, et al. FK-506, a novel immunosuppressant isolated from a streptomyces. II. Immunosuppressive effect of FK-506 in vitro. *J Antibiot.* 1987; 40:1256–1265.

51. Sawada S, Suzuki G, Kawase Y, et al. Novel immunosuppressive agent, FK506 in vitro effects on the cloned T-cell activation. *J Immunol.* 1987; 139:1797–1803.

52. Zeevi A, Duquesnoy R, Eiras G, et al. Immunosuppressive effect on FK-506 on in vitro lymphocyte alloactivation: synergism with cyclosporine A. *Transplant Proc.* 1987; 19(suppl 6):40–44.

53. McDiarmid SV, Colonna JO, Shaked A, et al. Differences in oral FK506 dose requirements between adult and pediatric liver transplant patients. *Transplantation.* 1993; 55(6):1328–1332.

54. Venkataramanan R, Jain A, Cadoff E, et al. Pharmacokinetics of FK506 preclinical and clinical studies. *Transplant Proc.* 1990; 22(1):52–56.

55. Starzl TE, Todo S, Fung JJ, et al. FK-506 for liver, kidney and pancreas transplantation. *Lancet.* 1989; 2:1000–1004.

56. Burke MD, Omar G, Thomson AW, et al. Inhibition of the metabolism of cyclosporine by human liver microsomes by FK506. *Transplantation.* 1990; 50(5):901–902.

57. First RM, Fitzsimmons WE. *Yonsei Medical Journal.* 2004; 25(6):1127–1131.

58. Newhaus P, Blumhardt G, Bechstein WO, et al. Comparison of FK506- and cyclosporine-based immunosuppression in primary orthotopic liver transplantation. *Transplantation.* 1995; 59:31–40.

59. Tamura K, Kobayashi M, Hashimoto K, et al. A highly sensitive method to assay FK-506 levels in plasma. *Transplant Proc.* 1987; 5(suppl 6): 23–29.

60. Backman L, Nicar M, Leve M, et al. FK506 trough levels in whole blood and plasma in liver transplant recipients: correlation with clinical events and side effects. *Transplantation.* 1994; 57(4):519–525.

61. Starzl TE, Abu-Elmagd K, Tzakis A, et al. Selected topics on FK506, with special references to rescue of extrahepatic whole organs grafts, transplantation of "forbidden organs," side effects, mechanisms and practical pharmacokinetics. *Transplant Proc.* 1991; 23(1):914–919.

62. Alessiani M, Kusne S, Martin M, et al. Infection in adult liver transplantation under FK-506 immunosuppression. *Transplant Proc.* 1991; 23(1):1501–1503.

63. McDiarmid SV, Colonna JO, Shaked A, et al. A comparison of renal function in cyclosporine- and FK506-treated patients after primary orthotopic liver transplantation. *Transplantation.* 1993; 56(4):847–853.

64. Steinmuller TM, Graf K, Schleicher J, et al. The effect of FK506 versus cyclosporine on glucose and lipid metabolism—a randomized trial. *Transplantation.* 1994; 58(6):669–674.

65. Reyes J, Gayoiski T, Fung JJ, et al. Expressive dysphasia possibly related to FK506 in two liver transplant recipients. *Transplantation*. 1990; 50(6):1043–1044.

66. Abu-Elmagd K, Fung JJ, Alessiani M, et al. The effect of graft function on FK-506 plasma levels, doses and renal function with particular reference to the liver. *Transplantation*. 1991; 52:81–87.

67. Mor E, Sheiner PA, Schwartz ME, et al. Reversal of severe FK506 side effects by conversion to cyclosporine-based immunosuppression. *Transplantation*. 1994; 58(3):380–382.

68. Taylor-Fishwick DA, Kahan M, Hiestand P, et al. Evidence that rapamycin has differential effects on IL-4 function. Multiple IL-4 signaling pathways and implications for in vivo use. *Transplantation*. 1993; 56(2):368–374.

69. Morris RE, Wu J, Shorthouse R, et al. A study of the contrasting effects of cyclosporine, FK506, and rapamycin on the suppression of allograft rejection. *Transplant Proc*. 1990; 22(4):1638–1641.

70. Wood RP, Katz SM, Kahan BD. New immunosuppressive agents. *Transplant Sci*. 1991; 1(1):34–46.

71. Kahan BD. Efficacy of sirolimus compared with azathioprine for reduction of acute renal allograft rejection: a randomised multicentre study. The Rapamune U.S. Study Group. *Lancet*. 2000; 356(9225):194–202.

72. Moses JW, Leon MB, Popma JJ, et al. SIRIUS Investigators. Sirolimus-eluting stents versus standard stents in patients with stenosis in a native coronary artery. *N Engl J Med*. 2003; 349(14):1315–1323.

73. Wu L, Birle DC, Tannock IF. Effects of the mammalian target of rapamycin inhibitor CCI-779 used alone or with chemotherapy on human prostate cancer cells and xenografts. *Cancer Research*. 2005; 65(7):2825–2831.

74. Schumacher G, Oidtmann M, Rueggeberg A, et al. Sirolimus inhibits growth of human hepatoma cells alone or combined with tacrolimus, while tacrolimus promotes cell growth. *World J Gastroenterol*. 2005; 11(10):1420–1425.

75. Heimberger AB, Wang E, McGary EC, et al. Mechanisms of action of rapamycin in gliomas. *Neuro-Oncology*. 2005; 7(1):1–11.

76. Dean PG, Lund WJ, Larsen TS, et al. Wound healing complications after kidney transplantation: a prospective, randomized comparison of sirolimus and tacrolimus. *Transplantation*. 2004; 77(10):1555–1561.

77. Vasquez EM. Sirolimus: A new agent for prevention of renal allograft rejection. *Am J Health-Syst Pharm*. 2000; 57:437–451.

78. Boratyska M, Banasik M, Patrzalek D, et al. Sirolimus delays recovery from posttransplant renal failure in kidney graft recipients. *Transplantation Proc*. 2005; 37(2):839–842.

79. Haydar AA, Denton M, West A, et al. Sirolimus-induced pneumonitis: three cases and a review of the literature. *Am J Transplant*. 2004; 4(1):137–139.

80. Lindenfeld JA, Simon SF, Zamora MR, et al. BOOP is common in cardiac transplant recipients switched from a calcineurin inhibitor to sirolimus. *Am J Transplant*. 2005; 5(6):1392–1396.

81. Lee S, Coco M, Greenstein SM, et al. The effect of sirolimus on sex hormone levels of male renal transplant recipients. *Clin Transplant*. 2005; 19(2):162–167.

82. Rogers CC, Hanaway M, Alloway RR, et al. Corticosteroid avoidance ameliorates lymphocele formation and wound healing complications associated with sirolimus therapy. *Transplant Proc*. 2005; 37(2):795–797.

83. Chapman TM, Perry CM. Everolimus. *Drugs*. 2004; 64(8):861–872.

84. Kirchner GI, Meier-Wiedenbach I, Manns MP. Clinical pharmacokinetics of everolimus. *Clinical Pharmacokinetics*. 2004; 43(2):83–95.

85. Vitko S, Margreiter R, Weimar W, et al. RAD B201 Study Group. Three-year efficacy and safety results from a study of everolimus versus mycophenolate mofetil in de novo renal transplant patients. *Am J Transplant*. 2005; 5(10):2521–2530.

86. Morice MC, Serruys PW, Sousa JE, et al. RAVEL Study Group. Randomized study with the sirolimus-coated Bx velocity balloon-expandable stent in the treatment of patients with de novo native coronary artery lesions. A randomized comparison of a sirolimus-eluting stent with a standard stent for coronary revascularization. *N Engl J Med*. 2002; 346(23):1773–1780.

87. Grube E, Sonoda S, Ikeno F, et al. Six- and twelve-month results from first human experience using everolimus-eluting stents with bioabsorbable polymer. *Circulation*. 2004; 109(18):2168–2171.

88. Eisen HJ, Tuzcu M, Dorent R, et al. RAD B253 Study Group. Everolimus for the prevention of allograft rejection and vasculopathy in cardiac transplant recipients. *N Engl J Med*. 2003; 349:847–858.

89. Farasati NA, Shapiro R, Vats A, et al. Effect of leflunomide and cidofovir on replication of BK virus in an in vitro culture system. *Transplantation*. 2005; 79(1):116–118.

90. Williams JW, Mital D, Chong A, et al. Experiences with leflunamide in solid organ transplantation. *Clin Transplantation*. 2002; 73(3):358–366.

91. Williams JW, Javaid B, Kadambi PV, et al. Leflunomide for polyomavirus type BK nephropathy. *N Engl J Med*. 2005; 352(11):1157–1158.

92. John GT, Manivannan J, Chandy A, et al. Leflunomide therapy for cytomegalovirus disease in renal allograft recipients. *Transplantation*. 2004; 77(9):1460–1461.

93. Kyles AE, Gregory CR, Griffey SM, et al. Immunosuppression with a combination of the leflunomide analog, FK778, and microemulsified cyclosporine for renal transplantation in mongrel dogs. *Transplantation*. 2003; 75(8):1128–1133.

94. Krieger NR, Emre S. Novel immunosuppressants. *Pediatric Transplantation*. 2004; 8(6):594–599.

95. Chan GL, Canafax DM, Johnson CA. The therapeutic use of azathioprine in renal transplantation. *Pharmacotherapy.* 1987; 7(5):165–177.

96. Van Scoik KG, Johnson CA, Porter WR. The pharmacology and metabolism of the thiopurine drugs 6-mercaptopurine and azathioprine. *Drug Metab Rev.* 1985; 16(1&2):157–174.

97. Odlind B, Grefberg N, Hartvig P, et al. Pharmacokinetics of azathioprine and 6-mercaptopurine: methodological aspects and preliminary results in uremic patients. *Scand J Urol Nephrol.* 1981; 64(suppl):213–219.

98. Odlind B, Hartvig P, Lindstrom B, et al. Serum azathioprine and 6-mercaptopurine levels and immunosuppression activity after azathioprine in uremic patients. *Int J Immunopharmacol.* 1986; 8:1–11.

99. Lin SN, Jessup K, Floyd M, et al. Quantitation of plasma azathioprine and 6-mercaptopurine levels in renal transplant patients. *Transplantation.* 1980; 29:290–294.

100. Maddocks JL. Clinical pharmacological observations on azathioprine in kidney transplant patients [abstract]. *Clin Sci Mol Med.* 1978; 55:20P.

101. Chan GL, Erdmann GR, Gruber SA, et al. Pharmacokinetics of 6-thiouric acid and 6-mercaptopurine in renal allograft recipients after oral administration of azathioprine. *Eur J Clin Pharmacol.* 1989; 36(3):265–271.

102. Chan GL, Gruber SA, Skjei KL, et al. Principles of immunosuppression. *Crit Care Clin.* 1990; 6(4):841–892.

103. Ding TL, Benet LZ. Determination of 6-mercaptopurine and azathioprine in plasma by high-performance liquid chromatography. *J Chromatogr.* 1979; 163:281–288.

104. Ding TL, Gamberatoglio JG, Amend WJC, et al. Azathioprine (AZA) bioavailability and pharmacokinetics in kidney transplant patients [abstract]. *Clin Pharmacol Ther.* 1980; 27(2):250.

105. Watts GF, Corston R. Hypersensitivity to azathioprine in myasthenia gravis. *Postgrad Med J.* 1984; 60:362–363.

106. Brooks RJ, Dorr RT, Durie BGM. Interaction of allopurinol with 6-mercaptopurine and azathioprine. *Biomedicine.* 1982; 36:217–222.

107. Coffey JJ, White CA, Lesk AB, et al. Effect of allopurinol on the pharmacokinetics of 6-mercaptopurine (MSC 775) in cancer patients. *Cancer Res.* 1972; 32:1283–1289.

108. Vetten KB. Immunosuppressive therapy and anesthesia. *South African Med J.* 1973; 47:767–770.

109. Dretchen KL, Morgenroth VH III, Standaert FG, et al. Azathioprine: effects on neuromuscular transmission. *Anesthesiology.* 1976; 45:604–609.

110. Spiers ASD, Mibashan PS. Increased warfarin requirement during mercaptopurine therapy: a new drug interaction. *Lancet.* 1974; 2:221–222.

111. Winklestein A. The effects of azathioprine and 6MP on immunity. *J Immunopharmacol.* 1979; 1:429–454.

112. Maddocks JL, Lennard L, Amess J, et al. Azathioprine and severe bone marrow depression [letter]. *Lancet.* 1986; 1:156.

113. Lennard L, Murphy MF, Maddocks JL, et al. Severe megaloblastic anaemia associated with abnormal azathioprine metabolism. *Br J Clin Pharmacol.* 1984; 17:171–172.

114. Old CW, Flannery EP, Grogan TM, et al. Azathioprine-induced pure red blood cell aplasia. *JAMA.* 1978; 240:552–554.

115. Rosman M, Bertino JR. Azathioprine. *Ann Intern Med.* 1973; 79:694–700.

116. Berne TV, Chatterjee SN, Craig JR, et al. Hepatic dysfunction in recipients of renal allografts. *Surg Gynecol Obstet.* 1975; 141:171–175.

117. Zarday Z, Veith FJ, Gliedman ML, et al. Irreversible liver damage after azathioprine. *JAMA.* 1972; 222:690–691.

118. McCormack JJ, Johns DG. Purine antimetabolites. In: Chabner B, ed. *Pharmacologic Principles of Cancer Treatment.* Philadelphia, PA: WB Saunders; 1982:213–218.

119. Nakashima Y, Howard JM. Drug-induced acute pancreatitis. *Surg Gynecol Obstet.* 1977; 145: 105–109.

120. Penn I. Cancer is a complication of severe immunosuppression. *Surg Gynecol Obstet.* 1986; 162:603–610.

121. Allison AC, Eugui EM. The design and development of an immunosuppressive drug, mycophenolate mofetil. *Springer Semin Immunopathol.* 1993; 14(4):353–380.

122. Allison AC, Eugui EM, Sollinger HW. Mycophenolate mofetil: mechanisms of action and effects in transplantation. *Transplant Rev.* 1993; 7(3):129–139.

123. Sollinger HW, Deierhoi MH, Belzer FO, et al. RS-61443 (mycophenolate mofetil)—a phase I clinical study and pilot rescue trial. *Transplantation.* 1992; 53:428–432.

124. Sollinger HW, Belzer FO, Deierhoi MH, et al. RS-61443 (mycophenolate mofetil)—a multicenter study for refractory kidney transplant rejection. *Ann Surg.* 1992; 216:513–519.

125. Klintmalm GB, Ascher NL, Busutill RW, et al. RS-61443 for the treatment of resistant human liver rejection. *Transplant Proc.* 1993; 25(pt 1):697.

126. Taylor DO, Ensley RD, Olsen SL, et al. Mycophenolate mofetil (RS-61443): preclinical, clinical and three year experience in heart transplantation. *J Heart Lung Transplant.* 1994; 13:571–582.

127. Budde K, Schmouder RL, Nashan B, et al. Pharmacodynamics of single doses of the novel immunosuppressant FTY720 in stable renal transplant patients. *Am J Transplant.* 2003; 3(7):846–854.

128. Salvadori M, Holzer H, de Mattos A, et al. The ERL B301 Study Groups. Enteric-coated mycophenolate sodium is therapeutically equivalent to mycophenolate mofetil in de novo renal transplant patients. *Am J Transplant.* 2004; 4(2):231–236.

129. Nashan B, Ivens K, Suwelack B, et al. myPROMS DE02 Study Group. LA01 Study Group. Conversion from mycophenolate mofetil to enteric-coated mycophenolate sodium in maintenance renal transplant patients: preliminary results from the myfortic prospective multicenter study. *Transplantation Proc.* 2004; 36(2 suppl): 521S–523S.

130. Sollinger HW. Mycophenolate mofetil for the prevention of acute rejection in primary cadaveric renal allograft recipients. U.S. Renal Transplant Mycophenolate Mofetil Study Group. *Transplantation.* 1995; 60(3):225–232.

131. European Mycophenolate Mofetil Cooperative Study Group. Placebo-controlled study of mycophenolate mofetil combined with cyclosporin and corticosteroids for prevention of acute rejection. *Lancet.* 1995; 345(8961):1321–1325.

132. Shaw LM, Nawrocki A, Korecka M, et al. Using established immunosuppressant therapy effectively: lessons from the measurement of mycophenolic acid plasma concentrations. *Therapeutic Drug Monitoring.* 2004; 26(4):347–351.

133. Okamoto M, Wakabayashi Y, Higuchi A, et al. Therapeutic drug monitoring of mycophenolic acid in renal transplant recipients. *Transplantation Proc.* 2005; 37(2):859–860.

134. CellCept® (Mycophenolate Mofetil) [package insert]. Nutley, NJ: Roche Laboratories; 2006.

135. Allison, AC, Euguie EM, Sollinger HW. Mycophenolate mofetil: mechanism of action and effects in transplantation. *Transplant Rev.* 1993; 14(4):353–380.

136. Alfieri C, Kieff E, Allison AC. Effect of mycophenolic acid on Epstein-Barr virus infection on human B lymphocytes. *Antimicrob Agents Chemother.* 1994; 38:126–129.

137. Woodruff MFA, Anderson NF. Effect of lymphocyte depletion by thoracic duct fistula and administration of anti-lymphocyte serum on the survival of skin homografts in rats. *Nature.* 1963; 200:702–704.

138. Delmonico FL, Auchincloss H, Rubin RH, et al. The selective use of antilymphocyte serum for cyclosporine treated patients with renal allograft dysfunction. *Ann Surg.* 1987; 206:649–654.

139. Fassbinder W, Scheuermann EH, Stutte HJ, et al. Improved graft prognosis by treatment of steroid-resistant rejections with ATG and plasmapheresis. *Proc Eur Dialysis Transplant Assn.* 1983; 20:362–367.

140. Hardy MA, Nowygrod R, Elberg A, et al. Use of ATG in treatment of steroid-resistant rejection. *Transplantation.* 1980; 29:162–164.

141. Kreis H, Mansoum R, Descamps JM, et al. Antithymocyte globulin in cadaver kidney transplantation: a randomized trial based on T-cell monitoring. *Kidney Int.* 1981; 19:438–444.

142. Nelson PW, Cosimi AB, Delmonico FL, et al. Antithymocyte globulin as the primary treatment for renal allograft rejection. *Transplantation.* 1983; 36:587–589.

143. Sheil GR, Mears D, Kelly GE, et al. A controlled trial of antilymphocyte globulin therapy (ALG) in man. *Transplant Proc.* 1972; 4:501–505.

144. Shield CF, Cosimi AB, Tolkoff-Rubin N, et al. Use of antithymocyte globulin for reversal of acute allograft rejection. *Transplantation.* 1979; 28:461–469.

145. Starzl TE, Marchioro TL, Porter KKA, et al. The use of heterologous antilymphoid agents in canine renal and liver homotransplantation and human renal homotransplantation. *Surg Gynecol Obstet.* 1967; 124(2):301–308.

146. Fries D, Hiesse C, Lantz O, et al. Optimization of antilymphocytes globulin in renal transplantation. *Transplant Proc.* 1990; 22(4):1793–1794.

147. Cosimi AB. Antilymphocyte globulin: a final (?) look. In: Morris PJ, Tilney NL, eds. *Progress in Transplantation.* Edinburgh: Churchill Livingstone; 1985:167–188.

148. Cosimi AB, Delmonico FL. Anti-lymphocyte antibody immunosuppressive therapy. In: Williams GM, Burdick JF, Solez K, eds. *Kidney Transplant Rejection.* New York, NY: Marcel Dekker; 1986:335–340.

149. Macdonald PS, Mundy J, Keogh AM, et al. A prospective randomized study of prophylactic OKT3 versus equine antithymocyte globulin after heart transplantation—increased morbidity with OKT3. *Transplantation.* 1993; 55(1):110–116.

150. Ormrod D, Jarvis B. Antithymocyte globulin (rabbit): A review of the use of thymoglobulin in the prevention and treatment of acute renal allograft rejection. *BioDrugs.* 2000; 14(4):255–273.

151. Goggins WC, Pascual MA, Powelson JA, et al. A prospective, randomized, clinical trial of intraoperative versus postoperative thymoglobulin in adult cadaveric renal transplant recipients. *Transplantation.* 2003; 76(5):798–802.

152. Atgam [package insert] Kalamazoo, MI: The Upjohn Company; 2006.

153. Clark KR, Forsythe JLR, Shenton BK, et al. Flow-cytometric monitoring of ATG therapy for steroid-resistant rejection. *Transplant Proc.* 1992; 24(1):315.

154. Cerilli G, Brastle L, Clarke J, et al. Correlation of cell reaction patterns and in vitro immunosuppression capabilities of six ATG products used clinically. *Transplant Proc.* 1985; 17:2760.

155. Clark KR, Forsythe JLR, Shenton BK, et al. Administration of ATG according to the absolute T-lymphocyte count during therapy for steroid-resistant rejection. *Transpl Int.* 1993; 6:18–21.

156. Lawley TJ, Bielory L, Gascon P, et al. A prospective clinical and immunologic analysis of patients with serum sickness. *N Engl J Med.* 1984; 311:1407–1413.

157. Vermnier I, Giraud P, Eche JP, et al. Hematologic side effects of antilymphocyte globulins: prevalence and impact on therapeutic protocol. *Transplant Proc.* 1985; 17:2765–2766.

158. Melosky B, Karim M, Chui A, et al. Lymphoproliferative disorders after renal transplantation in patients receiving triple or quadruple immunosuppression. *J Am Soc Nephrol*. 1992; 2(suppl 12):S290–294.

159. Chang TW, Kung PC, Gingras SP, et al. Does OKT3 monoclonal antibody react with an antigen-recognition structure on human T-cells? *Proc Natl Acad Sci USA*. 1981; 78(3):1805–1808.

160. Reinherz EL, Meuer S, Fitzgerald KA, et al. Antigen recognition by human T-lymphocytes is linked to surface expression of the T-3 molecular complex. *Cell*. 1982; 30:735–743.

161. Chatenoud L, Bandrihaye MF, Krefs H, et al. Human in vivo antigenic modulation induced by the anti-T-cell OKT3 monoclonal antibody. *Eur J Immunol*. 1982; 12:979–982.

162. Delmonico FL, Cosimi AB. Monoclonal antibody treatment of human allograft recipients. *Surg Gynecol Obstet*. 1988; 166(1):89–98.

163. Shield CF, Norman DJ. Immunologic monitoring during and after OKT3 therapy. *Am J Kidney Dis*. 1988; 11:112–119.

164. Miller RA, Maloney DG, McKillop J, et al. In vivo effects of murine hybridoma monoclonal antibody in a patient with T-cell leukemia. *Blood*. 1981; 58:78–86.

165. Rinnooy Kan EA, Wright SD, Welte K, et al. Fc receptors on monocytes cause OKT3-treated lymphocytes to internalize T3 and to secrete IL-2. *Cell Immunol*. 1986; 98:181.

166. Carreno M, Miller J, Fuller NL. Are OKT3 binding sites on T-cells modulated or merely converted (blind-folded) by OKT3 during therapy? *Transplant Proc*. 1989; 21(1):987–988.

167. Gedel H, Lebeck LL, Jensik FC. Discordant expression of CD3 and T-cell receptor antigen on lymphocytes from patients treated with OKT3. *Transplant Proc*. 1989; 21(1):1745–1746.

168. Kreis H, Legendre C, Chatenoud L. OKT3 in organ transplantation. *Transplant Rev*. 1991; 5:181–199.

169. Alloway R, Kotb M, Hathaway D, et al. The pharmacokinetic profile of standard and low-dose OKT3 induction immunosuppression in renal transplant recipients. *Transplantation*. 1994; 58(2):249–253.

170. Leone MR, Barry JM, Alexander SR, et al. Monoclonal antibody OKT3 therapy in pediatric kidney transplant patients. *J Pediatr*. 1990; 116(suppl 5):S86–91.

171. Schroeder TJ, Ryckman FC, Hurtubise PE, et al. Immunological monitoring during and following OKT3 therapy in children. *Clin Transplant*. 1991; 5:191–196.

172. Ryckman FC, Schroeder TJ, Pedersen SH, et al. Use of monoclonal antibody immunosuppressive therapy in pediatric renal and liver transplantation. *Clin Transplant*. 1991; 5:186–190.

173. Chatenoud L. Immunologic monitoring during OKT3 therapy. *Clin Transplant*. 1993; 7:422–430.

174. Colvin RB, Preffer FI. Laboratory monitoring of therapy with OKT3 and other murine monoclonal antibodies. *Clin Lab Med*. 1991; 11(3):693–714.

175. Henell KR, Norman DJ. Monitoring OKT3 treatment: pharmacodynamic and pharmacokinetic measures. *Transplant Proc*. 1993; 25(suppl 1):83–85.

176. Thistlethwaite JR, Stuart JK, Mayes JT, et al. Complications and monitoring of OKT3 therapy. *Am J Kid Dis*. 1988; 11:112–119.

177. Shield CF, Norman DJ. Immunologic monitoring during and after OKT3 therapy. *Am J Kid Dis*. 1988; 11:120–124.

178. Cosimi AB. Clinical development of orthoclone OKT3. *Transplant Proc*. 1987; 19(suppl 1):7–16.

179. Chatenoud L, Ferran C, Legendre C, et al. In vivo cell activation following OKT3 administration. Systemic cytokine release and modulation by corticosteroids. *Transplantation*. 1990; 49(4):697–702.

180. Abramowicz D, Schandene L, Goldman M, et al. Release of tumor necrosis factor, interleukin-2, and gamma-interferon in serum after injection of OKT3 monoclonal antibody in kidney transplant recipients. *Transplantation*. 1989; 47:606–608.

181. Rowe PA, Rocker GM, Morgan AG, et al. OKT3 and pulmonary capillary permeability. *Br Med J*. 1987; 255:1099.

182. Hosenpud JD, Norman DJ, Pantley GA, et al. OKT3-induced hypotension in cardiac allograft recipients treated for resistant rejection. *J Heart Transplant*. 1989; 8:159–166.

183. Emmons C, Smith J, Flanigan M. Cerebrospinal fluid inflammation during OKT3 therapy [letter]. *Lancet*. 1986; 2:510.

184. Martin MA, Massanaari RM, Nghiem DD, et al. Nosocomial aseptic meningitis associated with administration of OKT3. *JAMA*. 1988; 259:2002–2005.

185. Thomas DM, Nicholls AJ, Feest TG, et al. OKT3 and cerebral oedema. *Br Med J*. 1987; 295:1486.

186. Thistlethwaite JR, Gaber AO, Haag BW, et al. OKT3 treatment of steroid resistant renal allograft rejection. *Transplantation*. 1987; 43(2):176–184.

187. Norman W, Shield CF, Barry J, et al. A U.S. clinical study of orthoclone OKT3 in renal transplantation. *Transplant Proc*. 1987; 19(suppl 1):21–27.

188. Todd PA, Brogden RN. Muromonab CD3: a review of its pharmacology and therapeutic potential. *Drugs*. 1989; 37:871–899.

189. Ortho Multicenter Transplant Study Group. A randomized clinical trial of OKT3 monoclonal antibody for acute rejection of cadaveric renal transplants. *N Engl J Med*. 1985; 313:337–342.

190. Chatenoud L, Legendre C, Ferran C, et al. Corticosteroid inhibition of the OKT3-induced cytokine-related syndrome—dosage and kinetics prerequisites. *Transplantation*. 1991; 51(2):334–338.

191. Bemelman FJ, Buysman S, Surachno J, et al. Pretreatment with divided doses of steroids strongly decreases the side-effects of OKT3. *Kidney Int*. 1994; 46:1674–1679.

192. Alegre M, Gastaldello K, Abramowicz D, et al. Evidence that pentoxifylline reduces anti-CD3 monoclonal antibody-induced cytokine release syndrome. *Transplantation.* 1991; 52:674–679.

193. Chatenoud L. OKT3-induced cytokine-release syndrome: prevention effect of anti-tumor necrosis factor monoclonal antibody [review]. *Transplant Proc.* 1993; 25(2 suppl 1):47–51.

194. First MR, Schroeder T, Hariharan S, et al. The effect of indomethacin on the febrile response following OKT3 therapy. *Transplantation.* 1992; 53:91–94.

195. Kreis H. Adverse events associated with OKT3 immunosuppression in the prevention of allograft rejection. *Clin Transplant.* 1993; 7:431–446.

196. Krieger NR, Emre S. Novel immunosuppressants. *Pediatric Transplantation.* 2004; 8(6):594–599.

197. Gruessner RW, Kandaswamy R, Humar A, et al. Calcineurin inhibitor- and steroid-free immunosuppression in pancreas-kidney and solitary pancreas transplantation. *Transplantation.* 2005; 79(9):1184–1189.

198. Watson CJ, Bradley JA, Friend PJ, et al. Alemtuzumab (CAMPATH 1H) induction therapy in cadaveric kidney transplantation-efficacy and safety at five years. *Am J Transplant.* 2005; 5(6):1347–1353.

199. Becker YT, Becker BN, Pirsch JD, et al. Rituximab as treatment for refractory kidney transplant rejection. *Am J Transplant.* 2004; 4(6):996–1001.

200. Ganne V, Siddiqi N, Kanaplath B, et al. Humanized anti-CD20 monoclonal antibody (Rituximab) treatment for post-transplant lymphoproliferative disorder. *Clin Transplant.* 2003; 17:417–422.

201. Sonnenday CJ, Warren DS, Cooper M, et al. Plasmapheresis, CMV hyperimmune globulin, and anti-CD-20 allow ABO-incompatible renal transplantation without splenectomy. *Am J Transplant.* 2004; 4(8):1315–1322.

202. Berard JL, Velez RL, Freeman RB, et al. A review of interleukin-2 receptor antagonists in solid organ transplantation. *Pharmacotherapy.* 1999; 19(10):1127–1137.

203. Wiseman LR, Faulds D. Daclizumab: a review of its use in the prevention of acute rejection in renal transplant recipients. *Drugs.* 1999; 58(6):1029–1042.

204. Chapman TM, Keating GM. Basiliximab: a review of its use as induction therapy in renal transplantation. *Drugs.* 2003; 63(24):2803–2835.

205. Webster AC, Playford EG, Higgins G, et al. Interleukin 2 receptor antagonists for renal transplant recipients: a meta-analysis of randomized trials. *Transplantation.* 2004; 77(2):166–176.

206. Vincenti F, Pace D, Birnbaum J, et al. Pharmacokinetic and pharmacodynamic studies of one or two doses of daclizumab in renal transplantation. *Am J Transplant.* 2003; 3(1):50–52.

207. Stratta RJ, Alloway RR, Lo A, et al. PIVOT Study Group. One-year outcomes in simultaneous kidney-pancreas transplant recipients receiving an alternative dosing regimen of daclizumab. *Transplantation Proc.* 2004; 36(4):1080–1081.

208. Halloran PF. Immunosuppressive drugs for kidney transplantation. *N Engl J Med.* 2004; 351(26):2715–2729.

209. Saemann MD, Zeyda M, Diakos C, et al. Suppression of early t-cell receptor-triggered cellular activation by the janus kinase 3 inhibitor WHI-P-1541. *Transplantation.* 2003; 75(11):1783–1785.

210. Kovarik JM, Schmouder RL, Slade AJ. Overview of FTY720 clinical pharmacokinetics and pharmacology. *Therapeutic Drug Monitoring.* 2004; 26(6):585–587.

211. Brinkmann V, Pinschewer DD, Feng L, et al. FTY-720: altered lymphocyte traffic results in allograft protection. *Transplantation.* 2001; 72(5):764–769.

212. Ferguson R. FTY720 immunomodulation: optimism for improved transplant regimens. *Transplant Proc.* 2004; 36(suppl 2S):549S–553S.

213. Tedesco H, Kahan B, Mourad G, et al. FTY720 combined with Neoral(r) and corticosteroids is effective and safe in prevention of acute rejection in renal allograft recipients (interim data). *Am J Transplant.* 2001; 1(suppl 1):342. Abstract 429.

214. Kahan B, Chodoff L, Leichtman A, et al. Safety and pharmacodynamics of multiple doses of FTY720 in stable renal transplant recipients. *Am J Transplant.* 2001; 1(suppl 1):300. Abstract 654.

215. Salvadori M, Budde K, Charpentier B, et al. FTY720 0124 Study Group. FTY720 versus MMF with cyclosporine in de novo renal transplantation: a 1-year, randomized controlled trial in Europe and Australasia. *Am J Transplant.* 2006; 6(12):2912.

216. Halloran PF. Immunosuppressive drugs for kidney transplantation. *N Engl J Med.* 2004; 351(26):2715–2729.

217. Larsen CP, Pearson TC, Adams AB, et al. Rational development of LEA29Y (belatacept), a high-affinity variant of CTLA4-Ig with potent immunosuppressive properties. *Am J Transplant.* 2005; 5(3):443–453.

218. Larsen CP, Knechtle SJ, Adams A, et al. A new look at blockade of T-cell costimulation: a therapeutic strategy for long-term maintenance immunosuppression. *Am J Transplant.* 2006; 6 (5, pt 1):876–883.

219. Borie DC, Changelian PS, Larson MJ, et al. Immunosuppression by the JAK3 inhibitor CP-690,550 delays rejection and significantly prolongs kidney allograft survival in nonhuman primates. *Transplantation.* 2005; 79(7):791–801.

220. Venkataramanan R, Habucky K, Burckart GJ, et al. Clinical pharmacokinetics in organ transplant patients. *Clin Pharmacokin.* 1989; 116(3):134–161.

221. Cantarovich M, Fitchett D, Latter DA. Cyclosporine trough levels, acute rejection and renal dysfunction after heart transplantation. *Transplantation.* 1995; 59(3):444–447.

222. Modry DL, Stinson EB, Oyer PE, et al. Acute rejection and massive cyclosporine requirements in heart transplant recipients treated with rifampin. *Transplantation.* 1985; 39:313–314.

223. Offermann G, Keller F, Molzahn M. Low cyclosporine A blood levels and acute graft rejection in a renal transplant recipient during rifampin treatment. *Am J Nephrol.* 1985; 5:385–387.

224. Wassner SJ, Pennisi AJ, Malekzadeh MH, et al. The adverse effect of anticonvulsant therapy on renal allograft survival. *J Pediatr.* 1976; 88(1):134–137.

225. Nelson DR, Kamataki T, Waxman DJ, et al. The P450 superfamily: update on new sequences, gene mapping, accession numbers, early trivial names of enzymes, and nomenclature. *DNA Cell Biol.* 1993; 112(1):1–51.

226. Kronbach T, Fischer V, Meyer UA. Cyclosporine metabolism in human liver: identification of a cytochrome P-450III gene family as the major cyclosporine-metabolizing enzyme with other drugs. *Clin Pharmacol Ther.* 1988; 43:630–635.

227. Vincent SH, Karanam BV, Painter SK, et al. In vitro metabolism of FK-506 in rat, rabbit, and human liver microsomes; identification of a major metabolite and of cytochrome P450 3A as the major enzymes responsible for its metabolism. *Arch Biochem Biophys.* 1992; 294:454–460.

228. Peters DH, Fitton A, Plosker GL, et al. Tacrolimus; a review of its pharmacology, and therapeutic potential in hepatic and renal transplantation. *Drugs.* 1993; 46(4):746–794.

229. Lo A, Burckart GJ. P-glycoprotein and drug therapy in organ transplantation. *J Clin Pharmacol.* 1999; 39(10):995–1005.

230. Kaminsky LS, Fasco MJ. Small intestinal cytochromes P450 [review]. *Crit Rev Toxicol.* 1991; 21(6):407–422.

231. Kolars JC, Schmiedlin-Ren P, Schuetz JD, et al. Identification of rifampin-inducible P450IIIA4 (CYP3A4) in human small bowel enterocytes. *J Clin Invest.* 1992; 90(5):1871–1878.

232. Watkins PB, Wrighton SA, Schuetz EG, et al. Identification of glucocorticoid-inducible cytochromes P-450 in the intestinal mucosa of rats and man. *J Clin Invest.* 1987; 80(4):1029–1036.

233. Jain AB, Venkataramanan R, Fung J, et al. Pharmacokinetics of cyclosporine and nephrotoxicity in orthotopic liver transplant patients rescued with FK506. *Transplant Proc.* 1991; 23(6):2777–2779.

234. Rowland M, Gupta SK. Cyclosporine-phenytoin interaction: re-evaluation using metabolite data. *Br J Clin Pharmacol.* 1987; 24:329–334.

235. Hebert MF, Roberts JP, Preuksaritanont T, et al. Pharmacokinetics and drug disposition: bioavailability of cyclosporine with concomitant rifampin administration is markedly less than predicted by hepatic enzyme induction. *Clin Pharmacol Ther.* 1992; 52:453–457.

236. Van Buren D, Wideman CA, Ried M, et al. The antagonistic effect of rifampin upon cyclosporine bioavailability. *Transplant Proc.* 1984; 16:1642–1645.

237. McAllister WAC, Thompson PJ, Al-Habet SM, et al. Rifampicin reduces effectiveness and bioavailability of prednisolone. *Br Med J.* 1983; 286(6369):923–925.

238. Wadhwa NK, Schroeder TJ, O'Flaherty E, et al. Pharmacokinetics and drug interactions of cyclosporine and erythromycin. *Clin Res.* 1986; 34:638A.

239. Wadhwa NK, Schroeder TJ, O'Flaherty E, et al. Interaction between erythromycin and cyclosporine in a kidney and pancreas allograft recipient. *Ther Drug Monit.* 1987; 9(1):123–125.

240. Gupta SK, Bakran A, Johnson RWG, et al. Cyclosporine-erythromycin interaction in renal transplant patients. *Br J Clin Pharmacol.* 1989; 27:475–481.

241. Cakaloglu Y, Tredger JM, Devlin J, et al. Importance of cytochrome P-450IIIA activity in determining dosage and blood levels of FK506 and cyclosporine in liver transplant recipients. *Hepatology.* 1994; 20(2):309–316.

242. Bailey DG, Arnold JMO, Spence JD. Grapefruit juice and drugs: how significant is the interaction? *Clin Pharmacokinet.* 1994; 26:91–98.

243. Ducharme MP, Provenzano R, Dehoorne-Smith M, et al. Trough concentrations of cyclosporine in blood following administration with grapefruit juice. *Br J Clin Pharmacol.* 1993; 36:457–459.

244. Yee GC, Stanley DL, Pessa LJ, et al. Effect of grapefruit juice on blood cyclosporin concentration. *Lancet.* 1995; 345:955–956.

245. Ducharme PM, Warbasse LH, Edwards DJ. Disposition of intravenous and oral cyclosporine after administration with grapefruit juice. *Clin Pharmacol Ther.* 1995; 57(5):485–491.

246. Doble N, Hykin P, Shaw R, et al. Pulmonary mycobacterium tuberculosis in acquired immune deficiency. *Br Med J.* 1985; 291:849–850.

247. Watkins PB. Drug metabolism by cytochromes P450 in the liver and small bowel. *Gastroenterol Clin North Am.* 1992; 21(3):511–526.

248. Ding TL, Gamberatoglio JG, Amend WJC, et al. Azathioprine (AZA) bioavailability and pharmacokinetics in kidney transplant patients. *Clin Pharmacol Ther.* 1980; 27(2):250.

249. Chan GL, Canafax DM, Johnson CA. The therapeutic use of azathioprine in renal transplantation. *Pharmacotherapy.* 1987; 7(5):165.

250. Yee GC, Self SG, McGuire TR, et al. Serum cyclosporine concentrations and risk of acute GVHD after allogeneic marrow transplantation. *N Engl J Med.* 1988; 319:65–70.

251. Burke JF, Pirsch JD, Ramos EF, et al. Long-term efficacy and safety of cyclosporine in renal-transplant recipients. *N Engl J Med.* 1994; 331(6):358–363.

252. Beutler D, Molteni S, Zeugin T, et al. Evaluation of instrumental, nonisotopic immunoassays (fluorescence polarization immunoassay and enzyme-multiplied immunoassay technique) for cyclosporine monitoring in whole blood after kidney and liver transplantation. *Ther Drug Monit.* 1992; 14:424–432.

253. Moran M, Mozes MF, Maddux MS, et al. Prevention of acute graft rejection by the prostaglandin E1 analogue misoprostol in renal-transplant recipients

treated with cyclosporine and prednisone. *N Engl J Med*. 1990; 322(17):1183–1188.

254. Bianco JA, Almgren, J, Kern DE, et al. Evidence that oral pentoxifylline reverses acute renal dysfunction in bone marrow transplant recipients receiving amphotericin B and cyclosporine. *Transplantation*. 1991; 51:925–927.

255. Dawidson I, Rooth P, Fry WR, et al. Prevention of acute cyclosporine-induced renal blood flow inhibition and improved immunosuppression with verapamil. *Transplantation*. 1989; 48(4):575–580.

256. Morales JM, Andres A, Alvarez C, et al. Calcium channel blockers and early cyclosporine nephrotoxicity after renal transplantation: a prospective randomized study. *Transplant Proc*. 1990; 22(4):1733–1735.

257. Watschinger B, Ulrich W, Vychytil A, et al. Cyclosporine A toxicity is associated with reduced endothelin immunoreactivity in renal endothelium. *Transplant Proc*. 1992; 24(6):2618–2619.

258. Horton CM, Freeman CD, Nolan PE Jr., et al. Cyclosporine interactions with miconazole and other azole-antimycotics: a case report and review of the literature. *J Heart Lung Transplant*. 1992; 11(6):1127–1132.

259. First MR, Schroeder TJ, Weiskittel P, et al. Concomitant administration of cyclosporine and ketoconazole in renal transplant patients. *Lancet*. 1989; 2(8673):1198–1201.

260. Nanez R, Martin M, Venkataramanan R, et al. Fluconazole therapy in transplant recipients receiving FK506. *Transplantation*. 1994; 57(10):1521–1523.

261. Venkataramanan R, Jain A, Warty VS, et al. Pharmacokinetics of FK506 in transplant patients. *Transplant Proc*. 1991; 23(6):2736–2740.

262. Vasquez EM, Shin GP, Sifontis N, et al. Concomitant clotrimazole therapy more than doubles the relative oral bioavailability of tacrolimus. *Therapeutic Drug Monitoring*. 2005; 27(5):587–591.

263. Kumar MSA, Sierka DR, Damask AM, et al. Safety and success of kidney transplantation and concomitant immunosuppression on HIV-positive patients. *Kid Internation*. 2005; 67:1622–1629.

264. Freeman DJ, Laupacis A, Keown PA, et al. Evaluation of cyclosporine-phenytoin interaction with observations on cyclosporine metabolites. *Br J Clin Pharmacol*. 1984; 18:887–893.

265. Keown PA, Laupacis A, Carruthers G, et al. Interaction between phenytoin and cyclosporine following organ transplantation. *Transplantation*. 1984; 38(3):304–306.

266. Brockmoller J, Neumayer HH, Wagner K, et al. Pharmacokinetic interaction between cyclosporin and diltiazem. *Eur J Clin Pharmacol*. 1990; 38(3):237–242.

267. Grino JM, Sebate I, Castelao AM, et al. Influence of diltiazem on cyclosporine clearance. *Lancet*. 1986; 1:1387.

268. Kohlhaw K, Wonigeit K, Frei U, et al. Effect of the calcium channel blocker diltiazem on cyclosporine A blood levels and dose requirements. *Transplant Proc*. 1988; 20:572–574.

269. Renton KW. Inhibition of hepatic microsomal drug metabolism by the calcium channel blockers diltiazem and verapamil. *Biochem Pharmacol*. 1985; 34:2549–2553.

270. Bourbigot B, Guiserix J, Airiau J, et al. Nicardipine increases cyclosporine blood levels. *Lancet*. 1986; 1:1447.

271. Cantarovich M, Hiesse C, Lockiec F, et al. Confirmation of the interaction between cyclosporine and the calcium channel blocker nicardipine in renal transplant patients. *Clin Nephrol*. 1987; 28:190–193.

272. McNally P, Mistry N, Idle J, et al. Calcium channel blockers and cyclosporine metabolism. *Transplantation*. 1989; 48:1071.

273. Miller LW, Schlant RC, Kobashigawa J, et al. Task Force 5: complications. *J Am Coll Cardiol*. 1993; 22(1):41–53.

274. Maurer JR. Therapeutic challenges following lung transplantation. *Clin Chest Med*. 1990; 11(2):279–290.

275. Fabrega AJ, Lopez-Boado M, Gonzalez S. Problems in the longterm renal allograft recipient. *Crit Care Clin*. 1990; 6(4):979–1005.

276. Kiok MC. Neurologic complications of pancreas transplants. *Neurol Clin*. 1988; 6(2):367–376.

277. Van Thiel DH, Dindzans VJ, Gavaler JS, et al. The postoperative problems and management of the liver transplant recipient. *Prog Liver Dis*. 1990; 9:657–685.

278. Slavis SA, Novick AC, Steinmuller DR, et al. Outcome of renal transplantation in patients with a functioning graft for 20 years or more. *J Urol*. 1990; 144(1):20–22.

279. Braun WE. Long-term complications of renal transplantation. *Kidney Int*. 1990; 37(5):1363–1378.

280. Fischer SA. Infections complicating solid organ transplantation. *Surg Clin North Am*. 2006; 86:1127–1145.

281. Rubin RH, Tolkoff-Rubin NE. The impact of infection on the outcome of transplantation. *Transplant Proc*. 1991; 23(4):2068–2074.

282. McCarthy JM, Karim MA, Kruger H, et al. The cost impact of cytomegalovirus disease in renal transplant recipients. *Transplantation*. 1993; 55:1277–1282.

283. Pouteil-Noble C, Ecchard R, Landrivon G, et al. Cytomegalovirus infection—an etiologic factor for rejection. *Transplantation*. 1993; 55: 851–857.

284. Ho M. Epidemiology of cytomegalovirus infections. *Rev Infect Dis*. 1990; 12(suppl 7):S701–710.

285. Rubin RH. Impact of cytomegalovirus infection on organ transplant recipients. *Rev Infect Dis*. 1990; 12(suppl 7):S754–766.

286. Boland GJ, Hene RJ, Ververs C, et al. Factors influencing the occurrence of active CMV infections after organ transplantation. *Clin Exp Immunol*. 1993; 94:306–312.

287. Balfour HH, Chace BA, Stapleton JR, et al. A randomized, placebo-controlled trial of oral acyclovir for the prevention of cytomegalovirus disease in recipients of renal allografts. *N Engl J Med.* 1989; 21:1381–1387.

288. Anonymous. Cytomegalovirus. *Am J Transplant.* 2004; 4(suppl 10):51–58.

289. Nalesnik MA, Locker J, Jaffe R, et al. Clonal characteristics of posttransplant lymphoproliferative disorders. *Transplant Proc.* 1988; 20(suppl 1): 280–283.

290. Hanto DW, Frizzera G, Gajl-Peczalska KJ, et al. Epstein-Barr virus-induced B-cell lymphoma after renal transplantation: acyclovir therapy and transition from polyclonal to monoclonal B-cell proliferation. *N Engl J Med.* 1982; 306:913–918.

291. Penn I. The changing patterns of posttransplant malignancies. *Transplant Proc.* 1991; 23(1):1101–1103.

292. Hibberd PL, Rubin RH. Antiviral therapy—an antimalignancy strategy for transplant recipients? *Clin Transplant.* 1992; 6(special issue):240–245.

293. Brumbaugh J, Baldwin JC, Stinson EB, et al. Quantitative analysis of immunosuppression in cyclosporine-treated heart transplant patients with lymphoma. *J Heart Transplant.* 1985; 4:307–311.

294. Penn I. Cancers after cyclosporine therapy. *Transplant Proc.* 1988; 20(suppl 1):276–279.

295. Emery RW, Lake KD. Post-transplantation lymphoproliferative disorder and OKT3 [letter]. *N Engl J Med.* 1991; 324(20):1437.

296. Cosimi AB, Rubin RH. Post-transplantation lymphoproliferative disorder and OKT3 [letter]. *N Engl J Med.* 1991; 324(20):1438.

297. Abramowicz D, Goldman M, De Pauw L, et al. Post-transplantation lymphoproliferative disorder and OKT3 [letter]. *N Engl J Med.* 1991; 324(20):1439.

298. Swinnen LJ, Costanzo-Nordin MR, Fisher SG, et al. Increased incidence of lymphoproliferative disorder after immunosuppression with the monoclonal antibody of OKT3 in cardiac transplant recipients. *N Engl J Med.* 1990; 323:1723–1728.

299. Anonymous. Epstein-Barr virus and lymphoproliferative disorders after transplantation. *Am J Transplant.* 2004; 4(suppl 10):59–65.

300. Loren AW, Tsai DE. Post-transplant lymphoproliferative disorder. *Clin Chest Med.* 2005; 26:631–645.

301. Opelz G, Dohler B. Lymphomas after solid organ transplantation: a collaborative transplant study report. *Am J Transplant.* 2003; 4:222–230.

302. Svoboda J, Kotloff R, Tsai D. Management of patients with post-transplant lymphoproliferative disorder: the role of rituximab. *Transplant International.* 2006(19):259–269.

303. Petterson E, Hovi T, Ahonen T, et al. Prophylactic oral acyclovir after renal transplantation. *Transplantation.* 1985; 39:279–281.

304. Rubin RH, Tolkoff-Rubin NE. Antimicrobial strategies in the care of organ transplant recipients. *Antimicrob Agents Chemother.* 1993; 37(4):619–624.

305. Lynfield R, Herrin JT, Rubin RH. Varicella in pediatric renal transplant recipients. *Pediatrics.* 1992; 90:216–220.

306. Josephson MA, Williams JW, Chandraker A, et al. Polymavirus-associated nephropathy: update on antiviral strategies. *Transplant Inf Disease.* 2006; 8:95–101.

307. Anonymous. BK virus. *Am J Transplant.* 2004; 4(suppl 10):89–91.

308. Randhawa P, Brennan DC. BK virus infection in transplant recipients: and overview and update. *Am J Transplant.* 2006; 6:2000–2005.

309. Hirsch HH. Polyomavirus BK nephropathy: a re-emerging complication in renal transplantation. *Am J Transplant.* 2002; 2:25–30.

310. Mylonakis E, Goes N, Rubin RH, et al. BK virus in solid organ transplant recipients: an emerging syndrome. *Transplantation.* 2001; 72(10):1587–1592.

311. Hibberd PL, Rubin RH. Clinical aspects of fungal infection in organ transplant recipients. *Clin Infect Dis.* 1994; 19(suppl 1):S33–40.

312. Collins LA, Samore MH, Roberts MS, et al. Risk factors for invasive fungal infections complicating orthotopic liver transplantation. *J Infect Dis.* 1994; 170(3):544–552.

313. Tollemar J, Andersson S, Ringden O, et al. A retrospective clinical comparison between antifungal treatment with liposomal amphotericin B (AmBisome) and conventional amphotericin B in transplant patients. *Mycoses.* 1992; 35(9-10):215–220.

314. Anonymous. Fungal infections. *Am J Transplant.* 2004; 4(suppl 10):110–134.

315. Paya CV. Fungal infections in solid organ transplantation. *Clin Infec Dis.* 1993; 16:677–688.

316. Anonymous. *Pneumocystis jiroveci* (formerly *Pneumocystis carinii*). *Am J Transplant.* 2004; 4(suppl 10):135–141.

317. Magee C, Pascual M. The growing problem of chronic renal failure after transplantation of a nonrenal organ. *N Engl J Med.* 2003; 349(10): 994–996.

318. Lake KD. Management of post-transplant obesity and hyperlipidemia. In: Emery RW, Miller L, eds. *Handbook of Cardiothoracic Transplantation.* Philadelphia, PA: Hanley & Belfus; 1995:147–164.

319. Pirsch JD, D'Alessandro AM, Sollinger HW, et al. Hyperlipidemia and transplantation: etiologic factors and therapy. *J Am Soc Nephrol.* 1992; 2(12 suppl):S238–242.

320. Pirsch JD, Friedman R. Primary care of the renal transplant patient. *J Gen Intern Med.* 1994; 9(1):29–37.

321. Johnson CP, Gallagher-Lepak S, Zhu YR, et al. Factors influencing weight gain after renal transplantation. *Transplantation.* 1993; 56(4):822–827.

322. Palmer M, Schaffner F, Thung SN. Excessive weight gain after liver transplantation. *Transplantation.* 1991; 51(4):797–800.

323. Rubin S, Dale J, Santamaria C, et al. Weight change in cardiac transplant patients. *Can J Cardiovasc Nurs.* 1991; 2(2):9–13.

324. Buchanan C, Smith L, Corbett J, et al. A retrospective analysis of ezetimibe treatment in renal transplant recipients. *Am J Transplant.* 2006; 6(4):770–774.

325. Bergman AJ, Burke J, Larson P, et al. Interaction of single-dose ezetimibe and steady-state cyclosporine in renal transplant patients. *J Clin Pharmacol.* 2006; 46(3):328–336.

326. Jindal RM. Posttransplant diabetes mellitus—a review. *Transplantation.* 1994; 58(12):1289–1298.

327. Keown PA, Shackleton CR, Ferguson BM. Long-term mortality, morbidity, and rehabilitation in organ transplant recipients. In: Paul LC, Solez K, eds. *Organ Transplantation: Long-Term Results.* New York, NY: Marcel Dekker; 1992:57–84.

328. Ost L. Effects of cyclosporine on prednisolone metabolism. *Lancet.* 1984; 1:451.

329. Tyden G, Brattstrom C, Gunnarsson R, et al. Metabolic control at 2 months to 4.5 years after pancreatic transplantation, with special reference to the role of cyclosporine. *Transplant Proc.* 1987; 19:2294.

330. Ried M, Gibbons S, Kwok D, et al. Cyclosporine levels in human tissues of patients treated for one week to one year. *Transplant Proc.* 1983; 15:2434.

331. Jindal RM, Popsecu I, Schwartz ME, et al. Diabetogenicity of FK506 versus cyclosporine in liver transplant recipients. *Transplantation.* 1994; 58:370.

332. Cunningham J. Posttransplantation bone disease. *Transplantation.* 2005; 79(6):629–634.

333. Cohen A, Shane E. Osteoporosis after solid organ and bone marrow transplantation. *Osteoporos Int.* 2003; 4(8):617–630.

SELF-ASSESSMENT QUESTIONS

1. Which of the HLA antigens are considered most important for a successful outcome in transplantation?

   A. HLA- A, B, and C
   B. HLA-DP, DQ, DR
   C. HLA-A, B, and DR
   D. All of the above

2. Which of the following types of rejection episodes usually present within a week to 6 months posttransplant, are characterized by histological biopsy findings consistent with lymphocyte infiltrates, and typically respond to antirejection therapy?

   A. Hyperacute rejection
   B. Acute rejection
   C. Accelerated acute rejection
   D. Chronic rejection

3. The usefulness of corticosteroids in organ transplantation results from which of the following actions?

   A. Direct inhibitory effect on circulating lymphocytes
   B. Modulation of specific cellular immune functions
   C. Specific anti-inflammatory action in the transplanted organ
   D. A and B only

4. Which of the following is improved by switching from cyclosporine to tacrolimus-based immunosuppression?

   A. Hirsutism
   B. Tremors
   C. Diabetes
   D. Hepatotoxicity

5. Which of the following are common adverse effects of mycophenolate mofetil?

   A. Seizures
   B. Leukopenia
   C. Gastrointestinal distress
   D. Nephrotoxicity
      i. A only
      ii. A and B
      iii. B and C
      iv. All of the above

6. The adverse effects of OKT3 during the first several doses (including fever, hypotension, nausea and/or vomiting, and headaches) are related to:

   A. An allergic reaction to the murine component of OKT3
   B. Cytokine release secondary to T-cell activation
   C. Sepsis
   D. Serum sickness

7. Which of the following can result in decreased cyclosporine blood concentrations?

   A. Grapefruit juice
   B. Verapamil
   C. Fluconazole
   D. Phenytoin

8. Acute renal transplant rejection is initially treated with which therapy?

   A. ATG/OKT3 and/or prednisone
   B. Steroid pulse and/or prednisone
   C. CsA
   D. Quadruple therapy

9. The most common viral infection after transplantation is:

    A. Cytomegalovirus
    B. Herpes simplex virus
    C. Epstein-Barr virus
    D. Hepatitis C virus

10. What is the most common postoperative complication for kidney transplant patients?

    A. Hypertension
    B. Allograft rejection
    C. Viral infections
    D. New onset diabetes

CHAPTER 10

Bone Marrow Transplantation

Brad L. Stanford, Karen M. Fancher

CHAPTER OUTLINE

INTRODUCTION

Bone marrow transplantation (BMT) is the process of introducing hematopoietic stem cells from a donor into a compatible recipient. BMT is performed to reestablish marrow function in a patient whose bone marrow is defective or damaged, usually the result of high doses of chemotherapy or disease. The transfer of hematopoietic stem cells rescues the recipient from potentially fatal hematologic toxicity by ultimately creating new blood elements.

BMT is primarily used to treat malignant hematologic diseases, including acute and chronic leukemias, lymphomas, and multiple myeloma. It may also be used to treat immune system disorders. A list of diseases potentially treated with BMT is found in **Table 10.1**.

LEARNING OBJECTIVES

After completing this chapter, the reader should be able to:

Table 10.1. Indications for Bone Marrow Transplantation

Autologous BMT Preferred	Autologous BMT Controversial
Breast cancer	Autoimmune disorders
Ewing's sarcoma/rhabdomyosarcoma	Multiple sclerosis
Hodgkin's disease	Rheumatoid arthritis
Multiple myeloma	Systemic lupus
Non-Hodgkin's lymphoma	Acute leukemias
Ovarian cancer	Chronic myelogenous leukemia
Testicular cancer	Chronic lymphocytic leukemia
	Neuroblastoma
Allogenic BMT Preferred	**Allogeneic BMT Controversial**
Acute leukemias	Chronic lymphocytic leukemia
Aplastic anemia (severe)	Hereditary immune system disorders
Chronic myelogenous leukemia	Idiopathic thrombocytopenia purpura
Myelodysplastic syndromes	Inborn errors of metabolism
Myeloproliferative disorders	Severe combined immunodeficiency
	Hodgkin's disease
	Multiple myeloma
	Neuroblastoma
	Non-Hodgkin's lymphoma
	Sickle cell disease

Source: Horowitz MM. Uses and growth of hematopoietic cell transplantation. In: Blume KG, Forman SJ, Appelbaum FR, eds. *Thomas' Hematopoietic Stem Cell Transplantation*. 3rd ed. Malden, MA: Blackwell Publishing; 2004:9–15.[1]

1. Discuss the different types of bone marrow transplantation and the rationale for using each type.
2. Explain how bone marrow patients and their donors are matched using the HLA system.
3. Describe the preparative regimens for patients undergoing bone marrow transplantation.
4. Understand the concept of nonmyeloablative BMT.
5. Describe the pathophysiology of acute GVHD.
6. Discuss various management strategies for the prophylaxis and treatment of GVHD.
7. Describe the potential infectious complications of BMT and methods of prophylaxis and treatment.

TYPES OF BMT

There are four sources of marrow for BMT. In an autologous transplant, the patient serves as his own donor and receives his own hematopoietic stem cells that have been previously collected and stored. In a syngeneic transplant, the patient receives hematopoietic stem cells from an identical twin sibling. Allogeneic bone marrow transplantation involves infusing hematopoietic stem cells from a genetically distinct donor: a relative, usually a sibling (match-related donor, MRD), or an unrelated person (match-unrelated donor, MUD). The fourth source of stem cells is umbilical cord blood (UCB). Initially, UCB was used for match-related transplants but is now widely used in unrelated BMT.

Each type of transplant has advantages and disadvantages. Donor availability is low for allogeneic, syngeneic, and UCB transplants, but this is not an issue in autologous BMT. Autologous transplants usually result in fewer immunologic complications because the donor receives his own cells. But an autologous transplant risks the reinfusion of malignant cells, offers no immunologic effect against the patient's underlying disease (graft-versus-leukemia effect, GVL), and is associated with high rates of relapse. An allogeneic or UCB BMT offers a GVL effect, but also risks rejection of the donor marrow by the patient (graft rejection) as well as an attack of the donor's T lymphocytes on the recipient (graft-versus-host disease, GVHD). Which type of BMT is appropriate is often based on many factors, including the type of malignancy, donor availability, the patient's age, comorbid conditions, and other issues. A summary of the different types of BMT is found in **Table 10.2**.

Table 10.2. Advantages and Disadvantages of the Various Types of BMT

Donor Type	Donor Source	Advantages	Disadvantages
Autologous	Self	Donor availability No GVHD	Potential reinfusion of malignant cells (increased risk of relapse)
Syngeneic	Identical twin	No malignant cells in infusion Decreased rates of GVHD	Donor availability Limited GVL
Allogeneic	Related HLA match Unrelated HLA match	No malignant cells in infusion GVL	Potential GVHD Potential graft rejection Donor availability Process limited by age and co-morbidities
Umbilical cord blood	Related HLA match Unrelated HLA match	No malignant cells in infusion Decreased rates of GVHD Potential GVL	Potential GVHD Potential graft rejection Donor availability Limited volume of collected cells Increased rates of infection post-BMT

GVHD = graft versus host disease; GVL = graft versus leukemia effect; HLA = human leukocyte antigen.

COLLECTION OF HEMATOPOIETIC STEM CELLS

Hematopoietic stem cells are found in the bone marrow, peripheral blood, and umbilical cord blood. Stem cells are abundant in the bone marrow; they can be harvested through aspirations from the iliac crests of the pelvis in a procedure that typically requires general anesthesia. In the umbilical cord, stem cells are collected from the placental blood after birth, with no risk to the mother or baby.[2]

Peripheral blood stem cell (PBSC) transplantation is the transplantation of only peripheral blood stem cells (instead of bone marrow). Stem cells are normally present in very low numbers in the peripheral blood. But stem cells in the marrow can be mobilized into the peripheral blood using colony-stimulating factors (such as granulocyte colony-stimulating factor, GCSF) or chemotherapy. Mobilized PBSCs can then be collected in an outpatient leukapheresis procedure and stored for later use.

Using PBSCs instead of bone marrow has several advantages. Patients who receive mobilized PBSCs have more rapid engraftment of the hematopoietic system, especially in the platelet lineage.[3,4] PBSC collection may be less likely to be contaminated with malignant cells compared to bone marrow stem cells, and thus may reduce relapse rates in patients whose disease has spread to the bone marrow.[3,4] And PBSC transplantation spares the donor the discomfort associated with marrow aspirations and does not require general anesthesia.

PBSC transplantation is the preferred method of autologous BMT, and is gaining popularity in allogeneic transplants. There were initial concerns that some of the numerous peripheral T lymphocytes would contaminate the infusion and cause an increased incidence of acute GVHD. Early studies have not shown an increased risk of acute GVHD, but some studies have reported an increased risk of chronic GVHD.[5,6] Disease-free and overall survival rates in patients receiving PBSC transplantation are at least equivalent to those patients who received bone marrow.[7]

TISSUE TYPING

For allogeneic donors, the degree of compatibility between donor and recipient tissue types is of critical importance. An appropriate match reduces the risk of graft rejection as well as the incidence of GVHD.

HLA System

The compatibility of a potential donor is evaluated by studies of a cluster of genes on the short arm of chromosome six.[8] This group of genes—the major histocompatibility complex (MHC)—encodes for cell surface proteins responsible for differentiating self from nonself. In humans, this region is known as the human leukocyte antigen (HLA) complex.

Genes in the HLA system are subdivided into class I, class II, and class III loci. Class I and class II antigens are most important in organ transplantation, while class III antigens have other functions within the immune system. The major function of class I and II antigens is to present foreign antigens to T lymphocytes. Class I antigens (HLA-A, HLA-B, and HLA-C) are the primary targets for cytotoxic T lymphocytes, and are found on all nucleated cells in the human body. The major class II antigen (HLA-D, specifically HLA-DR) is the primary target for helper T lymphocytes, and is found only on the surface of B lymphocytes, macrophages, and activated T lymphocytes. When there is a mismatch between donor and recipient marrow at HLA-A, HLA-B, or HLA-DR, the recipient appears foreign to the donor T lymphocytes, which can result in GVHD.

Minor histocompatibility antigens are also present, but their characteristics are not well defined. T-lymphocyte response against minor histocompatibility antigens is mediated by an MHC class I process, and thus may also play a role in the development of GVHD. Due to uncertainty of function and importance, minor antigens are not typically matched prior to transplant.

Donor/Recipient Matching

Serologic or molecular testing is performed at each of the three loci (HLA-A, -B, and -DR). Because every child receives a set of HLA genes from both parents, each patient has two phenotypes on each locus. Accordingly, a "perfectly" matched donor is a six-of-six antigen match. The most common donor for an allogeneic BMT is an HLA-identical sibling. The probability of siblings being HLA-matched follows classical Mendelian genetics and is one in four. Because American families are relatively small, only about 30% of Americans have an HLA-identical sibling donor.[8,9]

For patients who do not have a compatible sibling donor, an unrelated individual may be identified. Organizations such as the National Marrow Donor Program (NMDP) have registered millions of HLA types for potential MUD transplants. The likelihood of finding an unrelated individual with HLA-identical marrow is about 1 in 10,000–20,000,[10] but varies widely based on the frequency of the patient's HLA type in the general population and ethnic background. Unfortunately, most minorities are not as well represented in donor programs as whites, making the probability of finding a match in certain ethnic groups much lower.

If a completely matched donor cannot be identified, a sibling who is mismatched at one locus may be considered. Patients who receive single-antigen mismatched BMT from a sibling

are at increased risk of incidence and severity of GVHD, but overall survival does not appear to be affected[11,12]; the lack of difference in survival may be due to the GVL effect. More than a single-antigen mismatch usually results in an unacceptable incidence of GVHD and mortality.

PREPARATIVE REGIMEN

Chemotherapy and Radiation

Patients undergoing allogeneic BMT receive myeloablative doses of chemotherapy, with or without radiation, before receiving the donor's hematopoietic stem cells. This intensive conditioning has three main goals: to provide a sufficient degree of immunosuppression and avoid destruction of the graft by the patient's immune system; to destroy any residual malignant cells; and to provide physical space in which the new marrow will grow.[8] The ideal conditioning regimen has activity against the patient's malignancy, along with significant immunosuppressive properties to ensure that the donor's marrow is not rejected by the patient's residual immune system.

The choice of chemotherapy agents in BMT is restricted, since the dose-limiting toxicities of most chemotherapy agents are not hematological and would be fatal if given in high doses. Chemotherapy agents used in BMT are typically alkylating agents, which have a steep dose–response curve and whose primary toxicity is myelosuppression. These agents have varying degrees of immunosuppression and minimal non-hematologic toxicities; examples include cyclophosphamide, busulfan, etoposide, carmustine, and melphalan. These agents' common nonhematologic side effects are found in **Table 10.3**. Most conditioning regimens consist of several chemotherapy agents that are non-cross-resistant and have nonoverlapping toxicities.

Some conditioning regimens include total body irradiation (TBI), which increases the regimen's immunosuppressive effects and penetrates sites inaccessible to chemotherapy. Common toxicities from TBI include pulmonary toxicity, mucositis, infertility, and growth retardation in children.[9,13]

Targeted radiation may be achieved with the use of monoclonal antibodies and radiolabeled isotopes. This method may allow delivery of increased doses of radiation directly to the marrow, while sparing non-hematologic toxicities.[9,13] Standard conditioning regimens have been combined with radiolabeled monoclonal antibodies in small clinical trials, but this approach is not yet universally accepted.

Table 10.3. Chemotherapy Agents Commonly Used in BMT

Drug	Non-Hematologic Toxicities
Busulfan (Busulfex, Myleran)	Pulmonary fibrosis Seizures Veno-occlusive disease
Carboplatin (Paraplatin)	Peripheral neuropathy Renal dysfunction
Carmustine (BCNU)	Hepatotoxicity Pulmonary fibrosis
Cyclophosphamide (Cytoxan, Neosar)	Hemorrhagic cystitis Cardiomyopathy Mucositis
Etoposide (VP-16, VePesid)	Hypotension Mucositis
Fludarabine (Fludara)	Neurotoxicity Pulmonary hypersensitivity
Ifosfamide (Ifex)	Hemorrhagic cystitis Neurotoxicity Renal toxicity
Melphalan (Alkeran)	Mucositis GI toxicity
Thiotepa (TESPA, Thioplex)	Dermatologic toxicity Neurotoxicity Mucositis
Total body irradiation (TBI)	GI toxicity Mucositis Pulmonary toxicity

Sources: Adapted from Armitage JO. Bone marrow transplantation. *N Engl J Med*. 1994; 300(12):827–838; Bensinger WI, Spielberger R. Preparative regimens and modification of regimen-related toxicities. In: Blume KG, Forman SJ, Appelbaum FR, eds. *Thomas' Hematopoietic Stem Cell Transplantation*. 3rd ed. Malden, MA: Blackwell Publishing; 2004:158–177.[8,13]

Pretransplant Immunosuppression

Patients receiving an unrelated BMT have an increased risk of graft rejection compared to patients receiving a related BMT, because of the residual immune function of the recipient mounting a response against the donor. Lymphocyte immune globulin (ATG, Atgam) or antithymocyte globulin (Thymoglobulin) may be added to the conditioning regimen to increase the suppression of the patient's residual immune function and decrease the risk of graft rejection.

Time Course of Transplantation

Patients undergoing BMT receive their conditioning regimen with chemotherapy or radiation prior to receiving the hematopoietic stem cell infusion. The day of stem cell infusion is commonly known as "day 0." So the days preceding the transplant are known as the "negative days" (i.e., "day −4") and the days after transplant are the "positive days" (i.e., "day +3"). Patients typically receive chemotherapy, radiation, or both for several days and then have several days of rest before the stem cell infusion. This allows the chemotherapy to be metabolized and eliminated prior to the infusion of new cells.

Donor Lymphocyte Depletion

Because GVHD is the most significant complication of allogeneic BMT, eliminating (purging) the T lymphocytes from the donor marrow can minimize the development of acute GVHD. Several methods are available to deplete the donor marrow. T lymphocytes can be physically separated from the stem-cell product by ex vivo negative selection or ex vivo positive selection of hematopoietic stem cells.[14] T-lymphocyte depletion can also be accomplished with in vivo monoclonal antibodies specifically directed against T lymphocytes.[14]

Because T lymphocytes also facilitate engraftment and mount an immune response against the patient's malignancy, mortality from graft failure or disease relapse may exceed that of acute GVHD when purged products are used.[15] The role of lymphocyte depletion is currently undefined, but may be considered in patients at high risk for GVHD or those with comorbid conditions that would preclude conventional GVHD prophylaxis[14] (see GVHD section).

NONMYELOABLATIVE BMT

Traditional BMT is performed by giving large, myeloablative doses of chemotherapy and then "rescuing" the patient from these toxicities by reestablishing marrow function with the infusion of new hematopoietic cells. This results in a high incidence of treatment-related morbidity and mortality, so older or debilitated patients are often not suitable for such a toxic procedure. Nonmyeloablative BMT (NMT, or "mini-transplant") is being explored to provide this potentially curative treatment option to a greater number of patients. NMT is based on the concept that the majority of antitumor activity in an allogeneic BMT is from the GVL effect of the donor T cells, instead of from the

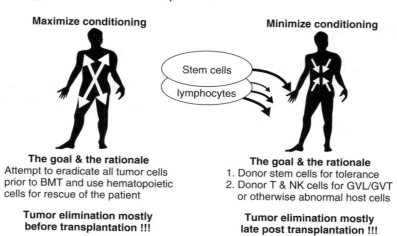

Figure 10.1. Goals and rationales for traditional hematopoietic stem cell transplantation compared to nonmyeloablative stem cell transplantation. BMT = bone marrow transplantation; NK = natural killer cells; GVL/GVT = graft-versus-leukemia/graft-versus-tumor. (Source: Slavin S, Morecki S, Weiss L, et al. Nonmyeloablative stem cell transplantation: reduced-intensity conditioning for cancer immunotherapy—from bench to patient bedside. *Semin Oncol.* 2004; 31:9; with permission.)

elimination of malignant cells with myeloablative doses of chemotherapy. Patients receiving an NMT receive a lower-intensity conditioning regimen that avoids the toxicity of a myeloablative BMT, yet is immunosuppressive enough to allow donor engraftment and GVL[2,11,16,17] (**Figure 10.1**). In the small numbers of patients who have received NMTs to date, treatment-related morbidity and mortality have been low.[2,11,16] However, since the GVL and GVHD processes cannot yet be separated, GVHD is a major clinical problem in NMT.[2,11,17] NMT remains an option under investigation, and may be considered for patients normally excluded from conventional BMT.

COMPLICATIONS OF BMT

Long-term outcomes following BMT may be compromised by posttransplant complications. Both autologous and allogeneic transplant patients may experience bacterial, fungal, and viral infections. In addition, patients receiving allogeneic transplantation may also experience both acute GVHD (aGVHD) and chronic GVHD (cGVHD). The time course of these toxicities is summarized in **Figure 10.2** and is discussed in the following sections.

Acute GVHD and GVL Effect

Historically, aGVHD appears in the first 100 days following transplantation, although this is now known to be arbitrary since cGVHD may appear

prior to day 100. The incidence of aGVHD is about 30% to 60% in HLA-matched sibling donors, but varies according to certain risk factors (**Table 10.4**) and the prophylactic regimen used.[20] The risk is significantly higher in single-mismatched transplant recipients and in MUD transplants. And a recent meta-analysis found the risk of both aGVHD and cGVHD may be higher in patients receiving PBSC transplants instead of BMT.[21]

Pathophysiology of Acute GVHD

aGVHD arises when alloreactive donor T lymphocytes attack and damage host tissues. Although differences in MHC antigens play a role in the pathogenesis of aGVHD, disparities in the minor histocompatibility antigens have also been recently identified to play a key role.[22] This explains the incidence of aGVHD despite HLA-identity between a donor and recipient. The pathophysiologic basis for aGVHD was recently described as a three-phase process (**Figure 10.3**).[23]

The first two phases are collectively known as the afferent phase. The first phase is a result of a "cytokine storm" of inflammatory cytokines, such as interleukin-1 (IL-1), tumor necrosis factor α (TNF-α), and interferon γ (IFN-γ), released early in the preparative regimen due to direct mucosal tissue damage. These cytokines up-regulate adhesion molecules and MHC antigens, which sensitize the recognition of host MHC and minor histocompatibility antigens by donor T cells.[24] The second phase is the result of recipient and donor

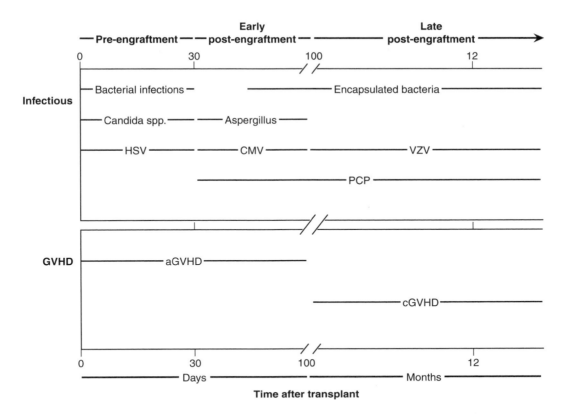

Figure 10.2. Summary of immunologic and infectious complications after bone marrow transplantation. HSV = herpes simplex virus; CMV = cytomegalovirus; VZV = varicella zoster virus; PCP = *Pneumocystis jiroveci*; aGVHD = acute graft-versus-host disease; cGVHD = chronic graft-versus-host disease. (Source: Adapted from McCune JS, Winter LL, Dix SD. Hematopoietic cell transplantation. In: Koda-Kimble MA, Young YL, eds. *Applied Therapeutics: The Clinical Use of Drugs*. 8th ed. Baltimore, MD: Lippincott Williams & Wilkins; 2005; with permission.)

Table 10.4. Risk Factors for Acute Graft-versus-Host Disease (aGVHD)

Risk Factor	aGVHD Risk
HLA-matching	One mismatch—70%–75% 2–3 mismatches—up to 90%
Age	Pediatric—~20% Age 20–50 years—30% Age 51–62 years—70%
Sex	Increased with gender mismatch Highest in females donating to males
Parity	Decreased in nulliparous women
Host microenvironment	Decreased in patients with aplastic anemia with the use of antibiotics, gut and skin decontamination
Umbilical cord blood source	Decreased risk
Number of donor T cells infused	Increased risk with higher dose

HLA = human leukocyte antigen.
Source: Adapted from Flowers MED, Kansu E, Sullivan KM. Pathophysiology and treatment of graft-versus-host disease. *Hematol Oncol Clin North Am*. 1999; 13:1091–1112.[19]

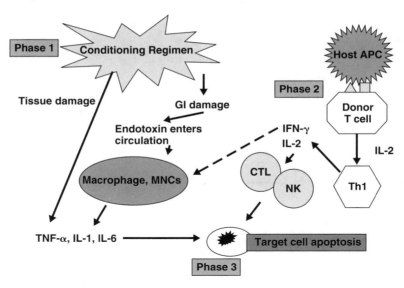

Figure 10.3. Pathophysiology of acute graft-versus-host disease. APC = antigen presenting cell; CTL = cytotoxic T lymphocyte; GI = gastrointestinal; IL-1& IL-6 = interleukins 1 & 6; IFN = interferon; MNCs = mononuclear cells; NK = natural killer cells; TH1 = T-helper cell type 1; TNF = tumor necrosis factor. (Source: Couriel D, Caldera H, Champlin R, et al. Acute graft-versus-host disease: pathophysiology, clinical manifestations, and management. *Cancer.* 2004; 101(9):1937; with permission.)

antigen-presenting cells (APCs), along with the cytokines, inducing donor-derived T lymphocytes to clonally expand and differentiate into effector cells. The activated T cells are of the T-helper 1 (Th1) phenotype and produce IL-2 and IFN-γ, which leads to the third (efferent) phase. This phase is mediated by inflammatory cytokines produced by damaged tissue and activated donor T cells driving cytotoxicity against target host cells through cytotoxic T cells (CD8⁺ lymphocytes), macrophages, and natural killer (NK) cells. Along with the activated T cells, these cells secrete TNF-α and other cytokines—causing further damage to host tissues and the subsequent release of additional cytokines that continue the destructive cycle in a positive feedback loop. So the clinical effects that occur during aGVHD result from both direct effects of activated T cells and indirect effects of inflammatory cytokines on host tissues.

Staging and Grading

aGVHD is the primary cause of both early and late mortality in patients receiving allogeneic BMT. Death is typically caused by infection, hemorrhage, or organ dysfunction. The primary organs affected by aGVHD are the skin, liver, and gastrointestinal (GI) tract, and the usual manifestations include rash, increased liver function tests, and secretory diarrhea. A clinical staging and grading system

(**Table 10.5**) used by most transplant centers considers the number of organs involved, the extent of organ involvement, and Eastern Cooperative Oncology Group (ECOG) performance status. aGVHD is graded on a scale from 0–IV, and mortality increases with worsening GVHD as indicated in **Table 10.6**.[25] The poor survival of grade II–IV aGVHD is not surprising given the destructive cycle of continued T-cell activation, the subsequent tissue destruction followed by cytokine release, further T-cell activation, and so on. An extensive discussion of the clinical manifestations of aGVHD is beyond the scope of this chapter; excellent reviews have been published on this subject.[19,23,26]

Mechanisms of GVL

Historically, high-dose chemotherapy was thought to be the most important mediator of long-term survival in allogeneic BMT patients. But studies from the early 1990s showed that recipients of syngeneic BMT or T-cell-depleted allogeneic BMT had a higher risk of leukemic relapse.[27,28] This led to the finding that the GVL effect is important for tumor eradication. It is also demonstrated by the efficacy of donor lymphocyte infusions for inducing durable remissions in patients with chronic myeloid leukemia (CML).[29] As previously discussed, this discovery serves as the basis for nonmyeloablative ("mini-allo") allogeneic transplants.

Table 10.5. Organ Staging of Acute Graft-versus-Host Disease

Stage	Skin	Liver	Gut
0	No rash	Bilirubin <2 mg/dL	No diarrhea
I	Rash <25% of BSA without symptoms	Bilirubin 2–3 mg/dL	Diarrhea >500–1000 mL/day; nausea & emesis
II	Rash ≥25% & <50% of BSA or erythema with pruritis	Bilirubin 3–6 mg/dL	Diarrhea >1000–1500 mL/day; nausea & emesis
III	Rash ≥50% BSA or generalized erythema	Bilirubin 6–15 mg/dL	Diarrhea >1500 mL/day; nausea & emesis
IV	Generalized exfoliative or ulcerative dermatitis or bullous formation	Bilirubin ≥15 mg/dL	Severe abdominal pain ± ileus

BSA = body surface area.
Source: Adapted from Przepiorka D, Weisdorf D, Martin P, et al. 1994 Consensus conference on acute GVHD grading. *Bone Marrow Transplant*. 1995; 15:825–828.[25]

The GVL effect is mediated by donor immune cells (including CD8+ and CD4+ T lymphocytes) and NK cells.[30] CD4+ T cells secrete IL-2, resulting in the clonal expansion of cytotoxic CD8+ T cells. Unfortunately, these cells recognize both the host

malignancy and normal tissue as foreign, so the positive GVL effects must be balanced with the negative GVHD effects. This paradox complicates the posttransplant management of allogenic BMT patients since the elimination of disease relapse is the primary goal of the transplant, and the GVL effects cannot be separated from the GVHD effects. The graft-versus-tumor effect is also under active investigation for nonhematological malignancies such as renal cell carcinoma and melanoma.[31]

The ideal model would eliminate deleterious GVHD effects while retaining beneficial GVL effects, as illustrated in **Figure 10.4**. It has been suggested that different subsets of T-cell populations are responsible for GVL and GVHD. This may be mediated by differences in minor histocompatibility antigens between the host leukemia cells and normal cells. As discussed previously, nonselective methods for donor lymphocyte depletion use anti-CD52 monoclonal antibodies (alemtuzumab, Campath), anti-CD3, and anti-CD5. But these methods result in a higher risk of graft failure and disease relapse. Recent investigations have shown it may be possible to selectively purge the donor marrow of T cells specifically responsible for GVHD. A randomized controlled trial demonstrated that CD8+ T-cell depletion using a monoclonal antibody combined with complement could achieve equivalent survival outcomes with decreased incidence and severity of aGVHD.[32] A population of regulatory CD4+CD25+ T lymphocytes has been identified that may selectively inhibit the T-cell population responsible for GVHD.[33] Ricin-conjugated antibodies and immunotoxin-conjugated monoclonal antibodies directed against CD25+ (IL-2 receptor) cells have also been studied.[34,35] Early data suggest a strategy of delayed donor lymphocyte infusions

Table 10.6. Clinical Grading of Acute Graft-versus-Host Disease

Grade	Skin	Liver	Gut	ECOG Performance Status*	Mortality Rates
0 (None)	0	0	0	0	10%
1 (Mild)	1–2	0	0	0	10%
2 (Moderate)	1–3	1	1	1	60%
3 (Severe)	2–3	2–3	2–3	2	60%
4 (Life threatening)	2–3	2–3	2–3	2–4	100%

ECOG = Eastern Cooperative Oncology Group.
*Grade 0 = Fully active; Grade 1 = restricted activity; Grade 2 = ambulatory >50%; Grade 3 = ambulatory <50%; Grade 4 = bedbound
Source: Adapted from Przepiorka D, Weisdorf D, Martin P, et al. 1994 Consensus conference on acute GVHD grading. *Bone Marrow Transplant*. 1995; 15:825–828.[25]

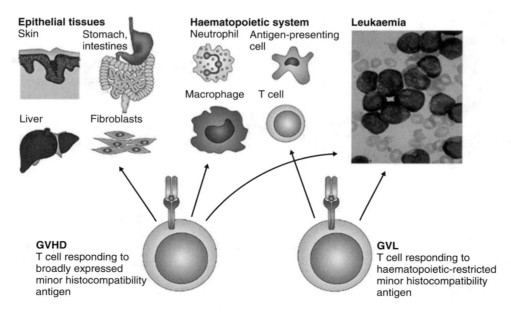

Nature Reviews | Cancer

Figure 10.4. Separating the GVL effect from the GVHD effect. Donor T cells specific for minor histocompatibility antigens that are broadly expressed by both hematopoietic and epithelial cells of the recipient are believed to cause graft-versus-host disease (GVHD). These T cells could also contribute to the graft-versus-leukemia (GVL) effect if leukemic cells express the minor histocompatibility antigens that are recognized by the T cells. Donor T cells specific for minor histocompatibility antigens that are selectively expressed by hematopoietic cells could induce a GVL response without GVHD. (Source: Bleakley M, Riddell SR. Molecules and mechanisms of the graft-versus-leukemia effect. *Nat Rev Cancer.* 2004; 4:376; with permission.)

(DLI) following T cell depletion (the so-called "add-back" strategy) may allow the early benefits of T cell depletion (decreased aGVHD and toxicity) while later restoring the GVL effect.[36]

POSTTRANSPLANT IMMUNOSUPPRESSIVE AGENTS

Patients who receive allogeneic BMT require immunosuppression to circumvent GVHD. Nonspecific agents (ATG, corticosteroids, methotrexate) and specific agents (cyclosporine, tacrolimus, mycophenolate) are used for both prophylaxis and treatment, although modern prophylaxis regimens typically delete corticosteroids to preserve them for use as initial treatment of aGVHD (**Table 10.7**). One limitation of these agents is that they often give rise to significant toxicity. Various anti-cytokine antibodies have also been used in recent years, primarily in the treatment of steroid-refractory aGVHD. Detailed discussion of the pharmacology and toxicity of these agents may be found in Chapter 9; a brief discussion of their role in BMT follows.

ATG

ATG is a polyclonal immunoglobulin mixture derived from horses (lymphocyte immune globulin, Atgam) or rabbits (antithymocyte globulin, Thymoglobulin) immunized with human thymocytes. This agent is a potent mediator of T-cell clearance from the circulation and modifier of T-cell activity, including homing and cytotoxicity. It is most often used as part of GVHD prophylaxis for MUD transplants, which reduces the incidence of aGVHD. However, using ATG in this type of BMT did not reduce transplant-related mortality because of the increased risk of infection seen with the use of ATG.[37] A recent paper compared two studies using different total doses (7.5 mg/kg vs. 15 mg/kg) and different schedules (day −4, −3 vs. day −5, −4, −3, −2), respectively.[38] The higher dose and schedule trial significantly decreased grade III–IV aGVHD compared to the non-ATG arm, whereas the low dose and schedule trial did not. These trials reveal that dose and timing of ATG surrounding the day of transplant is critical. Though ATG may also be used for the treatment of steroid-refractory

Table 10.7. Typical aGVHD Prophylaxis Regimens

Regimen	Dosing	Notes
Methotrexate (MTX) +	15 mg/m² IV day +1, 10 mg/m² days +3, +6, +11	Monitor liver & renal function; third spacing
Cyclosporine (CSA)	3–5 mg/kg IV day −1 to day +180	Slow taper if no GVHD; convert to PO 1:3 ratio in 2 divided doses as tolerated Check for drug interactions
Methotrexate (MTX) +	15 mg/m² IV day +1, 10 mg/m² days +3, +6, +11	As above
Tacrolimus (FK506)	0.03 mg/m² CIV day −1 to day +180	Slow taper if no GVHD; convert to PO 1:4 ratio in 2 divided doses as tolerated Check for drug interactions
Mini-dose MTX +	5 mg/m² IV day +1, +3, +6, +11	Studied primarily in MUD transplants
Tacrolimus (FK506)	0.03 mg/m² CIV day −2 to day +180	As above (MTX/FK506)

PO = by mouth; IV = intravenous; CIV = continuous intravenous infusion; MUD = matched unrelated donor.

aGVHD, considerable variation in the formulation and doses used[39] (as well as questionable outcomes) make use in this area difficult.[40]

Corticosteroids

Corticosteroids are the initial treatment of choice for aGVHD. These agents function by a complex, multifactorial mechanism involving direct lymphotoxicity and inhibition of inflammatory cytokines such as IL-1, IL-2, IL-6, and TNF-α. Oral prednisone or intravenous methylprednisolone are the agents typically used at doses ranging from 1–2 mg/kg/day to 1 g/m² of methylprednisolone with a slow taper. These high doses result in apoptosis of lymphocytes involved in tissue damage associated with aGVHD. Although response rates for patients initially treated with corticosteroids for aGVHD are 50% to 60%,[41] many who respond to corticosteroid therapy will experience GVHD-related infection and other complications from long-term corticosteroid use. Patients who do not respond will require salvage therapy for steroid-refractory aGVHD, which has an extremely poor prognosis. Almost all patients who survive will eventually develop cGVHD.

Cyclosporine and Tacrolimus

Cyclosporine (CSA, Neoral, Sandimmune, Gengraf) and tacrolimus (FK506, Prograf) reversibly bind to cytoplasmic immunophilins known as cyclophilin and FK-binding protein 12 (FKBP), respectively, in T lymphocytes. The resulting complex inhibits the activity of calcineurin (a calcium-dependent phosphatase), leading to decreased synthesis of IL-2 and other cytokines critical for continued T-cell activation and proliferation. Tacrolimus is 10–100 times more potent than cyclosporine, which, combined with the difference in immunophilin binding, may explain limited activity (response rate <20%) in patients who are refractory to cyclosporine.[42]

Randomized phase III trials in both HLA-identical sibling BMT[43] and unrelated-donor BMT[44] comparing tacrolimus with cyclosporine, both combined with methotrexate, revealed decreased incidences of aGVHD with tacrolimus. Despite these results, widespread adoption of tacrolimus as the standard-of-care for aGVHD prophylaxis has not occurred, perhaps due to the higher mortality seen in patients with advanced disease in the HLA-identical sibling BMT trial.[43]

Cyclosporine and tacrolimus cause similar patterns of toxicity. The primary side effects from these agents are nephrotoxicity, hypertension, neurotoxicity, infection, and hyperglycemia. Many of these toxicities are more severe in BMT patients than in solid-organ transplant patients because of concomitant toxicity of the preparative regimen. Both agents are also substrates of cytochrome P450 3A4, so multiple drug interactions may occur with other medications frequently used in BMT (i.e., azole antifungals, phenytoin).

Antimetabolites

The folate antagonist methotrexate is a critical component of typical prophylactic regimens for aGVHD with the use of a short-course schedule (Table 10.7). This agent down-regulates T lymphocytes by inhibiting proliferation and induces tolerance following BMT. Side effects such as myelosuppression, renal and hepatic toxicity, and mucositis make the replacement of methotrexate with potentially less toxic medications a priority. Caution must be exercised when using methotrexate in patients with pleural effusions or ascites because of significant third-spacing.

Pentostatin (Nipent) is a nucleoside analog and a potent inhibitor of adenosine deaminase, a key enzyme in T-lymphocyte cell division. Lymphocytes are particularly sensitive to the effects of pentostatin because the metabolism of 2′-deoxyadenosine is blocked, leading to accumulation and lymphocyte apoptosis.[45] A promising recent phase I trial demonstrated a 76% overall response rate in steroid-refractory aGVHD with little effect on neutrophil counts.[46]

MMF

Mycophenolate mofetil (MMF, CellCept) is an antiproliferative agent that reversibly inhibits the enzyme inosine monophosphate dehydrogenase (IMPDH), the rate-limiting enzyme in de novo guanosine nucleotide synthesis. Because T lymphocytes are exquisitely dependent on this pathway for their synthesis, cell death occurs. MMF has been studied most extensively in nonmyeloablative BMT settings where promising activity has been noted with reduced toxicity, especially in older adults.[47] A recent retrospective trial comparing CSA + MTX versus CSA + MMF found no differences in overall survival, relapse rate, or acute or chronic GVHD with shortened myeloid recovery time in the CSA + MMF arm.[48] This may result in a lower incidence of infection in widespread use. Myelosuppression and GI complaints (diarrhea, nausea, abdominal pain) are the most common toxicities seen with MMF.

Anticytokine Antibodies

Inflammatory cytokines responsible for mediating the effects of GVHD are ideal targets for monoclonal antibody intervention. Antibodies directed against the IL-2 receptor (humanized anti-TAC, daclizumab, Zenapax), TNF-α (infliximab, Remicade), and a recombinant IL-1 receptor antagonist have all been investigated. A 47% CR rate with 53% survival on day 120 was demonstrated using daclizumab in steroid-refractory patients with aGVHD.[49] In contrast, significantly increased mortality was shown in the combination arm of a trial comparing corticosteroids + daclizumab to corticosteroids alone for the initial treatment of aGVHD.[50] Daclizumab is currently confined to treatment of steroid-refractory aGVHD. Infliximab exhibits significant activity in steroid-refractory aGVHD,[51] though the incidence of invasive fungal infections in this and another cohort series limits its utility.[52] Finally, while a recombinant IL-1 antagonist appears to have activity in steroid-refractory aGVHD with limited toxicity,[53] a recent randomized trial in combination with CSA + MTX for prophylaxis of aGVHD did not reduce the incidence of aGVHD or improve survival.[54]

These and other monoclonal antibodies under investigation appear to have significant activity in steroid-refractory aGVHD, though infusion reactions and infectious complications limit their widespread use. Another role for monoclonal antibodies is in vivo T-cell purging, as previously discussed. Alemtuzumab (Campath) is directed against CD52, which is abundantly expressed on all human lymphocytes. One study using this agent for T-cell depletion showed lower incidences of both aGVHD and cGVHD compared to historic controls.[55] Alemtuzumab is also being incorporated into the preparative regimen for nonmyeloablative transplants, although a higher incidence of cytomegalovirus (CMV) reactivation has been found, and patients receiving alemtuzumab may require DLI to achieve tumor control.[56] This suggests that while alemtuzumab decreases the incidence of both aGVHD and cGVHD, the GVL effect is also decreased.

Chronic GVHD (cGVHD)

cGVHD is a complication of allogeneic BMT that occurs in about 40% to 60% of long-term survivors. Though poorly understood, cGVHD is theoretically caused by alloreactive T-cell destruction of host tissues as well as thymus dysfunction, leading to retention of peripheral autoreactive T cells. It is typically defined as occurring after the first 100 days following BMT, and the incidence is rising because of the increasing age of recipients and the expanded use of mismatched-sibling donors and MUD transplants.[57] Previous aGVHD is a key risk factor for development of cGHVD. cGVHD generally manifests in a manner resembling autoimmune disorders where almost any organ—skin, liver, mouth, eyes, GI tract, respiratory tract, nervous system, and hematopoietic system—may be affected.

cGVHD also results in profound immunodeficiency from impaired T- and B-cell production, altered T-cell function, impaired antibody production, and functional asplenia.[58] Consequently, infection is the chief cause of death in these patients.

Staging for cGVHD consists of a limited stage characterized by localized skin involvement or evidence of liver dysfunction, whereas extensive stage cGVHD consists of extensive skin involvement or involvement of other organs. The treatment of choice for cGVHD consists of alternate-day CSA and prednisone. Because there is no standard of therapy for cGVHD in refractory cases, many other agents (MMF, sirolimus, thalidomide, hydroxychloroquine, pentostatin, cyclophosphamide, and various topical agents for skin lesions) may be used.[59] Prophylaxis for infection with anti-infectives and vaccinations is also critical.

MANAGEMENT OF INFECTIOUS COMPLICATIONS

Infectious complications are a primary cause of morbidity and mortality in patients who have received allogeneic BMT. Three primary phases directly linked to risk factors have been identified: pre-engraftment (up to day 15–30), early postengraftment (postneutrophil engraftment to day 100), and late post-engraftment (day 100 to normal immunity).[60] The time-course of various infections (bacterial, fungal, viral) associated with BMT is illustrated in Figure 10.2. The primary risk period for patients receiving autologous BMT is the preengraftment period because of the associated neutropenia. Immunodeficiency (resulting from immunosuppressive drugs and the effects of GVHD) is the primary etiology postengraftment in allogeneic BMT. Guidelines for the prevention of infectious complications have been published by the Centers for Disease Control and Prevention (CDC) and are summarized in **Table 10.8**.[61]

Bacterial and Fungal Infections

Bacterial infections are most common during the neutropenic phase, before engraftment occurs. Infection must be assumed when fever occurs in this setting, and empiric broad-spectrum antibacterials must be initiated promptly with bacteriocidal activity against gram-negative microbes.[62] The pattern of bacterial isolates in BMT has changed in the past 15 years from primarily gram-negative to gram-positive, so empiric vancomycin may be added to the regimen. This has been attributed to increasing use of prophylactic fluoroquinolones, use of more

intensive preparative regimens leading to severe mucositis, and the presence of indwelling central catheters in these patients. Although prophylactic antibacterials have been shown to decrease the incidence of bacteremia, overall survival is not improved so routine use is not recommended.[61]

Invasive fungal infections in allogeneic BMT carry extremely high rates of morbidity and mortality and present difficulty in management. These infections may occur after prolonged neutropenia and immunosuppression. In fact, prolonged corticosteroid use for GVHD has been found to be a significant risk factor for fungal infections.[63] The mortality from *Candida* sp. has steadily fallen since the advent of routine fluconazole prophylaxis, though the emergence and increased incidence of non-*albicans* species (*Candida glabrata*, *Candida krusei*) that are typically fluconazole-resistant is of concern.[64] Importantly, fluconazole does not have significant activity against molds, so *Aspergillus* sp. are increasingly common fungal pathogens in allogeneic BMT and prophylactic fluconazole. These infections are often treated with amphotericin B, voriconazole, and caspofungin, all of which have moderate activity against *Aspergillus*. Because mortality from these infections continues to be high, strategies using voriconazole as prophylaxis are under investigation. Finally, the risk of infection with non-*Aspergillus* mold species such as *Fusarium* sp. and *Zygomycetes* has also increased in recent years.[65] These pathogens are of particular concern since they lead to high mortality and are highly resistant to modern antifungals.

Viral Infections

Viral infections in allogenic BMT may be caused by organisms such as herpes simplex virus (HSV), CMV, and varicella zoster virus (VZV). These infections usually result from reactivation of prior exposure, not the development of a new infection. Significant morbidity is common in patients with HSV infection, which is complicated by mucositis from the preparative regimen. This complication is preventable in the majority of HSV-seropositive individuals using prophylactic acyclovir (Table 10.8). Newer congeners of acyclovir with improved oral bioavailability (valacyclovir, famciclovir) may also be used for prophylaxis and treatment of HSV in patients who can tolerate oral therapy.[66]

Until the last few years, CMV infection was the leading cause of death in allogeneic BMT patients, and the prognosis remains extremely poor. The usual time to onset is during the early postengraftment period (prior to day 100), and the most common presentation is interstitial

Table 10.8. Summary of Recommended Infection Prophylaxis Regimens for Adults Receiving Bone Marrow Transplantation by the Centers for Disease Control and Prevention

Pathogen	Indication	Regimen	Notes
Bacterial			
General prophylaxis	Prevention in allogeneic BMT patients with severe hypogammaglobulinemia (serum IGG <400 mg/dL <100 days post-BMT)	IV immunoglobulin 500 mg/kg/wk	Monitor for anaphylactic reactions & fluid overload
Pneumocystis jiroveci or *Toxoplasma gondii* in seropositive allogenic BMT patients	Prophylaxis in allogeneic BMT or certain autologous BMT recipients*: Start time of engraftment for ≥6 months post-BMT; give during immunosuppression or cGVHD	Trimethoprim/sulfamethoxazole one double-strength tablet by mouth daily or 3 times/wk	Monitor renal function, allergy, myelosuppression
Fungal			
Fluconazole-susceptible *Candida* spp.	Prophylaxis in allogeneic BMT or certain autologous BMT recipients*: Start day 0 until engraftment (day 30)	Fluconazole 400 mg PO or IV every day	Monitor liver function tests, fever, renal function
Viral			
CMV	Preemptive CMV treatment administered <100 days after allogeneic BMT at risk: Start ganciclovir at any level of antigenemia or viremia or has ≥2 consecutive positive CMV-DNA PCR tests	Ganciclovir 5 mg/kg/dose IV every 12 hours for 5–7 days, followed by 5–6 mg/kg IV daily for 5 days/week until day 100 or minimum of 3 weeks	Antigenemia or PCR should be negative when therapy stops. Monitor renal function, fever, myelosuppression
HSV	Prevention of HSV in seropositive adult BMT patients: Acyclovir at beginning of preparative regimen & continue until engraftment or mucositis resolves (day 30)	Acyclovir 200 mg PO 3 times daily *or* 250 mg/m^2/dose IV over 1 hour every 12 hours	Monitor renal function

CMV = cytomegalovirus; BMT = bone marrow transplant; PCR = polymerase chain reaction; IV = intravenous; HSV = herpes simplex virus; PO = by mouth; IGG = immunoglobulin G; cGVHD = chronic graft-versus-host disease.

*Patients with leukemia or lymphoma who have or will have prolonged neutropenia and mucosal damage from intense conditioning regimens or graft manipulation or who have recently received fludarabine or cladribine.

Source: Centers for Disease Control and Prevention (CDC). CDC/IDSA/ASBMT guidelines for the prevention of opportunistic infections (OIs) in hematopoietic stem cell transplantation (HSCT) patients. *MMWR Morb Mortal Wkly Rep.* 2000; 49:1–128.[61]

pneumonitis with mortality of 40% to 50%. Other manifestations, including gastroenteritis, retinitis, and encephalitis, may also occur. Primary risk factors for CMV include intensive preparative regimens, donor/recipient HLA mismatches, age, intensive immunosuppression, and GVHD.[67] BMT patients who are seropositive for CMV have the highest risk. So the best preventative strategy for CMV seronegative patients is using a seronegative donor, which is often difficult given the prevalence of CMV seropositivity in the general population (about 70%). Seronegative or leukocyte-depleted blood products should also be used; these com-

bined strategies result in an extremely low rate of CMV transmission to seronegative patients.

Additional attempts to decrease morbidity and mortality from CMV disease are derived from two strategies using ganciclovir: prophylaxis and preemptive treatment. Prophylaxis typically results in almost complete elimination of CMV disease, but is limited by side effects including myelosuppression (30%) and increased rates of fungal infection.[68] Many centers have adopted the preemptive approach using serial monitoring of CMV antigen or DNA-polymerase chain reaction in seropositive patients (preexisting or from seropositive donors). This preemptive approach demonstrated similar efficacy in preventing CMV disease compared to prophylaxis in a randomized trial, sparing unnecessary toxicity in many patients.[69] In mild cases, or cases of viremia only, the oral agent valganciclovir may be considered. Other agents have been developed (foscarnet, cidofovir) for patients who are intolerant or refractory to ganciclovir, though they are limited by severe renal toxicity and electrolyte wasting.

VZV infection occurs in 20% to 50% of allogeneic BMT patients and is often severe, as a result of immunosuppression or immunodeficiency.[60] It most frequently occurs in the late postengraftment period (around 5 months) as disseminated cutaneous involvement, although visceral lesions may occur in 10% to 15% of cases. The treatment of choice is high-dose intravenous acyclovir, although valacyclovir and famciclovir offer attractive oral alternatives. These agents have not yet been studied for VZV infection in BMT patients, so they cannot be considered standard therapy.

Long-Term Risk of Infection

Long-term survivors of BMT continue to have an increased risk of various infections, particularly allogeneic BMT patients who develop cGVHD or need prolonged immunosuppressive therapy.[70] T-lymphocyte depletion and dysfunction often persist, leading to possible infection with encapsulated bacteria (*Streptococcus pneumoniae, Haemophilus influenzae*), *Pneumocystis jiroveci* (PCP), VZV, and *Aspergillus*. Prophylaxis for PCP generally consists of trimethoprim–sulfamethoxazole for 6 months post-BMT, and is used in patients with cGVHD or on immunosuppressants. Dapsone, pentamidine, atovaquone, or penicillin may be used in sulfa-allergic patients. Finally, vaccinations are imperative after autologous or allogeneic BMT since immunity is lost after transplant. Live virus vaccines should not be administered to patients on immunosuppressive therapy because of the risk of infection. Refer to immunization guidelines that have been published by the CDC for specific recommendations.[61]

SUMMARY

Bone marrow transplantation (BMT) is a complex procedure that is a critical component of the treatment of many malignant and nonmalignant diseases. Allogeneic BMT may be curative in chronic myeloid leukemia, acute myeloid leukemia, and aplastic anemia. Much of the success of allogeneic BMT has been attributed to the graft-versus-leukemia (GVL) effect, serving as the impetus for nonmyeloab-

lative transplants that avoid the toxicity of intensive preparative regimens and allow transplantation in older patients. Unfortunately, the GVL effect must be balanced with the damaging effects of GVHD since there are currently no standard means to separate these effects. Nonetheless, promising research continues in this area to increase accessibility of this procedure to more patients. Infection continues to be a major cause of morbidity and mortality in allogeneic BMT patients during all phases of the posttransplant period. Novel, more effective, and less toxic anti-infectives will be needed in the coming years to improve the outcomes for these patients.

REFERENCES

1. Horowitz MM. Uses and growth of hematopoietic cell transplantation. In: Blume KG, Forman SJ, Appelbaum FR, eds. *Thomas' Hematopoietic Stem Cell Transplantation*. 3rd ed. Malden, MA: Blackwell Publishing; 2004:9–15.
2. Perkins JB, Yee, GC. Hematopoietic stem cell transplantation. In: DiPiro J, Talbert RL, Yee GC, et al., eds. *Pharmacotherapy: A Pathophysiologic Approach*. 4th ed. Norwalk, CT: Appleton and Lange; 2000:2425–2443.
3. Beyer J, Schwella N, Zingsem J, et al. Hematopoietic rescue after high-dose chemotherapy using autologous blood progenitor cells or bone marrow: a randomized comparison. *J Clin Oncol.* 1995; 13:1328–1335.
4. Schmitz N, Linch DC, Dreger P, et al. Filgrastim-mobilized peripheral blood progenitor cell transplantation in comparison with autologous bone marrow transplantation: results of a randomized phase III trial in lymphoma patients. *Lancet.* 1996; 347:353–357.
5. Van Hoef MEHM. HLA-identical sibling peripheral blood progenitor cell transplants. *Bone Marrow Transplant.* 1999; 24:555–560.
6. Storek J, Gooley T, Siadek M, et al. Allogeneic peripheral blood stem cell transplantation may be associated with a high risk of chronic graft-versus-host disease. *Blood.* 1997; 90:4705–4709.
7. Bensinger WI, Martin PJ, Storer B, et al. Transplantation of bone marrow as compared with peripheral blood cells from HLA-identical relatives in patients with hematologic cancers. *N Engl J Med.* 2001; 34:175–181.
8. Armitage JO. Bone marrow transplantation. *N Engl J Med.* March 24, 1994; 300(12):827–838.
9. Negrin RS, Blume KG. Allogeneic and autologous hematopoietic stem cell transplantation. In: Buetler E, Lichtman M, Coller S, et al., eds. *Williams Hematology.* 6th ed. New York, NY: McGraw-Hill; 2004:209–245.
10. Leukemia Society of America. Bone marrow transplantation and peripheral blood stem cell

transplantation. New York, NY: Leukemia Society of America; 1997.

11. Childs RW. Allogeneic stem cell transplantation. In: DeVita VT, Hellma S, Rosenberg SA, eds. *Cancer: Principles & Practice of Oncology.* 6th ed. Philadelphia, PA: Lippincott Williams & Wilkins; 2001:2779–2814.

12. Anasetti C, Amos D, Beatty PG, et al. Effect of HLA compatibility on engraftment of bone marrow transplants in patients with leukemia or lymphoma. *N Engl J Med.* 1989 Jan 26; 320(4):197–204.

13. Bensinger WI, Spielberger R. Preparative regimens and modification of regimen-related toxicities. In: Blume KG, Forman SJ, Appelbaum FR, eds. *Thomas' Hematopoietic Stem Cell Transplantation.* 3rd ed. Malden, MA: Blackwell Publishing; 2004:158–177.

14. Soiffer RJ. T-cell depletion to prevent graft-versus-host disease. In: Blume KG, Forman SJ, Appelbaum FR, eds. *Thomas' Hematopoietic Stem Cell Transplantation.* 3rd ed. Malden, MA: Blackwell Publishing; 2004:244–253.

15. Martin PJ, Hansen JA, Buckner CD, et al. Effects of in vitro depletion of T cells in HLA-identical allogeneic marrow grafts. *Blood.* 1985; 66:664–672.

16. Slavin S, Nagler A, Naparstek E, et al. Nonmyeloablative stem cell transplantation and cell therapy as an alternative to conventional bone marrow transplantation with lethal cytoreduction for the treatment of malignant and nonmalignant hematologic diseases. *Blood.* 1998; 91(3):756–763.

17. Slavin S, Morecki S, Weiss L, et al. Nonmyeloablative stem cell transplantation: reduced-intensity conditioning for cancer immunotherapy—from bench to patient bedside. *Semin Oncol.* 2004; 31:4–21.

18. McCune JS, Winter LL, Dix SD. Hematopoietic cell transplantation. In: Koda-Kimble MA, Young YL, eds. *Applied Therapeutics: The Clinical Use of Drugs.* 8th ed. Baltimore, MD: Lippincott Williams & Wilkins; 2005:92–114.

19. Flowers MED, Kansu E, Sullivan KM. Pathophysiology and treatment of graft-versus-host disease. *Hematol Oncol Clin North Am.* 1999; 13:1091–1112.

20. Lazarus HM, Vogelsang GB, Rowe JM. Prevention and treatment of acute graft-versus-host disease: the old and the new. A report from the Eastern Cooperative Oncology Group (ECOG). *Bone Marrow Transplant.* 1997; 19:577–600.

21. Cutler C, Giri S, Jeyapalan S, et al. Acute and chronic graft-versus-host disease after allogeneic peripheral-blood stem-cell and bone marrow transplantation: a meta-analysis. *J Clin Oncol.* 2001; 19:3685–3691.

22. Goulmy E, Schipper R, Pool J, et al. Mismatches of minor histocompatibility antigens between HLA-identical donors and recipients and the development of graft-versus-host disease after bone marrow transplantation. *N Engl J Med.* 1996; 334:281–285.

23. Couriel D, Caldera H, Champlin R, et al. Acute graft-versus-host disease: pathophysiology, clinical manifestations, and management. *Cancer.* 2004; 101:1936–1946.

24. Ferrera JLM, Cooke KR, Pan L, et al. The immunopathophysiology of acute graft-versus-host disease. *Stem Cells.* 1996; 14:473–489.

25. Przepiorka D, Weisdorf D, Martin P, et al. 1994 Consensus conference on acute GVHD grading. *Bone Marrow Transplant* 1995; 15:825–828.

26. Vogelsang GB, Lee L, Bensen-Kennedy DM. Pathogenesis and treatment of graft-versus-host disease after bone marrow transplant. *Annu Rev Med.* 2003; 54:29–52.

27. Horowitz MM, Gale RP, Sondel PM, et al. Graft-versus-leukemia reactions after bone marrow transplantation. *Blood.* 1990; 75:555–562.

28. Marmont AM, Horowitz MM, Gale RP, et al. T-cell depletion of HLA-identical transplants in leukemia. *Blood.* 1991; 78:2120–2130.

29. Kolb HJ, Schattenberg A, Goldman JM, et al. Graft-versus-leukemia effect of donor lymphocyte transfusions in marrow grafted patients. *Blood.* 1995; 86:2041–2050.

30. Bleakley M, Riddell SR. Molecules and mechanisms of the graft-versus-leukemia effect. *Nat Rev Cancer.* 2004; 4:371–380.

31. Srinivasan R, Barrett J, Childs R. Allogeneic stem cell transplantation as immunotherapy for nonhematological cancers. *Semin Oncol.* 2004; 31:47–55.

32. Nimer SD, Giorgi J, Gajewski JL, et al. Selective depletion of CD8+ cells for prevention of graft-versus-host disease after bone marrow transplantation. A randomized controlled trial. *Transplantation.* 1994; 57:82–87.

33. Edinger M, Hoffmann P, Ermann J, et al. CD4+CD25+ regulatory T cells preserve graft-versus-tumor activity while inhibiting graft-versus-host disease after bone marrow transplantation. *Nat Med.* 2003; 9:1144–1150.

34. Datta AR, Barrett AJ, Jiang YZ, et al. Distinct T cell populations distinguish chronic myeloid leukemia cells from lymphocytes in the same individual: a model for separating GVHD from GVL reactions. *Bone Marrow Transplant.* 1994; 14:517–524.

35. Mavroudis DA, Dermime S, Molldrem J, et al. Specific depletion of alloreactive T cells in HLA-identical siblings: a method for separating graft-versus-host and graft-versus-leukemia reactions. *Br J Hematol.* 1998; 101:565–570.

36. Ho VT, Soiffer RJ. The history and future of T-cell depletion as graft-versus-host disease prophylaxis for allogeneic hematopoietic stem cell transplantation. *Blood.* 2001; 98:3192–3204.

37. Bacigalupo A. Antilymphocyte/thymocyte globulin for graft versus host disease prophylaxis: efficacy and side effects. *Bone Marrow Transplant.* 2005; 35:225–231.

38. Bacigalupo A, Lamparelli T, Bruzzi P, et al. Antithymocyte globulin for graft-versus-host disease prophylaxis in transplants from unrelated donors: two randomized studies from Gruppo Italiano Trapianti Midollo Osseo (GITMO). *Blood.* 2001; 98:2942–2947.

39. Hsu B, May R, Carrum G, et al. Use of antithymocyte globulin for treatment of steroid-refractory acute graft-versus-host disease: an international practice survey. *Bone Marrow Transplant.* 2001; 28:945–950.
40. Arai S, Margolis J, Zahurak M, et al. Poor outcome in steroid-refractory graft-versus-host disease with antithymocyte globulin treatment. *Biol Blood Marrow Transplant.* 2002; 8:155–160.
41. Martin PJ, Schoch G, Fisher L, et al. A retrospective analysis of therapy for acute graft-versus-host disease: initial treatment. *Blood.* 1990; 76:1464–1472.
42. Kanamaru A, Takemoto Y, Kakishita E, et al. FK506 treatment of graft-versus-host disease developing or exacerbating during prophylaxis and therapy with cyclosporine and/or other immunosuppressants. *Bone Marrow Transplant.* 1995; 15:895–899.
43. Ratanatharathorn V, Nash RA, Przepiorka D, et al. Phase III study comparing methotrexate and tacrolimus (Prograf, FK506) with methotrexate and cyclosporine for graft-versus-host disease prophylaxis after HLA-identical sibling bone marrow transplantation. *Blood.* 1998; 92:2303–2314.
44. Nash RA, Antin JH, Karanes C, et al. Phase 3 study comparing methotrexate and tacrolimus with methotrexate and cyclosporine for prophylaxis of acute graft-versus-host disease after marrow transplantation from unrelated donors. *Blood.* 2000; 96:2062–2068.
45. Margolis J, Vogelsang G. An old drug for a new disease: pentostatin (Nipent) in acute graft-versus-host disease. *Semin Oncol.* 2000; 27(suppl. 5):72–77.
46. Bolanos-Meade J, Jacobsohn DA, Margolis J, et al. Pentostatin in steroid-refractory acute graft-versus-host disease. *J Clin Oncol.* 2005; 23:2661–2668.
47. Vogelsang GB, Arai S. Mycophenolate mofetil for the prevention and treatment of graft-versus-host disease following stem cell transplantation: preliminary findings. *Bone Marrow Transplant.* 2001; 27:1255–1262.
48. Neumann F, Graef T, Tapprich C, et al. Cyclosporine A and mycophenolate mofetil vs. cyclosporine A and methotrexate for graft-versus-host disease prophylaxis after stem cell transplantation from HLA-identical siblings. *Bone Marrow Transplant.* 2005; 35:1089–1093.
49. Przepiorka D, Kernan NA, Ippoliti C, et al. Daclizumab, a humanized anti-interleukin-2 receptor alpha chain antibody, for treatment of acute graft-versus-host disease. *Blood.* 2000; 95:83–89.
50. Lee SJ, Zahrieh D, Agura E, et al. Effect of upfront daclizumab when combined with steroids for the treatment of acute graft-versus-host disease: results of a randomized trial. *Blood.* 2004; 104:1559–1564.
51. Couriel D, Saliba R, Hicks K, et al. Tumor necrosis factor-α blockade for the treatment of acute GVHD. *Blood.* 2004; 104:649–654.
52. Marty FM, Lee SJ, Fahey MM, et al. Infliximab use in patients with severe graft-versus-host disease and other emerging risk factors for non-*Candida* invasive fungal infections in allogeneic hematopoietic stem cell transplant recipients: a cohort study. *Blood.* 2003; 102:2768–2776.
53. Antin JH, Weinstein HJ, Guinan EC, et al. Recombinant human interleukin-1 receptor antagonist in the treatment of steroid-resistant graft-versus-host disease. *Blood.* 1994; 84:1342–1348.
54. Antin JH, Weisdorf D, Neuberg D, et al. Interleukin-1 blockade does not prevent acute graft-versus-host disease: results of a randomized, double-blind, placebo-controlled trial of interleukin-1 receptor antagonist in allogeneic bone marrow transplantation. *Blood.* 2002; 100:3479–3483.
55. Hale G, Zhang MJ, Bunjes D, et al. Improving the outcome of bone marrow transplantation by using CD52 monoclonal antibodies to prevent graft-versus-host disease and graft rejection. *Blood.* 1998; 92:4581–4590.
56. Perez-Simon JA, Kottaridis PD, Martino R, et al. Non-myeloablative transplantation with or without alemtuzumab: comparison between two prospective studies in patients with lymphoproliferative disorders. *Blood.* 2002; 100:3121–3127.
57. Higman MA, Vogelsang GB. Chronic graft versus host disease. *Br J Haematol.* 2004; 125:435–454.
58. Maury S, Mary JY, Rabian C, et al. Prolonged immune deficiency following allogeneic stem cell transplantation: risk factors and complications in adult patients. *Br J Haematol.* 2001; 115:630–641.
59. Lee SJ. New approaches for preventing and treating chronic graft-versus-host disease. *Blood.* 2005; 105:4200–4206.
60. Leather HL, Wingard JR. Infections following hematopoietic stem cell transplantation. *Infect Dis Clin North Am.* 2001; 15:483–520.
61. Centers for Disease Control and Prevention (CDC). CDC/IDSA/ASBMT guidelines for the prevention of opportunistic infections (OIs) in hematopoietic stem cell transplantation (HSCT) patients. *MMWR Morb Mortal Wkly Rep.* 2000; 49:1–128.
62. Hughes WT, Armstrong D, Bodey GP, et al. 2002 Guidelines for the use of antimicrobial agents in neutropenic patients with cancer. *Clin Infect Dis.* 2002; 34:730–751.
63. De La Rosa GR, Champlin RE, Kontoyiannis DP. Risk factors for the development of invasive fungal infections in allogeneic blood and marrow transplant recipients. *Transpl Infect Dis.* 2002; 4:3–9.
64. Marr KA, Seidel K, White TC, et al. Candidemia in allogeneic blood and marrow transplant recipients: evolution of risk factors after the adoption of prophylactic fluconazole. *J Infect Dis.* 2000; 181:309–316.
65. Marr KA, Carter RA, Crippa F, et al. Epidemiology and outcome of mould infections in hematopoietic stem cell transplant recipients. *Clin Infect Dis.* 2002; 34:909–917.
66. Eisen D, Essell J, Broun ER, et al. Clinical utility of oral valacyclovir compared with oral acyclovir for the prevention of herpes simplex virus mucositis

following autologous bone marrow transplantation or stem cell rescue therapy. *Bone Marrow Transplant.* 2003; 31:51–55.

67. Zaia JA. Prevention and management of CMV-related problems after hematopoietic stem cell transplantation. *Bone Marrow Transplant.* 2002; 29:633–638.

68. Goodrich JM, Bowden RA, Fisher L, et al. Ganciclovir prophylaxis to prevent cytomegalovirus disease after allogeneic marrow transplant. *Ann Intern Med.* 1993; 118:173–178.

69. Boeckh M, Gooley TA, Myerson D, et al. Cytomegalovirus pp65 antigenemia-guided early treatment with ganciclovir versus ganciclovir at engraftment after allogeneic marrow transplantation: a randomized double-blind study. *Blood.* 1996; 88:4063–4071.

70. Wingard JR. Opportunistic infections after blood and marrow transplantation. *Transpl Infect Dis.* 1999; 1:3–20.

SELF-ASSESSMENT QUESTIONS

1. The purpose of a bone marrow transplant is to:

   A. Repair weakened bone marrow
   B. "Boost" the immune system during an infection
   C. Reconstitute marrow function after damage from disease or high doses of chemotherapy
   D. Replace bone marrow in aplastic anemia

2. Advantages of an allogeneic bone marrow transplant include:

   A. Increased GVHD
   B. Increased GVL
   C. No malignant cells in the infusion
   D. High donor availability
   E. B and C
   F. A, C, and D

3. Which of the following results in increased risk of disease relapse after BMT?

   A. An autologous BMT
   B. Donor lymphocyte depletion
   C. Using bone marrow instead of peripheral blood stem cells
   D. All of the above

4. Which of the following is a characteristic of acute graft-versus-host disease?

   A. Time of onset is typically after day 100.
   B. Occurs more commonly in MUD transplants than matched-sibling donor BMT.
   C. A primary mediator appears to be cytokine release.
   D. Production of antibody by B cells drives the tissue destruction.

5. Which of the following organ systems is *not* typically affected by acute graft-versus-host disease?

   A. Kidney
   B. Liver
   C. Gastrointestinal tract
   D. Skin

6. Which of the following is a potential complication for the use of cyclosporine in allogeneic BMT patients?

   A. Myelosuppression
   B. Drug interactions
   C. Renal toxicity
   D. B and C

7. Which of the following agents may *not* used in the treatment of chronic graft-versus-host disease?

   A. Thalidomide
   B. 6-Mercaptopurine
   C. Prednisone
   D. Mycophenolate

8. Which of the following statements regarding infectious complications surrounding BMT is *true*?

   A. Bacterial infections tend to occur primarily in the late postengraftment phase following BMT.
   B. Fluconazole is the drug of choice for treating *Aspergillus* infections.
   C. Acyclovir is the agent of choice for prophylaxis of herpes simplex virus infection.
   D. The primary toxicity of ganciclovir is renal toxicity.

9. Which of the following is a viable prevention strategy for cytomegalovirus infection in a CMV seropositive BMT recipient?

   A. Prophylactic acyclovir
   B. Preemptive ganciclovir
   C. Prophylactic ganciclovir
   D. B or C

CHAPTER 11

The Immunotherapy of Cancer

Douglas Smith, Rowena Schwartz, Gina Peacock, Lindsay Corporon

CHAPTER OUTLINE

Learning objectives
Cancer and the immune system
Oncogenes, tumor suppressor genes, and
cancer induction
    Function of cancer-associated genes
    Mutations in cancer-associated genes
    Induction of cancer: a multistep process
Tumor antigens
    Tumor antigen classification
    Tumor markers
    Immune response to tumors

Tumor evasion of the immune
system
Cancer immunotherapy
    Mechanisms of manipulating the immune
system
    Immunomodulators of biological response
modifiers
    Colony-stimulating factors
    Cytokine therapy
    Monoclonal antibodies as cancer therapy
    Others

LEARNING OBJECTIVES

After completing this chapter, the reader should
be able to:

1. Briefly describe the process of the development
   of cancer.
2. Describe the types of tumor antigens.
3. Describe the roles of immune system cells in
   response to tumors.
4. Discuss the theory of immunosurveillance and
   immunoediting.
5. Describe the biologic effects of interferons and the
   applications of these effects in cancer therapy.
6. Discuss the clinical applications of interferon
   in the treatment of melanoma, hairy cell leukemia, and chronic myelogenous leukemia.
7. Outline the immunologic changes seen with
   the administration of interleukin-2.

8. Discuss the complications seen in patients
   receiving high-dose interleukin therapy.
9. Compare and contrast the erythropoietin
   products epoetin alfa and darbepoetin alfa.
10. List potential applications of the white cell
    growth factors: granulocyte colony-stimu-
    lating factor and granulocyte-macrophage
    colony-stimulating factor.
11. Describe the advantages and disadvantages of
    monoclonal antibody-based cancer therapy.
12. List the various targets of currently approved
    monoclonal antibodies and explain the
    mechanisms of action.
13. Use standard nomenclature rules to identify
    the antibody source and tissue target for a
    given oncologic monoclonal antibody.
14. Predict the risk for hypersensitivity re-
    actions based on monoclonal antibody
    nomenclature.

15. Describe the rationale for antibody immuno-conjugates in the management of cancer.
16. Outline the rationale for the use of vaccines in cancer treatment and prevention.
17. Discuss the clinical applications of thalidomide and lenolidamide in the treatment of cancer.

CANCER AND THE IMMUNE SYSTEM

Cancer is one of the leading causes of death in industrialized nations. In 2006, more than 560,000 Americans will die of cancer and another 1.4 million will be diagnosed with cancer.[1] Because cancer is a major problem globally, there has been substantial research regarding its prevention and treatment.

The idea that tumors may be recognized and destroyed by the host immune system is not a new one. In the early 1900s Ehrlich first proposed that the host immune system may be able to identify tumors as nonself and eliminate them.[2] Many years later, Burnet developed this idea into the theory of immune surveillance—that a normal function of the host immune system is to survey the body for altered cells and destroy them.[3] This theory has been revised to include the idea that tumor cells do not just wait to be destroyed; they have developed ways not only to circumvent the immune system, but also to cause destruction of immune system cells. The relationship between the immune system and the development and progression of cancer is indeed very complex and is influenced by the local microenvironment. And recent evidence shows that some inflammatory and immunological host responses to tumors may lead to tumor progression as well as contribute to the anti-tumor effects previously described.[4]

ONCOGENES, TUMOR SUPPRESSOR GENES, AND CANCER INDUCTION

Function of Cancer-Associated Genes

The size of a cell population is determined by the rates of cellular proliferation (cell division), differentiation (cell specialization), and apoptosis (programmed cell death). These processes are normally well regulated to maintain a balance between the number of cells leaving a population (through apoptosis or differentiation) and the number being produced. Control of these processes involves genes encoding proteins that induce or inhibit cellular proliferation, function in the damage control system, or induce apoptosis. In the development of cancer, mutations in these genes disrupt the control of these regulatory processes, leading to uncontrolled proliferation, genetic instability, and finally invasion and metastasis.

Induction and control of cellular proliferation. Cellular proliferation is the process by which the body generates new cells to replace cells that have died, or produces additional cells when they are needed. Some types of cells (such as epithelial cells) divide very rapidly, while others (such as adult neural cells) do not divide at all. The cell cycle is the sequence of events through which a cell moves when growing and dividing. It can be divided into four phases: a growth phase (G1); a synthesis phase (S); a second growth phase (G2); and mitosis (M), the phase in which cell division occurs. In normal cells, the decision to enter the cell cycle is determined by positive and negative growth signals released from neighboring cells and from cells in endocrine glands. Transitions through the phases of the cell cycle are controlled by proteins called cyclins, cyclin-dependent kinases (CDKs), and cyclin-dependent kinase inhibitors. A simplified example of this process is shown in **Figure 11.1**. A growth factor binds to a receptor on the cell membrane. The receptor is then activated and, in turn, activates signal-transducing proteins that pass the signal to the nucleus. When the signal reaches the nucleus, it stimulates cyclin production. When the concentration of cyclins is high enough, they bind to CDKs and the cyclin-CDK combination molecules activate molecules that drive the cell cycle. Different cyclins and CDKs are responsible for regulating the transition through each phase of the cell cycle. Once the job is completed, the cyclins disengage from the CDKs; those particular cyclins are destroyed and others take over. This process may be described as a relay race in which different cyclin–CDK combinations are responsible for different legs of the race (see Figure 11.1).

Inhibition of cellular proliferation. Whereas growth-promoting pathways induce cellular proliferation, there are growth-inhibiting pathways that balance these by telling cells when not to divide (see Figure 11.1). The process is similar to the growth-stimulating pathway in that growth-inhibitory factors are released by neighboring cells and bind to the receptors on the surface of a cell. A signaling cascade is then activated, with cytoplasmic relay proteins

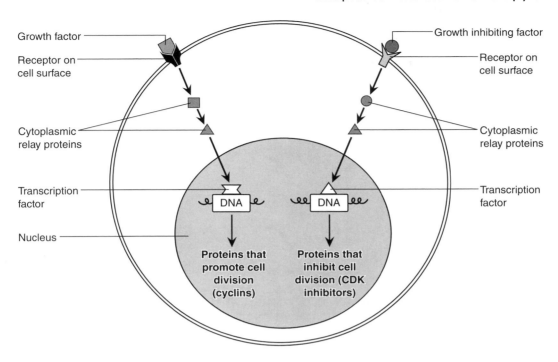

Figure 11.1. Stimulating and inhibitory pathways of cellular proliferation.

transmitting the growth-inhibitory signal to the nucleus. Then proteins, such as CDK inhibitors, are synthesized. These CDK inhibitors bind to and inactivate the cyclin–CDK complexes and halt progression of the cell cycle. The cell cycle has internal checkpoints at which the cell decides whether to proceed through the cycle. At these checkpoints, the cell determines if there is any DNA damage; if so, the cell cycle is halted and DNA repair initiated. If the DNA cannot be repaired, the normal cell initiates apoptosis or "cell suicide" so that mutations are not passed on to future cells.

Regulation of apoptosis. Apoptosis, or programmed cell death, is a process by which damaged cells can be destroyed and removed from the system. **Figure 11.2** is a simplified depiction of the two major mechanisms of apoptosis: external pathway and internal pathway. Apoptosis involves the activation of a chain of caspases, enzymes that cause cell death through the fragmentation of nuclear material and the breakdown of the cell's cytoskeleton. Phagocytic cells engulf the fragmented cells and clear them away, making apoptosis a very efficient process that leaves no cell fragments to cause necrosis and inflammation. One way to induce apoptosis is by the binding of specific ligands, such as FasL, to death receptors (CD95) located on the cell surface; this activates the

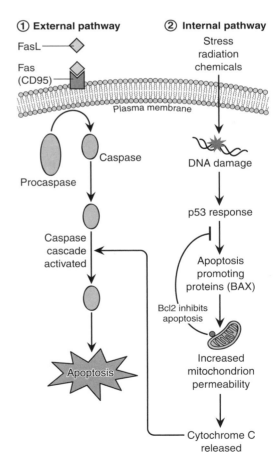

Figure 11.2. External and internal pathways of apoptosis.

Table 11.1. Examples of Protooncogenes/Oncogenes

Function of Gene Product (protein)	Protooncogene	Mode of Activation of Oncogene
Growth factor	TGFα	Overexpression
Growth factor receptors	ERB-B1 (HER1)	Overexpression
	ERB-B2 (HER-2/neu)	Amplification
Signal-transducing proteins	K-RAS H-RAS N-RAS	Point mutation
	ABL	Translocation
Nuclear regulatory proteins	C-MYC	Translocation
	N-MYC L-MYC	Amplification

Modified from: Kumar V, Abbas AK, Fausto N. Neoplasia. In: *Robbins & Cotran Pathologic Basis of Disease.* 7th ed. Philadelphia, PA: Elsevier Saunders; 2005:295.

initiation caspases (external pathway). These initiation caspases activate the executioner caspases, which, in turn, activate the proteases responsible for breaking down the cell. Another factor that can promote apoptosis is the exposure to agents that directly injure the cell, such as chemicals or radiation. This process (internal pathway) involves the tumor-suppressor gene *p53*. This gene encodes a protein (p53) that accumulates in response to DNA damage, and is responsible for halting the cell cycle and initiating DNA repair. If the repair fails, p53 induces apoptosis by triggering production of pro-apoptotic molecules (such as BAX) that favor the release of cytochrome c and APAF-1, activating the caspases that are instrumental in causing cell death. Genes that encode anti-apoptosis proteins, such as BCL2, protect cells from apoptosis by preventing the release of cytochrome c.

Cell death also occurs when cytotoxic T lymphocytes in the immune system induce apoptosis in cells containing foreign surface antigens. They do this by facilitating the entry of granzyme B (a serine protease) into the cell, activating the caspases that mediate apoptosis. Cytotoxic T lymphocytes can also initiate apoptosis through the death receptor (Fas or CD95) because they express FasL (Fas ligand) on their surfaces.

Gene mutations and the development of cancer. Nonlethal genetic damage to normal regulatory genes—such as protooncogenes, tumor suppressor genes, genes that control apoptosis, and genes involved in DNA repair—can lead to the development of cancer.

Protooncogenes (**Table 11.1**) are normal genes that promote cell proliferation. They code for proteins such as growth factors, growth factor receptors, signal-transducing proteins, nuclear regulatory proteins, and cell-cycle regulators that function in growth- and proliferation-promoting pathways. Gain of function mutations in protooncogenes produce oncogenes that can be instrumental in carcinogenesis. Oncogene activation can lead to the ability of cells to proliferate without external growth signals, either by synthesizing their own growth factor or by activating growth factor receptors (without the binding of growth factor). Some oncogenes produce mutated forms of oncoproteins. Others produce normal forms of gene products, such as growth factor receptors, that are overexpressed because of the increased transcription of the normal form of the gene. Other cancers exhibit oncogenes that are amplified forms of protooncogenes.

Tumor suppressor genes (**Table 11.2**) encode proteins, such as growth-inhibitory factors and their receptors, proteins involved in cell cycle regulation, proteins involved in apoptosis, signal-transducing proteins in growth-inhibitory pathways, and proteins that inhibit signal transduction in growth-promoting pathways. All these proteins are involved in growth inhibition. Loss of function mutations in tumor suppressor genes, coupled with gain of function mutations in protooncogenes, often leads to the development of cancer.

Table 11.2. Examples of Tumor Suppressor Genes

Tumor Suppressor Gene	Function of Gene Product (Protein)
TGF-β receptor	Growth inhibition receptor
APC/β-catenin NF-1	Inhibition of growth-promoting signal transduction
SMAD2 SMAD4	TGF-β (growth inhibition) signal transducing protein
RB	Regulator of the cell cycle (master brake)
p53	Cell cycle arrest and apoptosis in response to DNA damage
p16 (INK4a) p27	Regulation of cell cycle (inhibition of cyclin-dependent kinases)
BRCA-1 BRCA-2	DNA repair

Modified from: Kumar V, Abbas AK, Fausto N. Neoplasia. In: *Robbins & Cotran Pathologic Basis of Disease*. 7th ed. Philadelphia, PA: Elsevier Saunders; 2005:300.

Mutations in Cancer-Associated Genes

The genetic damage that leads to activation of oncogenes or inactivation of tumor-suppressor genes may be as small as a point mutation or may involve large portions of chromosomes or entire chromosomes. In the latter, the changes may become evident in the karyotype with parts of chromosomes, or even entire chromosomes, being gained or lost.

Translocations and inversions are two types of chromosomal rearrangements that can activate oncogenes, with translocations being the most common.[5] Translocations can activate oncogenes by promoting overexpression when they are removed from their regulatory elements. For example, in Burkitt lymphoma, the *MYC* protooncogene is moved from its normal position on chromosome 8 to a position on chromosome 14 (**Figure 11.3a**). In most cases, the coding sequence remains intact but the regulatory components are lost, resulting in overexpression. The other way translocations can activate oncogenes is by combining genetic sequences from two different chromosomes to form hybrid genes. An example of this type of translocation is found in chronic myelogenous leukemia. The Philadelphia chromosome is formed when the *c-ABL* gene is translocated from chromosome 9 to chromosome 22 where it fuses with the *BCR* gene (**Figure 11.3b**).

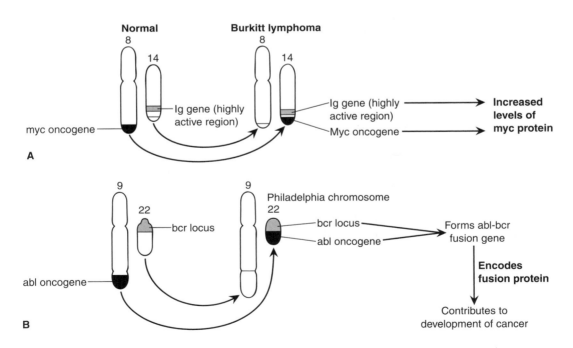

Figure 11.3. a. The myc oncogene becomes dysregulated when translocated from chromosome 8 to 14. This occurs in more than 90% of Burkitt lymphoma cases. **b.** Creation of the Philadelphia chromosome, which is present in approximately 95% of chronic myelogenous leukemia (CML) cases. There is a reciprocal translocation between chromosomes 9 and 22 that creates the abl-bcr fusion gene. This gene encodes a fusion protein with potent tyrosine kinase activity.

The protein product of this fused gene, BCR-ABL, has very potent tyrosine kinase activity and functions in a signal transduction pathway that promotes cell division.

Protein products of oncogenes can also be overexpressed by amplification of the genes that encode them. In these cases, a tumor cell may contain hundreds of copies of a given normal gene, which leads to the overproduction of normal protein products of that gene. An example of this occurs in breast cancer: *HER-2/neu,* a gene that codes for a growth factor receptor, is amplified.

Inactivation of tumor suppressor genes often occurs because of structural changes, such as deletions, but also may occur when the gene is "silenced by hypermethylation of promoter sequences that control the expression of the genes, without a change in DNA base sequence."[5,6] An example is *BRCA 1,* a tumor-suppressor gene involved in DNA repair, which has been found to be methylated in breast cancer as well as in other cancers.[7]

Induction of Cancer: A Multistep Process

Most human cancers exhibit a variety of genetic alterations, including activation of multiple oncogenes and inactivation of at least two tumor suppressor genes.[5] Because multiple mutations are required for the development of cancer and the incidence of cancer increases with age, there is evidence that carcinogenesis occurs through a series of steps.[8,9] This can be observed in both the phenotype and genotype.[5] At the phenotypic level, cancers exhibit such traits as the ability to generate their own growth-promoting signals, insensitivity to growth-inhibitory signals, the ability to replicate endlessly, the ability to evade apoptosis, the loss of DNA repair capabilities, the ability to sustain angiogenesis, and the ability to invade and metastasize.[8,9] There is evidence that the genetic changes facilitating development of these attributes likely occur stepwise. This process (progression) is best illustrated by the studies Fearson and colleagues conducted on the development of colorectal cancer. They determined that a majority of early adenomatous polyps carried an inactivated form of *APC* (tumor-suppressor gene), about half the adenomas studied contained mutant *RAS* (oncogene), and about half the advanced colon carcinomas contained an inactivated form of *p53* (tumor-suppressor gene also referred to as *TP53*).[8,10,11]

A tumor is formed from the proliferation of one transformed cell but multiple mutations are acquired along the way to the development of a malignancy. The malignant tumor is made up of a heterogeneous group of cells that evolved with attributes such as needing fewer or no growth factors, the ability to invade and metastasize, and the ability to evade the host immune system.[12]

TUMOR ANTIGENS

Tumor Antigen Classification

The theory that tumors contain unique antigens that somehow escape immune surveillance dates back to the early 1940s. Using inbred (syngeneic) mouse models, Gross was able to demonstrate an immune response to transplanted sarcoma.[13] Several investigators later were able to confirm tumor-specific antigens on methylcholanthrene-induced murine tumors.[14-16] Tumors transplanted to members of the same inbred strain of mice would grow and metastasize, eventually killing the animal. But if the tumor was removed before reaching a critical mass, the mice could survive and mount an immune response to subsequent tumor transplant. Because implantation of tumors into human hosts is unethical, other methods—including in vitro antibody-directed approaches and, more recently, T-cell antigen recognition techniques—have been developed to identify tumor antigens. In the ensuing decades, many antigens that elicit immune responses in animals and humans have been identified. These are classified as either tumor-specific or tumor-associated antigens. Tumor-specific antigens are expressed solely on tumor cells; tumor-associated antigens are found not only on tumor cells but also, to some extent, on normal cells. Because very few tumor-specific antigens have been identified in human tumors, a more appropriate classification for tumor antigens is based on molecular structure and source (**Figure 11.4**).[5]

Products of oncogenes and tumor suppressor genes as tumor antigens. As discussed previously, malignant transformation of proto-oncogenes and tumor suppressor genes results in the production of intracellular protein products. Some of these stimulate tumor growth, while others have no clearly defined role. In either case, these cytosolic proteins may undergo processing through major histocompatibility complex (MHC) pathways within the tumor cell and be recognized by corresponding T cells. Intracellular proteins processed through the class I MHC antigen pathway are recognized by CD8$^+$ cytotoxic T lymphocytes (CTLs), and are susceptible to their cytotoxic effects. Protein products processed through the class II MHC antigen pathway are recognized by

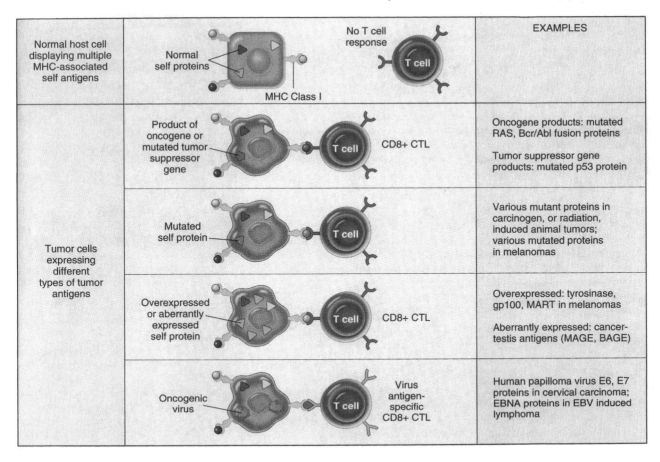

				EXAMPLES
Normal host cell displaying multiple MHC-associated self antigens	Normal self proteins / MHC Class I	No T cell response	T cell	
Tumor cells expressing different types of tumor antigens	Product of oncogene or mutated tumor suppressor gene		T cell — CD8+ CTL	Oncogene products: mutated RAS, Bcr/Abl fusion proteins Tumor suppressor gene products: mutated p53 protein
	Mutated self protein		T cell	Various mutant proteins in carcinogen, or radiation, induced animal tumors; various mutated proteins in melanomas
	Overexpressed or aberrantly expressed self protein		T cell — CD8+ CTL	Overexpressed: tyrosinase, gp100, MART in melanomas Aberrantly expressed: cancer-testis antigens (MAGE, BAGE)
	Oncogenic virus	Virus antigen-specific CD8+ CTL	T cell	Human papilloma virus E6, E7 proteins in cervical carcinoma; EBNA proteins in EBV induced lymphoma

Figure 11.4. Tumor antigens recognized by CD8$^+$ T cells. Reprinted, with permission, from Kumar V, Abbas AK, Fausto N. *Robbins & Cotran Pathologic Basis of Disease*. 7th ed. Philadelphia, PA: Elsevier Saunders; 2005.

CD4$^+$ T cells as phagocytosed tumor fragments via antigen presenting cells. (Please refer to Chapter 2 for an overview of major histocompatibility complex antigen pathways.) Examples of mutated oncogenes, tumor suppressors, and fusion proteins that can provide therapeutic targets include *RAS*, *p53*, and BCR/ABL, respectively.

Mutated gene products. Genetic instability and genomic damage associated with tumorigenesis can lead to production of numerous tumor-specific antigens. In the tumor transplantation studies of mice discussed previously, the tumor-specific antigens, so produced, fit into this category. Exposure to chemical or physical carcinogens, such as methylcholanthrene and radiation, respectively, can result in gene mutations of virtually any cell. These various mutated gene products are potential antigens; they are not recognized as self, and are therefore able to elicit a CTL response. Unfortunately, these do not make good targets for immune-directed therapy because each mutation is unique to the individual.

Overexpressed or aberrantly expressed cellular proteins. Proteins that are only expressed in certain tissues of the body may be abnormally expressed in some tumors. For example, tyrosinase, a melanoma antigen recognized by T cells (MART-1), and glycoprotein 100 (gp100) are nonmutated cellular proteins found only in normal melanocytes and retinal pigment epithelium. However, each has been found to be overexpressed in melanoma. The melanoma antigen (MAGE-1), another self-antigen normally found only in testis, has been identified in human melanoma and other tumors. Other tumor antigens with normal expression limited to testis—including GAGE, BAGE, and RAGE—have been found in melanoma and other tumors. Because these antigens are expressed in both tumors and testis, they are classified as cancer-testis antigens.

The *MAGE* gene family comprises several closely related genes believed to play a role in cell cycle regulation. *MAGE* is expressed in melanoma and also ovarian, breast, lung, prostate, bladder, and gastrointestinal carcinomas. Obviously, MAGE provides a good target for vaccine therapy and is currently under intensive investigation (see discussion later in this chapter).

Cellular proteins present at low levels in normal cells may be overexpressed in tumor cells. The *HER-2/neu* protein, mentioned earlier, is a member of the epidermal growth factor receptor family with low-level expression in normal tissues. Amplification of *HER-2/neu*, with resultant overexpression, is seen in various epithelial tumors, including breast and ovarian carcinoma. *HER-2/neu* provides an excellent target for immunotherapy and, in fact, one *HER-2/neu*-targeted monoclonal antibody is used clinically and at least one other is in late-stage development (see Monoclonal Antibodies as Cancer Therapy, later in this chapter).

Oncogenic viruses. Viruses have been causally linked to several cancers in animals and humans.[17,18] Antigens from the Epstein-Barr virus (EBV), hepatitis B virus (HBV), human T-cell leukemia virus type I (HTLV-1), and proteins E6 and E7 from human papillomavirus (HPV)-16 have been well characterized in human cancers. Epstein-Barr virus is associated with Burkitt's lymphoma and nasopharyngeal carcinoma. HTLV-1 is associated with adult T-cell leukemia/lymphoma. HPV causes 90% of cervical cancer (the most common cancer facing women worldwide), and HBV is linked with hepatocellular carcinoma.

Unlike chemical-induced tumors that appear to have limited cross-reactivity, viral-induced tumors tend to express tumor antigens that are shared by all tumors induced by the same virus. So the pursuit of immunotherapy for both prevention and treatment of viral-associated cancers is appealing. Vaccination programs have certainly helped reduce the incidence of hepatocellular carcinoma caused by hepatitis B, and HPV vaccination promises to greatly reduce the incidence of cervical cancer worldwide.

Tumor Markers

Tumor markers are specific substances unique to tumor type or tissue of origin; they are detectable in serum or body fluids. Although it is tempting to use tumor markers as screening tools, they generally lack the sensitivity and specificity needed to make a cancer diagnosis. Instead, they are used to help confirm a diagnosis, monitor treatment outcomes, and detect recurrence. Most tumor markers show a direct correlation with tumor burden and therefore disease course. Declining tumor marker levels after treatment indicates a good response to therapy. Increasing tumor marker levels ordinarily signifies lack of therapeutic effect or disease recurrence. Extreme elevations in tumor markers often reflect a heavy tumor burden and the need for aggressive treatment.

Tumor markers are considered tumor-associated antigens, but they are not generally used as immunotherapy targets. There are numerous tumor markers in use today; most laboratory tests for tumor markers are antibody-directed. New tumor markers are constantly being developed and investigated for diagnostic utility. A general discussion of the most common tumor markers follows.

Oncofetal antigens. Oncofetal antigens are proteins that are expressed in normally developing fetal tissues, but are not normally found in adult cells. They are also expressed to a high degree in certain tumor cells, hence the name oncofetal antigen. Two of the best known oncofetal antigens are carcinoembryonic antigen (CEA) and alpha-fetoprotein (AFP).

CEA is a membrane-bound glycoprotein expressed by embryonic gastrointestinal tissue, liver, and pancreas. About half of patients with early-stage colorectal cancer and most patients with late-stage colorectal cancer will have elevated serum CEA levels. Elevations are also seen in many patients with pancreatic, gastric, and lung cancer, and in nonmalignant diseases such as chronic obstructive airway disease, inflammatory bowel disease, and cirrhosis. CEA is used primarily to monitor colorectal cancer. Preoperative CEA level is recommended in all patients with colorectal cancer, with repeated measurements 1 month postoperatively and routinely thereafter, as indicated.[19,20]

AFP, another glycoprotein abundant early in fetal development, has tissue distribution similar to CEA. Serum AFP levels decline dramatically later in life, but abnormally high levels are seen in hepatocellular carcinoma and germ cell tumors of the ovaries and testis. As with CEA, elevations of serum AFP can also be seen in nonmalignant conditions such as toxic hepatic injury, ataxia telangiectasia, Wiskott-Aldrich syndrome, and pregnancy (particularly if there is fetal distress). Despite these problems with specificity, AFP (along with human chorionic gonadotropin [hCG]) is recommended for use as an aid in diagnosis, staging, monitoring, and detection of recurrent germ-cell tumors.[19]

Hormones. Human chorionic gonadotropin (hCG) is a glycoprotein heterodimer composed of two noncovalently bound subunits, α and β. It is produced by trophoblast tissue in pregnancy, and is responsible for many hormonal functions to support embryonic growth. Serum and urine concentrations rise exponentially in the first trimester and peak between 8 and 12 weeks of gestation. Elevated serum hCG levels later in life are abnormal, so hCG can be considered an oncofetal antigen. As mentioned, hCG has diagnostic and monitoring utility in germ-cell tumors. It is also a highly sensitive and specific marker for gestational trophoblastic neoplasia, and is used to accurately assess tumor volume and disease course.

Other glycoproteins. *Cancer antigen 125 (CA-125).* The murine monoclonal antibody OC 125 recognizes an epitope—cancer antigen 125 (CA 125)—that is expressed multiple times on a high-molecular-weight glycoprotein found in fetal coelomic epithelia. CA 125 is produced by normal epithelia of the peritoneum and endometrium and also by benign ovarian cysts. It is currently the best available tumor marker for epithelial ovarian cancer. Although not currently recommended for screening, most guidelines recommend using serum CA 125 for staging/prognosis, monitoring therapy, and detecting recurrence.[19]

Specific proteins. *Prostate-specific antigen (PSA).* Prostate-specific antigen (PSA) is a serine protease produced exclusively by epithelial prostate tissues. Physiologically, PSA is abundant in seminal fluid and functions to cleave proteins, which results in liquefaction. PSA is also present in the serum and can be detected by various antibody-directed assays. Serum levels rise with prostate malignancy, but elevations are also seen in nonmalignant conditions including benign prostatic hypertrophy (BPH), prostatitis, and acute urinary retention. PSA levels also increase with digital rectal examination, prostate biopsy, and cystoscopic examination of the prostate. Medications known to lower PSA include finasteride (Proscar and Propecia), dutasteride (Avodart), and some herbal preparations marketed for prostate health that contain saw palmetto.

PSA is the best known tumor marker, and its role in prostate cancer screening has been the subject of longstanding debate. Used alone, elevated PSA could lead to an unnecessary work-up for prostate cancer along with the expense and morbidity associated with ultrasonography and biopsy. A false positive or false negative test could also cause heightened anxiety or a false sense of comfort, respectively. Despite problems with specificity, PSA is a very sensitive tumor marker. In patients with confirmed prostate cancer, PSA accurately reflects tumor burden, and therefore becomes a very important monitoring tool. The American Cancer Society, American Urologic Association, and National Comprehensive Cancer Network all recommend monitoring PSA after prostate cancer diagnosis.[19-21] For early detection, all three organizations recommend offering PSA testing in conjunction with digital rectal examination, beginning at age 50 in patients with normal prostate cancer risk and life expectancy beyond 10 years.

Immune Response to Tumors

Immune responses to tumors can be humoral and cell mediated, with the latter playing the more important role.[22] Cytotoxic T lymphocytes, natural killer (NK) cells, and macrophages all play a role in tumor immunity. Even though evidence supports the idea that the host immune system recognizes tumors and produces a response to them, the immune response to tumor antigens is often very weak.[23,24] One reason for this decreased immune response is that there are very few antigens that are specific to cancer cells (tumor-specific antigens), and the host immune system often sees the tumor-associated antigens as self or altered self. Another barrier to antitumor immune responses is the production of immunoinhibitory factors by the tumor. The tumor does not passively wait to be eliminated by the immune system but, instead, fights back. In this section, we examine the roles of selected immune system cells in the immune response to tumors. We also examine the theory of immunosurveillance.

Role of CTLs, NK cells, and macrophages. *Cytotoxic T lymphocytes.* Cytotoxic T lymphocytes (CTLs), particularly CD8+ CTLs, have been shown to play a protective role against virus-associated neoplasms.[4,5] They contain antigen-specific receptors that recognize novel peptides bound to MHC class I antigens on the tumor cell surface. The CTL binds to the MHC-foreign antigen complex, and initiates a T-cell–mediated immune response. The immune response depends on the presence of both a self-component (MHC) and a foreign antigen; it is MHC-restricted. Though CD8+ CTLs also secrete cytokines, their greatest role is in directly killing tumor cells. On the other hand, CD4+ T cells (helper T cells) release cytokines, such as interleukin (IL)-2 and interferon gamma (IFN-γ), which stimulate the activity of other effector cells (CTLs, NK cells, and macrophages).

Natural killer (NK) cells. NK cells, also known as large granular lymphocytes, are found in the spleen, lymph nodes, bone marrow, and peripheral blood. NK cells are known to mediate innate immunity against pathogens as well as tumor cells. In mouse tumor models in which NK cells are absent, enhanced tumor formation has been observed.[25,26]

NK cells are regulated by a balance of signals from activating receptors and inhibitory receptors specific for MHC class I molecules.[26] In an effort to evade the immune system, many tumors exhibit a loss of MHC class I antigens (discussed later in this chapter). When these molecules are present, they have an inhibitory effect on NK cells, which is why NK cells do not normally lyse healthy cells. Therefore, NK cells may be more effective than

CD8$^+$ CTLs, which are dependent on the presence of MHC class I molecules in eliminating MHC-deficient tumor cells.[5,22] NK cells are stimulated by various agents including interferon alpha (IFN-α), IL-2, and tumor necrosis factor (TNF). One way in which NK cells act is through releasing apoptosis-inducing molecules from granules in the cells. NK cells bear FasL on their surfaces, and induce cell apoptosis through the Fas (CD95) receptor on target cells, too. NK cells may also destroy tumor cells through antibody-dependent cell-mediated cytotoxicity (ADCC) due to the presence of Fc receptors (CD16), which are receptors for the Fc region of immunoglobulin G (IgG) on their cell membranes. In addition, NK cells secrete IFN-γ, which activates other effector cells such as macrophages.

Macrophages. Macrophages are cytotoxic effector cells that may be activated by various agents, including endotoxins, immune complexes, and lymphokines (IL-1 and macrophage-activating factors [MAF] such as IFN-γ). As mentioned earlier, IFN-γ is produced by T cells as well as NK cells, and attracts macrophages to the site of the tumor. T cells can also release migration-inhibitory factor to prevent migration of macrophages away from the tumor-infiltrated area. Once activated, macrophages selectively kill tumor cells via cell lysis and phagocytosis. The secretion of TNF by activated macrophages may also contribute to their cytotoxicity. Like NK cells, macrophages also express Fc receptors, which enable them to attack antibody-coated target cells too. In addition to antitumor effects, macrophages present in tumors have been shown to play a role in the inflammatory process, promoting tumor cell progression, migration, and metastasis.[4]

Immunosurveillance and immunoediting. Certain types of cancer, especially cancers of the immune system, are known to occur more frequently in patients who are immunocompromised, either congenitally or because of immunosuppressive drugs or acquired immunodeficiency syndrome (AIDS); however, some types of cancer—such as breast, prostate, and lung—are not more prevalent in the immunocompromised host.

The concept of cancer immunosurveillance is not new but has been more recently expanded. The revised version now includes the concept that the immune system may actually promote the development of tumor cells that can effectively evade destruction.[27,28] This can be thought of as "survival of the fittest"; the traits that allow tumors to survive the host immune system are passed down, while the traits that make tumors more antigenic are eliminated from the population. In this revised theory, immunosurveillance is only

a part of the picture. The expanded idea is called immunoediting and includes three phases: elimination, equilibrium, and escape (**Figure 11.5**).[27,28] In this new theory of immunoediting, immunosurveillance fits into the first phase, elimination. The second phase, equilibrium, likely occurs just before the tumor is large enough to be clinically detected. The third stage, escape, is the period in which the tumor cells have evaded both the innate and the adaptive immune system.[28] The cells in the escape phase have survived the elimination and equilibrium phases, and thus have likely developed traits that allow them to effectively circumvent the host immune system. They not only proliferate in an uncontrolled manner, but also invade and metastasize. There is evidence that the immune system may also have protumor effects and may actually promote tumor growth and progression by producing growth factors or enzymes, such as matrix metalloproteinases (MMPs), that facilitate tumor invasion.[4,5]

TUMOR EVASION OF THE IMMUNE SYSTEM

Since cancer cells can be viewed as foreign to the body, it is expected that the body's own immune response would serve as a valuable mechanism for helping eradicate the foreign cancer cells. In fact, immune responses have been seen in vitro and in vivo for a number of malignancies, including melanoma and renal cell cancer. Conversely, every cancer cell that proliferates is an example of a cancer that has not been destroyed by the immune system. The reason these proliferating cancer cells can avoid the immune system is an active area of investigation; it may indicate potential aspects of the immune system that can be targeted for cancer therapy. If the cancer cell's lack of immunogenicity is a reason for its ability to proliferate, manipulation of the cell's immunogenicity may increase the body's immune response or increase the impact of immunotherapeutic strategies (interferon, monoclonal antibodies).

As described earlier, cancer cells often express antigens not present on nonmalignant cells. Unfortunately, these antigens are not always presented to the immune system in a microenvironment that favors activation of the immune response. One mechanism thought to contribute to poor tumor immunogenicity involves poor immune activation. For example, tumor cells do not express costimulatory molecules; without them, T lymphocytes may be less reactive.[29] Another difference observed between the environment

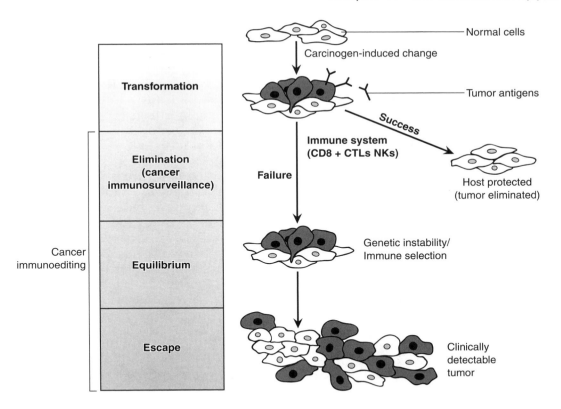

Figure 11.5. Cancer immunoediting: (1) normal cells exposed to carcinogen-induced damage become tumor cells; (2) tumor cells may express tumor-specific markers that activate the immune system; (3) if the immune system fails to destroy them, tumor cells may enter equilibrium and may produce new populations that may be even better at evading the immune system; and (4) in the escape phase, tumor becomes clinically detectable.

of a tumor and the environment of the immune responses (such as the site of an infection) is the lack of common inflammatory cells (monocytes, macrophages, and dendritic cells). These cells are important in triggering the immune system; when they are absent, or decreased, there is a decreased immune response.[29]

Another cause of poor tumor immunogenicity involves certain aspects of the cancer cell. Because tumors have unstable genomes, tumor cells can escape immune recognition because they mutate elements in antigen processing.[30] Certain tumor cells may produce proteins that mediate the immune response. For example, tumor cells may produce immunoinhibitory factors (such as transforming growth factor β and IL-10) that interfere with macrophage-mediated antigen presentation and other immune functions. This suggests that, as we evaluate the role of immunotherapy in select cancers, it is essential to evaluate the immunogenicity of the cancer type (e.g., melanoma), and perhaps the immunogenicity of individual patients, to determine the potential appropriateness of an immunotherapy strategy.

CANCER IMMUNOTHERAPY

Mechanisms of Manipulating the Immune System

The concept of using immunologic strategies to fight (or prevent) cancer has emerged over the past few decades. The evolving understanding of the basic science of immunity and the discovery of many important proteins and cells that coordinate the immune response have led to the successful application of immunotherapy. Very early attempts at immunotherapy were often broadly based; for example, use of bacterial products administered directly into tumors. The many applications of immunotherapy today extend broadly in cancer therapy, including strategies to prevent cancer, to treat cancer, and to eradicate micrometastases that may lead to recurrence of cancer (e.g., adjuvant setting). The rationale for the use of immunoprevention of cancer is the idea that the immune system is able to recognize transformed cells and destroy them before they develop into a clinically apparent cancer. Individuals with increased risk of cancer or who have a preneoplastic condition are targeted for immunoprevention.[31] As described later in this chapter, the exploitation of immune manipulation has also affected patient care, during the course of cancer treatment (e.g., white and red blood cell factors) or at the time of cancer progression.

The strategies, as well as the potential applications, range widely; biologic therapies include use of cytokines, monoclonal antibodies, vaccines that focus on tumor-specific or tumor-associated antigens, and combinations of these therapies. Many of these strategies are discussed below, but because this is a rapidly evolving field, new data are available daily.

Immunomodulators of Biologic Response Modifiers

Interferons. The interferons (IFNs) are a family of complex proteins with diverse biological functions. IFNs are induced by a viral infection and inhibit, or interfere with, the replication of other viruses. The physiologic actions of IFNs are closely tied to the network of cytokines that are important in the immune response, for IFNs are potent immunomodulators. The therapeutic potential of IFNs is broad, and extends beyond oncology. Therapeutic application of IFNs depends on the specific IFN, dose, schedule, duration of therapy, and potential combination.

Three interferons have been identified in humans: IFN-α, IFN-β, and IFN-γ. IFN-α and IFN-β are classified as type I IFNs, and IFN-γ is classified as a type II IFN. Type I IFNs are structurally related proteins coded by genes on chromosome 9, and they act through a common receptor. The IFN-α family consists of more than 20 structurally related proteins encoded by distinct genes. IFN-α-2a, -2b, and -2c differ slightly in amino acid sequence. IFN-β is from a single distinct gene. IFN-γ is coded by a gene on chromosome 12, and has a receptor distinct from type I interferons. IFN-γ is produced by T lymphocytes and NK cells after activation with immune and inflammatory stimuli.

Interferons have potent effects on cell proliferation, immunomodulation, and apoptosis. IFN activities include enhancement of the production and cytotoxic activity of NK and lymphokine-activated killer (LAK) cells, stimulation of other immunomodulating cytokines, and an increased expression of major histocompatibility antigens on the cell surface. These effects are believed to be at least partially responsible for the antitumor activity of IFNs.[32]

The toxicities seen with IFN are likely secondary to the effects they have on the immune system, and appear to be similar to what would be seen with a hyperimmune response. It follows that the clinical manifestation and severity may depend on the activity of the IFN regimen on the immune system. Indeed, the side effect profile of IFNs depends on many factors, including type of interferon, dose/regimen, route of administration, and patient factors such as comorbidities. The most common side effect of IFN is the cascade of symptoms often called constitutional symptoms or flu-like syndrome, because they mimic influenza. These can include acute symptoms such as fever, chills, myalgia, and fatigue, but may (with prolonged use) also include more chronic toxicities such as fatigue, anorexia, and depression.[33] Acetaminophen may prevent or minimize acute dose-related symptoms such as fever, myalgia, and chills. Opiates, most often the short-acting meperidine, are used to manage severe chills or rigors most commonly seen with high-dose intravenous IFN-α. Nonsteroidal anti-inflammatory drugs (NSAIDs) have been used to manage interferon-related myalgia, but their side effects may overlap with IFN side effects, such as decreased renal blood flow or nausea. Fatigue is one of the most frequently observed dose-limiting toxicities of interferon therapy.[33] Anorexia was reported in about 70% of patients receiving adjuvant interferon therapy for melanoma; it is thought to be mediated through direct effects on hypothalamic neurons, modification of normal hypothalamic neurotransmitters/neuropeptides, or effects from the stimulation of other cytokines.[33,34] Depression is common; its cause(s) may be multifactorial, including IFN-induced hypothyroidism and/or concomitant interferon symptoms (e.g., nausea and fatigue). Other toxicities, such as hematologic or hepatic toxicities, require monitoring and appropriate dose modification.

Interferon-α: clinical applications. Many of the initial uses of IFN-α in the treatment of certain malignancies have been replaced over time with alternative treatment strategies involving newer agents. For example, IFN-α was initially marketed in the United States in the mid-1980s for the treatment of hairy cell leukemia (HCL), but because of the advent of other effective treatment options, IFN-α is rarely used first line for HCL at this time. The activity of IFN-α in some of the malignancies discussed is included, as it remains a therapeutic option in these malignancies for patients who cannot receive, or have disease progression through, other therapies.

Hairy cell leukemia. IFN-α is an effective treatment for patients with hairy cell leukemia, and was, before cladribine, the treatment of choice.

IFN-α was found to eradicate hairy cells from both the peripheral blood and the bone marrow. Results from early trials demonstrated response rates as high as 80% with IFN-α. But most of the responses with interferon were partial responses, and the discontinuation of treatment resulted in relapse in most patients.[35] The dose regimen for HCL is 2 million units subcutaneously 3 times weekly for 12 months. Toxicities with this regimen included the constitutional symptoms described above, which are significant considering the duration of therapy.

Chronic myelogenous leukemia (CML). Until the advent of imatinib, IFN-α was the cornerstone of treatment for patients with CML who could not receive definitive treatment with high-dose chemotherapy followed by hematopoetic stem cell transplant. The dose regimen of IFN-α used in the management of CML is 5×10^6 units/m^2 subcutaneous 3 times weekly; the responses, both cytogenetic and hematologic, have resulted in increased survival.[36] The incidence of cytogenetic responses has varied greatly in clinical studies, as have the types of response. In randomized trials, the impact of IFN-α on survival was confirmed, and was thought to result from the delay of disease progression to blast crisis.[37] Combination therapy has been evaluated to exploit the benefit of IFN-α in CML. The combination of IFN and cytarabine has been shown to increase the rate of major cytogenetic response and to prolong survival in patients with chronic-phase CML.[38] The 3-year survival rate was 86% with the combination cytarabine and IFN-α. Toxicities associated with IFN-α in this regimen included myalgia, arthralgia, asthenia, weight loss, depression, and headache.[38] The addition of cytarabine increased toxicities, as would be expected, which include hematologic side effects such as thrombocytopenia.

Though there are many options for the management of CML, IFN-α remains an appropriate choice for some patients. Despite optimization of imatinib therapy, the role of IFN-α in management of CML has progressed. Patients with CML who cannot tolerate imatinib or who have poor responses to treatment may be potential candidates for IFN-α. The emergence of multitargeted tyrosine kinase inhibitors such as dasatinib, a BCR–ABL inhibitor that targets many of imatinib-resistant BCR–ABL mutations, may force the role of IFN-α in CML to be further redefined. For example, strategies for the use of IFN-α in patients with minimal residual disease, after other partially successful treatments, is a potential application to be evaluated.

Melanoma. IFN-α has been extensively evaluated in cutaneous melanoma. Initial studies of IFN-α in patients with metastatic disease showed highest response rates in patients with minimal disease burden. Encouragingly, responses were seen in all sites of disease, but the most frequent disease responses were seen in subcutaneous, lymph node, and pulmonary metastases. Strategies to optimize the responses in metastatic disease include high-dose IFN regimens, combination therapy with chemotherapy and/or immunotherapy, and regional administration of interferon.

A number of studies have evaluated various doses and schedules of recombinant interferon for treatment of metastatic melanoma, but no standard strategy is recommended.[39] Response rates in metastatic melanoma range from 10% to 30%, and overall response rates are about 15% for IFN-α. Unfortunately, the optimal dose, treatment schedule, and treatment combination/regimens have not been established for the management of metastatic melanoma. Single-agent recombinant IFN-α has demonstrated clinical response rates of about 15%, with durable responses in about a third of those patients. Response rates appear to be higher in patients with doses maximized, though a wide range of dosages has been shown to be effective: 10 million units/m^2/day to 50 million units/m^2 subcutaneously 3 times weekly. IFN-α given as a continuous therapy appears to be associated with better response rates than when given as a cyclic regimen.[39,40]

The combination of IFN-α with chemotherapy or other cytokines—biochemotherapy—has also been evaluated in melanoma in an attempt to exploit the unique mechanism of action of each drug in combination. The combination of IFN-α and dacarbazine has yielded mixed results and some controversy. A large randomized trial addressed biochemotherapy in metastatic melanoma, and demonstrated that response rates, time to treatment failure, and survival were not improved with the combination. Toxicity was increased with the combination therapy.[41]

IFN-α has been combined with aldesleukin (rIL-2), alone or with chemotherapy, in an attempt to increase the responses seen with either agent alone. The hope was that the up-regulation of histocompatibility antigens by IFN-α would increase susceptibility of cancer cells to IL-2. Unfortunately, response rates of the combination have not demonstrated any substantial advantage, and the risks of increased adverse effects seen with the combination do not appear to warrant its use at this time.[42]

As noted previously, response rates of IFN-α in clinical trials were highest in patients with minimal tumor burden. Based on the responses in metastatic melanoma, and the perceived benefit in patients with minimal disease, IFN-α has been evaluated in patients after curative surgery for treatment of any residual disease. The focus of this research has been in patients with a high risk of recurrence (those with large tumors or lymph node involvement) after primary surgery for melanoma. One of the challenges of the studies is trying to determine which patients are most likely to benefit from IFN-α adjuvant therapy, especially in light of cost and toxicity.

IFN-α-2b has been extensively studied as an adjuvant therapy after surgical resection in locally advanced melanoma in a variety of doses, schedules, and combinations. Initial excitement from the positive results of a multicenter trial comparing IFN-α-2b, at maximally tolerated doses, to observation in high-risk patients after surgical resection of melanoma has been tempered over recent years. The high-dose regimen, including an initial high dose intravenous induction phase of IFN-α for 4 weeks, was followed by a 48-week low-dose subcutaneous maintenance phase of IFN-α. The rationale for the induction phase was to provide peak levels of interferon sufficient to inhibit tumor growth and provide both anti-angiogenesis and immunomodulatory effects, while avoiding production of anti-interferon antibodies. Results from the initial study comparing a high-dose regimen (often referred to as high-dose interferon or HDI) to placebo demonstrated a significant improvement in relapse-free survival and overall survival in patients with high-risk melanoma; unfortunately, the response was coupled with significant toxicity.[43] Dose modifications were needed in about half the patients during the clinical trial. Toxicities included constitutional symptoms, hematologic toxicity, and hepatic toxicities, but 74% of the patients were able to complete the year of therapy in an outpatient setting. A subsequent report from the cooperative group study demonstrated a quality-of-life benefit with interferon therapy based on the quality-of-life-adjusted survival analysis.[44] This analysis calculates the quality-of-life-adjusted years gained as a result of IFN-α treatment or the clinical benefit of time without toxicities and without disease; the benefit demonstrated in this study in terms of life without disease outweighed the time with treatment-related toxicity. In an individual patient, this risk assessment should be considered and weighed against the individual's tolerance.

Because of the associated toxicity and adverse effects seen with IFN-α therapy, there is a worldwide concern about its usefulness for melanoma despite the possible benefits in relapse-free and overall survival.[45] One of the strategies evaluated to improve tolerability of IFN-α has been to look at more tolerable doses and dose schedules that still maintain the benefit of the drug in the adjuvant treatment of melanoma. The optimal dose of IFN-α in the adjuvant setting is not clear. A subsequent Eastern Cooperative Oncology Group (ECOG) trial designed to evaluate the impact of lower doses of interferon (LDI; 3 million units per dose subcutaneous 3 times weekly) for 24 months compared to the HDI and observation did not demonstrate a survival advantage of HDI versus observation.[39] An overall survival benefit was not seen for HDI or LDI compared to the observation arm, although the investigators speculated that this analysis of survival was affected by the number of patients in the observation arm that received interferon therapy after disease progression.

The current status of IFN-α as adjuvant treatment of cutaneous melanoma is being further evaluated to determine if improvement can be made in responses, patient selection, toxicity prevention or management, and place in therapy.

Other cancers. The antitumor effects of IFN-α—regulating cell proliferation, immunomodulation, and apoptosis—have provided a basis for evaluating the role of this agent in a variety of both solid and hematologic malignancies. Though the activity of the drug in different cancers has been demonstrated, the application in management is always evaluated with consideration of other treatments. For example, numerous clinical trials have confirmed clinical activity in metastatic renal cell cancer, with an objective response rate of about 15%. The effect of IFN-α on the survival of patients with metastatic renal cell carcinoma (RCC) is unclear because of a conservative estimate that about 3% of patients treated with IFN-α have a sustained clinical response lasting longer than a year.[46] At this time, IFN-α is not standard care for patients with metastatic RCC because there are other agents that have activity, convenience, and possibly improved tolerability. The question, then, is if there is a place for IFN-α in combination with newer evolving therapies.

IFN-α has been evaluated in a number of hematologic malignancies beyond HCL and CML. The applications of IFN-α in multiple myeloma and lymphomas have been extensively reviewed elsewhere.[36]

Interferon-γ. IFN-γ is unrelated to the type I interferons at both a genetic and protein level, and its biological activities appear to differ from the type I IFNs. IFN-γ is a major macrophage-activating factor and appears to play a critical role in promoting host-defense mechanism against a number of pathogens. IFN-γ also appears to play an important role in promoting host defense to tumors.[47] Despite great enthusiasm that IFN-γ would have a role in the treatment of a variety of cancers, clinical trials of IFN-γ with a number of solid and hematologic malignancies have not yielded any true successes.

An approach that has been considered is to combine IFN-γ with type I IFNs, based on the potential synergism of IFNs acting via two separate receptors. Though this strategy has led to clinical trials, the approach has not proven successful enough to warrant evaluation in treatment of a specific cancer. Researchers hope the exploitation of the both antiproliferative and tumor immunity activity may someday be translated into a clinical role for IFN-γ in cancer prevention or treatment.

Interleukin-2. Interleukin-2 (IL-2), originally known as T-cell growth factor, is a glycoprotein produced by activated lymphocytes. Aldesleukin, the only commercially available recombinant IL-2 (rIL-2), is approved for human use in the United States. Unlike the natural IL-2 protein, aldesleukin is nonglycosylated and has some amino acid modification. IL-2 is rapidly cleared from the circulation after intravenous administration, though there is a longer beta clearance of about 60–85 minutes consistent with a two-compartment model. Subcutaneous administration appears to achieve constant plasma concentrations for about 8 hours.[48]

The precise mechanism of the cytotoxicity of IL-2 is unknown. In vitro and in vivo, IL-2 stimulates the production and release of many secondary monocyte-derived and T-cell–derived cytokines, including IL-4, IL-5, IL-6, IL-8, TNF-α, granulocyte macrophage-colony stimulating factor (GM-CSF), and IFN-γ, which may have direct or indirect antitumor activities. In addition, IL-2 appears to stimulate the cytotoxic activities of NK cells, monocytes, LAK cells, and CTLs. High concentrations of IL-2 have not been shown to have a direct antitumor effect on cancer cells in vitro.

Immunologic changes are noted almost immediately after administration of rIL-2. Lymphopenia develops within minutes, and is thought to be secondary to margination of lymphocytes into the extravascular space. After discontinuation of the drug, there is a rebound lymphocytosis. With repetitive IL-2 administration, lymphocytes become activated and the expression of adhesion molecules increases. There is an antigen-specific clonal expansion of T cells and the stimulation of nonspecific immune cells such as NK and LAK cells. Lymphocytic infiltration into tumors may occur. B cells are also affected by IL-2. Many cytokines are produced through the activation of lymphocytes;

they appear to be important in the mechanisms by which rIL-2 mediates tumor regression.

Preclinical trials with IL-2 demonstrated a clear dose–response relationship between rIL-2 and tumor response. Based on these data, initial clinical trials of aldesleukin in patients with melanoma used relatively high doses of the drug as a single agent or in combination with LAK cells. The response rates seen in these trials ranged from 15% to 25%, and about 2% to 5% of patients achieved complete responses. The patients with melanoma who achieved a complete response, although small in number, had very durable responses (years). Responses were also seen at a number of metastatic sites such as lung, liver, bone, lymph nodes, and subcutaneous tissue. Based on the reevaluation of early clinical trials, rIL-2 (aldesleukin) was approved by the Food and Drug Administration (FDA) for treatment of metastatic melanoma. Overall, objective response rates were about 16%, but in some cases there were durable responses, and responses were seen in patients with large tumor burdens. Response rates occurred in a variety of disease sites including lung, liver, lymph nodes, soft tissue, and adrenals, as well as in bone disease.[49]

The results of phase II trials with rIL-2 also led to FDA approval of aldesleukin for treatment of metastatic RCC, and high-dose IL-2 by bolus administration has endured as a therapy for the disease. Although (as with melanoma) the responses may be only 15% to 20%, some of these responses are durable. Because of recent advances in the treatment of metastatic RCC using oral multitargeted tyrosine kinase inhibitors such as sunitinib and sorafenib, the role of high-dose IL-2 will need to be redefined.

The high aldesleukin doses used in initial clinical trials are associated with significant toxicities that limit its practicality for certain individuals as well as its broad application in certain health care systems. The high-dose aldesleukin regimen is 600,000 international units per kg per dose every 8 hours for 14 doses maximum; it is approved for treatment of metastatic melanoma and metastatic RCC. Successful treatment depends largely on the management of acute toxicities. One common and expected complication of therapy is cytokine-induced capillary leak syndrome (CLS).

CLS is caused by cytokine-induced increased permeability of capillary walls, which allows a shift of fluid from the intravascular space into extravascular space and tissue. As a patient becomes intravascularly dehydrated, hypotension may occur and precipitate reflex tachycardia and/or arrhythmias. The decrease in blood volume may also result in decreased renal perfusion and a subsequent decrease in urine output. The renal effects may manifest as an increase in blood urea nitrogen, serum creatinine, edema, weight gain, and a significant decrease (<50 mL/hour) in urine output. Visceral edema can result in pulmonary congestion, pleural effusions, and bowel and general edema. Patients receiving high-dose aldesleukin require careful toxicity monitoring and management similar to that of a critical care setting. Although some institutions manage patients receiving high-dose aldesleukin in an intensive care unit, most patients can be successfully managed in an inpatient oncology unit.

Other toxicities associated with IL-2 are similar to those seen with other cytokine therapy. Constitutional symptoms, including fevers, chills, anorexia, myalgias, and arthralgias, are relatively common. High-dose r-IL2 regimen side effects also include facial flushing, rashes, and nausea/vomiting. A more complete review of toxicities and strategies for prevention and management are available.[50]

As with the IFNs, an attempt to provide the benefit of aldesleukin therapy without the toxicity has resulted in a number of trials using a variety of treatment regimens and strategies. Studies have evaluated continuous-infusion aldesleukin therapy and lower dose aldesleukin alone or combined with chemotherapy and interferon therapy. Lower doses of aldesleukin given subcutaneously can be administered to patients in an outpatient setting, but this has not demonstrated the same response as those of patients receiving higher dose regimens. Direct head-to-head comparisons of various dosing schedules and regimens are needed to determine the optimum approach to aldesleukin therapy in metastatic melanoma.

The coadministration of LAK cells with aldesleukin does not appear to significantly improve clinical response. Though some studies have suggested improved response with co-administration of tumor infiltrating lymphocytes (TIL) with recombinant IL-2, the therapy is technically difficult and costly, and the overall clinical benefit has not been clearly demonstrated.

Colony-Stimulating Factors

Hematopoietic colony-stimulating factors (CSFs) are a group of growth factors that offer a variety of uses in oncology. The CSFs have a role in the production and differentiation of cells for all three hematopoietic cell lines, and can be used as a supportive measure for neutropenia, anemia, and thrombocytopenia. The growth factors are essential for proliferation, differentiation, maturation, and the functional activity of various hematopoietic stem cells. The CSFs manufactured by recombinant DNA technology include granulocyte macrophage colony-stimulating factors (GM-CSF), granulocyte colony-stimulating factor (G-CSF), macrophage colony-stimulating factor (M-CSF), multipotential CSF (multi-CSF or IL-3), IL-1, IL-4, IL-5, IL-6, IL-11, and erythropoietin (EPO).[51] Currently available CSFs are GM-CSF, G-CSF, and EPO. This section will review the appropriate use of hematopoetic CSFs in the oncology setting based on evidence in the current literature.

Erythropoietin. Erythropoietin (EPO) is a glycoprotein growth factor that binds to and activates erythroid progenitor cells in the bone marrow.[52] The progenitor cells then proliferate, differentiate, and mature, becoming mature functional erythrocytes. EPO plasma levels do not increase in response to anemic hypoxia in patients with chronic renal disease. Initial studies were done to see if EPO could decrease the number of transfusions in anemic patients on dialysis.[53,54] The intravenous administration of EPO in doses ranging from 25–500 units/kg 3 times a week caused a dose-dependent rise in the hematocrit, and decreased or eliminated the need for transfusion. Patients were also found to have improved quality of life and increased energy levels. Trials have also looked at EPO in patients with chronic renal disease who are not on dialysis. These patients, however, did not have severe anemia, and they were usually not transfusion-dependent; although improvement was seen, it was not dramatic. The amounts of EPO currently administered to patients with chronic renal failure are lower than those found to be effective in the early clinical trials. A recombinant EPO (rEPO) product, epoetin alfa, was the first CSF to be approved by the FDA. It was approved for the treatment of anemia of chronic renal failure at a dose of 50–100 units per kilogram of body weight, subcutaneously or intravenously, 3 times per week. Epoetin alfa contains the amino acid sequence identical to endogenous human EPO, and has a plasma half-life of about 3–10 hours in healthy volunteers after intravenous administration.

Darbepoetin alfa is another rEPO approved by the FDA. It is unique for the addition of two N-glycosylation sites that produce a molecule with a half-life about 3 times longer than epoetin alfa. Initial studies assessed the safety and efficacy of darbepoetin alfa in patients with chronic renal failure (CRF) who had not received prior treatment with rEPO. The first trial evaluated CRF patients receiving dialysis. The starting dose for patients receiving darbepoetin alfa was 0.45 µg/kg once weekly, and the starting dose for patients receiving epoetin alfa was 50 units/kg 3 times weekly.[55] When necessary, dosage adjustments were made to maintain hemoglobin in the study target range of 11–13 g/dL. The primary efficacy end point was the proportion of patients who experienced at least 1 g/dL increase in hemoglobin concentration to a level of at least 11 g/dL at the end of 20 weeks. The hemoglobin target was achieved by 72% of the 90 patients with darbepoetin alfa and 84% of the 31 patients treated with epoetin alfa. For patients with CRF, the FDA approved the starting dose of darbepoetin alfa 0.45 μg/kg body weight, administered subcutaneously or intravenously once weekly. Doses should be titrated to not exceed a target hemoglobin concentration of 12 g/dL. Predialysis patients may require lower maintenance doses. Some patients have been treated with darbepoetin alfa administered every 2 weeks.

Anemia is a common side effect of cancer and cancer therapy. Anemia associated with cancer and chemotherapy has also been linked to inappropriately low serum EPO concentrations in relation to hemoglobin concentration. Anemia due to malignancy may be related to a number of factors, including bone marrow involvement by the cancer, an impaired production of red blood cells directly related to the cancer treatment, or other nonspecific processes such as the inhibitory effect of tumor necrosis factor, iron deficiency, or low endogenous erythropoietin levels.[56] Initial studies looked at the use of EPO in a variety of clinical oncology settings, testing various doses and schedules. The trials were initially small, so some failed to demonstrate significant benefit. Larger trials, often cited in review of anemia, demonstrate the clinical benefits of EPO based on the reduction of red blood cell transfusion requirements, increase in hemoglobin, and improved quality of life.[56–59] Epoetin alfa was initially studied at a dose of 150 units/kg 3 times weekly, with the possibility of dose escalation to 300 units/kg in those who did not respond to the initial dose. Since patients may be reluctant, or unable, to receive therapy 3 times a week based on practical issues such as convenience, transportation, or time commitment, clinical trials have evaluated the use of EPO as a weekly regimen. In a nonrandomized trial, EPO was evaluated at 40,000 units once weekly by subcutaneous injection.[60] The study found patients undergoing chemotherapy had increases in hemoglobin levels, decreases in transfusion requirement, and improvement in quality of life similar to those observed with the 3-times weekly dosage schedule. Clinical practice has evolved to weekly dosing (for the convenience of cancer patients), administering 40,000 units

subcutaneously once weekly, and increasing the dose to 60,000 units once weekly in patients who do not initially respond.[61]

The efficacy of darbepoetin alfa in the treatment of cancer-related anemia in patients receiving chemotherapy has been investigated in several comparative[62–66] and noncomparative[67] studies. The most commonly evaluated efficacy endpoints in trials included (1) the incidence of red blood cell transfusion, (2) the proportion of patients needing red blood cell transfusion or reaching transfusion trigger (hemoglobin ≤8 g/dL), (3) the rate of hemoglobin response (≥2 g/dL increase in hemoglobin or hemoglobin level ≥12 g/dL, with no red blood cell transfusion in the preceding 28 days), and (4) the change in hemoglobin levels from baseline. Several different dose regimens have been used in clinical practice and clinical trials. Initial phase III trials evaluated the efficacy of darbepoetin alfa dosed 2.25 μg/kg once weekly in the treatment of anemia in patients with lung cancer[66] or lymphoproliferative malignancies[64] receiving chemotherapy. The dosage was doubled to 4.5 μg/kg once weekly for patients with an inadequate response. Darbepoetin alfa was found more effective than placebo in decreasing blood transfusion requirements, increasing hemoglobin concentration, and decreasing fatigue. Darbepoetin studies at a dosage of 200 μg every 2 weeks have been shown to be as effective as epoetin alfa at 40,000 units weekly.[68] Since darbepoetin has a long half-life, a once-every-3-week regimen of darbepoetin alfa (300 μg or 500 μg) has been evaluated in randomized, double-blind[62] or noncomparative[67] multicenter trials. After 15 weeks of treatment, darbepoetin alfa at the dosage of 500 μg every 3 weeks was deemed noninferior in efficacy to once-weekly dosing in patients with nonmyeloid malignancies.[62] An exploratory analysis of this study showed that 74% of patients receiving darbepoetin alfa at 500 μg every 3 weeks had their dosages reduced to 300 μg every 3 weeks, mainly as a result of rapid increases in hemoglobin levels. These reports supported investigation of the efficacy of darbepoetin alfa at a lower dosage. Darbepoetin alfa was also effective at a dosage of 300 μg every 3 weeks in cancer patients with chemotherapy-induced anemia. In a large single-arm trial, 79% of patients receiving darbepoetin alfa at the dose of 300 μg every 3 weeks for 13 weeks achieved a hemoglobin target of ≥11 g/dL; 73% of these patients were able to maintain hemoglobin within the range of 11–13 g/dL.[66]

The most commonly experienced side effects with rEPO are hypertension, thrombosis, seizures, and pure red cell aplasia. Blood pressure should be controlled in patients before initiating therapy with rEPO drugs, and monitored regularly. Because seizures have been reported in chronic renal failure patients, their hemoglobin levels should be monitored regularly. Hemoglobin levels should be targeted to 11–12 g/dL to decrease the risk of thrombosis.

In the United States, the recommended starting regimen of subcutaneous darbepoetin alfa in cancer patients with anemia is 2.25 μg/kg once weekly. Alternatively, the drug may be administered at a dosage of 200 μg every 2 weeks or 500 μg every 3 weeks.[61] rEPO therapy should be considered in asymptomatic anemia with risk factors for appearance of symptoms and symptomatic anemia when hemoglobin levels are 9–11 g/dL.[61] The aim is to maintain a hemoglobin level of 11–12 g/dL. Patients should have iron studies conducted, because evidence suggests that patients with iron deficiency respond better to rEPO if started on iron supplementation.

White cell growth factors: granulocyte colony-stimulating factor and granulocyte-macrophage colony-stimulating factor.
Granulocyte colony-stimulating factor (G-CSF) is a nonglycosylated Escherichia coli-derived recombinant protein that specifically and selectively acts to stimulate neutrophil production.[69] G-CSF initially received FDA approval for the treatment of neutropenia associated with myelosuppressive chemotherapy drugs at a dose of 5 μg/kg per day.[70] It has a relatively short serum half-life of about 3.5 hours, so it must be administered daily. Since the original approval of G-CSF, there are a number of new indications. G-CSF is also indicated for chronic administration in patients with idiopathic neutropenia, congenital neutropenia, and cyclic neutropenia. It is also approved for patients with nonmyeloid malignancies who are undergoing nonmyeloablative chemotherapy followed by transplantation to reduce the duration of neutropenia. G-CSF has also received approval for the mobilization of hematopoetic progenitor cells in the peripheral blood for collection by leukapheresis. The recommended dosage is 10 μg/kg per day, to be started at least 4 days before the first leukapheresis and continued until leukapheresis is completed.[71]

Pegylated filgrastim (pegfilgrastim) was created by attaching a polyethylene glycol (PEG) molecule to the G-CSF protein at the N-terminal methionine residue.[72] Pegfilgrastim has the advantage of having a longer half-life ranging from 15 to 80 hours after subcutaneous injection. In the initial dose finding trials for pegfilgrastim, doses were weight-based: 30, 100, or 300 μg/kg given every 2 weeks, compared to daily filgrastim. A trial including 13 patients with non-small cell lung cancer found that after chemotherapy, median absolute neutrophil count (ANC) nadirs were similar in the filgrastim and pegfilgrastim 30 μg/kg cohorts.[73] The ANC nadirs were highest in the pegfilgrastim 100 and 300 μg/kg cohorts. These results indicated the clearance of pegfilgrastim was based on neutrophil receptor binding, and the serum clearance was directly related to the number of neutrophils. Since clearance was related to the patient's own hematopoetic recovery, pegfilgrastim was considered to have patient-specific pharmacokinetics. Pegfilgrastim was then studied to compare a single fixed dose of pegfilgrastim of 6 mg with a dose of filgrastim 5 μg/kg daily. A single fixed dose of pegfilgrastim was found to be comparable to multiple daily injections of filgrastim.[74] The dose regimen in the FDA-approved labeling for pegfilgrastim is a single 6 mg fixed dose per chemotherapy cycle to begin 24–72 hours following the end of chemotherapy.[75] Because of the long half-life of the drug, it is currently recommended that 14 days be allowed following pegfilgrastim dosing until the next chemotherapy cycle. Pegfilgrastim is not indicated for the mobilization of hematopoetic progenitor cells.

GM-CSF is derived from three different sources: yeast (Saccharomyces cerevisiae), bacteria (E coli), and mammalian cells (Chinese hamster ovary cells). GM-CSF has a broader activity than G-CSF. It acts to stimulate the production and activity of neutrophils, basophils, eosinophils, monocytes, and early erythroid and megakaryocytic progenitor cells.[76] The effects of GM-CSF on multiple cell lineages have led to research on immunomodulatory effects of GM-CSF. GM-CSF enhances macrophage chemotaxis and phagocytosis, and stimulates cytokine release from the monocytes that enhance the function of NK cells. GM-CSF has also been found to expand and activate dendritic cells and to increase their migration to lymph nodes, stimulate naïve T cells, and activate eosinophils.[77] GM-CSF is being investigated for various applications, including use as an antitumor vaccine.

GM-CSF has FDA approval for the acceleration of myeloid engraftment in patients undergoing autologous transplant for the treatment of acute lymphoblastic leukemia, non-Hodgkin's lymphoma (NHL), and Hodgkin's lymphoma. The recommended dose for GM-CSF is 250 μg/m² per day.

Neutropenia.
Neutropenia and its infectious complications often lead to morbidity and mortality in patients receiving chemotherapy. Signs and symptoms of infection in the neutropenic patient should be carefully assessed, as some common

signs of infection are often absent in the patient with low white blood levels. Febrile neutropenia (FN) can result in hospitalization for the evaluation and initiation of intravenous antibiotics, leading to reduced quality of life, increased hospitalization costs, and possible complications. Options for reducing the incidence of FN associated with chemotherapy include the use of CSFs, prophylactic antibiotics, and chemotherapy dose reduction or delay. The use of prophylactic antibiotics is limited because of the risk of promoting the growth of resistant organisms; CSFs and dose reduction of chemotherapy are the most frequently used options.

Based on review of medical literature, the American Society of Clinical Oncology (ASCO) has published clinical practice guidelines for the use of CSFs.[71] The guidelines for primary prophylaxis (i.e., white blood cell growth factor administered after the first cycle of chemotherapy before any occurrence of neutropenia) support the use of a CSF when the risk of FN for a specific chemotherapy regimen is about 20% or higher.[71] Primary prophylaxis use of CSF may be warranted in select patients with a high risk of chemotherapy-induced infectious complications associated with other patient- or disease-specific factors. Certain clinical factors predispose to increased complications from prolonged neutropenia: patient age >65 years, poor performance status, previous episodes of FN, extensive prior treatment including large radiation ports, administration of combined chemoradiotherapy, cytopenias due to bone marrow involvement by tumor, poor nutritional status, presence of open wounds or active infections, more advanced cancer, and other serious comorbidities.[75] In such situations, primary prophylaxis with CSF is appropriate even with regimens with FN rates less than 20%.

Secondary prophylaxis (i.e., white blood cell growth factor administered after subsequent cycles of chemotherapy to reduce the risk of FN after prior occurrence of FN) is recommended for patients for whom a reduction in chemotherapy dose (e.g., dose reduction or delay) may compromise disease-free, overall survival or treatment outcome.

Therapeutic use of CSFs (i.e., administering white blood cell growth factors to treat a patient with severe neutropenia or FN) should not be routine for patients with neutropenia who are afebrile. But CSFs should be considered for patients with fever and neutropenia who are at high risk for infection-associated complications or who have prognostic factors associated with complications that predict poor clinical outcomes.[71] High-risk features include expected prolonged (>10 days)

and profound neutropenia (ANC <0.1 × 10^9/L), uncontrolled primary disease, age >65 years, pneumonia, hypotension and multiorgan dysfunction (sepsis syndrome), invasive fungal infection, or hospitalization at the time of fever.

Dose density. There is an increasing focus on dose-dense chemotherapy for a variety of different tumor types. Dose intensity is defined as the chemotherapy dose per unit time over which the treatment is given. Data suggest a survival benefit from the use of dose-dense or dose-intensive regimens with CSF support in a few specific settings. Node-positive breast cancer data has shown that dose-dense chemotherapy is more effective than standard-dose chemotherapy in achieving disease-free and overall survival.[78] A trial including young patients with diffuse aggressive NHL compared the combination chemotherapy regimen CHOP (cyclophosphamide, doxorubicin, vincristine, and prednisone) given every 21 days to CHOP given every 14 days with CSF support, with or without etoposide.[79] The primary end point of the study was event-free survival. The addition of CSF to CHOP displayed a statistically significant improvement, while the addition of CSF to the etoposide arm showed no difference in event-free survival. Additional trials are still needed, although their results will not be able to be generalized to other disease settings or regimens. Another study with a similar trial design evaluated the impact of dose density in older patients with diffuse aggressive lymphoma. A greater benefit was seen with the cycle length reduction to 2 weeks from 3 weeks, facilitated by the addition of CSF (CHOP every 14 days), than with the standard CHOP every 21 days, with improvements in event-free survival and overall survival.[80] Further studies are needed to develop more data on dose density.

Acute myeloid leukemia (AML). For treatment of acute myeloid leukemia (AML), CSFs have been used after both induction (initial chemotherapy used to induce a complete response) and consolidation chemotherapy (chemotherapy given after the complete response is obtained as an attempt to eliminate any residual undetectable disease). Generally, primary prophylaxis post-CSF use has resulted in a decreased time to neutrophil recovery by 2–6 days, and shorter hospitalization and antibiotic use. No consistent effects on complete response rates or patient survival have been demonstrated, nor evidence of leukemia stimulation or enhanced drug resistance. There is debate on the economic benefit of CSFs in this setting. CSF use after initial induction therapy has not been shown to have a favorable impact on survival, remission rate, or survival. Patients older than 55 may be the most likely to benefit. Postconsolidation CSF (use of CSF after the consolidation therapy) has resulted in decreased duration of severe neutropenia with reduced infection rates but no effect on survival or complete response rates. Two large randomized trials have evaluated the role of G-CSF after completion of consolidation therapy.[81,83] Both demonstrated decreases in the duration of severe neutropenia, with elimination of severe neutropenia in a small portion of patients. A decreased rate of infection requiring antibiotic therapy was also seen. There was no effect on duration of complete response or overall survival. This indicates that CSF can be used after consolidation chemotherapy is completed.

Acute lymphoblastic leukemia (ALL). Data for CSFs in acute lymphoblastic leukemia (ALL) are variable in supporting the clinical benefits.[83,84] No improvements in disease-free survival or overall survival have been demonstrated. CSFs have not been able to show a consistent impact on the duration of hospitalization or the incidence of neutropenia in patients with ALL. A large randomized study of children with high-risk ALL who received intensive induction and consolidation therapy failed to show any differences in the duration of hospitalization, incidence of FN, or incidence of severe infection between patients receiving G-CSF and those not receiving CSF despite an improvement in the time to neutrophil recovery of 2.5 days.[85] Despite the variability in studies, CSFs are routinely used after the completion of the initial first few days of induction chemotherapy therapy or the first postremission therapy as recommended by the ASCO guidelines.[71]

Myelodysplastic syndrome. ASCO guidelines recommend that CSFs may be used in a subset of patients with severe neutropenia and recurrent infections,[71] although data supporting the long-term use of CSFs in these patients is lacking. GM-CSF has been evaluated in myelodysplastic syndrome (MDS) and was found to increase the numbers of circulating neutrophils, eosinophils, monocytes, and lymphocytes. It has only minimal effect in increasing platelet counts and does not appear to reduce platelet or red blood cell transfusion requirements. G-CSF has also been evaluated; it demonstrated the ability to increase the absolute neutrophil count in a majority of patients and increase the reticulocyte count in a smaller number of patients. Results of a long-term study (3–16 months) of G-CSF for treatment of MDS showed that 10 out of 11 patients had increases in leukocyte and absolute neutrophil counts.[86] Patients who maintained an absolute neutrophil count above 1,500 neutrophils/mm³ had a sig-

nificantly lower incidence of bacterial infections. Three patients progressed to acute leukemia while on maintenance G-CSF. It is difficult to determine if this was related to the G-CSF or was simply the natural history of the disease.

Stem cell transplantation. CSFs have been investigated for use in patients undergoing allogeneic or autologous transplantation. They can be used for mobilizing peripheral blood stem cells (PBSCs) into the circulation for autologous transplants and healthy-donor allogeneic PBSC transplants. Over the last decade, PBSC transplantation has almost completely replaced bone marrow transplantation (BMT) because it results in an earlier hematopoietic recovery.[87] The optimal timing and protocols for using CSF to facilitate mobilization of stem cells or white blood cell recovery after marrow transplantation remains under investigation. Both GM-CSF and G-CSF have been investigated for use in patients undergoing either autologous or allogeneic transplantation, and several articles have been published on the use of hematopoietic growth factors in stem cell transplantation.[88–91] Initial trials were relatively small, nonrandomized studies that compared the results to historical controls. Both GM-CSF and G-CSF were found to have a significant impact on neutrophil recovery after autologous transplantation.[92] A marked reduction in the median duration of neutropenia (days of ANC <500/mm³) was observed, and G-CSF was also found to reduce the duration of severe neutropenia (defined as days of ANC <200/mm³). No effect was observed on the nadir (ANC <100/mm³) or the initial period of agranulocytosis. This indicated that early marrow progenitor cells are not affected by recombinant GM- or G-CSF. The initial trials also demonstrated a reduction in the number of documented infection, febrile days, and days in the hospital.[93,94]

Pretreatment with GM or G-CSF has been shown to increase the number of hematopoetic stem cells circulating in the peripheral blood, which reduces the number of leukapheresis treatments needed. The use of GM- or G-CSF-mobilized PBSCs reduces the time to neutrophil recovery when compared to bone marrow as a stem cell source. The time to recover platelets to 20,000 platelets/mm³ was almost 2 weeks shorter with mobilized PBSCs than with infused bone marrow. A randomized trial evaluated G-CSF after autologous PBSC to determine whether G-CSF could further decrease time to neutrophil engraftment after stem cell transplantation.[95] Patients who received G-CSF were found to have a reduction in the median time to a neutrophil count >500 neutrophils/mm³ compared to the control group.

The G-CSF treatment group also demonstrated significant reductions in the median duration of posttransplant hospitalization and the median number of days on nonprophylactic antibiotics. Statistically insignificant differences were found in the time it took for platelet engraftment, number of febrile days, progression-free survival, and overall survival. It was determined that G-CSF could enhance the neutrophil recovery associated with PBSC transplantation.

PBSCs are also being used in allogeneic transplantation. Initially, there was concern that PBSCs (which contain about 10 times more T cells than bone marrow) would increase the incidence of graft-versus-host disease (GVHD). In a pilot study evaluating the use of G-CSF-mobilized PBSCs for allogeneic transplantation,[96] eight patients with hematologic malignancies received unmodified PBSCs from HLA-identical siblings. The donors received G-CSF 16 μg/kg per day subcutaneously for the 5 days preceding PBSC collection; it was well tolerated by all donors. All the patients had engraftment of the stem cells; 7 of the 8 had a rapid neutrophil recovery (500 neutrophils/mm^3) before day 18 and a platelet recovery to 20,000 platelets/mm^3 by day 12 posttransplant. The incidence of acute GVHD was similar to that seen with allogeneic BMT; two patients experienced grade 2 acute GVHD, and another patient progressed to grade 3 GVHD.

A trial was done to evaluate the optimal dose of G-CSF to be given to donors. Three different cohorts were divided according to dosage: 3 μg/kg/day, 6 μg/kg/day, and 10 μg/kg/day administered daily for a maximum of 10 days, with leukapheresis starting on day 6.[97] All CD34$^+$ cells collected in the 10 μg/kg/day cohort on the sixth day were sufficient for allogeneic transplantation. Further studies are needed to evaluate whether the cells collected with this regimen produce rapid and sustained engraftment in the allogeneic recipients.

GM-CSF has also been used to stimulate hematopoeisis in patients with marrow graft failure after BMT. Marrow graft failure is defined as either a failure to reach 100 neutrophils/mm^3 by day 28 after transplant or a drop in neutrophils to <500 neutrophils/mm^3 for longer than 7 days after initial engraftment. In one trial, patients with marrow failure after autologous, allogeneic, or syngeneic BMT were pretreated with GM-CSF doses of 60 to 1000 μg/m^2 per day.[98] Fifty-seven percent (21 of 37) of the patients obtained an absolute neutrophil count of 500 neutrophils/mm^3 or more within 2 weeks after starting treatment. Survival at 100 days was 59% in patients treated with GM-CSF, compared with 32% in historic

controls, and survival at 1 year was 50% and 23%, respectively. None of the patients who received chemically purged bone marrow responded to the GM-CSF, whereas all patients who received non-purged bone marrow or bone marrow purged with monoclonal antibodies responded to treatment with GM-CSF. Another trial treated 140 patients with graft failure with GM-CSF 250 μg/m^2 per day for 15 days. Survival at 100 days for allogeneic BMT patients was 50% in the GM-CSF group and 28% in the historical control group. In autologous BMT patients, survival to day 100 was 72% in the GM-CSF group, compared with 59% for historical controls.

Colony-stimulating factors in older patients. As the population of older individuals with cancer increases, aging is one of the indications for which prophylactic growth factors are used regardless of the threshold risk for neutropenia. Many studies performed in breast cancer have found the risk of neutropenia following chemotherapy increases with age.[99-101] The threshold, which varies with different studies, has been ages over 60, 65, and 70.[100,101] This has also been shown in older patients with lymphoma.[102] In a retrospective study within community practice, the incidence of neutropenic fever was 34% in patients over 65 years and 21% for those younger; most of the episodes of FN occurred after the first course of treatment.[103] The average hospitalization was longer for the group of older patients in this study.

The benefits of CSFs have been shown when drug is administered 24–72 hours after chemotherapy. In the setting of high-dose therapy and autologous stem-cell rescue, the CSFs can be given between 24 and 120 hours after the administration of the high-dose therapy. Pegfilgrastim should not be administered in the period from 14 days before and 24 hours after administration of cytotoxic chemotherapy.

Monoclonal Antibodies as Cancer Therapy

Until recently, cancer treatment has primarily consisted of nonspecific and highly toxic chemotherapeutic agents. The consequence of cytotoxic chemotherapy is damage to cancer cells along with collateral damage to normal, rapidly proliferating tissues, such as mucosa, bone marrow, and hair. Clearly there was a need to develop more targeted, less toxic agents. With the approval of rituximab in 1997, monoclonal antibodies (mAbs) have begun to meet this demand. The success and rapidly expanding investigation into new antibody treatments for cancer has come after decades of work. Early disappointment resulted from using fully murine antibodies; these caused allergic reactions, showed inefficient host effector response, and lacked specific antigen targets. Patients developed neutralizing human antimurine antibodies (HAMA), which limited their ability to receive multiple doses, and shortened the circulating half-life of the antibody. Today these problems have been largely overcome by the use of chimeric (human/murine) and humanized antibodies. About two thirds of the chimeric molecule is from a human gene sequence; a humanized antibody contains about 95% human protein (**Figure 11.6**). Fully human mAbs are in development, and should offer the lowest risk for hypersensitivity reactions. Please refer to Chapter 2 for a review of monoclonal antibody structure and synthesis.

All currently approved mAbs for cancer treatment use the IgG backbone, and most use the specific subtype IgG1, the most potent activator of complement and immune effector cells. The average size of oncologic antibodies is 150 kD; this is much larger than the 1-kD size of most chemotherapeutic agents. This large size is a disadvantage, making it difficult for mAbs to distribute to, and penetrate, solid tumors.[104] But because these macromolecules exceed the renal threshold, they avoid first-pass renal clearance, prolonging half-life. Smaller antibody fragments can be used to improve tumor distribution, but they typically undergo first-pass renal clearance and more rapid elimination.

Chapter 3 provides an in-depth review of guidelines established by the U.S. Adopted Names (USAN) Council for naming mAbs.[105] **Table 11.3** summarizes nomenclature specific to oncologic mAbs.

The utility of mAbs in cancer treatment depends to a large extent on the targeted tumor antigen. As discussed earlier in this chapter, tumor-specific antigens make ideal targets for mAb

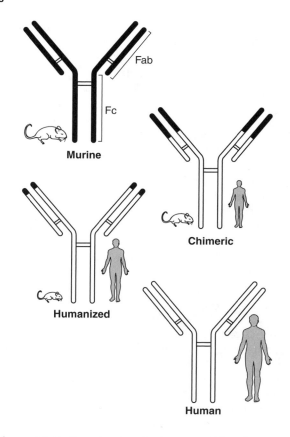

Figure 11.6. Monoclonal antibody source. Fab = fragment-antibody binding; Fc = fragment-crystalline.

therapy because the cytotoxic effects are focused on tumor cells. Effects of therapy directed at tumor-associated antigens spill over to antigen-expressing normal tissues. Unfortunately, the identification of tumor-specific antigens is rarely accomplished. Another quality of target antigens is their propensity to internalize, once bound by the therapeutic antibody. For mAbs that depend on complement-dependent cytotoxicity (CDC) or antibody-dependent cellular cytotoxicity (ADCC), internalization prevents binding of complement and effector cells. Finally, antigens that shed from tumor cell surfaces are problematic because the mAb becomes saturated with free antigens and cannot bind tumor targets.

Therapeutic mAbs with oncology application can employ unconjugated ("naked") molecules, or they can be joined or conjugated with various toxins, radionuclides, enzymes, or other compounds to form immunoconjugates. The antibody in this case provides a vehicle for carrying cytotoxic therapy to specific tumor targets. Currently there are eight mAbs approved for cancer treatment (**Table 11.4**). Five of them are unconjugated antibodies, one is toxin-conjugated, and two are radiolabeled. A discussion of these agents follows.

Table 11.3. Nomenclature of Monoclonal Antibodies in Cancer Treatment

mAb Source	Identifier	Tumor Type/ Target	Identifier
human	u	colon	-col-
mouse	o	melanoma	-mel-
rat	a	mammary	-mar-
humanized	zu	testis	-got-
hamster	e	ovary	-gov-
primate	i	prostate	-pr(o)-
chimera	xi	miscellaneous	-tum-
		cardiovascular	-cir-

Bevacizumab is a humanized mAb with cardiovascular target.

Table 11.4. Monoclonal Antibodies in Cancer Treatment

Year Approved	Name	Antibody Source	Antibody Structure	Target	FDA-Approved Indication
1997	rituximab (Rituxan®)	chimeric (human/mouse)	unconjugated	CD20	low-grade NHL
1998	trastuzumab (Herceptin®)	humanized	unconjugated	HER2	HER2 overexpressing MBC
2000	gemtuzumab ozogamicin (Mylotarg®)	humanized	toxin conjugated	CD33	AML
2001	alemtuzumab (Campath®)	humanized	unconjugated	CD52	CLL
2002	yttrium-90 ibritumomab tiuxetan (Zevalin®)	murine	radiolabeled	CD20	low-grade NHL
2003	iodine-131 tositumomab (Bexxar®)	murine	radiolabeled	CD20	low-grade NHL
2004	bevacizumab (Avastin®)	humanized	unconjugated	VEGF	metastatic CRC
2004	cetuximab (Erbitux®)	chimeric (human/mouse)	unconjugated	EGFR1	metastatic CRC

NHL = non-Hodgkin's lymphoma; HER2 = human epidermal growth factor receptor 2; MBC = metastatic breast cancer; AML = acute myeloid leukemia; CLL = chronic lymphocytic leukemia; VEGF = vascular endothelial growth factor; CRC = colorectal cancer; EGFR1 = epidermal growth factor receptor 1.

Rituximab. In 1997, rituximab became the first mAb approved by the FDA for cancer treatment. It is a chimeric IgG1 mAb directed against the CD20 antigen, which is present on the cell surface of 90% of normal and neoplastic B lymphocytes.[106] The transmembrane protein CD20 is thought to be involved in cell-cycle initiation and differentiation, and may also function as a calcium channel.[107,108] CD20 is an attractive target because it is not shed into the blood, nor does it internalize or change conformation upon antibody binding.[109] Furthermore, CD20 is not found on progenitor stem cells, normal plasma cells, or nonhematopoietic cell lines.[106] Although the in vivo effects are not well understood, rituximab has been shown to effect cell death by at least three different mechanisms: ADCC, CDC, and induction of apoptosis. In the process of ADCC, the Fab portion of rituximab binds to CD20 on target B cells, and the Fc domain binds Fcγ receptors (FCγR) on effector cells (NK cells and macrophages). When this complex is complete, effector cells become activated, resulting in B-cell lysis (**Figure 11.7**). Evidence for ADCC comes from studies showing failure to deplete B cells with use of anti-CD20 mAbs with inefficient Fc effector binding, and by using synthesized antibody fragments that lack Fc domains.[110] Further clinical evidence comes from data that show a correlation between Fc receptor subtype and therapeutic success with rituximab in patients with NHL.[111-113] Since the IgG1 subclass is known to be extremely efficient at fixing complement, CDC

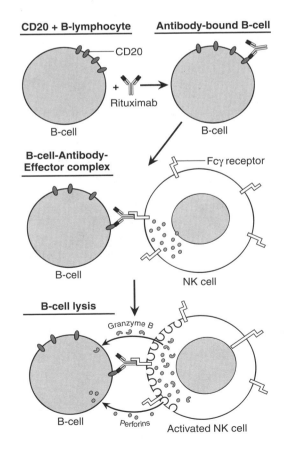

Figure 11.7. Rituximab-induced antibody-dependent cellular cytotoxicity (ADCC).

has also been demonstrated (see Complement-Dependent Cytotoxicity in Chapter 2).[114] Finally, there is in vitro evidence that rituximab binding to CD20 induces apoptosis.[115–118]

Rituximab clinical trials. Non-Hodgkin's lymphomas (NHLs) comprise a broad spectrum of diseases of the lymph node. The Working Formulation, developed in the 1980s, is one of the most commonly used classification systems for NHL today.[119] Accordingly, three grades of lymphoma are designated based on morphologic lymph node features: low-, intermediate-, and high-grade. Intermediate- and high-grade are considered aggressive, rapidly fatal lymphomas; low-grade predicts a less aggressive, indolent disease course. Ironically, low-grade lymphomas are generally incurable, whereas intermediate- and high-grade lymphomas are curable.

In a pivotal phase III trial of 166 patients with relapsed low-grade or follicular NHL, rituximab dosed at 375 mg/m² weekly x 4 weeks resulted in a 48% overall response rate (ORR) with 6% complete responses and a median time to progression of 13.2 months.[120] Results from this trial led to the approval of rituximab, and its utility in various settings of NHL has been extensively studied. With the more difficult to treat "bulky" NHL (tumor >10 cm), rituximab showed efficacy, but response rates were lower than those with nonbulky disease. The question of repeat dosing with disease relapse has also been addressed, and rituximab has proven safe and effective. Next, the combination of rituximab with CHOP chemotherapy was assessed in two phase II trials, and shown to enhance efficacy in patients with indolent and aggressive NHL.[121,122] Finally, the utility of rituximab combined with chemotherapy (R-CHOP) compared to chemotherapy alone (CHOP) as first-line therapy, was studied in 398 elderly patients with diffuse large B-cell lymphoma. An interim analysis showed statistical superiority of the combination arm versus chemotherapy alone in complete response rate (76% versus 63%), 24-month event-free survival (57% versus 39%), and 24-month overall survival (70% versus 57%), respectively.[123]

Safety of rituximab. In the pivotal trial, most adverse events were components of an infusion-related complex, typically occurring within the first few hours after starting the first rituximab infusion. These primarily consisted of fever (43%), chills/rigors (28%), nausea (18%), asthenia (13%), headache (14%), and hypotension (10%).[120] In most cases, events were short lived and responded to infusion interruption and careful rate titration. Diphenhydramine and acetaminophen pretreatment may prevent or lessen the severity of infusion reactions. The

manufacturer also recommends considering withholding antihypertensives, starting 12 hours before administration of rituximab, to reduce the risk for hypotension. After the first dose, 55% of patients completed therapy without further adverse events. Less frequent adverse effects include bone marrow toxicity, with leukopenia (7%), neutropenia (4%), thrombocytopenia (3%), and anemia (1%) reported; mostly grades 1 and 2. Severe, and sometimes fatal, infusion reactions, tumor lysis syndrome (TLS), and mucocutaneous reactions are life-threatening adverse effects reported rarely; they appear as black box warnings in product labeling.[124] Patients with large numbers of circulating lymphoma cells are at higher risk for infusion reactions and TLS. Underlying pulmonary and/or cardiac disease increase the risk for severe infusion reactions.

Rituximab is indicated for the treatment of relapsed or refractory low-grade or follicular, CD20⁺, B-cell NHL. It has recently received approval as either a 4-dose or an 8-dose weekly regimen, to be used in patients who have previously responded to rituximab and in patients who have bulky tumors.

Trastuzumab. Human epidermal growth factor receptor 2 (HER2) is one of four identified transmembrane tyrosine kinase receptors (**Figure 11.8**). Amplification of the oncogene *HER2* (also known as *HER2/neu* or *c-erbB-2*) results in overexpression of HER2 cell-surface receptors up to 100-fold.[125] HER2 overexpression is observed in about 25% to 30% of women diagnosed with breast cancer. It conveys a negative prognostic factor associated with aggressive, rapidly growing, and metastasizing tumors; negative hormone receptor status; relative chemotherapy insensitivity; and inferior survival.[126] Although there is no known ligand for HER2, it is known to dimerize with other

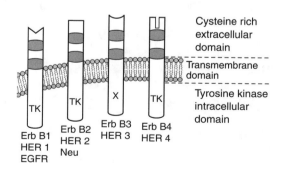

Figure 11.8. Four human epidermal growth factor receptor tyrosine kinases have been identified in epithelium and a variety of other tissues. They are composed of three basic domains: two cysteine-rich extracellular clusters, a hydrophobic transmembrane portion, and an intracellular tyrosine kinase (TK) component. ErbB3 lacks tyrosine kinase activity (X).

HER family receptors (HER1, HER3, and HER4) to form heterodimers (**Figure 11.9**).[127] Dimerization leads to tyrosine kinase activation, intracellular signal propagation, and ultimately cell growth and differentiation.[128]

Trastuzumab (Herceptin) is a humanized IgG1 monoclonal antibody developed to target HER2-overexpressing breast cancer. In vitro studies have shown that binding of trastuzumab to overexpressed HER2 receptors leads to ADCC,[129] CDC,[130] and down-regulation of HER2 from tumor cell surfaces.[131] Restoration of the adhesion molecules E-cadherin and α2 integrin has also been demonstrated, which may prevent metastatic progression.[132] In addition, cell cycle interruption has been shown as a consequence of induction of the tumor suppressors *p27KIP1* and *p130*.[132] Finally, trastuzumab may inhibit angiogenesis through decreased vascular endothelial growth factor production.[133]

Women most likely to benefit from trastuzumab are those with *HER2* gene amplification, as determined by fluorescence in-situ hybridization

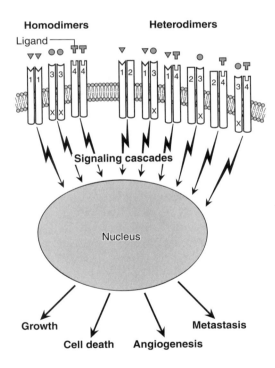

Figure 11.9. Ligand binding leads to HER dimerization and subsequent activation of the intracellular tyrosine kinase domain. Autophosphorylation of the tyrosine moiety follows with a cascade of signaling pathways from the cytoplasm to the nucleus. The end result is a wide range of possibilities including cell division, motility, angiogenesis, and cell death. Note that HER2 does not have an identified ligand and does not homodimerize in response to known ligands. HER3 relies on adjacent kinases for activation since it lacks tyrosine kinase activity (X).

(FISH) or 3+ overexpression of HER2 protein, as determined by immunohistochemistry (IHC). Current treatment guidelines recommend HER2 testing in all patients with invasive breast cancer.[134]

In a large multinational open-label trial, trastuzumab was administered to 222 women with HER2-overexpressing metastatic breast cancer (MBC).[135] All patients had disease progression following at least one prior chemotherapy regimen. Trastuzumab was dosed at 4 mg/kg loading dose, followed by weekly doses of 2 mg/kg. The overall response rate was 15% (4% complete recovery) with a median response duration of 9.1 months. Based on this trial, trastuzumab was approved for second-line, single-agent treatment of patients with MBC whose tumors overexpress HER2 protein.

Trastuzumab has been evaluated in combination with several cytotoxic chemotherapeutic agents. In a large pivotal trial, trastuzumab plus chemotherapy was compared to chemotherapy alone in first-line treatment for MBC.[136] A total of 469 patients were randomized to 1 of 4 treatment arms, depending on their prior anthracycline exposure (e.g., as part of their adjuvant therapy). Those with prior exposure were randomized to paclitaxel plus or minus trastuzumab. Patients without prior anthracycline exposure were randomized to doxorubicin or epirubicin plus cyclophosphamide (AC or EC), plus or minus trastuzumab. Chemotherapy was given once every 3 weeks for at least 6 cycles, and trastuzumab was given weekly until disease progression. Women assigned to chemotherapy-alone arms were allowed to receive trastuzumab upon disease progression as part of a separate extension study. Response rates, response duration, and survival all favored the trastuzumab arms over chemotherapy-alone arms. Consequently, trastuzumab was approved as first-line therapy in combination with paclitaxel for treatment of patients with HER2 overexpressing MBC and who have not yet received chemotherapy.

Four large phase III trials have been conducted to assess the utility of trastuzumab in the adjuvant setting for patients with HER2-overexpressing early breast cancer. The Herceptin Adjuvant (HERA) trial enrolled more than 5000 patients with HER2-overexpressing tumors of ≥1 cm.[137] After receiving approved neoadjuvant or adjuvant chemotherapy, patients were randomized to one of three groups: trastuzumab once every 3 weeks for 1 year (group A), trastuzumab once every 3 weeks for 2 years (group B), or observation only (group C). An interim analysis at 2 years showed a statistically significant improvement in disease-free survival for group A versus group C (85.8% versus 77.4%). The benefit of 2 years of adjuvant trastuzumab (group B) is not known at the time of this writing. The other three trials were designed to assess the benefit of trastuzumab given concurrently with, or following, adjuvant chemotherapy. The combined results of two of these trials (The National Surgical Adjuvant Breast and Bowel Project trial B-31 and The North Central Cancer Treatment Group trial N9831) showed an absolute difference in disease-free survival of 12% at a median follow-up of 2 years.[138] The Breast Cancer International Research Group (BCIRG) trial is the fourth phase III study of adjuvant trastuzumab in early breast cancer.[139] Interim results of BCIRG have not been published at the time of this writing.

Trastuzumab is generally well tolerated, with mild to moderate infusion reactions (fever and chills) occurring in 40% of patients during the initial infusion. This reaction responds to treatment with acetaminophen and or meperidine. More severe infusion reactions (including anaphylaxis) and pulmonary events are also reported, and fatalities have occurred. Nausea, vomiting, and pain (sometimes at the tumor site) occur infrequently. The incidence of bone marrow suppression, including grade 3 and 4 neutropenia and infection, is noted to be higher in patients receiving trastuzumab in combination with chemotherapy.

Cardiac toxicity was observed in trastuzumab clinical trials, both alone and in combination with chemotherapy. In the combination chemotherapy pivotal trial, cardiac dysfunction was observed in 7% of patients randomized to trastuzumab monotherapy.[140] New York Heart Association (NYHA) class III to IV heart failure accounted for 5% of these cases. A dramatic increase in the incidence of cardiac dysfunction was observed in the group randomized to trastuzumab plus anthracycline and cyclophosphamide; where the overall incidence of cardiac dysfunction was 25%, 19% was NHYA class III to IV. So the use of trastuzumab in combination with anthracyclines is not currently recommended. Routine baseline and periodic left ventricular function and symptom monitoring is recommended for patients undergoing trastuzumab therapy.[141] Most patients who develop trastuzumab-associated heart failure respond well to treatment and can continue the antibody.

Alemtuzumab. Chronic lymphocytic leukemia (CLL) is the most common adult leukemia, accounting for one third of all leukemias. B-lymphocyte abnormalities occur in 95% of all CLL cases. Treatment is normally reserved for late-stage, or symptomatic early-stage, disease, and consists of oral alkylators with or without prednisone and purine analogs (cladribine or fludarabine). Combination chemotherapy may be used for pal-

liation of late-stage (III to IV) disease. Antibody therapy includes rituximab, which can be used alone or in combination with chemotherapy, and alemtuzumab.

Alemtuzumab, or Campath-1H, is a humanized murine (rat) IgG1 antibody that binds CD52, an antigen found on the cell surface of virtually all B and T lymphocytes and most monocytes, macrophages, and NK cells. CD52 is found to a lesser extent on granulocytes and cells of the male genital tract, and is not expressed on erythrocytes or hematopoietic stem cells. Upon binding to CD52, alemtuzumab is proposed to cause cell death by three different mechanisms: ADCC, CDC, and apoptosis.[142,143]

The development of alemtuzumab typifies the challenges for development of safe and effective antibody therapy for cancer.[144] Originally developed as Campath-1M, this purely murine IgM antibody was very effective in preventing GVHD by in vitro purging of T cells from donor bone marrow.[145] In vivo use in combating hematologic malignancy was less rewarding, and the molecule underwent two subsequent changes. First, the antibody was changed to a murine IgG2b isotype, which had the ability to activate human Fc-receptors and broaden cytotoxicity to include ADCC. The second involved changing to a humanized antibody, which overcame problems with the development of HAMA and allowed for repeat dosing. The current antibody, Campath-1H, has been used in B-chronic lymphocytic leukemia (B-CLL), T-prolymphocytic leukemia, and low-grade NHL. It also shows promise in treating patients with refractory autoimmune cytopenias.[146]

In 2001, after over two decades in development, alemtuzumab received accelerated approval for third-line treatment of B-CLL in patients who have failed alkylators and fludarabine. Approval was based on results of three multicenter, open label, noncomparative studies involving 149 patients with B-CLL.[147-149] The largest trial enrolled 93 patients who were refractory to both alkylators and fludarabine. Alemtuzumab was slowly titrated up to 30 mg given intravenously 3 times weekly for up to 12 weeks.[147] Overall response rate was 33%, with 31% partial and 2% complete responses. An additional 59% of patients experienced disease stabilization. Median time to response was 1.5 months, and median duration of response was 8.7 months. Overall, 42 of 93 patients survived more than 18 months, with 68% of responders alive at the end of the study (35 months). Of those patients who presented with B symptoms (night sweats, chills, and weight loss) or fatigue, 52.5% experienced resolution of symptoms. Hepatomegaly completely resolved in 52% of patients, and another

23% of patients had at least a 50% reduction in size. Splenomegaly resolved in 54% of patients, and another 28% showed at least a 50% reduction in size. Lymphadenopathy resolved completely in 27% of patients, and at least a 50% reduction in node size was reported in another 47%. Treatment failure was directly correlated with lymph node size; no complete responses were noted in patients with lymph nodes >5 cm. In those who presented with cytopenias, neutropenia improved in 50%, thrombocytopenia improved in 39%, and anemia improved in 44% of patients following alemtuzumab treatment.

Infusion-related toxicity was reported by most patients in the above clinical trials; most were grade 1 or 2 in severity. Rigors, fever, nausea, vomiting, and rash were all components of the infusion reaction occurring in the first week, with a decrease in incidence and severity upon continued treatment. Careful dosage escalation and pretreatment with diphenhydramine and acetaminophen is recommended for preventing or blunting infusion reactions.[150]

Bone marrow suppression following alemtuzumab is profound. In clinical trials, the incidence of grade 3 or 4 neutropenia, thrombocytopenia, and anemia were reported at 70%, 52%, and 47%, respectively.[150] Median time to neutrophil recovery was 28 days; platelet recovery was 21 days. Grade 4 lymphopenia was universal with median CD4$^+$ count of 2 cells/μL 4 weeks into alemtuzumab treatment. Median CD4$^+$ count was 207 cells/μL at 2 months and 470 cells/μL at 6 months post treatment. CD8$^+$ lymphocyte counts fluctuated in a pattern similar to that of CD4$^+$ cells.

Infectious complications are the most significant adverse event associated with alemtuzumab use. The manufacturer recommends prophylaxis with trimethoprim–sulfamethoxazole and famciclovir at initiation of alemtuzumab and for 2 months after completion, or until CD4$^+$ count is $\geq$200 cell/μL, whichever occurs later. In the study by Keating et al., mild to moderate infections occurred in 28% of patients, and severe infections occurred in 27% of patients during the 3-month treatment period.[147] Septicemia occurred in 15% of patients with two patient deaths. Opportunistic infections developed in 19% of patients during the study and the 6-month follow-up period. Infections included *Pneumocystis carinii* pneumonia, *Aspergillus* pneumonia, rhinocerebral mucormycosis, systemic candidiasis, cryptococcal pneumonia, herpes zoster, pulmonary aspergillosis, invasive aspergillosis, and Listeria meningitis. Cytomegalovirus (7.5%) and herpes simplex (6.5%) reactivation and superficial moniliasis (10%) were noted

during the study period. Five deaths due to infection were noted during and up to 1 month after treatment and an additional six infection-related deaths occurred in the next 5 months.

In summary, alemtuzumab immunotherapy provides a treatment option for patients with refractory B-CLL. Hematologic and symptomatic improvement is seen, even in patients who have failed several prior chemotherapy treatments. Infusion reactions and infectious morbidity complicate the routine use of this agent. In an effort to improve efficacy and lessen toxicity, several small studies have shown promising results when using alemtuzumab administered subcutaneously and as first-line treatment of B-CLL.[151,152]

Bevacizumab. Angiogenesis or neovascularization is the process of creating new blood vessels. Normal body growth and repair is dependent on timely initiation and cessation of angiogenesis. To the growing fetus, new vasculature is needed to supply nutrients to developing tissue. Likewise, wound healing demands neovascularization for proper recovery. The process of angiogenesis is controlled by a balance between molecules that promote and molecules that inhibit angiogenesis.[153] Unregulated angiogenesis occurs in certain pathologic conditions, including diabetic retinopathy, macular degeneration, arthritis, psoriasis, and cancer.[154] Uncontrolled angiogenesis results in increased, tortuous, leaky microvessels and allows tumors to grow and spread or metastasize.[154]

Vascular endothelial growth factor (VEGF) is a potent stimulus for angiogenesis; it is overexpressed in most solid tumors and is associated with aggressive tumor growth and poor prognosis.[155] Since the discovery of VEGF-A in the late 1970s, five other VEGF family members have been identified.[156] Likewise, four different VEGF cell-surface receptors have been identified. Several excellent review articles have been published on this topic.[157-159] Most angiogenic activity is mediated by VEGF-A. Originally named vascular permeability factor (VPF), VEGF-A causes a profound increase in vascular permeability, leading to protein leakage and fibrin gel formation. This fibrin gel anchors endothelial cells and forms the foundation for new blood vessels. VEGF also provides protection for immature blood vessels by upregulating the anti-apoptotic Bcl-2 and A1 proteins in endothelial cells.[160]

Bevacizumab is a humanized IgG1 monoclonal antibody that binds VEGF-A and prevents the interaction between the VEGF-A ligand and its endothelial cell surface receptors, VEGFR-1 (Flt-1) and VEGFR-2 (KDR/Flk-1).[161] In colorectal cancer, this results in blockade of endothelial mitosis, decreased vascular permeability, and halted angiogenesis.[162] Encouraged by the demonstration of efficacy in preclinical animal models and safety in two phase I studies, investigators evaluated bevacizumab in a randomized phase II trial comparing bevacizumab plus fluorouracil (FU)/leucovorin (LV) with FU/LV alone in patients with metastatic colorectal cancer.[163] In this trial of first-line therapy, patients were randomized to one of three treatment arms: FU/LV alone, FU/LV plus bevacizumab 5 mg/kg every 2 weeks (low dose), and FU/LV plus bevacizumab 10 mg/kg every 2 weeks (high dose). Response rates, time to disease progression, and median survival time all favored the bevacizumab arms. This trial led to two concurrent phase III studies of first-line therapy and a third phase III study of second-line bevacuzumab in metastatic colorectal cancer (**Table 11.5**).

Hurwitz et al.[164] randomly assigned 815 patients to one of two treatment arms: irinotecan, fluorouracil, and leucovorin (IFL) alone or IFL plus bevacizumab. The addition of bevacizumab improved response rates and time to disease progression, and it increased median survival by 4.7 months. In a study by Kabbinavar and colleagues, 209 patients with metastatic colorectal cancer were allocated to FU/LV alone or in combination with bevacizumab.[165] These patients were poor candidates for first-line irinotecan because of performance status or age. Results of this trial showed a trend toward increased response rate and time to progression and a statistically and clinically significant 3.7-month increase in median survival with the addition of bevacizumab to FU/LV. The combination of bevacizumab and oxaliplatin-based chemotherapy was studied in 828 patients with advanced colorectal cancer who had failed first-line treatment with fluorouracil-based chemotherapy and irinotecan.[166] Patients were randomized to one of three treatment arms: bevacizumab alone, FU/LV/oxaliplatin (FOLFOX4) alone, or bevacizumab plus FOLFOX4. Randomization to the single-agent bevacizumab arm was stopped early because of suspected inferiority. A 17% improvement in median overall survival was reported in patients randomized to the bevacizumab/FOLFOX4 arm. During clinical trials of bevacizumab combined with chemotherapy, overlapping toxicities were minimal. The most common adverse effects with bevacizumab were asthenia, pain, abdominal pain, hypertension, headache, diarrhea, nausea, vomiting, stomatitis, anorexia, constipation, upper respiratory infection, epistaxis, dyspnea, exfoliative dermatitis, and proteinuria.[161] Infusion reactions were infrequent, with an incidence of less than 3%. Serious, and sometimes fatal, adverse events associated with bevacizumab included gastrointestinal perforation, wound dehiscence, and hemorrhage; all are boxed warnings in product labeling. Arterial thromboembolic events, hypertensive crisis, proteinuria/nephrotic syndrome, and congestive heart failure were also reported.

In February 2004, bevacizumab was approved by the FDA for use (in combination with intravenous 5-fluorouracil-based chemotherapy) for first-line therapy in patients with metastatic colorectal cancer. The use of bevacizumab in combination with paclitaxel has been recently reported with good results in patients with metastatic breast cancer and will likely lead to an expanded indication.[167] Clinical trials of bevacizumab in combination with other agents, and several other tumor types, are currently under way.

Table 11.5. Trials of Bevacizumab in Metastatic Colorectal Cancer

Study	Protocol	RR	TTP (mo)	Survival (mo)	(P Value)
Kabbinavar et al.[163]	FU/LV	17%	5.2	13.8	–
	FU/LV + BEV 5 mg/kg	40%	9	21.5	(0.137)
	FU/LV + BEV 10 mg/kg	24%	7.2	16.1	(0.582)
Hurwitz et al.[162]	IFL	34.8%	6.2	15.6	–
	IFL + BEV	44.8%	10.6	20.3	(<0.001)
Kabbinavar et al.[163]	FU/LV	15%	5.5	12.9	–
	FU/LV + BEV	26%	9.2	16.6	(0.16)
Giantonio et al.[164]*	FOLFOX4	NR	NR	10.7	–
	FOLFOX4 + BEV	NR	NR	12.5	(0.0024)

RR = response rate; TTP = time to progression; FU/LV = fluorouracil/leucovorin; BEV = bevacizumab; IFL = irinotecan, fluorouracil, and leucovorin; FOLFOX4 = folinic acid, fluorouracil, and oxaliplatin; NR = not reported.
* Second-line treatment.

Cetuximab. Epidermal growth factor receptor (EGFR), also known as HER1, is a member of the HER tyrosine kinase growth factor receptor family (Figure 11.9). It is a 170,000-kDa glycoprotein composed of an extracellular ligand-binding region, a transmembrane portion, and an intracellular tyrosine kinase domain.[168] Overexpression of EGFR by up-regulation of the proto-oncogene c-*erb*-B is known to occur in many solid tumors, including 60% to 80% of colorectal cancer cases.[169] Epidermal growth factor and transforming growth factor α (TGF-α) are two known ligands for EGFR; upon binding, EGFR forms homodimers or heterodimers with other HER family members (Figure 11.9). Dimerization leads to activation and autophosphorylation of the intracellular tyrosine kinase. The final result is signal propagation leading to cell growth and survival.

Cetuximab (C225) is a recombinant, chimeric IgG1 monoclonal antibody that binds the extracellular domain of EGFR. The Fv regions on the molecule are murine with human IgG1 heavy- and kappa light-chain constant regions. In preclinical studies, cetuximab has been shown to effectively block epidermal growth factor and TGF-α binding at EGFR receptors, leading to growth inhibition of tumor cell lines expressing high levels of EGFR.[170,171] While most of the preclinical data established cetuximab as a cytostatic agent, studies combining the drug with various chemotherapeutic agents demonstrated synergy and marked tumor response. In a study of irinotecan-resistant human tumor xenografts, cetuximab plus irinotecan showed good synergistic activity, but neither of these agents alone halted tumor growth.[172]

With this background, a phase II study was conducted in 121 patients with colorectal cancer refractory to fluorouracil and irinotecan, whose tumors tested positive for EGFR by immunohistochemistry.[173] In this noncomparative study, patients received a cetuximab 400 mg/m^2 intravenous (IV) loading dose followed by 250 mg/m^2 IV weekly, plus irinotecan at the patient's previous dosage. The overall response rate was 17% (all partial responses), while an additional 31% of patients had either a minor response or disease stabilization. In a phase II follow-up study, the same investigators sought to determine whether the results of the previous study were due to cetuximab alone.[174] Fifty-seven similar patients with EGFR-expressing metastatic colorectal cancer were given cetuximab as single-agent therapy at the same dosage and schedule. In the final analysis, six patients (10.5%) obtained a partial response and an additional 20 patients (35%) had either a minor response or disease stabilization. Finally, in

a larger comparative trial, 329 patients with irinotecan-refractory advanced colorectal cancer were randomized to either cetuximab plus irinotecan or cetuximab alone.[175] The results were similar to the two earlier trials with a response rate of 22.9% in the combination-therapy arm and 10.8% in the cetuximab-alone arm. Median time to progression and median survival time favored the combination-therapy arm (4.1 versus 1.5 months and 6.9 versus 8.6 months, respectively).

Based on these data, cetuximab received FDA approval in February 2004 for use in combination with irinotecan for treatment of patients with EGFR-expressing, metastatic colorectal cancer that is refractory to irinotecan-based chemotherapy. It was also approved as single-agent treatment of EGFR-expressing, metastatic colorectal cancer in patients who cannot tolerate irinotecan-based chemotherapy. Although patients enrolled in clinical trials were required to have immunohistochemical evidence of EGFR expression, there was no correlation with positive cells or the intensity of expression with the response rate. This raises the question of whether other targets are involved and whether overexpression of EGFR should actually be a requirement for cetuximab treatment of colorectal cancer.

In March 2006, cetuximab was granted FDA approval for first-line treatment of locally advanced squamous cell carcinoma (SCC) of the head and neck. Cetuximab was also approved for treatment of recurrent SCC of the head and neck. Approval for first-line therapy was based on a phase III, multinational study in which 424 patients with newly diagnosed SCC of the head and neck were randomized to radiation therapy alone or radiation combined with weekly cetuximab.[176] An interim analysis at 38 months showed that the addition of cetuximab improved local disease control and median overall survival (49 months versus 29.3 months, $P = 0.03$), more than radiation alone. The indication for single-agent treatment of recurrent SCC of the head and neck was based on results of a phase II, single-arm, multicenter trial of 103 patients with recurrent or metastatic SCC of the head and neck.[177] The objective response rate was 13%, with a median response duration of 5.8 months.

Cetuximab was generally well tolerated in clinical trials. Overlapping toxicities were minimal when combined with irinotecan-based therapies. Adverse events reported in over 20% of patients receiving cetuximab monotherapy include asthenia/malaise, abdominal pain, fever, infusion reaction, headache, diarrhea, nausea, vomiting, constipation, and acneform rash.[176] The occurrence of rash in almost all patients receiving cetuximab likely correlates with known EGFR expression on normal epithelium, including skin. Interestingly, the appearance and severity of rash has been correlated with drug efficacy.[178,179] Infusion reactions consisting of fever, chills, dyspnea, and other allergic symptoms may be prevented or blunted by pretreatment with antihistamine, as recommended by the manufacturer. Severe infusion reactions occurred in about 3% of cetuximab patients, with fatalities reported rarely; a boxed warning appears on product labeling. There have also been a few reports of interstitial lung disease with one fatality reported.

Gemtuzumab ozogamicin. The most common acute leukemia in adults is AML. The risk for AML increases with age with an incidence of 0.7–3.9 cases per 100,000 up to 60 years and 6.7–19.2 cases per 100,000 above 60 years.[180] Older patients are less able to tolerate standard induction chemotherapy, and also appear to be more treatment refractory than their younger counterparts. Even with excellent prognostic factors, only half of elderly patients achieve remission and only 20% of those are alive and leukemia-free at 2 years. Most elderly patients present with comorbid conditions, poor performance status, cytogenetic abnormalities, and drug resistance, making their chance for remission and survival particularly dismal. Most patients who achieve a remission will relapse, and the probability of attaining a second, durable remission in this population is very low. The morbidity and mortality associated with further treatment precludes many, if not most, of the elderly population from undergoing a second course of cytotoxic chemotherapy. Gemtuzumab ozogamicin was developed to offer an alternative therapy for elderly patients confronting relapsed AML.

Gemtuzumab ozogamicin (CMA676) is an immunodrug conjugate that binds the CD33 surface antigen. CD33 is expressed on more than 80% of AML blasts; it is also expressed on immature myeloid cells, megakaryocytes, and to a lesser extent on mature myeloid cells.[181] CD33 is not expressed on pluripotent hematopoietic stem cells or nonhematopoietic cells. Gemtuzumab ozogamicin is a recombinant humanized IgG4 antibody conjugated via a hydrolysable bifunctional linker with the antitumor antibiotic calicheamicin.[182] The antibody contains humanized framework and constant regions with a murine CD33-binding Fab fragment. Calicheamicin is derived from fermentation of the bacterium *Micromonospora echinospora* ssp. *calichensis*. About half the antibody is linked with 4–6 moles calicheamicin per mole of antibody. Upon binding to CD33, the complex is internalized via endocytosis. Calicheamicin is then believed to be released inside myeloblast lysosomes where it migrates to the nucleus and binds to DNA in the minor groove. This causes double-strand breaks and death.[183]

In preclinical study, gemtuzumab ozogamicin demonstrated highly specific targeting and destruction of AML cells. A phase I dose-escalation trial followed, enrolling 40 patients with relapsed or treatment-refractory CD33-positive (CD33+) AML.[184] Complete disappearance of leukemic blast cells from peripheral blood and bone marrow occurred in eight patients (20%) with complete blood count recovery in three patients (8%).

Three concurrent phase II multicenter studies of gemtuzumab ozogamicin were conducted in the United States, Canada, and Europe (201, 202, 203).[185] A total of 142 patients with CD33+ AML, in their first relapse, were given two doses of gemtuzumab ozogamicin 9 mg/m² by intravenous infusion over 2 hours, allowing at least 14 days between doses. Patients 60 years of age and older made up 56% of the study population. The primary endpoint, complete remission (CR), was defined as complete disappearance of peripheral myeloblasts with ≤5% blasts in bone marrow and normal peripheral blood counts (hemoglobin ≥9 g/dL, absolute neutrophil count ≥1500/μL, platelets ≥100,000/μL). They also had to be transfusion-independent. Secondary endpoints were the number of complete remissions with incomplete platelet recovery (CRps), and overall remission (OR), which combined CR and CRp. Results of pooled data from the three trials showed a CR rate of 16.2% with 13.4% CRps for an overall remission rate of 29.6%.

The most common adverse events reported in clinical trials with gemtuzumab ozogamicin were fever, chills, dyspnea, nausea and vomiting, myelosuppression, infection, liver enzyme abnormalities, and bleeding. Severe NCI grade 3 or 4 toxicity, reported in over 5% of patients, included thrombocytopenia (99%), neutropenia (98%), anemia (47%), hyperbilirubinemia (23%), AST elevations (17%), sepsis (16%), hypertension (9%), dyspnea (9%), hypotension (8%), neutropenic fever (7%), and pneumonia (7%).[186] Dose-limiting thrombocytopenia and neutropenia occurred in half the patients in phase I study. Infusion reactions (fever and chills) occurred in most patients. The onset of symptoms was usually within 6 hours of gemtuzumab ozogamicin infusion, and tended to be less frequent and severe with subsequent doses. Pretreatment with antihistamine (diphenhydramine 50 mg) and acetaminophen (650–1000 mg) is recommended for all patients. It appears that corticosteroids may also be helpful in preventing infusion reactions.[187]

Numerous spontaneous reports of severe hypersensitivity reactions, pulmonary toxicity, and hepatotoxicity led to early FDA review of postmarketing data and subsequent boxed warnings in gemtuzumab ozogamicin labeling.[182] Severe infusion reactions temporally related to gemtuzumab ozogamicin were reported in nine patients, four of whom died. At least two of the three following organ systems were involved: respiratory, cardiovascular, and skin. All but one case occurred during or after the first infusion, usually within 2 hours of receiving the dose. Eight cases of acute pulmonary toxicity occurred with five deaths reported. Five of these cases were reported as adult respiratory distress syndrome and three cases were reported as pulmonary edema. The risk for severe hypersensitivity and pulmonary reactions is increased in patients with large numbers of circulating myeloid blasts. The manufacturer recommends cytoreduction with hydroxyurea or leukapheresis in patients with peripheral blast counts greater than 30,000/μL. This, too, is included as a boxed warning in package labeling.

Both gemtuzumab ozogamicin and calicheamicin were found to cause hepatotoxicity in preclinical testing. As noted above, liver enzyme elevations are frequent and usually reversible. Many cases of hepatic veno-occlusive disease (VOD) and overt liver failure, with several fatalities, have been reported. Most cases of VOD occurred in patients who received gemtuzumab ozogamicin either before or after hematopoietic stem cell transplantation (HSCT). Although the precise mechanism for gemtuzumab ozogamicin-associated hepatotoxicity is not known, it may be due to the existence of CD33$^+$ cells in the liver sinusoids.[188]

Gemtuzumab ozogamicin (Mylotarg; Wyeth Labs) was given accelerated FDA approval in May 2000. It is indicated for use in patients with CD33$^+$ AML in first relapse who are 60 years of age or older and not candidates for cytotoxic chemotherapy. Most patients in clinical trials who achieved remission with gemtuzumab ozogamicin received further therapy, including HSCT. Because there have been no comparative studies, it is difficult to compare the safety and survival benefit of gemtuzumab ozogamicin versus cytotoxic chemotherapy. Ongoing studies of gemtuzumab ozogamicin alone and in combination with other chemotherapeutic agents in younger patients in the setting of HSCT will provide much-needed safety and efficacy data.

Yttrium-90 ibritumomab tiuxetan and iodine-131 tositumomab. Radioimmunotherapy (RIT) is accomplished by attaching a radioactive isotope to a monoclonal antibody.

The radionuclide-antibody conjugate created is designed to deliver a toxic payload to specific (antigen-bearing) targets. One therapeutic advantage to this strategy is that tumor cells that may evade "naked" antibody effects (because of inadequate antigen expression or tumor encasement) are less likely to escape penetrating radiation. From a toxicity standpoint, the targeted delivery of radiation damage to tumor cells limits collateral damage to normal tissues. Though there are only two radioimmunoconjugates currently approved, many more will likely follow in the years to come.

The first radioimmunoconjugate to gain FDA approval was yttrium-90 (^{90}Y) ibritumomab tiuxetan (Zevalin; Biogen Idec Pharmaceuticals), approved in 2002. The second, iodine-131 (^{131}I) tositumomab (Bexxar; GlaxoSmithKline), was approved in 2003. Both radioimmunoconjugates employ entirely murine antibodies that carry β-emitting radionuclides to target CD20$^+$ B lymphocytes of NHLs. In most cases nonhuman antibodies are disadvantageous because of rapid immune clearance, increased risk for allergic reactions, and the development of HAMA. In the case of these two radioimmunoconjugates, however, rapid clearance from the circulation helps decrease persistent radiation damage to healthy tissues. During clinical trials with these agents, HAMA responses were rare.[189,190]

Ibritumomab is a murine IgG1 anti-CD20 antibody that is the rituximab parent antibody. Yttrium-90, the therapeutic radioisotope, is conjugated to ibritumomab via the linker-chelator tiuxetan. The radioimmunotherapy process involves two steps: a biodistribution and dosimetry procedure followed 1–2 weeks later by the therapeutic radioimmunoconjugate dose. In the first step, the unlabeled antibody rituximab is given to saturate peripheral blood B cells and optimize biodistribution of the radiolabeled antibody that follows. Yttrium-90 is a pure β emitter and as such cannot be used for imaging. Therefore, indium-111 (^{111}In), which emits both β and γ radiation, is used for imaging, and provides a surrogate for yttrium-90 biodistribution. Indium-111 is conjugated with ibritumomab via the tiuxetan linker to form ^{111}In ibritumomab tiuxetan. In the second step, whole body gamma imaging is performed at prescribed time intervals. If biodistribution is acceptable, the therapeutic dose of 0.4 mCi/kg ^{90}Y ibritumomab tiuxetan is given 7–9 days later. This, again, is preceded by rituximab, which binds circulating CD20$^+$ cells.

Tositumomab is a murine IgG2a anti-CD20 antibody that directly chelates iodine-131, and so does not require a linker molecule. The procedure for administration of ^{131}I tositumomab is similar to the process for ^{90}Y ibritumomab tiuxetan. But because iodine-131 emits both β and γ radiation, ^{131}I tositumomab can be used for biodistribution and dosimetry as well as for therapeutic purposes. Oral iodide must be used, starting 24 hours before and continuing for 14 days after the ^{131}I tositumomab treatment to block uptake by the thyroid.

In phase I/II studies of ^{90}Y ibritumomab tiuxetan in patients with low-grade or intermediate-grade B-cell NHL, the maximum tolerated dose was found to be 0.4 mCi/kg (0.3 mCi/kg for baseline platelet counts of 100,000 to 149,000/μL).[191,192] Overall response rates in these patients with relapsed or treatment refractory disease ranged from 64% to 67%. Hematologic toxicity was the primary adverse event reported in these studies, with thrombocytopenia being the most common. Low platelet counts at baseline and a higher degree of disease involvement in bone marrow predicted an increased risk for severe thrombocytopenia.

^{90}Y ibritumomab tiuxetan plus rituximab was compared to rituximab alone in a pivotal phase III trial of 143 patients with relapsed or refractory low-grade, follicular, or transformed NHL.[193] Rituximab again was used as part of the therapeutic ^{90}Y ibritumomab tiuxetan regimen. Patients were randomized to either one dose of ^{90}Y ibritumomab tiuxetan 0.4 mCi/kg or 4 weekly doses of rituximab 375 mg/m². The overall response rate was 80% with ^{90}Y ibritumomab tiuxetan and 56% with rituximab alone ($P = .002$). Both median time to progression (11.2 versus 10.1 months) and median duration of response (14.2+ versus 12.1+ months) favored the radioimmunoconjugate but did not reach statistical significance. The utility of ^{90}Y ibritumomab tiuxetan in patients with rituximab-refractory low-grade B-cell NHL was studied in 54 patients.[194] Rituximab failure was defined as no response, progressive disease, or disease relapse within 6 months of treatment. The overall response rate in these patients was 74%, with 16% CR, and a median duration of response ≥7.7 months. Hematologic toxicity was frequent and severe in many patients, with four patients (8%) requiring hospitalization for infection. This was not unexpected because one third of these patients had bone marrow involvement of their lymphoma and a median of four prior chemotherapy regimens. This was an important finding because it showed that ^{90}Y ibritumomab tiuxetan was a viable option for patients who had no good treatment alternatives.

Iodine-131 tositumomab was studied in several phase II noncomparative trials of patients with NHL. Overall response rates ranged between 39% to 81% with 25% to 38% complete responses and a median duration of response between 9.9 and 14 months.[194-196] Patients in these studies had relapsed or refractory B-cell lymphoma, most with low-grade or transformed low-grade histology; however, some had the more aggressive intermediate- and high-grade classifications. Patients with low-grade or transformed low-grade NHL responded better to treatment than did patients with more aggressive histologies. Iodine-131 tositumomab was also studied in patients with rituximab-refractory indolent B-cell NHL.[197] The results of this trial were very similar to those reported above for ^{90}Y ibritumomab tiuxetan in this patient population. The complete response rate was actually higher with ^{131}I tositumomab, but this was probably because of a higher percentage of patients with bulky disease in the ^{90}Y ibritumomab tiuxetan study. Outcomes of a phase I/II trial showed encouraging results of ^{131}I tositumomab used in combination with chemotherapy and autologous stem cell transplantation.[198,199]

The adverse effects of ^{90}Y ibritumomab tiuxetan and ^{131}I tositumomab were essentially the same, with dose-limiting bone marrow suppression and infusion reactions being the most common.[200] Marrow suppression tended to be delayed, reaching nadir counts between 7 and 9 weeks after the dose and recovery 2–4 weeks later. A minority of patients needed blood product and/or growth factor support. In some cases cytopenias were prolonged. Infusion reactions occurred most frequently with the first dose of unlabelled antibody and did not typically occur with the subsequent dose or radiolabeled antibody. Severe infusion reactions with fatality were reported. All precautions associated with rituximab applied to the ^{90}Y ibritumomab tiuxetan protocol, since rituximab was part of the regimen. Asthenia, nausea, fever, chills, sweats, abdominal pain, headache, vomiting, throat irritation, cough, pruritus, and rash were the most common nonhematologic adverse events reported, and most of these were part of the infusion reaction complex. Development of HAMA occurred rarely in clinical trials of these agents.[201] Although both therapeutic radioimmunoconjugates used murine antibodies, HAMA was more likely to occur with the ^{131}I tositumomab regimen, because the unconjugated antibody (tositumomab) used to determine biodistribution and dosimetry was fully murine, and the unconjugated antibody (rituximab) used in the ^{90}Y ibritumomab tiuxetan regimen was chimeric. Most antibody exposure in these regimens comes from the unconjugated antibodies. The amount of antibodies used to deliver the radioactive payload is much smaller.

Both Yttrium-90 ibritumomab tiuxetan and ^{131}I tositumomab are indicated for treatment of patients with relapsed or refractory low-grade, follicular, or transformed B-cell NHL, including patients with rituximab-refractory disease. Several radiation safety precautions apply to both radioimmunoconjugates. Patients should use appropriate contraception for 1 year after treatment, regardless of patient gender.[189,190] Although there have been no trials comparing these agents, they appear to have equivalent efficacy and safety. Other applications for these radioimmunoconjugates are under investigation.

Oncologic mAbs in the pipeline. Nearly half the current FDA-approved antibody products are used to treat cancer. Over 25% of new drug development efforts involve antibodies; most of these agents will bear oncology indications.[202,203] Two new agents are in early clinical testing for lympho-proliferative disorders. HuMax-CD20 is a fully human, high-affinity mAb that targets CD20-positive B lymphocytes. It is currently undergoing phase I/II testing in patients with NHL and CLL. Siplizumab (MEDI-507) is a humanized mAb that binds to CD2 receptors found on T cells and NK cells; it may, therefore, be useful in treating T-cell lymphomas and leukemias. Pertuzumab is a promising mAb that binds HER-2 at a different epitope than trastuzumab, and prevents HER-2 dimerization with other epidermal growth factor receptors. Pertuzumab has potential application in several solid tumors, including those that do not overexpress HER-2. Another interesting antibody in development is the angiogenesis inhibitor IMC-IC11. In contrast to bevacizumab, this chimeric antibody binds VEGF-2 receptors, rather than binding VEGF. Phase I trials are under way using IMC-IC11 in patients with colorectal cancer.

The future holds great promise for mAbs as cancer therapy. Improvements to the unconjugated antibody and the use of a wide array of antibody-linked immunoconjugates will result in more effective, better tolerated treatment for patients facing cancer.

Others

Bacillus calmette-guérin (BCG) vaccine. BCG is a lyophilized preparation of live, attenuated organisms of the Calmette-Guérin strain of *Mycobacterium bovis* used to stimulate cell-mediated immunity to tuberculosis in countries where tuberculosis is epidemic and prophylaxis is not possible. BCG vaccine is a potent stimulator of host immunity, including NK cell and macrophage activity. The relatively nonspecific immunostimulant effect has led to many attempts to use BCG with cancer. Clinical trials of BCG in a variety of malignancies, such as melanoma, RCC, and colorectal cancer, have not demonstrated a role for this agent. Of interest is the inflammatory response seen when the drug is administered locally (e.g., intravesical administration in bladder cancer).[204] It is now believed this inflammatory response at the site of disease contributes to the immunogenicity of the cancer and increases the antitumor response. For example, intravesical BCG appears to induce inflammatory response at the bladder resulting in destruction of the cancer cells and sloughing of tissue. This local inflammatory effect is one of the reasons that BCG is used in some cancer vaccine therapies. BCG is included in tumor antigen-containing vaccines to enhance the vaccine's induction of host immunity to the antigen. These therapies are currently being investigated in a variety of malignancies.

Current use of BCG in cancer is commonly limited to intravesical administration as adjuvant therapy for the treatment of superficial bladder cancer. Transurethral resection (TUR) plus intravesical BCG has been shown to be superior to TUR alone or TUR and chemotherapy for delaying time to recurrence in patients with superficial bladder cancer.[205] Unfortunately, the optimal dose regime for adjuvant therapy has not been well established. Common toxicities include dysuria and urinary frequency following therapy. Hematuria may occur, usually after multiple treatments.[206] Less common side effects include granulomatous prostatitis, epididymo-orchitis, hepatitis, and pneumonitis.[207] In a small group of patients, BCG sepsis was seen and was thought to be caused by systemic absorption of BCG.

Notably, the commercial source of BCG contains viable attenuated mycobacteria. A black box warning in the FDA-approved labeling cautions that BCG infections have been reported in health care workers who had exposure during preparation or from accidental needle stick.[208] Also, nosocomial infections have been reported in patients who received parenteral drugs prepared in areas in which the BCG was prepared. All material used for drug manipulation, preparation, and administration should be considered biohazardous. After preparation, it is important to clean the preparation area, including the biological safety cabinet, before preparation of any other product. It is essential that when this drug is prepared in nonpharmacy areas, such as a physician's office, the same care be given to decontamination of the preparation area. It is also recommended that urine voided within 6 hours of administration be handled as infectious waste.

Because BCG contains viable attenuated mycobacteria, there is valid concern in using this agent for immunocompromised patients, including patients with HIV infection. This may be an appropriate concern in patients who have received immunosuppressive therapies.

Thalidomide and immunomodulatory analogs (IMiDs). One of the most exciting, and perhaps surprising, developments in the past decade is the revival of thalidomide.[209] Thalidomide and IMiDs (such as lenalidomide) have numerous effects on the body's immune system. These agents inhibit cytokines such as TNFα, GM-CSF, and a number of interleukins (IL-1β, IL-6, IL-12). These agents also stimulate T lymphocytes, causing the proliferation, production, and activation of cytokines that increase T-cell anticancer activity. IL-2-mediated primary T-cell production increases the production of IFN-γ and decreases the density of TNF-α-induced cell surface adhesion molecules. Additionally, these agents possess anti-angiogneic and pro-apoptotic properties.[210]

Thalidomide was approved by the FDA in late 1998 for treatment of chronic erythema nodosum leprosum. The anti-inflammatory and immunomodulatory effects of the drug provided a basis to further evaluate its use in management of a variety of cancers and inflammatory conditions (e.g., GVHD). The challenge of this agent continues to be toxicity. Historically, teratogenicity when taken between days 27 and 40 of gestation, has made this an agent with limitations.[211] Fetal abnormalities include malformed shortened extremities (phocomelia) and deformities of the eyes, ears, and gastrointestinal tract. The marketing of the drug with a very restrictive program, STEPS, was done to prevent prescribing to women of child-bearing potential.

Thalidomide has a number of other problematic complications that can be challenging in some patients.[212] Sedation and fatigue are common. Skin rashes manifest as skin eruptions. Severe dermatologic reactions, such as Stevens-Johnson syndrome, have rarely occurred with this agent.[213] Neuropathy, often presenting as severe constipation or peripheral neuropathy, can be dose limiting in some patients. High-risk patients include the elderly and patients with neuropathy secondary to chemotherapy, diabetes, or other comorbidities. Prevention strategies, such as prophylactic bowel regimens, can help prevent this complication. Thromboembolic events are increased with thalidomide, and seem to be increased in patients receiving thalidomide in combination with chemotherapy and/or corticosteroids.[214]

Multiple myeloma. The revival of thalidomide can be attributed, in part, to its success in patients with relapsed or refractory myeloma. Initial studies of thalidomide, with or without dexamethasone, in heavily pretreated patients with relapsed or refractory myeloma demonstrated an exciting effect, with overall response rates from 25% to 60%.[215-217] The dose of thalidomide varied in trials, but dose escalation beyond 400 mg per day was, and is, often limited secondary to toxicities. It was hypothesized that the toxicity profile might be higher in this patient population, which had received significant chemotherapy (often including autologous stem cell transplantation).

The success in relapsed myeloma led to the evaluation of thalidomide, combined with dexamethasone, as front-line therapy in myeloma.[218,219] Response rates between 60% to 70% were reported in noncomparative trials. In a comparative trial of thalidomide and dexamethasone versus dexamethasone as a single agent in newly diagnosed patients with multiple myeloma, combination therapy demonstrated an advantage.[220] The response rates of the combination were over 60% (versus 40% with dexamethasone alone) and led to the approval of this agent for front-line therapy in myeloma in 2006. It is important to note that thalidomide did not compromise stem cell mobilization; it could, therefore, be used as an induction therapy in patients who were eventually planned to receive autologous stem cell transplantation. Toxicity could be significant, including neuropathy, sedation, and increased risk of venous thromboembolism.

In elderly patients with myeloma, thalidomide has been combined with oral melphalan and prednisone (MP). In a phase III randomized trial, thalidomide at lower doses (100 mg per day) were combined with six monthly courses of oral melphalan (daily × 7 each month) and prednisone (daily × 7 each month).[221] Interim response rates of 80% were a significant improvement of response rates with MP alone (48%). This strategy of treatment is an important advance for patients who are not candidates for transplantation.

Lenalidomide is a second-generation analog of thalidomide, with a similar chemical structure. This analog appears to be a more potent immunomodulator than thalidomide and has the benefit of less constipation, neuropathy, and sedation when compared to thalidomide.[222] Of note, toxicities may be higher when the dose/dose schedule is escalated.[223] Preclinical work indicates that lenalidomide targets the tumor and the tumor microenvironment via caspase-8-mediated apoptosis. Additionally, lenalidomide was not teratogenic in the New Zealand rabbit model.[224] This agent, approved by the FDA in 2006 for treatment of a subset of myelodysplastic syndrome and myeloma, shows great promise in a number of malignancies, including CLL, AML, and NHL.

Lenalidomide was initially approved for the treatment of a group of patients with myelodyplastic syndrome. In a relatively small trial, 43 patients with transfusion-dependent or symptomatic anemia received lenalidomide (10 or 25 mg) orally each day for 21 days every 28 days.[225] Response rates were highest in patients with a clonal interstitial deletion involving chromosome 5q31.1. Lenalidomide improved anemia and decreased the routine use of red blood cell transfusions in over half the patients. Toxicities included bone marrow suppression, specifically neutropenia (65%) and thrombocytopenia (74%). Dose adjustments are recommended based on hematopoetic parameters.

Recently, lenalidomide was approved for treatment of relapsed multiple myeloma. In phase I dose-escalation studies, patients with refractory myeloma were treated with lenalidomide. As with the initial studies in myeloma with thalidomide, many of these patients were heavily pre-treated. Most of the responses seen in this study were at doses of 25–50 mg per day. Dose-limiting toxicity was myelosuppression. Initial reports of phase II and III trials demonstrated that the activity of this drug was superior to high-dose dexamethasone in relapsed myeloma.[226, 227] It is likely that clinical trials will evaluate more fully the role in myeloma beyond that of refractory disease.

The role of thalidomide and related agents is just beginning to be defined. The translation of the basic research to clinical trials has occurred rapidly, and there are many questions to answer. As the mechanism(s) of action of these agents are clarified, clinical applications are likely to expand. For example, lenalidomide appears to increase ADCC, and, therefore, may be an appropriate agent to combine with mAb therapy. The combination with chemotherapy and immunotherapy will need to be evaluated in specific cancers, and perhaps in select subsets of patients with those cancers.

Cancer vaccines. *Vaccines.* Despite a multidisciplinary approach combining surgery, chemotherapy, and radiation that has led to a dramatic improvement in survival for patients with cancer, there still remain many patients who are resistant to standard therapies. New strategies are needed to improve overall survival. Immunotherapy represents an appealing approach, and vaccination is an important strategy because of its ability to actively recognize and kill the malignant cells. The goal of cancer immunotherapy is to establish an effective antitumor response through the immune system. A large number of cancer vaccine clinical trials involving different tumor types and various vaccine strategies are under way.

The rationale behind immunization and the use of various types of vaccines is discussed extensively in Chapter 6. Tumor-associated antigens (TAAs), which are recognized by T cells, serve as attractive targets for cancer vaccines.[228] TAAs can be isolated, identified, and characterized. For a particular TAA to be used as a target, it must be expressed in the tumor and not in normal cells. For the cellular immune system to recognize it, the TAA must be either expressed on the cell surface or presented by MHC proteins. T cells should be available to recognize and respond to the TAA. Ideally, the TAA should be expressed in more than one type of cancer to be more broadly applicable. Once a target is identified, a platform that can induce the immune response is needed. Platforms may be highly specific or they may be less specific; current platforms include tumor cell-based vaccines, peptides/proteins, dendritic cells (DCs), and recombinant viral vectors.

Characteristics of a good tumor vaccine include the ability to target delivery to professional antigen-presenting cell (APC), direct activation of the APC/DC, ready access of vaccine/antigen to cross-presentation pathways, ability to induce effector T-cell responses without significant reliance on multiple components of the immune system, availability to generate from public/universal antigens instead of deriving from each individual tumor for individual patients, and resistance to the generation of autoimmunity.[229]

Autologous whole-cell vaccines appeal because they contain TAAs that are potentially targeted by the immune system, including TAAs specific to the patient. The main disadvantages of this approach are the difficulty of obtaining malignant cells from patients and limited availability of tumor source in the adjuvant setting. Allogeneic preparations made in vitro overcome this drawback. Both autologous and allogeneic tumor cells have been genetically engineered with cytokines such as GM-CSF and IL-2 to recruit and activate APCs at the vaccination site. This favors the uploading of TAAs and their presentation of T cells in secondary lymphoid organs.[230] The efficacy of whole-cell tumor vaccines has not been confirmed by phase III trials in the therapeutic or adjuvant setting. One reason for disappointing results is the insufficient immunization rate of the vaccination regimen. Heat-shock proteins can be isolated and used as a polyvalent, autologous cancer-vaccine preparation with undefined tumor-associated antigens. This removes the need to identify epitopes of tumor-associated antigens that are recognized by cytotoxic T lymphocytes. A major challenge for heat-shock protein-based cancer vaccines is that they bind peptides with low affinity and are generally believed to be unique to the individual's tumor and, therefore, not effective in another patient. Though individual efficacy may be greater, the logistics of having to produce a personalized vaccine for each person makes it more difficult to conduct large-scale clinical trials.[229] Vaccine trials with heat-shock proteins are ongoing. Overall, the clinical responses have been modest; two complete responses were seen in the first melanoma trial,[231] but results from the second trial were less promising.[232]

Another avenue for tumor vaccines is to target the cause of the malignancy, and use vaccination as prevention. Human papillomavirus (HPV) infection causes many of the cases of cervical cancer. A prophylactic HPV vaccine is now available for immunizing girls or women before they become sexually active. The vaccination is to be given in a series of three vaccines at 0, 2, and 6 months.[233]

Cancer vaccines are a nontoxic therapeutic approach to cancer. The therapeutic benefits of cancer vaccines are still limited, and no vaccination treatment regimen should be considered outside clinical trials, as phase III trials have not shown a significant improvement in overall survival compared to patients who have received standard therapies. Vaccine trials are ongoing in individuals with a variety of cancers including, but not limited to, melanoma,[234] non-small cell lung cancer,[235] breast cancer,[236] prostate cancer,[237] ovarian cancer, and renal cell and gastrointestinal malignancies.[238]

REFERENCES

1. American Cancer Society (ACS). *Cancer Facts and Figures—2006.* Atlanta, GA; 2006.
2. Ehrlich P. Ueber den jetzigen Stand der Karzinomforschung. *Ned Tijdschr Geneeskd.* 1990; 273–290.
3. Burnet FM. Immunological surveillance in neoplasia. *Transplant Rev.* 1971; 7:3–25.
4. Hanahan D, Lanzavecchia A, Mihich E. Fourteenth Annual Pezcoller Symposium: The Novel Dichotomy of Immune Interactions with Tumors. *Cancer Res.* 2003; 63(11):3005–3008.
5. Kumar V, Abbas AK, Fausto N. *Robbins & Cotran Pathologic Basis of Disease.* 7th ed. Philadelphia, PA: Elsevier Saunders; 2005:269–342.
6. Esteller M. Relevance of DNA methylation in the management of cancer. *Lancet Oncol.* 2003; 4(6):351–358.
7. Herman JG, Baylin S. Gene silencing in cancer in association with promoter hypermethylation. *N Engl J Med.* 2003; 349(21):2042–2054.
8. Hahn WC, Weinberg RA. Rules for making human tumor cells. *N Engl J Med.* 2002; 347(20):1593–1603.
9. Hanahan D, Weinberg RA. The hallmarks of cancer. *Cell.* 2000; 100(1):57–70.
10. Fearon ER, Vogelstein B. A genetic model for colorectal tumorigenesis. *Cell.* 1990; 61(5):759–767.
11. Kinzler KW, Vogelstein B. Lessons from hereditary colon cancer. *Cell.* 1996; 87:159–170.
12. Weinberg RA. How cancer arises. *Sci Am.* 1996; 275(3):62–70.
13. Gross L. Intradermal immunization of C3H mice against a sarcoma that originated in an animal of the same line. *Cancer Res.* 1943; 3:326–333.
14. Foley EJ. Antigenic properties of methylcholanthrene-induced tumors in mice of the strain of origin. *Cancer Res.* 1953; 13:835–837.
15. Prehn RT, Main JM. Immunity to methylcholanthrene-induced sarcomas. *JNCI.* 1957; 18:769–778.
16. Klein G, Sjogren HO, Klein E, et al. Demonstration of resistance against methylcholanthrene-induced sarcomas in the primary autochthonous host. *Cancer Res.* 1960; 20:1561–1572.
17. Chang C, Martin RG, Livingston DM, et al. Relationship between T-antigen and tumor specific transplantation antigen in simian virus 40-transformed cells. *J Virol.* 1979; 29:69–75.
18. Livingston DM, Bradley MK. The simian virus 40 large T antigen. A lot packed into a little. *Mol Biol Med.* 1987; 4:63.
19. Sturgeon C. Practice guidelines for tumor marker use in the clinic. *Clin Chem.* 2002;48(8):1151–1159.
20. Bast R, Ravdin P, Hayes D, et al. 2000 Update of recommendations for the use of tumor markers in breast and colorectal cancer: clinical practice guidelines of the American Society of Clinical Oncology. *J Clin Oncol.* 2001; 19(6):1865–1878.
21. National Comprehensive Cancer Network (NCCN) Clinical Practice Guidelines in Oncology—v.1. 2005. www.nccn.org/professionals/physician–gls/pdf/prostate.pdf. Accessed November 28, 2005.
22. Whiteside TL. Immunologic disorders: Immune responses to malignancies. *J Allergy Clin Immunol.* 2003; 111(2 Suppl):S677–686.
23. Renkvist N, Castelli C, Robbins PF, et al. A listing of human tumor antigens recognized by T cells. *Cancer Immunol Immunother.* 2001; 50:3–15.
24. Golsby RA, Kindt TJ, Osborne BA, et al, eds. *Immunology.* 5th ed. New York, NY: W.H. Freeman and Company; 2003:499–522.
25. Janeway CA, Travers P, Walport M, et al. *Immunobiology: The Immune System in Health and Disease.* 6th ed. New York, NY: Garland Science; 2005:630–642.
26. Cerwenka A, Lanier LL. Natural killer cells, viruses, and cancer. *Nature Reviews Immunology.* 2001; 1(1):41–49.
27. Smyth MJ, Godfrey DI, Trapani JA. A fresh look at tumor immunosurveillance and immunotherapy. *Nature Immununol.* 2001; 2(4):293–299.
28. Dunn GP, Old LJ, Schreiber RD. The immunobiology of cancer immunosurveillance and immunoediting. *Immunity.* 2004; 21(2):137–148.

29. Matzinger P. An innate sense of danger. *Semin Immunol.* 1998; 10:399.

30. Restifo NP. Cancer vaccines: basic principles. General concepts and preclinical studies. In: Rosenberg SA, ed. *Biologic Therapy of Cancer.* 3rd ed. Philadelphia, PA: J.B. Lippincott Company; 2000:571–572.

31. Spisek R, Dhodapkar MV. Immunoprevention of cancer. *Hematol Oncol Clin N Am.* 2006; 20:735–750.

32. Talpaz M , Kantarjian H, Kurzrock R, et al. Interferon-alpha produces sustained cytogenetic response in chronic myelogenous leukemia: Philadelphia chromosome-positive patients. *Ann Intern Med.* 1991; 114:532–539.

33. Kirkwood JM, Bender C, Agarwala S, et al. Mechanisms and management of toxicities associated with high-dose interferon alfa-2b therapy. *J Clin Oncol.* 2002; 20:3703–3718.

34. Plata-Salaman CR. Cytokines and anorexia: A brief overview. *Semin Oncol.* 1998; 25(Suppl 1):64–72.

35. Grever M, Kopecky K, Foucar MK, et al. Randomized comparison of pentostatin versus interferon alfa-2a in previously untreated patients with hairy cell leukemia. Final report from the Italian Cooperative Group for HCL. *Ann Oncol.* 1994; 5(8):725–731.

36. Talpaz M, Ravandi F, Kurzrock, et al. Interferon-α and -β: Clinical applications. Leukemias, lymphoma, and multiple myeloma. In: Rosenberg SA, ed. *Biologic Therapy of Cancer.* 3rd ed. Philadelphia, PA: J.B. Lippincott Company; 2000:209–224.

37. Italian Cooperative Study Group on Chronic Myeloid Leukemia. Interferon alfa-2a compared with conventional chemotherapy for the treatment with chronic myeloid leukemia. *N Engl J Med.* 1994; 330(12):820–825.

38. Guilhot F, Chastang C, Michallett M, et al. Interferon alfa-2b combined with cytarabine versus interferon alone in chronic myelogenous leukemia. *N Engl J Med.* 1997; 337(4):223–229.

39. Kirkwood JM. Interferon-α and β: clinical applications: melanoma. In: Rosenberg SA, ed. *Biologic Therapy of Cancer.* 3rd ed. Philadelphia, PA: J. B. Lippincott Company; 2000:224–251.

40. Creagan ET, Ahmann DL, Frytak S, et al. Phase II trials of recombinant leukocyte A interferon in disseminated malignant melanoma: results in 96 patients. *Cancer Treat Rep.* 1986; 70:619–624.

41. Falkson CI, Ibrahim J, Kirkwood JM, et al. Phase III trial of dacarbazine versus dacarbazine with interferon alfa 2b versus dacarbazine with tamoxifen versus dacarbazine with interferon alfa 2b and tamoxifen in patients with metastatic melanoma: an Eastern Cooperative Oncology Group Study (E3690). *J Clin Oncol.* 1998; 16:1743–1751.

42. Marincola FM, White DE, Wise AP, et al. Combination therapy with interferon alfa-2a and interleukin-2 for the treatment of metastatic cancer. *J Clin Oncol.* 1995; 113:1110–1122.

43. Kirkwood JM, Straderman MH, Ernstoff MS, et al. Interferon alfa-2b adjuvant therapy of high-risk resected cutaneous melanoma: The Eastern Cooperative Oncology Group Trial EST 1684. *J Clin Oncol.* 1996; 14:7–17.

44. Cole BF, Gelber RD, Kirkwood JM, et al. A quality-of-life-adjusted survival analysis of interferon alfa-2b adjuvant treatment for high-risk resected cutaneous melanoma: an Eastern Cooperative Oncology Group Study (E1684). *J Clin Oncol.* 1996; 14:2666–2673.

45. Moschos SJ, Kirkwood JM. Present status and future prospects for adjuvant therapy of melanoma: Time to build upon the foundation of high-dose interferon alfa-2b. *J Clin Oncol.* 2004; 22:11–14.

46. Minasian LM, Motzer RJ, Gluck L, et al. Interferon alfa-2a in advanced renal cell carcinoma: treatment results and survival in 159 patients with long-term follow-up. *J Clin Oncol.* 1993; 11:1368–1375.

47. Shankaran V, Schreibre RD. Interferon-γ: Basic principles and clinical applications. In: Rosenberg SA, editor. *Biologic Therapy of Cancer.* 3rd ed. Philadelphia, PA: J.B. Lippincott Company; 2000:286–301.

48. Konrad MW, Hemstreet G, Hersh EM, et al. Pharmacokinetics of recombinant interleukin-2 in humans. *Cancer Res.* 1990; 50:2009–2017.

49. Atkins MB, Lotze M, Dutcher JP, et al. High-dose recombinant interleukin-2 therapy for patients with metastatic melanoma: analysis of 270 patients treated from 1985–1003. *J Clin Oncol.* 1999; 17:2105–2116.

50. Schwartz RN, Stover L, Dutcher J. Managing toxicities of high-dose interleukin-2. *Oncology.* 2002; 16(Suppl 13):11–20.

51. Metcalf D. Haemopoietic growth factors 1. *Lancet.* 1989; 1(8642):825–827.

52. Oates JA, Wood AJ. Erythropoietin. *N Engl J Med.* 1991; 324(19):1339–1344.

53. Winearls CG, Oliver DO, Pippard MJ, et al. Effect of human erythropoietin derived from recombinant DNA on the anaemia of patients maintained by chronic heamodialysis. *Lancet.* 1986; 2(8517):1175–1178.

54. Eschbach JW, Egrie JC, Downing MR, et al. Correction of the anemia of end-stage renal disease with recombinant human erythropoietin: Results of a combined phase I and II clinical trial. *N Engl J Med.* 1987; 316(2):73–78.

55. Coyne D, Ling BN, Toto R, et al. Novel erythropoiesis stimulating protein (NESP) correct anemia in dialysis patients when administered at reduced dose frequency compared with recombinant-human erythropoietin (r-HuEPO) [Abstr SU624], 33rd Annual Meeting of the American Society of Nephrology, October 13–16, 2000, Toronto, Canada.

56. Rizzo JD, Lichtin AE, Woolf SH, et al. Use of epoetin in patients with cancer: evidence-based clinical practice guidelines of the American Society of

Clinical Oncology and the American Society of Hematology. *Blood*. 2002; 100(7):2303–2320.

57. Siedenfeld J, Piper M, Flamm C, et al. Epoetin treatment of anemia associated with cancer therapy: a systematic review and meta-analysis of controlled clinical trials. *J Natl Cancer Inst*. 2001; 93(16):1204–1214.

58. Bohilius J, Langensiepen S, Schwarzer G, et al. Recombinant human erythropoietin and overall survival in cancer patients: results of a comprehensive meta-analysis. *J Natl Cancer Inst*. 2005; 97(7):489–498.

59. Hellstrom LE. Efficacy of erythropoietin in the myelodysplastic syndromes: a meta-analysis of 205 patients from 17 studies. *Br J Haematol*. 1995; 89:67–71.

60. Gabrilove JL, Cleeland CS, Livingston RB, et al. Clinical evaluation of once-weekly dosing of epoetin alfa in chemotherapy patients: improvements in hemoglobin and quality of life are similar to three-times-weekly dosing. *J Cin Oncol*. 2001; 19(11):2875–2882.

61. Clinical Practice Guideline in Oncology—v.2.2006 Cancer- and Treatment-Related Anemia. NCCN, 2006. Available at: http://www.nccn.org/. Accessed May 15, 2006.

62. Canon JL, Vansteenkiste J, Bodoky G, et al. Randomized, double-blind, active-controlled, randomized phase III trial of every-3-week darbepoetin alfa for the treatment of chemotherapy-induced anemia. *J Natl Cancer Inst*. 2006; 98(4):273–284.

63. Glaspy J, Henry D, Patel R, et al. Effects of chemotherapy on endogenous erythropoietin levels and the pharmacokinetics and erythropoietic response of darbepoetin afla: A randomized clinical trial of synchronous versus asynchronous dosing of darbepoetin alfa. *Eur J Cancer*. 2005; 41:1140–1149.

64. Hedenus M, Adriansson M, San Miguel J, et al. Efficacy and safety of darbepoetin alfa in anaemic patients with lymphoproliferative malignancies: a randomized, double-blind, placebo-controlled study. *Br J Haematol*. 2003; 122(3):394–403.

65. Kotasek D, Steger G, Faught W, et al. Darbepoetin alfa administered every 3 weeks alleviates anaemia in patients with solid tumours receiving chemotherapy; results of a double-blind, placebo-controlled, randomized study. *Eur J Cancer*. 2003; 39(14):2026–2034.

66. Vansteenkiste J, Pirker R, Massuti B, et al. Double-blind, placebo-controlled, randomized phase III trial of darbepoetin alfa in lung cancer patient receiving chemotherapy. *J Natl Cancer Inst*. 2002; 94(16):1211–1220.

67. Boccia R, Malik IA, Raja V, et al. Darbepoetin alfa administered every three weeks is effective for the treatment of chemotherapy-induced anemia. *Oncologist*. 2006; 11:409–417.

68. Schwartzberg LS, Yee LK, Senecal FM, et al. A randomized comparison of every-2-week darbepoetin alfa and weekly epoetin alfa for the treatment of chemotherapy-induced anemia in patients with

breast, lung, or gynecologic cancer. *Oncologist*. 2004; 9:696–707.

69. Dale DD. Colony-stimulating factors for the management of neutropenia in cancer patients. *Drugs*. 2002; 62 Suppl.1:1–15.

70. Heuser M, Ganser A. Colony-stimulating factors in the management of neutropenia and its complications. *Ann Hematol*. 2005; 84:697–708.

71. Smith T, Khatcheressian J, Lyman GH, et al. 2006 Update of recommendations for the use of white blood cell growth factors: an evidence-based clinical practice guideline. *J Cin Oncol*. 2006; 24(19):1–19.

72. Curran MP, Goa KL. Pegfilgrastim. *Drugs*. 2002; 62(8):1207–1213.

73. Johnston E, Crawford J, Blackwell S, et al. Randomized, dose-escalation study of SD/01 compared with daily filgrastim in patients receiving chemotherapy. *J Cin Oncol*. 2000; 18(13):2522–2528.

74. Green M, Koelbl H, Baselga J, et al. A randomized double-blind multicenter phase III study of fixed-dose single-administration pegfilgrastim versus daily filgrastim in patients receiving myelosuppressive chemotherapy. *Ann Oncol*. 2003; 14:29–35.

75. Clinical Practice Guideline in Oncology—v.1.2006 Myeloid Growth Factors. NCCN, 2006. Available at: http://www.nccn.org/. Accessed June 15, 2006.

76. Groopman J, Molina J, Scadden D. Hematopoietic growth factors. *N Eng J Med*. 1989; 321(21):1449–1459.

77. Meijer E, Dekker AW, Rozenberg-Arska M, et al. Influence of cytomegalovirus seropositivity on outcome after T cell-depleted bone marrow transplantation: contrasting results between recipients of grafts from related and unrelated donors. *Clin Infect Dis*. 2002; 35(6):703–712.

78. Citron ML, Berry DA, Cirrincione C, et al. Randomized trial of dose-dense versus conventionally scheduled and sequential versus concurrent combination chemotherapy as postoperative adjuvant treatment of node-positive primary breast cancer: first report of Intergroup Trial C9741/Cancer and Leukemia Group B Trial 9741. *J Clin Oncol*. 2003; 21(8):1431–1439.

79. Pfreundschuh M, Truemper L, Kloess M, et al. Two-weekly or 3-weekly CHOP chemotherapy with or without etoposide for the treatment of young patients with good-prognosis (normal LDH) aggressive lymphomas: results of the NHL-B1 trial of the DSHNHL. *Blood*. 2004; 104(3):626–633.

80. Pfreundschuh M, Truemper L, Kloess M, et al. Two-weekly or 3-weekly CHOP chemotherapy with or without etoposide for the treatment of elderly patients with aggressive lymphomas: results of the NHL-B2 trial of the DSHNHL. *Blood*. 2004; 104(3):634–641.

81. Harousseau JL, Witz B, Lioure B, et al. Granulocyte colony-stimulating factor after intensive consolidation chemotherapy in acute myeloid leukemia: Results of a randomized trial of the Groupe Ouest-

Est Leucemias Aigues Myeloblastiquest. *J Clin Oncol.* 2000; 18:780–787.

82. Heil G, Hoelzer D, Sanz MA, et al. The International Acute Myeloid Leukemia Study Group: A randomized, double-blind, placebo-controlled phase III study of filgrastim in remission induction and consolidation therapy for adults with de novo acute myeloid leukemia—The International Acute Myeloid Leukemia Study Group. *Blood.* 1997; 90:4710–4718.

83. Larson RA, Dodge RK, Linker CA, et al. A randomized controlled trial of filgrastim during remission induction and consolidation chemotherapy for adults with acute lymphoblastic leukemia: CALGB study 9111. *Blood.* 1998; 92(5):1556–1564.

84. Pui C, Boyett JM, Hughes WT, et al. Human granulocyte colony-stimulating factor after induction chemotherapy in children with acute lymphoblastic leukemia. *New Engl J Med.* 1997; 336(25):1781–1787.

85. Heath J, Steinherz P, Altman A, et al. Human granulocyte colony stimulating-factor in children with high-risk acute lymphoblastic leukemia: A Children's Cancer Group Study. *J Clin Oncol.* 2003; 21:1612–1617.

86. Negrin R, Haeuber D, Nagler A, et al. Maintenance treatment of patients with myelodysplastic syndromes using recombinant human granulocyte colony-stimulating factor. *Blood.* 1990; 76(1):36–43.

87. Lemoli R, deVivo A, Damiani D, et al. Autologous transplantation of granulocyte colony-stimulating factor-primed bone marrow is effective in supporting myeloablative chemotherapy in patients with hematologic malignancies and poor peripheral blood stem cell mobilization. *Blood.* 2003; 102(5):1595–1600.

88. Lazarus H. Recombinant cytokines and hematopoietic growth factors in allogeneic and autologous bone marrow transplantation. *Cancer Treat Res.* 1997; 77:255–301.

89. Nimer SD, Champlin RE. Therapeutic use of hematopoietic growth factors in bone marrow transplantation. *Cancer Treat Res.* 1990; 50:141–164.

90. Singer JW, Nemunaitis J. Recombinant growth factors in bone marrow transplantation. *Bone Marrow Transplant.* 1991;7 suppl 1:10–12.

91. Nemunaitis J, Singer JW, Sanders JE. The use of recombinant human granulocyte macrophage colony-stimulating factor in autologous bone marrow transplantation. *Bone Marrow Transplant.* 1991; 7 suppl 3:24–27.

92. Jansen J, Thompson EM, Hanks S, et al. Hematopoietic growth factor after autologous peripheral blood transplantation: comparison of G-CSF and GM-CSF. *Bone Marrow Transplant.* 1999; 23(12):1251–1256.

93. Nemunaitis J, Buckner CD, Dorsey KS, et al. Retrospective analysis of infectious disease in patients who received recombinant human granulocyte-macrophage colony-stimulating factor versus patients not receiving a cytokine who underwent autologous bone marrow transplantation for treatment of lymphoid cancer. *Am J Clin Oncol.* 1998; 21(4):341–346.

94. Nemunaitis J, Rosenfeld CS, Ash R, et al. Phase III randomized, double-blind, placebo-controlled trial of rhGM-CSF following allogeneic bone marrow transplantation. *Bone Marrow Transplant.* 1993; 15(6):949–954.

95. Klumpp TR, Mangan KF, Goldberg SL, et al. Granulocyte colony-stimulating factor accelerates neutrophil engraftment following peripheral-blood stem-cell transplantation: a prospective, randomized trial. *J Clin Oncol.* 1995; 13(6):1323–1327.

96. Bensinger W, Appelbaum F, Rowley S, et al. Transplantation of allogeneic peripheral blood stem cells mobilized by recombinant human granulocyte colony-stimulating factor. *Blood.* 1995; 85(6):1655–1658.

97. Grigg AP, Roberts A, Raunow H, et al. Optimizing dose and scheduling of filgrastim (granulocyte colony-stimulating factor) for mobilization and collection of peripheral blood progenitor cells in normal volunteers. *Blood.* 1995; 86(12):4437–4445.

98. Nemunaitis J, Singer J, Buckner C, et al. Use of recombinant human granulocyte-macrophage colony-stimulating factor in graft failure after bone marrow Transplantation. *Blood.* 1990; 76(1):245–253.

99. Crivellari D, Bonetti M, Castigilione-Gertsch M, et al. Burdens and benefits of adjuvant cyclophosphamide, methotrexate, and fluorouracil and tamoxifen for elderly patients with breast cancer: the International Breast Cancer Study Group Trial VII. *J Clin Oncol.* 2000; 18(7):1412–1422.

100. Dees E, O'Reilly S, Goodman S, et al. A prospective pharmacologic evaluation of age-related toxicity of adjuvant chemotherapy in women with breast cancer. *Cancer Invest.* 2000; 18:521–529.

101. Kim Y, Rubenstein EB, Rolston KV, et al. Colony-stimulating factors (CSFs) may reduce complication and death in solid tumor patients with fever and neutropenia. *Proc Am Soc Clin Oncol.* 2000; 19:612a. Abstract 2411.

102. Gomez H, Mas L, Casanova L, et al. Elderly patients with aggressive non-hodgkin's lymphoma treated with CHOP chemotherapy plus granulocyte macrophage colony-stimulating factor: Identification of two age subgroups with differing hematologic toxicity. *J Clin Oncol.* 1998; 16:2352–2358.

103. Morrison VA, Picozzi V, Scott S, et al. The impact of age on delivered dose intensity and hospitalizations for febrile neutropenia in patients with intermediate-grade non-hodgkin's lymphoma receiving initial CHOP chemotherapy: a risk factor analysis. *Clin Lymphoma.* 2001; 2(1):47–56.

104. Cheng J, Adams G, Robinson M, et al. Monoclonal Antibodies. In: DeVita VT, Hellman S, Rosenberg SA, eds. *Cancer: Principles & Practice of Oncology.* 7th ed. Philadelphia, PA: Lippincott Williams & Wilkins; 2004:445–456.

105. Van Laan S. American Medical Association (USAN) Monoclonal antibodies; last updated May 2005. Available at: http://www.ama-assn.org/ama/pub/category/13280.html. Accessed June 6, 2005.

106. Anderson KC, Bates MP, Slaughenhoupt BL, et al. Expression of human B cell-associated antigens on leukemias and lymphomas: a model of human B cell differentiation. *Blood*. 1984; 63:1424–1433.

107. Tedder TF, Boyd AW, Freedman AS, et al. The B cell surface molecule B1 is functionally linked with B cell activation and differentiation. *J Immunol*. 1985; 135(2):973–979.

108. Tedder TF, Zhou LJ, Bell PD, et al. The CD20 surface molecule of B lymphocytes functions as a calcium channel. *J Cell Biochem*. 1990; 14D:195.

109. Einfeld DA, Brown JP, Valentine MA, et al. Molecular cloning of the human B cell CD20 receptor predicts a hydrophobic protein with multiple transmembrane domains. *EMBO J*. 1988; 7:711–717.

110. Cragg MS, Glennie MJ. Antibody specificity controls in vivo effector mechanisms of anti-CD20 reagents. *Blood*. 2004; 103:2738–2743.

111. Cartron G, Dacheux L, Salles G, et al. Therapeutic activity of humanized anti-CD20 monoclonal antibody and polymorphism in IgG Fc receptor FcγRIIIa gene. *Blood*. 2002; 99:754–758.

112. Anolik JH, Campbell D, Felgar RE, et al. The relationship of FcγRIIIa genotype to degree of B cell depletion by rituximab in the treatment of systemic lupus erythematosus. *Arthritis Rheum*. 2003; 48:455–459.

113. Weng W-K, Levy R. Two immunoglobulin G fragment C receptor polymorphisms independently predict response to rituximab in patients with follicular lymphoma. *J Clin Oncol*. 2003; 21:3940–3947.

114. Harjunpaa A, Junnikkala S, Meri S. Rituximab (anti-CD20) therapy of B-cell lymphomas: direct complement killing is superior to cellular effector mechanisms. *Scand J Immunol*. 2000; 51:634–641.

115. Deans JP, Li H, Polyak MJ. CD20-mediated apoptosis: signaling through lipid rafts. *Immunology*. 2002; 107:176–182.

116. Byrd JC, Kitada S, Flinn IW, et al. The mechanism of tumor cell clearance by rituximab in vivo in patients with B-cell chronic lymphocytic leukemia: evidence of caspase activation and apoptosis induction. *Blood*. 2002; 99:1038–1043.

117. Bannerji R, Kitada S, Flinn IW, et al. Apoptotic-regulatory and complement-protecting protein expression in chronic lymphocytic leukemia: relationship to in vivo rituximab resistance. *J Clin Oncol*. 2003; 21:1466–1471.

118. Janas E, Priest R, Wilde JI, et al. Rituxan (anti-CD20 antibody)-induced translocation of CD20 into lipid rafts is crucial for calcium influx and apoptosis. *Clin Exp Immunol*. 2005; 139(3):439–446.

119. The Non-Hodgkin's Lymphoma Pathologic Classification Project. National Cancer Institute-sponsored study of classifications of non-Hodgkin's lymphomas: summary and description of a working formulation for clinical usage. *Cancer*. 1982; 49:2112.

120. McLaughlin P, Grillo-López AJ, Link BK, et al. Rituximab chimeric anti-CD20 monoclonal antibody therapy for relapsed indolent lymphoma: half of patients respond to a four-dose treatment program. *J Clin Oncol*. 1998; 16:2825–2833.

121. Czuckman MS, Grillo-Lopez AJ, White CA, et al. Treatment of patients with low-grade B-cell lymphoma with the combination of chimeric anti-CD20 monoclonal antibody and CHOP chemotherapy *J Clin Oncol*. 1999; 17:268–276.

122. Vose JM, Link BK, Grossbard ML, et al. Phase II study of rituximab in combination with CHOP chemotherapy in patients with previously untreated, aggressive non-Hodgkin's lymphoma *J Clin Oncol*. 2001; 19:389–397.

123. Coiffier B, Lepage E, Briere J, et al. CHOP chemotherapy plus rituximab compared with CHOP alone in elderly patients with diffuse large-B-cell lymphoma. *N Engl J Med*. 2002; 346:235–242.

124. Rituxan [package insert]. San Francisco, CA: Genentech; December 2004.

125. Wang SC, Hung MC. HER2 overexpression and cancer targeting. *Semin Oncol*. 2001; 28(suppl. 16):115–124.

126. Seshadri R, Firgaira FA, Horsfall DJ, et al. Clinical significance of HER-2/neu oncogene amplification in primary breast cancer. The South Australian Breast Cancer Study Group. *J Clin Oncol*. 1993; 11(10):1936–1942.

127. Graus-Porta D, Beerli R, Daly J, et al. ErbB-2, the preferred heterodimerization partner of all ErbB receptors, is a mediator of lateral signaling. *EMBO J*. 1997; 16(7):1647–1655.

128. Olayioye M, Neve R, Lane H, et al. The ErbB signaling network: receptor heterodimerization in development and cancer. *EMBO J*. 2000; 19(13):3159–3167.

129. Lewis GD, Figari I, Frendly B, et al. Differential responses of human tumor cell lines to anti-p185HER2 monoclonal antibodies. *Cancer Immunol Immunother*. 1993; 37:255–263.

130. Sliwkowski M, Lofgren J, Lewis G, et al. Nonclinical studies addressing the mechanism of action of trastuzumab (Herceptin). *Semin Oncol*. 1999; 26:60–70.

131. Hudziak RM, Lewis GD, Winger M, et al. p185HER2 monoclonal antibody has antiproliferative effects in vitro and sensitizes human breast tumor cells to tumor necrosis factor. *Mol Cell Biol*. 1989; 9:1165–1172.

132. Oka H, Shiozaki H, Kobayashi K, et al. Expression of E-cadherin cell adhesion molecules in human breast cancer tissues and its relationship to metastasis. *Cancer Res*. 1993; 53:1696–1701.

133. Petit AM, Rak J, Hung MC, et al. Neutralizing antibodies against epidermal growth factor and ErbB-2/neu receptor tyrosine kinases downregulate vascular endothelial growth factor

production by tumor cells in vitro and in vivo: angiogenic implications for signal transduction therapy of solid tumors. *Am J Pathol.* 1997; 151:1523–1530.

134. National Comprehensive Cancer Network (NCCN) Clinical Practice Guidelines in Oncology—v.1. 2006. www.nccn.org/professionals/physician-gls/pdf/breast.pdf. Accessed June 19, 2006.

135. Cogleigh MA, Vogel CL, Tripathy D, et al. Multinational study of the efficacy and safety of humanized anti-HER2 monoclonal antibody in women who have HER2 overexpressing metastatic breast cancer that has progressed after chemotherapy for metastatic disease. *J Clin Oncol.* 1999; 17(9):2639–2648.

136. Slamon DJ, Leyland-Jones B, Shak S, et al. Use of chemotherapy plus a monoclonal antibody against HER2 for metastatic breast cancer that overexpresses HER2. *N Engl J Med.* 2001; 344(11):783–792.

137. Piccart-Gebhart MJ, Proctor M, Leyland-Jones B, et al. Trastuzumab after adjuvant chemotherapy in HER-2 positive breast cancer. *N Engl J Med.* 2005; 353:1659–1672.

138. Romond EH, Perez EA, Bryant J, et al. Trastuzumab plus adjuvant chemotherapy for operable HER-2 positive breast cancer. *N Engl J Med.* 2005; 353:1673–1684.

139. Slamon D, Eiermann W, Robert N, et al. Phase III randomized trial comparing doxorubicin and cyclophosphamide followed by docetaxel with doxorubicin and cyclophosphamide followed by docetaxel and trastuzumab with docetaxel, carboplatin and trastuzumab in HER 2 positive early breast cancer patients. BCIRG 006 study. *Breast Cancer Res Treat.* 2005; 94(suppl 1):S5.

140. Tan-Chiu E, Yothers G, Romond E, et al. Assessment of cardiac dysfunction in a randomized trial comparing doxorubicin and cyclophosphamide followed by paclitaxel, with or without trastuzumab as adjuvant therapy in node-positive, human epidermal growth factor receptor 2-overexpressing breast cancer: NASBPB-31. *J Clin Oncol.* 2005; 23:7811–7819.

141. Herceptin [package insert]. San Francisco, CA: Genentech; February 2005.

142. Dyer MJ, Hale G, Hayhoe FG, et al. Effects of campath-1 antibodies in vivo in patients with lymphoid malignancies: influence of antibody isotype. *Blood.* 1989; 73:1431–1439.

143. Rowan W, Tite J, Topley P, et al. Cross-linking of the CAMPATH-1 antigen (DC52) mediates growth inhibition in human B- and T-lymphoma cell lines, and subsequent emergence of CD52-deficient cells. *Immunology.* 1998; 95:427–436.

144. Stern M, Herrmann R. Overview of monoclonal antibodies in cancer therapy: present and promise. *Crit Rev Oncol Hematol.* 2005 Apr; 54(1):11–29.

145. Heit W, Bunjes D, Wiesneth M, et al. Ex vivo T-cell depletion with the monoclonal antibody campath-1 plus human complement effectively prevents acute graft-versus-host disease in allogeneic bone marrow transplantation. *Br J Haematol.*1986; 64:479–486.

146. Willis F, Marsh JC, Bevan DH, et al. The effect of treatment with campath-1H in patients with autoimmune cytopenias. *Br J Haematol.* 2001 Sep; 114(4):891–898.

147. Keating M, Flinn I, Jain V, et al. Therapeutic role of alemtuzumab (campath-1H) in patients who have failed fludarabine: results of a large international study. *Blood.* 2002; 99(10):3554–3561.

148. Osterborg A, Dyer MJ, Bunjes D, et al. Phase II multicenter study of human CD52 antibody in previously treated chronic lymphocytic leukemia. European study group of campath-1H treatment in chronic lymphocytic leukemia. *J Clin Oncol.* 1997; 15(4):1567–1574.

149. Osterborg A, Fassas AS, Anagnostopoulos A, et al. Humanized CD52 monoclonal antibody campath-1H as first-line treatment in chronic lymphocytic leukaemia. *Br J Haematol.* 1996; 93:151–153.

150. Campath [package insert]. Richmond, CA: Berlex Laboratories; November 2004.

151. Bowen AL, Zomas A, Emmett E, et al. Subcutaneous campath-1H in fludarabine-resistant/relapsed chronic lymphocytic and B-prolymphocytic leukaemia. *Br J Haematol.* 1997; 96:617–619.

152. Lundin J, Kimby E, Bjorkholm M, et al. Phase II trial of subcutaneous anti-CD52 monoclonal antibody alemtuzumab (campath-1H) as first-line treatment for patients with B-cell chronic lymphocytic leukemia (B-CLL). *Blood.* 2002; 100(3):768–773.

153. Folkman J, Shing Y. Angiogenesis. *J Biol Chem.* 1992; 267:10931–10934.

154. Carmeliet P, Jain RK. Angiogenesis in cancer and other diseases. *Nature.* 2000; 407:249–257.

155. Verheul HMW, Pinedo HM. Vascular endothelial growth factor and its inhibitors. *Drugs Today.* 2003; 39(suppl C):81–93.

156. Dvorak HF, Orenstein NS, Carvalho AC, et al. Induction of a fibrin-gel investment: An early event in line 10 hepatocarcinoma growth mediated by tumor-secreted products. *J Immunol.* 1979; 122:166–174.

157. Neufeld G, Cohen T, Gengrinovitch S, et al. Vascular endothelial growth factor (VEGF) and its receptors. *FASEB.* 1999; 13:9–22.

158. Dvorak H. Vascular permeability factor/vascular endothelial growth factor: A critical cytokine in tumor angiogenesis and a potential target for diagnosis and therapy. *J Clin Oncol.* 2002; 20:4368–4380.

159. Ferrara N, Gerber H, LeCouter J. The biology of VEGF and its receptors. *Nat Med.* 2003; 9(6):669–676.

160. Gerber HP, Dixit V, Ferrara N. Vascular endothelial growth factor induces expression of the antiapoptotic proteins Bcl-2 and A1 in vascular endothelial cells. *J Biol Chem.* 1998; 273(21):13313–13316.

161. Avastin [package insert]. South San Francisco, CA: Genentech; February 2004.

162. Fernando NH, Hurwitz HI. Inhibition of vascular endothelial growth factor in the treatment of colorectal cancer. *Semin Oncol.* 2003; 30(3 suppl 6):39–50.

163. Kabbinavar F, Hurwitz HI, Fehrenbacher L, et al. Phase II, randomized trial comparing bevacizumab plus fluorouracil (FU)/leucovorin (LV) with FU/LV alone in patients with metastatic colorectal cancer. *J Clin Oncol.* 2003; 21:60–65.

164. Hurwitz H, Fehrenbacher L, Novotny W, et al. Bevacizumab plus irinotecan, fluorouracil, and leucovorin for metastatic colorectal cancer. *N Engl J Med.* 2004; 350(23):2335–2342.

165. Kabbinavar FF, Schulz J, McLeod M, et al. Bevacizumab (Avastin), a monoclonal antibody to vascular endothelial growth factor, prolongs progression-free survival in first-line colorectal cancer in subjects who are not suitable candidates for first-line CPT-11 [abstract]. *J Clin Oncol.* 2004; 22(suppl):3516.

166. Giantonio BJ, Catalano P, Meropol N, et al. High-dose bevacizumab in combination with FOLFOX4 improves survival in patients with previously treated advanced colorectal cancer: Results from the Eastern Cooperative Oncology Group (ECOG) study E3200. Paper presented at Gastrointestinal Cancers Symposium, Hollywood, FL; January 27–29, 2005.

167. Genentech. Interim analysis of Phase III trial shows avastin plus chemotherapy improved progression-free survival in patients with first-line metastatic breast cancer. Available at: http://www.gene.com/gene/news/press-releases/display.do?method=detail&id=8307. Accessed May 17, 2005.

168. Carpenter G, Cohen S. Epidermal growth factor. *J Biol Chem.* 1990; 265:7709–7712.

169. Porebska I, Harlozinska A, Bojarowski T. Expression of the tyrosine kinase activity growth factor receptors (EGFR, ERB B2, ERB B3) in colorectal adenocarcinomas and adenomas. *Tumour Biol.* 2000; 21:105–115.

170. Goldstein NI, Prewett M, Zuklys K, et al. Biological efficacy of a chimeric antibody to the epidermal growth factor receptor in a human tumor xenograft model. *Clin Cancer Res.* 1995; 1:1311–1318.

171. Gill GN, Kawamoto T, Cochet C, et al. Monoclonal anti-epidermal growth factor receptor antibodies which are inhibitors of epidermal growth factor binding and antagonists of epidermal growth factor binding and antagonists of epidermal growth factor-stimulated tyrosine protein kinase activity. *J Biol Chem.* 1984; 259:7755–7760.

172. Prewett M, Hooper A, Bassi R, et al. Enhanced antitumor activity of anti-epidermal growth factor receptor monoclonal antibody IMC-C225 in combination with irinotecan (CPT-11) against human colorectal tumor xenografts. *Clin Cancer Res.* 2002; 8:994–1103.

173. Saltz L, Rubin M, Hochster H, et al. Cetuximab 9IMC-C225) plus irinotecan (CPT-11) is active in CPT-11 refractory colorectal cancer (CRC) that expresses epidermal growth factor receptor (EGFR). Paper presented at ASCO Annual Meeting. San Francisco, CA; May 12–16, 2001.

174. Saltz L, Meropol N, Loehrer P, et al. Phase II trial of cetuximab in patients with refractory colorectal cancer that expresses the epidermal growth factor receptor. *J Clin Oncol.* 2004; 22:1201–1208.

175. Cunningham D, Humblet Y, Siena S, et al. Cetuximab monotherapy and cetuximab plus irinotecan in irinotecan-refractory metastatic colorectal cancer. *N Engl J Med.* 2004; 351:337–345.

176. Bonner JA, Harari PM, Giralt J, et al. Radiotherapy plus cetuximab for squamous-cell carcinoma of the head and neck. *N Engl J Med.* 2006; 354(6):567–578.

177. Erbitux [package insert]. Princeton, NJ: Bristol-Myers Squibb Company; March 2006.

178. Saltz I, Kies JL, Abbruzzese N, et al. The presence and intensity of the cetuximab-induced acne-like rash predicts increased survival in studies across multiple malignancies. *Proc Am Soc Clin Oncol.* 2003; 22:204. Abstract 817.

179. Perez-Solar R. Can rash associated with HER1/EGFR inhibition be used as a marker of treatment outcome? *Oncology (Huntingt).* 2003; 17(11 suppl 12):23–28.

180. Reis L, Kosary C, Hankey B, et al, eds. SEER Cancer Statistics Review, 1973–1996. NIH publication 99-2789. Bethesda, MD: National Cancer Institute; 1999.

181. Dinndorf P, Andrews R, Benjamin D, et al. Expression of normal myeloid-associated antigens by acute leukemia cells. *Blood.* 1986; 67:1048–1053.

182. Mylotarg [package insert]. Philadelphia, PA: Wyeth Laboratories; April 2005.

183. Ikemoto N, Kumar R, Ling T, et al. Calicheamicin-DNA complexes: Warhead alignment and saccharide recognition of the minor groove. *Proc Natl Acad Sci U S A.* 1995; 92:10506–10510.

184. Sievers E, Appelbaum F, Spielberger S, et al. Selective ablation of acute myeloid leukemia using antibody-targeted chemotherapy: a Phase 1 study of an anti-CD33 calicheamicin immunoconjugate. *Blood.* 1999; 93(11):3678–3684.

185. Sievers E, Larson R, Stadtmauer E, et al. Efficacy and safety of gemtuzumab ozogamicin in patients with CD33-positive acute myeloid leukemia in first relapse. *J Clin Oncol.* 2001; 19(13):3244–3254.

186. Bross P, Beitz J, Chen G, et al. Approval summary: gemtuzumab ozogamicin in relapsed acute myeloid leukemia. *Clin Cancer Res.* 2001; 7:1490–1496.

187. Giles F, Cortes J, Halliburton T, et al. Intravenous corticosteroids to reduce gemtuzumab ozogamicin infusion reactions. *Ann Pharmacother.* 2003; 37:1182–1185.

188. Rajvanshi P, Shulman H, Sievers E, et al. Hepatic sinusoidal obstruction after gemtuzumab ozogamicin (Mylotarg) therapy. *Blood.* 2002; 99(7):2310–2314.

189. Zevalin [package insert]. Cambridge, MA: Biogen Idec Inc; April 2005.
190. Bexxar [package insert]. Research Triangle Park, NC: GlaxoSmithKline; March 2005.
191. Knox S, Goris M, Trisler K, et al. Yttrium-90-labeled anti-CD20 monoclonal antibody therapy of recurrent B-cell lymphoma. *Clin Cancer Res.* 1996; 2:457–470.
192. Witzig T, White C, Wiseman G, et al. Phase I/II trial of IDEC-Y2B8 radioimmunotherapy for treatment of relapsed or refractory CD20⁺ B-cell non-Hodgkin's lymphoma. *J Clin Oncol.* 1999; 17(12):3793–3803.
193. Witzig T, Gordon L, Cabanillas F, et al. Randomized controlled trial of yttrium-90 labeled ibritumomab tiuxetan radioimmunotherapy versus rituximab immunotherapy for patients with relapsed or refractory low-grade, follicular or transformed B-cell non-Hodgkin's lymphomas. *J Clin Oncol.* 2002; 20(10):2453–2463.
194. Witzig TE, White CA, Flinn IW, et al. Zevalin™ radioimmunotherapy of rituximab-refractory follicular non-Hodgkin's lymphoma. *Blood.* 2000; 96:507a. Abstract 2183.
195. Zelentez AD, Vose JM, Knox S, et al. Iodine 131 tositumomab for patients with transformed low-grade non-Hodgkin's lymphoma: overall clinical trial experience. *Blood.* 1999; 94(suppl 1):632a. Abstract 2806.
196. Kaminski MS, Zasadny KR, Francis IR, et al. Iodine-131 anti-B1 radioimmunotherapy for B-cell lymphoma. *J Clin Oncol.* 1996; 14:1974–1981.
197. Vose J, Wahl R, Saleh M, et al. Multicenter phase II study of iodine-131 tositumomab for chemotherapy-relapsed/refractory low-grade and transformed low-grade B-cell non-Hodgkin's lymphomas. *J Clin Oncol.* 2000; 18(6):1316–1332.
198. Horning SJ, Lucas JB, Younes A, et al. Iodine-131 tositumomab for non-Hodgkin's lymphoma patients who progressed after treatment with rituximab: results of a multicenter phase II study. *Blood.* 2000 (abstr 2184); 96:508a. Abstract 2184.
199. Press O, Eary J, Gooley T, et al. A phase I/II trial of iodine-131-tositumomab (anti-CD20), etoposide, cyclophosphamide, and autologous stem cell transplantation for relapsed B-cell lymphomas. *Blood.* 2000; 96(9):2934–2942.
200. Leonard JP, Frenette G, Dillman RO, et al. Interim safety and efficacy results of Bexxar™ in a large multicenter expanded access study. *Blood.* 2001; 98:133a. Abstract 559.
201. Gordon LI, White CA, Leonard JP, et al. Zevalin™ radioimmunotherapy is associated with a low incidence of human anti-mouse antibody (HAMA) and human anti-Rituxan™ antibody (HACA) response. *Blood.* 2001; 98:228b. Abstract 4632.
202. Carter P. Improving the efficacy of antibody-based cancer therapies. *Nat Rev Cancer.* 2001; 1(2):118–129.
203. Reff ME, Kandasamy H, Braslawsky B, et al. Future of monoclonal antibodies in the treatment of hematologic malignancies. *Cancer Control.* 2002; 9(2):152–166.
204. Bohle A, Nowe CH, Ulmer AJ, et al. Elevations of cytokines interleukin-1, interleukin-2, and tumor necrosis factor in the urine of patients with intravesical bacillus Calmette-Guerin immunotherapy. *J Urol.* 1990; 144:59–64.
205. Shelley MD, Wilt TJ, Court J, et al. Intravesical bacillus Calmette-Guerin is superior to mitomycin C in reducing tumor recurrence in high-risk superficial bladder cancer: a meta analysis of randomized trials. *BJU Int.* 2004; 93:485.
206. Lamm DL, van der Meijden APM, Morales A, et al. Incidence and treatment of complications of bacillus Calmette-Guerin intravesical therapy in superficial bladder cancer. *J Urol.* 1992; 147:596.
207. Koya MP, Simon MA, Soloway MS. Complications of intravesical therapy for urothelial cancer of the bladder. *J Urol.* 2006; 175:2004–2010.
208. Bacillus of Calmette and Guerin Vaccine [package insert].
209. Raje N. Thalidomide—a revival story. *N Engl J Med.* 1999; 341(21):1606–1609.
210. Teo SK. Properties of thalidomide and its analogues: implications for anticancer therapy. *AAPSJ.* 2005; 7(1):E14–E19.
211. Lenz W. A short history of thalidomide embryopathy. *Teratology.* 1988; 38:203–215.
212. Ghobrial IM, Rajkumar SV. Management of thalidomide toxicity. *J Suppor Oncol.* 2003; 1:194–205.
213. Rajkumar SV, Gertz MA, Witzig TE. Life-threatening toxic epidermal necrolysis with thalidomide therapy for myeloma. *N Engl J Med.* 2000; 343:972–973.
214. Osman K, Gomenzo R, Rajkumar SV. Deep vein thrombosis and thalidomide therapy for multiple myeloma. *N Engl J Med.* 2001; 344:1951–1952.
215. Singhal S, Mehta J, Desikan R, et al. Anti-tumor activity of thalidomide in refractory multiple myeloma. *N Engl J Med.* 1999; 341:1565–1571.
216. Barlogie B, Spencer T, Tricot G, et al. Long term follow-up of 169 patients receiving a phase II trial of single agent thalidomide for advanced and refractory multiple myeloma. *Blood.* 2000; 96:514a.
217. Kumar S, Gertz MA, Dispenzieri A, et al. Response rate, durability of response, and survival after thalidomide therapy for relapsed multiple myeloma. *Mayo Clin Proc.* 2003; 78:34–39.
218. Weber D, Rankin K, Gavino M, et al. Thalidomide alone or with dexamethasone for previously untreated multiple myeloma. *J Clin Oncol.* 2003; 21(1):16–19.
219. Rajkumar SV, Hayman S, Gertz MA, et al. Combination therapy with thalidomide plus dexamethasone for newly diagnosed myeloma. *J Clin Oncol.* 2002; 20:4319–4323.
220. Rajkumar SV, Blood D, Vesole D, et al. Phase III clinical trial of thalidomide plus dexamethasone compared with dexamethasone alone in newly diagnosed multiple myeloma: a clinical trial co-

ordinated by the Eastern Cooperative Oncology Group. *J Clin Oncol.* 2006; 24:431–436.

221. Palumbo A, Bertola A, Musto P, et al. A prospective randomized trial of oral melphalan, prednisone, thalidomide (MPT) versus oral melphalon, prednisone (MP): An interim analysis. *Blood.* 2004; 104:207.

222. Dredge K, Horsfall R, Robinson SP, et al. Orally administered lenalidomide is anti-angiogenic in vivo and inhibits endothelial cell migration and Akt phosphorylation in vitro. *Microvascular Res.* 2005; 69:56–63.

223. Sharma RA, Steward WP, Daines CA, et al. Toxicity profile of the immunomodulatory thalidomide analogue, lenalidomide: Phase I clinical trials of three dosing schedules in patients with solid malignancies. *Eur J Cancer.* 2006; 42(14):2318–2325.

224. Bartlett JB, Dredge K, Dalgleish AG. The evolution of thalidomide and its IMiD derivatives as anticancer agents. *Nat Rev Cancer.* 2004; 4:314–322.

225. List A, Kurtin S, Roe DJ, et al. Efficacy of lenalidomide in myelodysplastic syndromes. *N Engl J Med.* 2005; 352:549–557.

226. Richardson PG, Jagannath S, Schlossman RL, et al. A multi-center, randomized, phase 2 study to evaluate the efficacy and safety of two CDC-5013 dose regimens when used alone or in combination with dexamethasone for the treatment of relapsed or refractory multiple myeloma. *Blood.* 2003; 102:235a.

227. Weber DM, Chen C, Niesvizky R, et al. Lenalidomide plus high-dose dexamethasone provides improved overall survival compared to high-dose dexamethasone alone for relapsed or refractory multiple myeloma (MM): Results of a North American phase III study (MM-009). *Proc Am Soc Clin Oncol.* 2006. Abstract 7521.

228. Berinstein N. Overview of therapeutic vaccination approaches for cancer. *Semin Oncol.* 2003; 30(3)suppl 8:1–8.

229. Lee KP, Raez LE, Podack ER. Heat shock protein-based cancer vaccines. *Hem Oncol Clin N Am.* 2006; 20:637–659.

230. Mocellin S, Mandruzzato S, Bronte V, et al. Part I: Vaccines for solid tumours. *Lancet.* 2004; 5:681–689.

231. Belli F, Testori A, Rivoltini L, et al. Vaccination of metastatic melanoma patients with autologous tumor-derived heat-shock protein peptide complexes: clinical and immunologic findings. *J Clin Oncol.* 2002; 20:4169–4180.

232. Pilla L, Patuzzo R, Rivoltini L, et al. A phase II trial of vaccination with autologous, tumor-derived heat-shock protein peptide complexes Gp96, in combination with GM-CSF and interferon-alpha in metastatic melanoma patients. *Cancer Immunol Immunother.* 2006; 55(8):958–968.

233. Lowy DR, Schiller JT. Prophylactic human papillomavirus vaccines. *J Clin Invest.* 2006; 116(5):1167–1173.

234. Faries MB, Morton DL. Therapeutic vaccines for melanoma. *Biodrugs.* 2005; 19(4):247–260.

235. O'Mahony D, Kummar S, Gutierrez ME. Non-small-cell lung cancer vaccine therapy: a concise review. *J Cin Oncol.* 2005; 23(35):9022–9028.

236. Deisseroth A, Tang Y, Maynard J, et al. Vaccine for prevention of breast cancer. ASCO Annual Meeting Proceeding Part I. *J Clin Oncol.* 2006; 24(18S):2580.

237. Tarassoff CP, Arlen PM, Gulley JL. Therapeutic vaccines for prostate cancer. *Oncologist.* 2006; 11:451–462.

238. Mosolits S, Ullenhag G, Mellstedt H. Therapeutic vaccination in patients with gastrointestinal malignancies. A review of immunological and clinical results. *Ann Oncol.* 2005:1–16.

SELF-ASSESSMENT QUESTIONS

1. Which of the following statements is/are *true* regarding the development of cancer?

   A. A "loss of function" mutation in a cancer suppressor gene often contributes to the development of cancer.
   B. A "gain of function" mutation in a proto-oncogene (oncogene) often contributes to the development of cancer.
   C. Growth factors and growth factor receptors are protein products of tumor suppressor genes.
      i. I only
      ii. III only
      iii. I and II only
      iv. II and III only
      v. I, II, and III

2. All of the following statements are *true* regarding the immune response to tumors *except*:

   A. Immune responses to tumors can be humoral and cell mediated.
   B. The immune system exhibits both protumor and antitumor effects.
   C. In the escape phase of immunoediting, the tumor cells have "learned" how to evade the innate and adaptive components of the immune system.
   D. Immune response is very efficient because tumor-specific antigens are prevalent in most types of cancer.

3. Select the true statement regarding interferons:

   A. Interferon-α is a type II interferon.
   B. Interferon activities include the enhancement of the production of natural killer cells.

C. The most common toxicity of interferon is rash.

D. Interferon-α is considered first-line therapy for individuals with hairy cell leukemia.

4. Which therapy listed below is associated with cytokine-induced capillary leak syndrome?

   A. Interferon-α
   B. Interleukin-2
   C. Thalidomide
   D. Granulocyte macrophage colony-stimulating factor

5. Which of the following statements is true regarding darbepoetin alfa?

   A. Darbepoetin alfa is chemically identical to erythropoietin.
   B. Darbepoetin should always be dosed on weight for the treatment of chemotherapy-induced anemia.
   C. Darbepoetin alfa should be titrated to a target hemoglobin concentration of 14 g/dL.
   D. Patients receiving darbepoetin alfa should be evaluated to ensure they do not require supplemental iron prior to initiation of therapy.

6. All of the following are advantages of monoclonal antibodies as cancer therapy *except*:

   A. The molecular size allows monoclonal antibodies to easily penetrate tumor cells.
   B. Monoclonal antibodies provide a targeted approach to cancer treatment.
   C. Monoclonal antibodies can serve as a vehicle to carry toxic payloads to specific tumor cells.
   D. The molecular size exceeds the renal threshold and increases half life.
   E. All of the above are advantages of monoclonal antibodies as cancer therapy.

7. Which statement most accurately describes the hypothetical monoclonal antibody curatumumab?

   A. Pretreatment antihistamine and antipyretic is necessary prior to infusion, and this antibody should be limited to one dose due to the risk of HAMA.
   B. Pretreatment antihistamine and antipyretic is probably unnecessary, but the

antibody should be limited to one dose due to the risk of HACA.

   C. Pretreatment antihistamine and antipyretic is probably unnecessary, and there are no restrictions on repeat dosing.
   D. Pretreatment antihistamine and antipyretic is necessary prior to infusion, and there are no restrictions on repeat dosing.
   E. None of the above statements accurately describes curatumumab.

8. The rituximab mechanism of action is best described as:

   A. Antibody-dependent cellular cytotoxicity
   B. Complement-dependent cytotoxicity
   C. Apoptosis induction
   D. A and B only
   E. A, B, and C

9. The rationale for the development of gemtuzumab ozogamicin was to create:

   A. An immunoconjugate that would deliver toxic radionuclide to malignant B lymphocytes.
   B. A "naked" antibody that would bind CD52 antigen on the cell surface of malignant B and T lymphocytes.
   C. An immunoconjugate that would bind epidermal growth factor receptors and block tyrosine kinase.
   D. A "naked" antibody that would bind vascular endothelial growth factor.
   E. An immunoconjugate that would deliver an antitumor antibiotic to malignant myeloblasts.

10. What is a true statement regarding thalidomide?

   A. Common side effects associated with thalidomide include sedation and fatigue.
   B. Thalidomide-induced neuropathy often presents as confusion and ataxia.
   C. Thalidomide toxicities are often only seen with initiation of the drug, and resolve with chronic therapy.
   D. Thalidomide has less neuropathy than the second-generation analogue, lenalidomide.

ANSWERS TO SELF-ASSESSMENT QUESTIONS

Chapter 1—Overview of the Immune System

1. C. Macrophages and neutrophils are two examples of innate or antigen non-specific cells. Lymphocytes (B cells and T cells) are the only antigen-specific cells in humans.

2. A. CD3 and CD7 are examples of "clusters of differentiation" molecules, and are completely unrelated to PRRs. TLR4 is a PRR, but it recognizes bacterial lipopolysaccharide rather than viral RNA.

3. C. C1q must bind to two adjacent Fc antibody fragments to activate the classical pathway. IgM circulates as a pentamer (five antibody monomers bound together in a ring-like structure), thereby easily providing the required Fc fragments for complement activation. IgG circulates as a monomer and is, therefore, not capable of activating complement unless a second IgG immune complex binds to C1q.

4. D. Immunologic memory, adaptation, and formation of an immune complex are all characteristics of the adaptive immune system. Each is performed by lymphocytes or the byproducts of lymphocytes.

5. B. T cells cannot process and present antigen since they do not express class II HLA molecules. The other three cells are known as "professional antigen-presenting cells" because they *do* express class II HLA.

6. D. Innate immunity is not capable of adaptation or clonal expansion. Only lymphocytes can do this (adaptive immunity). Transplant rejection is a normal adaptive immune response against a "foreign pathogen"—in this case, unfortunately, a transplanted organ.

7. C. Interleukin-2 has no role in helper T cell activation. Instead, IL-2 is involved in clonal expansion of an activated T cell.

8. A. Tregs are already activated when they enter the bloodstream. Therefore, they don't need any activation signals.

9. C. Cognate B cell activation against a particular antigen can only occur between the B cell and a helper T cell that has already been activated by the same antigen. Follicular dendritic cells are capable of "priming" B cells, but full activation cannot take place without helper T cell signaling.

10. B. Allergic rhinitis is Type I (mast cell degranulation). Immune thrombocytopenic purpura is Type II (immune complex bound to the surface of a circulating platelet), and contact dermatitis is Type IV (T cell mediated). Rheumatoid arthritis is Type III (immune complexes deposited in synovial fluid of joints).

Chapter 2—Monoclonal Antibodies and Antibody Fragments

1. D. The original mAbs were made by fusing murine (mouse) spleen cells and murine myeloma cells, resulting in the secretion of murine mAbs.

2. B. The response is a human against murine (mouse) antibody (HAMA).

3. A. The less deviation from the normal structure of human antibodies and, therefore, foreign protein, the less likely it is that a reactive immune response will be induced.

4. C. Chimeric mAbs use murine variable regions, while the rest of the mAb is of human origin.

Therefore, about 1/3 of the peptide sequence is typically of murine origin.

5. A. Production via genetic engineering for fragments is simpler and faster than that for whole mAbs.

6. D. Plasmids and bacteriophage display, both using bacterial expression systems, are used for synthesizing fragments. To date, bacterial chromosomal DNA has not been useful in propagating Ab fragments.

7. B. The variable fragment has been the most useful for delivery of toxins to target cells.

8. C. Each binding region is targeted to a unique conformation, making bispecific mAbs useful in bringing targets or target and toxin into close proximity.

9. C. ^{99m}Tc emits a gamma photon, ideal for imaging, while the others emit particles, ideal for therapy.

10. A. The "o" within the name indicates this antibody is of murine origin.

Chapter 3—Cytokines, Chemoattractants, and Adhesion Molecules

1. D. The ancient definition of the inflammatory response consists of redness (rubor), pain (dolor), swelling (tumor), and heat (calor). Therefore, the correct answer is both A (pain and redness) and C (swelling and heat).

2. C. The main cytokines mediating innate immune responses are also known as pro-inflammatory cytokines. These comprise IL-6, IL-1, and TNF-α.

3. A. Sepsis is due to a massive release of TNF-α by systemic tissues. The released TNF-α causes clot formation in the small vessels of vital organs such as the kidneys and liver. This leads to decreased perfusion and, eventually, multiple organ failure.

4. B. The three main functions of type I interferons are (1) inhibition of viral replication, (2) activation of NK cells, and (3) enhanced expression of MHC class I molecules on neighboring non-infected cells.

5. D. The function of Th1 cells is to activate macrophages to such an extent that they can destroy intravesicular microbes. The main function of Th2 cells is to activate B cells. The Th1 cells mainly produce IL-2 and IFN-γ, while Th2 cells mainly produce IL-4, IL-5, IL-10, and IL-13. The cells that are affected by Th1 cells are mainly macrophages, while those activated by Th2 cells are mainly B cells. Therefore, the correct answer is "all of the above."

6. E. The subset of CD4 T cells known as regulatory, or suppressor, T cells produce the anti-inflammatory cytokines IL-4, IL-10, and TGF-β. This profile of cytokines allows the regulatory T cells to inhibit pro-inflammatory responses such as those present in rheumatoid arthritis.

7. D. The activation of Th1 cells is necessary for defense against intravesicular pathogens that live in macrophages. The cytokines produced by the Th1 cells activate the macrophage to such an extent that it can then destroy the intravesicular microbes.

8. C. TNF-α is a pro-inflammatory cytokine that plays a role in the pathogenesis of rheumatoid arthritis. Treatment with antibodies against TNF-α has been used to improve symptoms of this autoimmune disease.

9. C. The structural classification of chemokines is based on the number and position of cysteines near the amino terminus.

10. A. CXCL8 has two important functions. One is to change the adhesive properties of leukocytes by changing expression of the cell surface molecules. The other is to guide the recruited leukocyte to the center of infection by a concentration-based gradient.

11. E. Adhesion molecules play a number of important roles in the immune response. These roles include interaction of antigen-presenting cells with T cells, extravasation of neutrophils to sites of inflammation, and homing of B cells and naïve T cells to secondary lymphoid tissue. Therefore, the correct answer is "all of the above."

12. C. GlyCAM-1 is a vascular addressin expressed on the high endothelial venules. It is important for the movement of naïve T cells into lymph nodes.

Chapter 4—Mechanisms of Hypersensitivity and Drug Allergy

1. D. Refer to Table 4.1.

2. A. Refer to Table 4.2.

3. B. The release of preformed mediators begins a physiologic response within minutes of allergen exposure.

4. C. The correct answer is often a late phase reaction (4–6 hours after allergen exposure).

5. B. Refer to Table 4.2. Beneficial aspects of the immune mechanisms underlying type I hypersensitivity include the expulsion of parasites.

6. C. Refer to Table 4.2.

7. A. Refer to Table 4.2; type II hypersensitivity defends the body against cellular pathogens such as extracellular bacteria.

8. A. Refer to Table 4.2.

9. C. Formation of immune complexes near the site of administration elicits a localized Arthus reaction.

10. D. Type IV relies on T lymphocytes and macrophages.

11. D. Contact dermatitis reactions are also seen after exposure to metals, cosmetics, plants, rubber, medications, resins, and some chemicals.

12. B. Refer to Table 4.2.

13. C. Topical administration presents the greatest risk.

14. D. Both sulfonamides and halothane are metabolized to haptens through P450-mediated metabolism.

15. B. The frequency of allergic reactions to cephalosporin administration is only 5.6%.

16. A. Quinine-induced thrombocytopenia is the correct answer.

17. D. Patient factors such as specific HLA alleles, slow acetylator status, and dose and duration of exposure increase the risk for developing drug-induced type III hypersensitivity.

18. D. Drugs applied topically, metabolized by keratinocytes, and drugs administered orally, metabolized by hepatocytes, are correct.

19. A. Physicians tell patients to carry an epinephrine syringe.

20. A. Antibiotics appear to be the class of drug with the greatest risk for fatality.

Chapter 5—Inflammatory Diseases and Immunization

1. B. Since histamine release is a major hallmark of IgE mediated Type I hypersensitivities, H1 antagonists are very effective in treating the Type I allergic response.

2. D. While epinephrine is a proven effective *treatment* for anaphylaxis, hyposensitization immunotherapy is a proven therapy for patients with seasonal allergic rhinitis, allergic asthma, or insect venom hypersensitivity. Omalizumab is indicated as a second-line therapy for moderate to severe persistent asthma patients who do not respond to combination therapy; avoidance of the trigger is the only proven effective prevention for anaphylaxis.

3. C. Ankylosing spondylitis has an almost absolute association with the HLA-B27 allele.

4. B. Predominate populations of Th2 CD4+ T cells lead to increased B cell activation, and subsequently to a robust humoral response.

5. D. Protein processing, cytokines, cytokine receptors, and other genes are all non-HLA genes.

6. A. Th1 CD4+ T cells activate professional antigen presenting cells, leading to the cellular response.

7. E. IFN-α, which increases levels of IL-10 and IL-4, has been shown to attenuate Th1 activity. Likewise, the T cell modifying peptide glatiramer acetate (Copaxone®) has been shown to bind both MHC and TCR, inducing IL-14, IL-10, and TGFβ-1 release from Th2/Treg cells and thus decreasing Th1/CTL cell activation.

8. See Table 5-2 for answers.

Chapter 6—Common Infectious Diseases and Immunization

1. E. Antibody is important for clearing extracellular organisms; these can be viruses (when they are not inside of cells), protozoans, or bacteria. Th1 cells are also called inflammatory T cells and are recruited to the site of an infection of intracellular bacteria (e.g., tuberculosis); these cells are able to recruit and activate macrophages to more successfully destroy this type of bacteria. Cytotoxic T cells are able to recognize cells that have a pathogen reproducing in the cytoplasm of the cell (generally viruses) and induce death in these cells.

2. D. Interferons are produced by both macrophages and virally infected cells. Macrophages produce interferon γ (IFN-γ, immune interferon), and the virally infected cells produce interferons α and β (IFN-α and IFN-β). Interferons can affect the function of cells throughout the body. The effects of IFNs on cells of the immune

system include activation of natural killer (NK) cells, stimulation of antigen presentation and costimulator (B7) expression by antigen-presenting cells, and enhancement of CD4$^+$ Th1 responses. The effect of IFNs on other cells acts to inhibit viral infection in susceptible cells. Viral infection is inhibited by decreasing cellular receptors for the virions, reducing virus entry into the host cell, inhibiting transcription of viral genes, and inhibiting production of viral DNA and RNA genomes. NK cells are able to recognize host cells that are infected by a virus and stimulate these cells to undergo apoptosis, thus inhibiting viral replication.

Interleukins are produced by many cells, but they serve to regulate cell responses, and in general are not important for clearing viral infections.

3. C. Perforin is a protein related to the C9 component of complement and functions by creating holes in the plasma membrane of an infected cell. These holes allow granzymes access to the cytoplasm of the cell, resulting in the induction of apoptosis.

Antibody and complement are only able to clear pathogens, which are outside cells; IFN-α and IFN-β are produced by cells, which are infected with a virus, not by cytotoxic T cells.

4. A. PAMP receptors recognize microbial products including glycolipids, lipoproteins, and flagella, and these receptors in cooperation with Toll receptors activate the phagocytic cell. Other receptors recognize bacterial polysaccharides, glycolipids, lipopolysaccharides, and lipoarabinomannans, and also aid in the phagocytosis of the bacteria.

5. D. IgA is important in protecting the gut against parasitic worms, helping to prevent their attachment to the gut wall. IgE mediates mast cell activation by binding to high affinity receptors on these cells. Once antigen has bound IgE, the mast cell degranulates, releasing toxic mediators including histamine and heparin that are toxic to the parasites. The activated mast cells also secrete cytokines and chemokines, which activate inflammation and recruit additional cells to the site of infection, and leukotrienes, which stimulate mucous production and smooth muscle contraction.

IgG may play a small role through activation of antibody-dependent cell-mediated cytotoxicity, but it does not have a role as important as the other classes of antibody.

6. A. Immunization is the introduction of a killed or weakened pathogen or components of the pathogen with the specific intent of stimulating an adaptive immune response to the antigen.

7. D. A live vaccine should not be able to establish a pathogenic infection that is severe and easily disseminated through the population. In addition, it should not be able to establish a latent infection that might recur in the individual at a later date. This is especially important because a vaccine that can establish a latent infection might be able to cause a severe infection if the recipient becomes immunocompromised.

8. C. Killed vaccines cannot replicate within the host; therefore, they cannot cause disease or revert to pathogenic variants and spread through the population. Because they cannot replicate, they generally require larger amounts (not less) of antigen than does an attenuated vaccine. The inclusion of large amounts of extraneous material means that there is an increased possibility of adverse reactions due to these materials.

9. D. The protective antigen in Hemophilus B is the purified polysaccharide. Pure polysaccharides are T-independent antigen. These antigens are unable to stimulate T cells and are unable to induce protective immunity in children less than 2 years old. By cross-linking the polysaccharide to protein (often tetanus toxoid), the vaccine is able to stimulate T cells (T dependent) and induce immune responses in children.

10. C. A toxoid is a chemically inactivated toxin, which has the same three dimensional structure as the active toxin and which, when used as an immunogen, will stimulate the production of neutralizing Ab. If activation is incomplete, the toxoid may revert to a biologically active toxin.

11. B. The tetanus vaccine is a chemically inactivated toxoid vaccine; the Hib vaccine is a conjugate of tetanus or diphtheria toxoid and purified polysaccharide. The measles vaccine is an attenuated viral vaccine. The hepatitis B vaccine is produced by expressing the hepatitis B surface antigen (HBsAg) in the yeast, *Saccharomyces cerevisiae*. Expression of HBsAg in this vector resulted in the formation of highly immunogenic particles containing this Ag, which resemble the immunogenic Dane particles that had been purified from human plasma.

12. E. Refer to Table 6.5.

13. E. Passive immunization transfers antibodies specific for certain toxins, venoms, and diseases. This passive transfer allows antibody to bind to the antigen and prevent antigen binding to the target cell. Antibody to toxins and venoms includes snake and spider venom as well as botulism, tetanus, and diphtheria toxin. Numerous diseases, such as hepatitis A, hepatitis B, herpes family viruses, and respiratory syncytial virus, can be treated with antibody. Finally, Rh-negative pregnant women with an Rh incompatibility with the fetus are treated to prevent the development of anti-Rh antibodies in the woman.

14. E. IVIG is used to replace antibody in patients who cannot produce their own antibody. These include both primary and secondary immunodeficiencies. Primary immunodeficiencies include primary agammaglobulinemias. Secondary immunodeficiencies may result from malignancy or treatment for the malignancy, certain viral and bacterial infections, and AIDS. In addition, IVIG has been shown to be able to inhibit B cell activation and production of autoantibodies in certain autoimmune diseases and thrombocytopenias.

15. B. Multivalent vaccines are vaccines that contain more than one purified antigen. The advantage of these vaccines is that, with a single injection, they stimulate an immune response to a number of different antigens. In other words, by including antigens from more than one pathogen, the one immunization induces immunity to more than one disease. Examples of multivalent vaccines include the diphtheria, pertussis, and tetanus vaccines as well as the measles, mumps, rubella vaccine.

Chapter 7—Immunology of HIV Infection and AIDS

1. C. When HIV is encountered, the immune response triggers both humoral and cellular factors. Because HIV is persistently replicating, the normal return to quiescence is not observed, and the immune system enters a state of chronic activation.

2. C. Three steps are necessary for HIV to enter cells, including attachment, co-receptor binding, and HIV fusion. The initial attachment between virus and cell is the coupling of the viral gp120 subunit to the CD4$^+$ T cell.

3. C. The proportion of cases occurring among women, racial, and ethnic minorities, and via heterosexual transmission, increased over the decade of 1993 to 2003. The largest decline in HIV cases is among perinatal transmission.

4. B. Persons with a CD4$^+$ T-cell count <200 cells/mm^3 or an AIDS indicator condition such as PCP pneumonia would be considered to have a diagnosis of AIDS.

5. B. Infants born to HIV-infected mothers have maternally acquired antibodies, which can be detected up to 18 months of age.

6. A. PCR is used to detect antibodies to HIV in the patient's blood.

7. D. Kaposi's sarcoma and non-Hodgkin's lymphoma are malignancies that are associated with HIV infection.

8. C. Treatment options for *Pneumocystis jiroveci* pneumonia include trimethoprim/sulfamethoxazole, atovaquone, and pentamidine. Dapsone is effective for prophylaxis of PCP, but is not recommended by itself for treatment.

9. E. Blood is the standard for HIV testing, however, alternative antibody testing has been developed for testing saliva and urine.

10. E. With adequate immune reconstitution from antiretroviral therapy, it is safe to discontinue chemoprophylaxis for select opportunistic infections, including *Pneumocystis jiroveci* pneumonia, toxoplasmosis, and cryptococcal meningitis.

11. D. Initial treatment for cryptococcal meningitis includes amphotericin B, combined with flucytosine, to decrease the risk of relapse for 2 weeks. This is then followed by consolidation treatment and secondary prophylaxis with fluconazole.

12. B. The majority of HIV-infected individuals harbor the chemokine coreceptor CCR5.

13. E. Transmission of HIV may occur through sexual, parenteral, and perinatal exposures.

14. D. HIV viremia can be quantified by polymerase chain reaction (PCR), nucleic acid sequence-based amplification (NASBA), and branched DNA signal amplification (bDNA).

15. A. Toxoplasmosis is the most common cause of focal encephalitis in patients with AIDS.

Chapter 8—HIV Treatment Strategies

1. C. Eradication of HIV infection or cure is not possible at this time. The goals of therapy are to achieve maximal and durable viral load suppression, restore and maintain immunologic function, reduce morbidity and mortality, and improve quality of life.

2. D. HIV therapy should be modified for treatment failure, toxicity, or nonadherence.

3. C. Women with CD4$^+$ T-cell counts >250 cells/mm^3 at the start of therapy, including pregnant women, are 12 fold more likely to develop severe, life-threatening, and sometimes fatal hepatoxicity. Risk in men with CD4$^+$ T-cell counts >400 cells/mm^3 at the start of therapy is 6.3% versus 1.2% in those with <400 cells/mm^3.

4. C. Drug toxicity has been shown to be a leading cause for nonadherence to antiretroviral therapy.

5. B. Public Health Force Task Force guidelines recommend triple combination regimens with zidovudine as a part of the regimen.

6. A. Currently FDA-approved antiretroviral drugs act by the following mechanisms: inhibition of fusion, reverse transcriptase, and protease.

7. B. Lipodystrophy syndrome describes morphologic changes (fat atrophy and hypertrophy) as well as metabolic complications (dyslipidemias and insulin resistance).

8. A. Stavudine is an NRTI. Enfuvirtide is a fusion inhibitor. Saquinavir and tipranavir are protease inhibitors.

9. A. The "prime-boost strategy" uses two vaccines, one after the other, to build a better immune response.

10. B. Recently published guidelines for the management of chronic kidney disease in HIV-infected patients recommend that all newly diagnosed patients have their kidney function evaluated by urinalysis and estimations of glomerular filtration rate (GFR) at baseline.

11. A. Approximately 8% of patients who start abacavir will develop a hypersensitivity reaction that involves non-specific gastrointestinal complaints, myalgias, fatigue, fever, shortness of breath, and rash.

12. C. Therapeutic immunization, corticosteroids, and IFN-α are potential immune-based therapies for HIV infection.

13. A. Strategies that either suppress or enhance the immune response to HIV infection are under evaluation.

14. B. False. The rationale for using therapeutic drug monitoring (TDM) is that subtherapeutic serum levels of protease inhibitors can lead to the development of resistance and hence failure of the regimen.

15. C. Immunologic adjuvants are used to increase the type, strength, and durability of the vaccine response.

Chapter 9—Solid Organ Transplantation

1. C. Class I and II HLAs serve as the primary activators of the helper T cell response in initiating the first steps of the immune response to foreign tissue. HLA-A, B, and C are classified as Class I proteins (found on the cell surface of most cells). HLA-DP, DQ, and DR are Class II proteins (more restricted; found mainly on antigen presenting cells, monocytes, and B lymphocytes). However, it is the combination of Class I and II HLA-A, B, and DR that is considered most important for a successful outcome in transplantation.

2. B. Hyperacute rejection occurs within minutes to a few hours posttransplant (essentially in the operating room). Accelerated acute rejection usually occurs within 6 days posttransplant and typically does not respond to antirejection therapy. Chronic rejection usually occurs beyond 6 months posttransplant with biopsy findings consistent with intimal thickening and fibrosis and also does not respond well to antirejection therapy.

3. D. Corticosteroids cause a rapid and profound drop in circulating T cells as a result of various pharmacologic effects, including a direct inhibitory effect on circulating lymphocyte, modulation of specific cellular immune functions, and *nonspecific, potent anti-inflammatory* effect—a result of the inhibition of arachidonic acid release and suppression of macrophage phagocytosis.

4. A. The most common side effects associated with cyclosporine include nephrotoxicity, hepatotoxicity, hypercholesterolemia, and cosmetic effects such as hirsutism and gingival hyperplasia. Tacrolimus can induce diabetes, hepatotoxicity, and CNS effects such as tremors. The most common cosmetic effect seen with tacrolimus is alopecia.

5. C. Mycophenolate mofetil is associated with dose-related gastrointestinal side effects such as diarrhea and bone marrow suppression. CNS effects and nephrotoxicity are not common side effects associated with mycophenolate mofetil.

6. B. OKT3 is a murine monoclonal antibody that binds to the CD3 receptor on circulating T cells, thus inhibiting the generation of cytotoxic T cells responsible for graft rejection. Most patients experience a mild to severe flu-like syndrome with the first several doses, which is related to the activation of T cells, resulting in release of cytokines such as IL2 and TNF. It is the production of these cytokines that result in these side effects.

7. D. Cyclosporine is metabolized by CYP3A4 and is a substrate and inhibitor of CYP3A4; the potential for drug interactions with other agents that are metabolized by this pathway remain high. Inhibitors of CYP3A4 such as verapamil and fluconazole may increase cyclosporine blood concentrations. Beverages like grapefruit juice have also been shown to inhibit gut metabolism of cyclosporine, resulting in increased cyclosporine drug concentrations. Inducers of CYP3A4 such as phenytoin results in decreased cyclosporine blood concentrations and potential allograft rejection.

8. B. Acute renal transplant rejection is initially treated with high dose pulse corticosteroid therapy, which can reverse 70% to 75% of these rejection episodes. Antilymphocyte preparations like ATG/OKT3 are reserved for severe acute rejection episodes or steroid resistant acute rejection episodes. CSA and quadruple therapy are maintenance agents that typically do not play a role in reversing acute rejection episodes.

9. A. Cytomegalovirus remains the most prevalent viral pathogen, causing symptomatic infection in up to 60% of the transplant population. Infections with herpes, Epstein Barr virus, and hepatitis C are generally confined to latent infections reactivated by immunosuppression or other stress factors.

10. A. In the era of modern immunosuppression, the incidence of acute allograft rejection is <20% at most centers. Prophylaxis and treatment of viral infections are fairly effective, and the incidence of new onset diabetes is largely dose related. However, cardiovascular disease, potentiated by hypertension and hypercholesterolemia, affects more that 80% of kidney transplant recipients, with cardiovascular disease being the primary cause of death within the first year in these patients.

Chapter 10—Bone Marrow Transplantation

1. C. Bone marrow transplantation is typically performed to allow for new bone marrow to grow after it has been destroyed by myeloablative chemotherapy or disease.

2. E. An allogeneic BMT provides an increased graft-versus-leukemia (GVL) effect, and the donor's marrow is free of malignancy, which both decrease the risk of disease relapse. However, because the donor is genetically distinct from the recipient, there is significant risk of graft-versus-host disease (GVHD). In addition, allogeneic donor availability is poor, with only 30% of Americans having a genetically matched sibling and widely variable rates of matching an unrelated donor.

3. D. Autologous BMT is associated with increased risk of disease relapse compared to other types of BMT, since malignant cells may be re-infused along with the new hematopoietic stem cells. Donor lymphocyte depletion is also associated with increased disease relapse, since the T lymphocytes that would typically destroy the host malignancy have been removed. Lastly, bone marrow transplantation is associated with greater risk of relapse when compared with peripheral blood stem cell transplantation, as the peripheral blood may be less likely to be contaminated with malignant cells.

4. C. The cytokine storm is in the first phase of a three-phase cascade of events leading to aGVHD. aGVGD typically begins prior to day 100 rather than after and is far more common in MUD transplants due to greater differences in minor histocompatibility antigens in unrelated donors than in matched-sibling donors. Cytotoxic and helper T cells drive the tissue damage associated with aGVHD.

5. A. The skin, liver, and gastrointestinal tract are the organ systems typically affected by aGVHD in patients receiving allogeneic BMT. Kidneys are not affected.

6. D. Drug interactions are very common with cyclosporine since it is a CYP450 3A4 substrate. Renal toxicity is one of the most common adverse effects of cyclosporine and manifests as rising serum creatinine and electrolyte

wasting. Myelosuppression is uncommon with cyclosporine, but does often occur with mycophenolate.

7. B. 6-Mercaptopurine is not typically used in the treatment of cGVHD. All of the other agents have been tested in limited studies for cGVHD with variable success.

8. C. Prophylactic acyclovir should be used for all BMT patients who are HSV seropositive. Fluconazole lacks coverage for mold infections, thus *Aspergillus* is not affected by fluconazole. Bacterial infections are most common during the pre-engraftment phase following BMT when the patient is neutropenic. The primary toxicity of ganciclovir is myelosuppression.

9. D. Both prophylactic and preemptive ganciclovir strategies have been utilized for CMV in BMT patients, although preemptive ganciclovir decreases toxicity with similar outcomes. Acyclovir has minimal activity against CMV and should not be used for prophylaxis.

Chapter 11—The Immunotherapy of Cancer

1. C. Statements I and II are true regarding the development of cancer. Statement III is false because growth factors and growth factor receptors are protein products of protooncogenes/oncogenes.

2. D. The first three statements are true, and option "D" is false because tumor-specific antigens are *not* very prevalent.

3. B. Interferon activities include the enhancement of the production of natural killer cells. Interferon α is a type I interferon. The most common toxicities seen with IFNs are constitutional symptoms, although rash can occur. At this time, IFN α is not considered first-line therapy for individuals with hairy cell leukemia.

4. B. Capillary leak syndrome is an expected side effect with interleukin-2 therapy. It may occur with other cytokines, but is not as common with doses used in clinical practice (e.g., GM-CSF and IFN).

5. D. Patients receiving darbepoetin alfa should be evaluated to assure they do not require supplemental iron prior to intitiation of therapy, as they will be producing red blood cells.

6. A. The molecular size allows monoclonal antibodies to easily penetrate tumor cells. The average size of a mAb is 150 kD, much too large to passively move through cell membranes.

7. C. Pretreatment antihistamine and antipyretic is probably unnecessary, and there are no restrictions on repeat dosing. According to the United States Adopted Names (USAN) Council for naming mAbs, curatumumab is a purely human source antibody. The risk for hypersensitivity reactions is minimal; therefore, the need for pretreatment with antihistamine and antipyretic is probably unnecessary. Likewise, the development of HAMA or HACA is not a concern and repeat dosing is feasible.

8. E. A, B, and C. Rituximab has been shown to demonstrate ADCC, CDC, and induction of apoptosis (see text for supporting information).

9. E. An immunoconjugate, which would deliver an antitumor antibiotic to malignant myeloblasts, is the correct answer. Gemtuzumab ozogamicin targets CD33 antigen present on leukemic myeloblasts. Once the antibody is bound to CD33, the complex internalizes via endocytosis. The antitumor antibiotic calicheamicin is then believed to be released inside myeloblast lysosomes where it migrates to the nucleus and binds to DNA in the minor groove. This causes double-strand breaks and cell death.

10. A. Common side effects associated with thalidomide include sedation and fatigue. Neuropathy also occurs, often increasing over time, and presents as peripheral neuropathy and constipation. Lenalidomide appears to have less neurotoxicity when compared to thalidomide.

Glossary

ABO system—the major blood grouping system in humans.

Active immunization—inducing immune system recognition and reactivity against harmful agents by exposure to antigens (also known as vaccination).

Adaptive (acquired) immunity—an antigen-specific immunity that develops as a result of exposure to an antigen.

Addressins—mucin-like vascular adhesion molecules expressed mainly by the endothelium and bound to L-selectin.

Adhesion molecules—a group of molecules that can be grouped into four structural classes. They play important roles in diverse immune responses such as interaction of leukocytes with the endothelial cells of blood vessels and homing of naïve T and B lymphocytes to secondary lymphoid tissues.

Adjuvant—material, usually an aluminum salt, capable of nonspecifically enhancing an immune response.

Adoptive immunotherapy—the transfer of active immunologic reagents to a tumor-bearing host (such as the transfer of cells with antitumor reactivity to mediate antitumor effects).

Affinity—the strength of attraction between a single binding site on an antibody and the corresponding binding site on its complementary antigen; an expression of strength of binding between two entities.

Affinity chromatography—a method used to isolate pure proteins by coupling either antibody or antigen to an inert solid phase, such as dextran beads in a column. A solution containing the antigen or the antibody of interest is run through the column, where the specific antigen or antibody will bind. The specific antigen or antibody can then be eluted from the column in a concentrated pure form.

Agammaglobulinemia—a deficiency of all classes of serum immunoglobulins.

Agglutination—the process by which particles (e.g., red blood cells or bacteria) complex to form clumps; specific immunoglobulins sometimes cause this effect.

AIDS-related complex—a term encompassing a variety of conditions, including unexplained weight loss, oral candidiasis, unexplained fever, extrainguinal lymphadenopathy, oral hairy leukoplakia, unexplained night sweats, herpes zoster, and unexplained diarrhea.

Allele—one of two or more alternate genes present at a given locus on a chromosome.

Allergen—an antigen capable of causing an allergic reaction.

Allergy—an immunologic hypersensitivity.

Alloantigens—allelic forms of antigens present in some, but not all, individuals in a given species.

Allogeneic or allogenic—molecules or cell types within a species that have identical functions but are antigenically distinct.

Allograft—grafted tissue of genetically nonidentical individuals of the same species.

Alloreactive—an immune response to a transplanted allograft.

Alpha-fetoprotein—an embryonic globulin, similar to serum albumin, that can be detected in the serum of adults with primary liver cancer tumors.

Anaphylatoxins—complement fragments C4a, C3a, and C5a, which can induce mast cell degranulation, resulting in increased vascular permeability and smooth muscle contraction.

Anaphylaxis—an immediate allergic reaction mediated by IgE-sensitized mast cells.

Anergy—diminished cell-mediated reactivity as shown by the inability to react to a battery of common skin-test antigens.

Antibody—an immunoglobulin produced by mature B cells or plasma cells in response to an antigenic stimulus and capable of binding with a specific antigen.

Antibody affinity—a measure of the strength of the bond between a single antigen-combining site (Fab) and an antigenic determinant.

Antibody avidity—a measure of the antigen-antibody binding strength that is dependent on the affinity to the epitope and the effective number of binding sites on the antibody. Avidity is enhanced by the number of bonds formed and is usually much greater than affinity.

Antibody-dependent cell-mediated cytotoxicity—a means of destroying target cells by coating them with antibody that attracts Fc receptor–bearing non-antigen-specific effector cells (natural killer cells, macrophages, and neutrophils).

Antigen—a molecule or the specific molecular sequence of a molecule recognized by the immune system (i.e., the target of an immune response).

Antigen-binding sites—locations on the antibody molecule that combine specifically with the corresponding antigenic determinant.

Antigenic modulation—a phenomenon in which cells lose or internalize their surface antigens after interactions with the immune system.

Antigen-presenting cell—a specific type of cell (e.g., macrophage, dendritic cell, or B cell) that activates an antigen-specific helper T lymphocyte by displaying processed antigen complexed to a major histocompatibility complex class II molecule.

Anti-idiotypic antibodies—antibodies directed against the surface determinants of the antigen-combining site of other antibodies.

Antilymphocyte globulins—antibodies directed against lymphocytes, usually used as an immunosuppressive agent. Commonly produced by hyperimmunizing animals with human lymphocytes.

Antiserum—serum from any animal that contains antibodies against a specific antigen.

Antithymocyte globulins—polyclonal antibodies directed against human thymus lymphocytes, typically used as an immunosuppressive agent. Commonly produced by hyperimmunizing horses with human thymocytes.

Antitoxin—an antibody or antiserum prepared in response to a toxin or toxoid.

Apoptosis—programmed cell death.

Ascites—serous fluid that collects in the peritoneum of an animal; this fluid may contain antibodies produced by an injected hybridoma.

Asplenia—impaired reticuloendothelial function of the spleen.

Atopy—the state of being allergic to normal environmental antigens.

Attenuated—made less virulent.

Attenuated vaccine—a preparation composed of live microbes of low virulence that can induce immunity against highly virulent microbes.

Autoantibody—an antibody to normal self antigens.

Autoantigen—a host's self antigen.

Autoimmunity—an immune response to autoantigens.

Autologous antigen—an antigen found in the host that does not normally elicit an immune response; also called a self antigen.

Avidity—the functional combined strength of all the interactions between an antigen and the entire antibody (multiple Fab sites). *See* **Antibody avidity.**

Azathioprine—a purine analogue converted to 6-mercaptopurine in vivo, useful as an immunosuppressant.

B lymphocytes—antigen-specific cells derived from the bone marrow in mammals that are the precursors of plasma cells, which respond to antigenic stimulation by secreting antibodies.

Bacillus Calmette-Guérin—a strain of live, attenuated *Mycobacterium bovis* that may induce resolution of some local tumors, probably through enhanced macrophage- or T cell–mediated activity.

Basophils—antigen non-specific granulocytic cells that release histamine and other inflammatory mediators during an inflammatory response.

Biological response modifiers—a heterogeneous group of substances that, in a specific or nonspecific manner, promote immune interactions with malignant cells.

Blotting—a technique of transferring DNA, RNA, or protein separated in gels onto a reactive membrane, such as nitrocellulose.

Bursa of Fabricius—lymphoid tissue found in the hind gut of birds that is responsible for B-lymphocyte maturation.

Cachectin—a monokine, also referred to as tumor necrosis factor, that is an endogenous pyrogen and catabolic substance.

Carcinoembryonic antigen—an antigen normally found in the fetal gut that may be present in the serum of patients with cancer (primarily of the colon or lung) as well as in smokers and patients with inflammatory conditions.

Cell-mediated immunity—antigen-specific immunity mediated by T lymphocytes.

Chemokines—a large family of molecules, which play a pivotal role in the migration of leukocytes to an area of damage. Different type of cells can produce chemokines in order to recruit leukocytes such as neutrophils and monocytes to the foci of infection. Chemokines also play a role in lymphocyte development and migration, adaptive immune responses, and angiogenesis.

Chemotaxis—the chemical attraction of antigen-non-specific phagocytic cells to the site of inflammation or infection; the attraction of living protoplasm to chemical stimuli.

Chimeric antibody—an antibody made up of fragments from different species (e.g., an antibody with mouse Fab and human Fc segments).

Class I genes—genes of the major histocompatibility complex responsible for compatibility of tissues and organs (also known as histocompat-ibility or transplantation genes); HLA-A, -B, and -C loci encode for the class I HLA molecules in humans.

Class II genes—genes of the major histocompatibility complex that participate in the immune response (also known as Ir genes); HLA-D loci encode for the class II HLA molecules in humans.

Class III genes—genes of the major histocompatibility complex that contribute to the complement system and tumor necrosis factor.

Clone—one of a group of genetically identical cells derived from a single original cell.

Clusters of differentiation (CD)—a nomenclature system that categorizes cell surface molecules of human leukocytes; also used to categorize monoclonal antibodies according to the antigens they recognize.

Codominance—equal expression of alleles inherited from each parent.

Colony-forming unit (CFU), granulocyte-monocyte—a term used to describe the in vitro production of a colony of cells of granulocytic and monocytic lineage within a semisolid medium, such as methylcellulose.

Colony-stimulating factors (CSFs)—a group of substances that increase production and activity of various types of hematologic cells. Granulocyte-macrophage CSF stimulates granulocytes and macrophages; granulocyte CSF stimulates primarily granulocytes (neutrophils).

Complement—a network of circulating and cell surface proteins that initiate and stimulate early antigen non-specific inflammatory responses via chemotaxis and opsonization.

Conjugate—a product obtained by joining two or more dissimilar molecules (e.g., radioisotopes, drugs, or toxins covalently coupled to an antibody).

Cytokines—a generic term for soluble substances produced by cells to communicate with other cells to trigger or suppress cellular activity after interaction with an antigen. *See also* **Soluble mediators** (synonym).

Cytotoxic T cell (Tc)—a T cell that expresses surface CD8; identifies self and non-self via MHC-I; and, when activated, differentiates into a "killer" cell that is effective against virally infected and cancerous cells.

Cytotoxicity—the process of killing cells.

Delayed hypersensitivity reactions—a specific inflammatory immune reaction elicited by an antigen and mediated by primed T cells; does not usually appear until 24 hours after contact with an antigen.

Demargination—the movement of cells from the endothelial walls of blood vessels into outlying tissue.

Determinant—a three-dimensional site on an antigen to which antibody is specifically able to become attached by its antigen-binding site. A single antigen may have several antigenic determinants (epitopes).

Diapedesis—the active amoeba-like movement of blood cells, including phagocytes, through the endothelial cells lining the walls of capillaries into the tissue.

Differentiation—a process during hematopoiesis in which cells take on functions and abilities different from their predecessors.

Effector cells—cells (lymphocytes, phagocytes) that directly function to achieve the end result, as opposed to regulatory cells.

Encephalitis—inflammation of the brain.

***Env* gene**—the gene that encodes for the envelope protein of human immunodeficiency virus.

Enzyme-linked immunosorbent assay (ELISA)—an immunoassay in which antibody or antigen is detected by the binding of an enzyme coupled to either anti-immunoglobulin or antibody specific for the antigen.

Enzyme-multiplied immunoassay technique (EMIT)—a quantitative competitive immunoassay that uses an enzyme detection system. The enzyme-coupled antigen retains its enzymatic activity when unbound but loses its activity when bound to the antibody. The enzyme activity is inversely proportional to the amount of antibody-antigen binding.

Eosinophils—antigen non-specific granulocytic cells capable of phagocytosis. Eosinophils also ingest immune complexes and clear parasitic organisms from the host.

Epitope—a single antigenic determinant; the specific molecular sequence of an antigen to its complimentary antibody attaches.

Fab—a fragment of antigen binding or the portion of an antibody that contains the antigen-binding sites.

F(ab')₂—a dimeric fragment that contains two antigen-binding sites formed by the cleaving of the antibody to fragments with pepsin.

Fc—a crystallizable fragment or the portion of an antibody that binds to macrophages, lymphocytes, and mast cells via Fc receptors. Also carries sites for fixation of complement.

Fc receptors—receptors located on cell surfaces that bind the Fc portion of an antibody molecule.

Fluorescence—the absorption of light at one wavelength and the emission of light at another wavelength.

Fluorescence immunoassay—an immunoassay technique that uses fluorescent-labeled antibodies or antigens to detect the presence of the antibody-antigen complex.

Fusion—a technique by which the cellular membranes of two or more cells are combined to form one cell; the resulting hybrid cell contains many of the chromosomes of the fusion partners.

***Gag* gene**—the gene that encodes for the core protein of human immunodeficiency virus.

Gastroenteritis—an acute inflammation of the lining of the stomach and intestines.

Gene—a unit of DNA that encodes for a single polypeptide chain.

Genotype—all alleles detected in a given individual; a genetic "portrait."

Graft-versus-host disease—a pathological reaction caused by the transplantation of competent donor T cells into an incompetent host (that is, one unable to reject them). This reaction occurs when the donor cells attack the host.

Graft-versus-leukemia effect—the decreased incidence of leukemic relapses seen in patients receiving allogenic transplants in comparison with autologous transplants.

Granulocytes—a group of antigen-nonspecific cells capable of phagocytosis. Granulocytes include neutrophils, eosinophils, and basophils.

Granulocytopenia—decreased numbers of granulocytes in the peripheral blood.

Group-specific—common to all the members of a group of viruses.

Haplotype—the set of genes present on any one chromosome; they are inherited as a unit. Each somatic cell will have two haplotypes, one of paternal origin and one of maternal origin.

Haptens—small antigenic molecules that are not immunogenic unless conjugated to a larger carrier molecule.

HAT—acronym for a selective cell culture medium containing hypoxanthine, aminopterin, and thymidine; used in monoclonal antibody technology to select for fused myeloma and B-lymphocyte cells (hybridomas).

Helper (CD4⁺) T cell—a subclass of T cells responsible for stimulating other T cells and B cells; also called helper T lymphocytes.

Hematopoiesis—the formation and development of blood cells.

Hematopoietic growth factor—*see* **Colony-stimulating factors.**

Hemolytic disease of the newborn—a disease of newborns characterized by anemia and jaundice and caused by incompatibilities of the Rh phenotype of mother and fetus (also known as erythroblastosis fetalis).

High endothelial venule—a section of the circulatory system in which the specific structure is designed to allow some lymphocytes to cross from the lymphatic system to the blood.

Histiocyte—a synonym for macrophage.

Histocompatibility—the ability to accept grafts between individuals.

Human antimurine antibody (HAMA) response—an antibody response produced in humans against infused immunogenic murine antibodies (usually monoclonal antibodies); also called human antibodies to mouse antibodies or human antimouse antibodies.

Human immunodeficiency virus (HIV)—believed by most investigators to be the cause of acquired immunodeficiency syndrome.

Human leukocyte antigens (HLA)—the major histocompatibility antigens in humans.

Humoral immunity—antigen-specific immunity mediated by antibody molecules, which are secreted by plasma cells and found in plasma, lymph, and other tissue fluids.

Hybridoma—a cell or cell line obtained by the fusion of two different cells. A hybridoma cell contains chromosomes from each of the fusion partners. A B-cell hybridoma results from the fusion of a B lymphocyte and a tumorous plasma cell. It is capable of prolonged survival and can secrete antibody.

Hyperchimeric antibody—a monoclonal antibody in which the hypervariable regions come from a non-human source (such as a mouse) and the rest of the antibody structure is derived from human sources. Also known as a humanized antibody.

Hypergammaglobulinemia—an excess of gamma globulin in the blood.

Hypervariable region—a subsection within the variable region of an antibody responsible for the antigen specificity of the antibody. Denoted for the high variance of amino acid sequences between antibodies of different specificity.

Idiotype—the particular antigen specificity of all antibody molecules produced by a given clone of B lymphocytes.

Immune complexes—antigen-antibody complexes.

Immunization—the process of inducing active or passive specific immunity by administering antigenic substances or antigen-specific antibodies.

Immunodeficiency—a partial or total deficiency of cellular immunity, humoral immunity, or both.

Immunogen—any substance able to provoke an immune response.

Immunoglobulin—an antigen-specific glycoprotein consisting of heavy chains and light chains linked together, often synthesized in response to the presence of a foreign substance. *See also* **Antibody.**

Immunomodulator—an agent capable of enhancing, suppressing, or restoring an immune system either directly or indirectly.

Immunosuppression—the prevention or diminution of the immune response by irradiation or administration of pharmacologic agents.

Immunotoxin—the conjugate of an antibody and a naturally occurring toxic substance, such as ricin.

Inflammation—a consequence of a nonspecific immune response causing tissue damage, characterized by tissue pain, swelling, and warmth.

Integrins—adhesion molecules expressed on leukocytes. They interact with ICAM molecules expressed on activated endothelial cells to allow extravasation of leukocytes into sites of inflammation or naïve lymphocytes into secondary lymphoid tissues.

Interferon—a glycoprotein that exerts virus-nonspecific but host-specific antiviral activity.

Interleukin—a soluble factor released from leukocytes or other cells with defined biological effects. Protein composition and DNA sequence of encoding gene are defined. (*See* Chapter 2 for specific interleukins.)

Interstitial pneumonitis—an insidious, slowly progressive interstitial lung disease marked by interstitial infiltration of the lungs by lymphocytes, plasma cells, and lymphoblasts.

J chain—a joining chain normally found in polymeric immunoglobulins (IgM and IgA).

Kupffer cells—mononuclear phagocytes that are fixed within the sinusoids of the liver.

Langerhans cell—a macrophage fixed in the skin responsible for antigen presentation to lymphocytes.

Leukotrienes—lipoxygenase metabolites of arachidonic acid with multiple biological activities.

Levamisole—an anthelmintic drug with possible immuno-stimulating effects.

Linkage-associated antigens—surface antigens, each of which is commonly associated with one or more specific diseases.

Lipopolysaccharide—any compound in which lipid is linked to polysaccharide. Often refers to an endotoxin derived from the cell wall of gram-negative bacteria.

Liposome—a spherical microstructure consisting of concentric phospholipid bilayers. Liposomes are hollow in the center and may be filled with drugs.

Locus—a position on the chromosome where a specific gene is found.

Lymphokine-activated killer (LAK) cells—an NK cell that develops an increased antitumor effect when activated by IL-2 or IFN-γ, which are secreted by T-cells.

Lymphokines—soluble secretory products of lymphocytes that stimulate or suppress the activity of other cells.

Lymphopoiesis—the development of lymphatic tissue.

Lysosomes—intracellular organelles containing digestive enzymes (lysozymes).

Lysozyme—a muramidase capable of hydrolyzing structural bonds in the cell walls of certain bacteria, particularly gram-positive cocci.

Macrophage—a phagocytic cell found in tissue and believed to be derived from blood monocytes; may act as an antigen-presenting cell.

Major histocompatibility complex (MHC)—a collection of genes found in all vertebrate species that encodes for the production of cell surface proteins associated with transplantation, immune response, and the complement system. In humans, the MHC is also known as the human leukocyte antigen complex. *See* **Human leukocyte antigens.**

Mast cells—granulocytic cells that leave the bone marrow more quickly than basophils, mature in connective tissue, and retain the capacity to differentiate. There are two types of mast cells: connective tissue–type mast cells and mucosal-type mast cells.

Mitogen—a substance that induces proliferation of lymphocytes.

Mixed lymphocyte reaction—the in vitro proliferative response of lymphocytes after exposure to lymphocytes of differing haplotypes.

Modulation—the disappearance of cell surface receptors after combining with specific antibodies.

Monoclonal antibodies (mAbs)—homogeneous antibodies produced by a single clone. mAbs can be of any class of antibodies; however, most murine MAbs are of the IgG or IgM class.

Monocytes and macrophages—mononuclear phagocytic cells. Monocytes mature (differentiate) into macrophages.

Monokines—biologically active substances secreted by monocytes and macrophages, such as interleukin 1 and tumor necrosis factor.

Mononuclear phagocyte system—mononuclear phagocytic cells found primarily in the reticular connective tissue of immune and other organs. *See also* **Reticuloendothelial system.**

Mucositis—inflammation of the mucosal membrane.

Mucus—a clear, viscid secretion of mucous membranes consisting of mucin, epithelial cells, and leukocytes.

Muramyl dipeptide—a substance derived from mycobacterial cell walls, used as an immunostimulant, similar to Bacillus Calmette-Guérin.

Myeloma cell line—a category of tumorous plasma cells with the sustained ability to grow in culture.

Natural killer cells—lymphocytes that preferentially kill virally infected or malignant cells in the absence of prior immunization.

Neutralization—the process by which antibody, either with or without complement, neutralizes the infectivity of microorganisms such as viruses.

Neutropenia—a decrease in the number of neutrophils in the blood.

Nude mice—a hairless strain of mice that congenitally lacks a thymus and has a marked deficiency in T lymphocytes but *does* possess natural killer cells.

Oncofetal antigens—cell surface markers normally present on fetal, but not adult, tissue that are also found on malignant cells.

Oncogene—a gene of mammalian or viral origin that is capable of causing neoplastic transformation of cells.

Ontogeny—the development of the individual organism.

Opsonin—a substance that binds to antigens and enhances phagocytosis by macrophages and neutrophils (e.g., complement and antibodies).

Opsonization—the process by which particles, microorganisms, or immune complexes become coated with complement or antibodies that make them more easily phagocytosed.

Paratope—a site on an antibody or a T-cell receptor that binds to the epitope of an antigen.

Passive immunization—providing temporary immunity by introduction of protective agents (e.g., preformed antibodies or specific cells) derived from extrinsic sources into a nonimmune host.

Perforins—proteins found in the cytoplasmic granules of natural killer cells that promote pore formation in nonself cells, leading to leakage of cell contents and cell death.

Peyer's patches—discrete colonies within gut mucosal-associated lymphoid tissue that contain mature B and T cells.

Phagocytes—cells capable of phagocytosis.

Phagocytosis—the process by which cells ingest and enzymatically destroy solid substances, such as bacteria and foreign particles.

Phagolysosome—a product of the fusion of a phagosome with a lysosome.

Phagosome—a vesicle that forms around a particle engulfed by a phagocyte.

Phenotype—a description of all the alleles detected in a given individual by serologic testing.

Plasma cell—the mature B lymphocyte, which is capable of secreting antibody.

Pluripotent stem cell—a primitive cell that has the potential to differentiate into any mature, functional cell.

Polyclonal activation—the activation of many clones of nonspecific lymphocytes.

Polymerase chain reaction (PCR)—a process that enables the amount of a particular DNA sequence or gene to be greatly amplified.

Prostaglandins—cyclooxygenase metabolites of arachidonic acid with many biological activities.

Proto-oncogene—a normal gene that is usually involved in cellular growth or regulation and that, when altered or mutated, can become an oncogene.

Regulatory cell—a cell that has the primary function of stimulating or suppressing the production or activation of other cells, such as effector cells.

Reticuloendothelial system—a term, perhaps antiquated, used to describe the mononuclear phagocyte system, a collection of cells that share the common function of phagocytosis and digestion of particulate material.

Retinitis—inflammation of the retina, typically due to infection.

Retrovirus—a virus capable of transcribing viral RNA to DNA by means of the enzyme reverse transcriptase.

Rh system—a blood grouping system based on Rh antigens.

Rheumatoid factor—an antibody directed at human IgG that is present in patients with rheumatoid arthritis and other connective tissue diseases.

Selectins—membrane glycoproteins induced on activated endothelial cells bind oligosaccharides (sulfated sialyl-Lewis moieties) on the cell surface of circulating leukocytes. They initiate the first interactions between the endothelium and immune-competent cells.

Self-renewal—a process by which some early bone marrow progenitor cells replenish their population rather than allowing all cells to undergo differentiation.

Serologic typing—a method of detecting cell surface antigens by using antisera.

Seropositive—showing positive results upon blood examination.

Serotherapy—the administration of antisera or specific immunoglobulins that are targeted for a specific antigen. *See also* **Passive immunization.**

Soluble mediators—secreted regulatory proteins, including all proteins or glycoproteins (such as interleukins, interferons, and cytokines) that mediate immune function.

Specificity—selective reactivity; the ability to distinguish among different determinants or sections of antigens.

Stem cell—a cell capable of self-replication and differentiation into various kinds of secondary cells.

Stroma—supporting cells within the bone marrow, including fibroblasts, endothelial cells, adipocytes, and macrophages. The stromal cells produce many of the growth factors that promote hematopoiesis.

Suppressor T cell (CD8$^+$)—a subclass of T cells responsible for suppressing the immune response to a stimulus; also called suppressor T lymphocytes.

Swine flu—the name given to a type of influenza that broke out in 1976 and stimulated a nationwide vaccination program.

Syngeneic—genetically identical (as in identical twins or inbred strains of animals).

T lymphocytes—cells derived from the bone marrow that differentiate within the thymus; they play a major role in the activity of the cell-mediated immune system. *See also* **Helper T cell** and **Suppressor T cell.**

T-cell receptor (TCR)—a molecule on the surface of T lymphocytes specifically capable of recognizing antigen in association with major histocompatibility complex molecules. TCRs consist of two polypeptide chains (alpha and beta or gamma and delta) associated with the CD3 complex.

Thymocyte—a lymphocyte found in the thymus, most of which are immature precursors.

Thymus—the small immunologic organ found in the anterior mediastinal cavity, responsible for T-cell growth and development.

Tolerance—an immunologic response of nonreactivity to a particular antigen, although responses to other antigens are normal.

Toxoid—a pharmacologically inactive toxin preparation that retains the ability to stimulate production of antitoxin.

Transfection—the process by which a DNA segment may be introduced into another cell, incorporated, and read to produce a protein.

Transfectoma—a continually renewing cell (e.g., a hybridoma or a myeloma cell) that has been transfected with a foreign DNA segment.

Tumor necrosis factor alpha (TNF-α)—a substance produced by host monocytes and macrophages that is capable of killing tumorous cells and eliciting inflammatory responses; also referred to as cachectin.

Type-specific—distinct for each virus within the group.

Vaccination—active immunization with antigenic material to provide resistance and to prevent disease (also known as active immunization).

Vaccine—a product consisting of attenuated or killed microbial agents used as an antigen to provide immunity.

Variolation—the injection of live smallpox virus from disease pustules to protect against smallpox.

Virion—formed virus particle.

Virulence—the degree of pathogenicity of various strains of organisms.

Visceral—any large interior organ in one of the three great cavities of the body, especially the abdomen.

Western blot—an immunoblotting method used for identifying specific proteins recognized by antibodies.

Wheal-and-flare—a cutaneous reaction in response to an injected antigen consisting of a raised edematous lesion surrounded by erythema.

Xenogenic—derived from tissues of individuals of different species. *See* **Allogenic.**

α_2-microglobulin—the protein that forms the light chain of HLA class I antigens.

Index

bone marrow transplants and, 220–23
cancer and, 258
dosing, monitoring, 176–77
drug allergy and, 68, 72
HIV/AIDS and, 160
inflammatory diseases and, 79, 83
organ transplants and, 170, 175, 178–79, 181–82, 186, 190, 196–97, 198
pharmacology, clinical uses, 176
side effects of, 177
Corynebacterium diphtheria, 100
Costimulatory pathways, 173–74
COX inhibitors, nonselective, 85
COX-2 inhibitors, 85
CroFab, 45
Cromolyn sodium, 79
Cross-presentation, 11
Crotalid snake venoms, 31
Crotalinae Polyvalent Immune Fab, 45
Cryptococcal meningitis, 143–44
Cryptococcus neoformans, 196
Crystalline aluminum oxyhydroxide, 108
CsA, drug interactions, 190–91, 192
CsA, pharmacodynamic interactions, 189–90
CsA, pharmacokinetic interactions, 189
Cyclic adenosine monophosphate (cAMP), 79
Cyclin-dependent kinases, 230, 231
Cyclins, 230, 231
Cyclophosphamide, 83, 170, 214, 215, 247, 253, 254
Cyclosporine (CsA)
adverse effects, toxicity, 178, 179, 180
bone marrow transplantation and, 221
dosing, monitoring, 178
HIV/AIDS and, 163
inflammatory diseases and, 83
organ transplantation and, 170, 175, 181–82, 184, 188, 193–94, 196–98
pharmacology, clinical uses, 177–78
Cytarabine, 241
Cytochrome P450, 178, 189–92, 221
Cytogam, 193
Cytokine(s), 49–50, 161–62, 240
answer key, 276
classification by effector mechanisms, 51
classification by structural characteristics, 51
inflammatory response and, 50
innate immune response and, 50, 52
mediating adaptive immunity, 52–54
mediators, 173
production of, 176
responsible for effector T-cell function, 53–54
storm, 216
Cytomegalovirus, 125, 145, 193, 222, 223–25
antigens, 224
Cytotoxic T cells, 96
effector functions of, 98
lymphocytes, 11, 237
Cytoxan, 83, 215

D

Dacarbazine, 241
Daclizumab, 38, 42, 185, 187–88, 222
Danazole, 180
Dapsone, 143, 159, 193, 196, 225
Darbopetin alfa, 244–45
Darunavir, 156, 160
Dasatinib, 241

Data and Safety Monitoring Boards, 165
Delabiridine, 156
Dendritic cells (DCs), 7
Department of Defense, 165
Department of Health and Human Services, 153
antiretroviral therapy guidelines, 154
Desensitization. *See* Hyposensitization
Desloratidine, 78
Dexamethasone, 262, 263
Diabetes mellitus, 81
insulin-dependent, 82
onset after organ transplant, 197–98
Diclofenac, 189
Didanosine, 156, 159
Dideoxynucleosides, 155
Di-dgA-RFB4, 44–45
DiGeorge syndrome, 20
Digibind, 40, 45
Digitoxin, 31
Digoxin Immune Fab, 40, 45
Diltiazem, 180, 189, 191, 192
Diphenhydramine, 78, 252, 255, 258
Diphtheria, 106, 115, 120
antitoxin, 125
toxin, 33
Diphtheria/tetanus/pertussis vaccine, 116, 120
Disease-modifying anti-rheumatologic drugs (DMARDs), 85
Diuretics, 71, 190, 197
DNA vaccine, HIV, 164, 165
DNA-polymerase chain reaction, 224
Docetaxel, 70
Donor lymphocyte
depletion, 215
infusions, 219–20
Donor/recipient matching, 214
Dose-density chemotherapy, 247
Doxorubicin, 247, 253
Drugs
allergies to, 63
allergies answer key, 276–77
contributing to type I hypersensitivity, 69–70
contributing to type II hypersensitivity, 70–71
contributing to type III sensitivity, 71–72
contributing to type IV sensitivity, 72
organ transplant interactions, 188–92
resistance assays, 154
toxicity of, 154
Dual-energy x-ray absorptiometry, 158
Dutasteride, 237
Dyslipidemias, 158

E

Eastern Cooperative Oncology Group, 218, 242
Ebola virus, 102
Echinocandins, 193, 196
Edrecolomab Mab17-1A, 39
Efalizumab, 39, 88
Efavirenz, 156
Emtricitabine, 156
Enbrel, 40, 44, 85, 90
Enfuvirtide, 155, 156, 157
Enisoprostil, 189
Enzyme immunoassay (EIA) tests, 142
Enzyme inducers, 190–91
Enzyme-linked immunosorbent assay (ELISA), 28, 139, 141, 179

Hepatitis A, 104, 105, 109, 125
  vaccine, 117, 120
Hepatitis B, 106, 125
  IMIG, 126
  vaccine, 117, 120–21
Hepatotoxicity, 158–59
HER family, 253
HER-2/neu, 234, 236, 252, 261
Herceptin, 38, 42, 251, 253
Herceptin Adjuvant (HERA) trial, 253–54
Herpes simplex virus, 195, 223
Herpes viruses, 145, 193–95
Highly active antiretroviral therapy (HAART), 143, 155,
  157–59, 190
Hippocrates, 122
Histamine release, 18
HIV. See also Human immunodeficiency virus
HIV Lipodystrophy Case Definition Study Group, 158
HIV Vaccine Trials Network, 165
HIV-1 p24 antigen test, 138
Home Access Express, 142
Hormones, 236–37
HRS-3/A9, 44
Human antimurine antibodies (HAMA), 28, 186, 250,
  254, 259–60
Human chorionic gonadotropin (hCG), 236–37
Human epidermal growth factor receptor 2, 252
Human immune system, 3
Human immunodeficiency virus (HIV), 19, 102, 133
  answer key, 279–80
  antiretroviral agents, 153–54, 155–60
  candidiasis, 144–45
  CDC HIV/AIDS classification, 140
  ELISA testing, 141
  etiology/epidemiology, 134
  herpesvirus/cytomegalovirus, 145
  home testing kits, 142
  immune suppression, 163
  immunologic therapy, 161–63
  immunopathogenesis, 136–38
  meningitis, 143–44
  natural history, diagnosis, stages, 139–40
  neoplasms, 145–46
  opportunistic infections, 143
  p24 antigen assay, 141–42
  parenteral exposure, 138–39
  perinatal exposure, 139
  pneumonia, 143
  polymerase chain reaction, 142
  rapid testing, 142
  resistance testing, 143
  RNA quantitation, 142–43
  saliva, urine tests, 142
  sexual exposure to, 138
  symptoms associated with seroconversion, 139
  testing generally, 140–41
  therapy modification, 154–55
  toxoplasmosis, 144
  transmission, prevention, 138–39
  treatment commencement, 154
  untreated history, 136
  vaccine development, 163–65
  viral replicative cycle, 135–36
  Western blot testing, 141
Human leukocyte antigen (HLA), 217
  complex, 172–73
  system, 213–14
Human papillomavirus (HPV), 106–7, 264
  vaccine, 117, 121
Human papillomavirus-16, 236

Human T-cell leukemia virus, 236
Humanized antibodies, 29
Humanized anti-TAC, 222
HuMax-CD20, 261
Humira, 39, 85, 90
Humoral immunity, 13–15, 99, 163–64
Hybrid genes, 233
Hybridomas, 27–28, 35
Hydralazine, 71, 72
Hydrochloroquine sulfate, 83
Hydroxyurea, 159, 259
Hygiene, 104
Hyperlipidemia, 197
Hypersensitivity, 17–18, 72–73
  answer key, 276–77
  drugs contributing to type I, 69–70
  drugs contributing to type II, 70–71
  drugs contributing to type III, 71–72
  drugs contributing to type IV, 72
  hapten hypothesis, 69
  reactions, 159–60
  responses, pharmaceutical compounds, 68–72
  risk groups for, 68–69
  treatment of, 72
Hypersensitivity mechanisms, 63
  type I, 64–67
  type II, 65, 66, 67
  type III, 65, 66, 67–68
  type IV, 65, 66, 68
Hypertension, 196–97
Hypogammaglobulinemia, 125
Hyposensitization, 80
Hypoxanthine guanine-phosphoribosyl transferase
  (HGPRT), 27
Hypoxanthine, 27

I

Ibritumomab, 259–60
Ibuprofen, 85, 189
Idiopathic thrombocytopenic purpura, 18
Ifex, 215
IFN-β, 84
  1a, 88
  1b, 88
Ifsofamide, 215
IgG backbone, 250
ImAb-14C5, 41
Imaging, monoclonal antibodies, 36
Imatinib, 241
IMC-IC11, 261
Immune complex-mediated hypersensitivity, 65, 66,
  67–68
Immune complex-mediated inflammation, 18
Immune globulin therapy, 172
Immune response, to tumors, 237–38
Immune suppression, HIV, 163
Immune surveillance, 230
Immune system, 22
  answer key, 275
  autoimmunity, 18–19
  components, 172–73
  human disease, inflammation, 17
  hypersensitivity, 17–18
  primary lymphoid organs, 15–16
  secondary lymphoid organs, 16–17
Immune thrombocytopenia, 127
Immune tolerance
  central, 19

J

K

L

M

N

Sorafenib, 243
Spingostine 1-phosphatase receptor agonists, 188
Spironolactone, 190
Spleen, 17
Squamous cell carcinoma, 257
Squamous cell skin carcinoma, 21
St. John's Wort, 180
Staphylococcus aureas, 100, 102, 125
Statins, 197
Stavudine, 156, 157, 159
Stem cell transplantation, 248–49
Steroids, 185, 186, 190, 193–94, 196
Stevens-Johnson syndrome, 160, 182, 262
Streptococcus
    agalctiae, 100
    pneumoniae, 100, 106, 122–23, 225
    pyogenes, 19, 100, 125
Streptomyces tsukubaensis, 178
Sulfadiazine, 144
Sulfadimidine, 180
Sulfamethoxazole, 72
Sulfamethoxazole/trimethoprim, 193
Sulfonamides, 70–71, 160
Sulindac, 189
Sunitinib, 243
Suppressor T lymphocytes, 12
"Swine flu" vaccine, 115
Sympathomimetic agents, 78–79
Synagis, 39, 43
Syngeneic transplant, 212, 213
Synthetic fragments, 30–33

T

T cells, 80–81
    activation, 173
    antigen recognition techniques, 234
    deficiencies, isolated, 19–20
    effector, 53–54
    inhibitors, early, 177–80
    inhibitors, late, 180–82
    proliferation of activated, 53
    receptors, 8–9, 173
    vaccination, 89
T helper cells, 96, 218
    effector functions of, 97
T lymphocytes, 4
    antigen presentation to, 8–9
    cytotoxic, 11
    helper, 9–10, 11
    memory, 11
    suppressor, 11
Tacrolimus, 181, 193–94, 196, 197–98, 221
    adverse effects, toxicity, 179, 180
    dosing, monitoring, 179
    drug interactions, 190–91, 192
    pharmacodynamic interactions, 189
    pharmacokinetic interactions, 189
    pharmacology, clinical use, 178–79
Tagamet, 78
Taxanes, 70
Tc-Mab170, 40
Tc-99m Arcitumomab, 41
Tc-99m Fanolesomab, 41
Tc-99m NeutroSpec, 41
Teniposide, 70
Tenofovir, 156, 159
TESPA, 215

Tetanus, 115, 120
    antitoxin, 125
Th1/Th2 (helper) cells, 80–81
Thalidomide, 262–63
    and immunomodulatory analogs, 262–63
Therapeutic drug monitoring, antiretroviral therapy, 160
Therapeutic immunization, HIV, 161
Thevetia, 31
Thiazide diuretics, 198
Thiazolidinediones, 158
Thimerosal, 72
Thioplex, 215
Thiotepa, 215
Thrombocytopenia, 71
Thymidine, 27
Thymoglobulin, 185, 193, 215, 220
Thymus, 16
Tienilic acid-induced hepatitis, 71
Tipranavir, 160
Tirofiban, 71
Tissue typing, 213–14
    techniques, 170
Tiuxetan, 259
Tolerance, organ transplant, 175
Toll-like receptors, 4
Topiramate, 159
Tositumomab, 38, 259–60
    and Iodine I-131, 40
Toxoid vaccines, 106
Toxoplasma gondii, 196, 224
Toxoplasmosis, 144
Tramadol, 159
Transforming growth factor, 51
Transforming growth factor α, 257
Translocations, 233
Trastuzumab, 38, 42, 251, 252–54, 261
Treatment, 192
    failure, 154
    interruption, 155
Trepomena pallidum, 100
Triamterene, 190
Triazoles, 193
Tricyclic antidepressants, 31, 159
Trimethoprim, 72
Trimethoprim/sulfamethoxazole (TMP/SMX), 143, 183, 190, 196, 224, 255
Troleandomycin, 180
Tru-Scint AD, 40
Tuberculin skin test, 18
Tuberculosis, 144
Tumor
    antigen classification, 234–36
    immune response to, 237–38
    immune system evasion, 238–39
    infiltrating lymphocytes, 244
    markers, 236–37
Tumor necrosis factor (TNF), 50–53, 216, 218, 238
Tumor necrosis factor α, 222
Tumor suppressor gene, 232, 233
Tumor suppressor gene *p53*, 232, 234
Tumor-associated antigens, 21, 234–35, 250, 263
Tumor-associated macrophages, 21
Tumor-specific antigens, 234–35, 250
2B1, 44
Tymidine analog agents, 157
Typhoid vaccine
    oral, 119, 124
    typhoid Vi, 119, 124
Tyrosinase, 235

Tyrosine kinase inhibitors, multitargeted, 243
Tysabri, 40, 87, 90

U

UDP-glucuronyltransferases, 189
Umbilical cord stem cells, 212, 213
Uni-Gold Recombigen HIV, 142
United Network for Organ Sharing, 171–72
United States Adopted Name Council, 36, 250
University of Pittsburgh, 178
Urine tests, 142

V

Vaccine
    adjuvants, 108–9
    attenuated live, 104–5
    boosting and schedules, 109
    DNA, 107
    HIV, 161
    -induced arthritis, 107
    initiative, 115–16
    killed/inactivated, 105
    multivalent subunit, 108
    purified macromolecules, 106–7
    recombinant-vector, 107
    risks and benefits of, 109, 114–15
    specific, 116–24
    synthetic-peptide, 107–8
"Vaccines for Children" program, 115
Vaccinia, 125
    vaccine, 123–24
Valacyclovir, 193, 195, 223, 225
Valganciclovir, 145, 193, 194
Vancomycin, 223
Varicella vaccine, 119, 124
Varicella zoster virus, 115, 125, 195, 223, 225
Varicella-zoster IMIG, 126
Vascular endothelial growth factor, 255–56
Venoglobulin-S, 127, 128
VePesid, 215
Verapamil, 180, 189, 191
Vibrio sp., 100

Vibro cholerae, 107
Vincristine, 247
Viral infections, 96, 98–99, 103, 223–25
Virologic failure, 154
Vitamin D, 198
Vitaxin, 38
Von Willebrand factor, 71
Voriconazole, 180, 223
VP-16, 215

W

Warfarin, 183
West Nile encephalitis, 102
Western blot test, 139, 141, 142
White cell growth factors, 246–47
White pulp, 17
Whole-cell tumor vaccines, 263
Whooping cough, 114
Working Formulation, 252
World Health Organization, 68, 105, 123, 127, 133

X–Y

Xolair, 38, 43, 80, 89
Y-DOTA-epratuzumab, 44
Yellow fever vaccine, 119, 124
Yttrium-90 ibritumomab tiuxetan, 37, 38, 41, 251, 259–61

Z

Zafirlukast, 78, 79
Zalcitabine, 156, 159
Zenapax, 38, 42, 185, 222
Zevalin, 37, 38, 41, 251
Zidovudine, 138, 155, 156, 160, 161–62
Zileuton, 78, 79
Zoster, 115
Zyflo, 78, 79
Zygomycetes, 223
Zyrtec, 78